Emergency Ultrasound

Emergency Ultrasound

O. John Ma, M.D.
Vice Chair
Department of Emergency Medicine
Truman Medical Center
Associate Professor of Emergency Medicine
University of Missouri – Kansas City School of Medicine
Kansas City, Missouri

James R. Mateer, M.D., R.D.M.S.
Clinical Professor of Emergency Medicine
Medical College of Wisconsin
Attending Staff Physician
Waukesha Memorial Hospital
Waukesha, Wisconsin

McGraw-Hill
Medical Publishing Division

New York Chicago San Francisco Lisbon London Madrid
Mexico City Milan New Delhi San Juan Seoul Singapore
Sydney Toronto

EMERGENCY ULTRASOUND

Copyright © 2003 by The **McGraw-Hill Companies**, Inc. All rights reserved.
Printed in the United States of America. Except as permitted under the United States Copyright Act of 1976, no part of this publication may be reproduced or distributed in any form or by any means, or stored in a data base or retrieval system, without the prior written permission of the publisher.

2 3 4 5 6 7 8 9 0 KGP KGP 0 9 8 7 6 5 4 3

ISBN: 0-07-137417-5

This book was set in Garamond by Circle Graphics.
The editors were Andrea Seils and Nicky Panton.
The production supervisor was Lisa Mendez.
The cover designer was Aimee Nordin.
The index was prepared by Coughlin Indexing Services, Inc.

Quebecor/Kingsport was the printer and binder.

This book is printed on acid-free paper.

Library of Congress Cataloging-in-Publication Data
Ma, O. John.
    Emergency ultrasound / O. John Ma, James R. Mateer.
       p. ; cm.
    Includes bibliographical references and index.
    ISBN 0-07-137417-5
    1. Diagnosis, Ultrasonic. 2. Emergency medicine. I. Mateer, James R. II. Title.
    [DNLM: 1. Emergencies. 2. Ultrasonography—methods. 3. Emergency Medical
Services—methods. WN 208 M111e 2003]
    RC78.7.U4 M32 2003
    616.07′543—dc21
                                                                2002016624

Completion of this book required tremendous sacrifice and patience from my family.
I am dedicating this book to Davis, Natasha, Gabrielle, and Elizabeth for their love and support.
— O. John Ma —

I also am dedicating this book to my family: Sean, Shannon, Kristen, and Jody.
In addition, I would like to thank all of those who have stimulated me to pursue
the clinical practice of limited emergency ultrasound, either directly by their
support and encouragement, or indirectly through their initial adversity.
—James R. Mateer —

CONTENTS

CONTRIBUTORS

Aaron E. Bair, M.D.
Assistant Professor
Division of Emergency Medicine
University of California–Davis Medical Center
Sacramento, California
(Chapter 15)

Katie Bakes, M.D., R.D.M.S.
Emergency Ultrasound Fellow
Department of Emergency Medicine
Harbor–UCLA Medical Center
Torrance, California
(Chapter 12)

Michael Blaivas, M.D., R.D.M.S.
Director, Emergency Ultrasound
Department of Emergency Medicine
North Shore University Hospital
Manhasset, New York
(Chapters 10 and 14)

Andreas Dewitz, M.D., R.D.M.S.
Director, Emergency Ultrasound
Department of Emergency Medicine
Boston Medical Center
Boston, Massachusetts
(Chapter 16)

William E. Durston, M.D.
Associate Professor of Medicine
University of California–Davis
Attending Staff Physician
Kaiser Foundation Hospital
Sacramento Medical Center
Sacramento, California
(Chapter 2)

J. Christian Fox, M.D., R.D.M.S.
Assistant Professor of Medicine
Director, Emergency Ultrasound
University of California–Irvine
Division of Emergency Medicine
Orange, California
(Chapter 13)

Bradley W. Frazee, M.D.
Assistant Professor of Emergency Medicine
Department of Emergency Medicine
Highland General Hospital
Oakland, California
(Chapters 12 and 16)

Michael J. Lambert, M.D., R.D.M.S.
Fellowship Director, Emergency Ultrasound
Department of Emergency Medicine
Resurrection Medical Center
Chicago, Illinois
(Chapters 1, 3, and 13)

O. John Ma, M.D.
Vice Chair
Department of Emergency Medicine
Truman Medical Center
Associate Professor of Emergency Medicine
University of Missouri–Kansas City School
  of Medicine
Kansas City, Missouri
(Chapter 4)

Diku Mandavia, M.D.
Attending Staff Physician
Department of Emergency Medicine
Cedars–Sinai Medical Center
and
Los Angeles County–USC Medical Center
Clinical Assistant Professor of Emergency Medicine
Keck School of Medicine of the University of Southern
    California
Los Angeles, California
(Chapter 9)

Marc L. Martel, M.D.
Attending Staff Physician
Hennepin County Medical Center
Minneapolis, Minnesota
(Chapter 11)

James R. Mateer, M.D., R.D.M.S.
Clinical Professor of Emergency Medicine
Medical College of Wisconsin
Attending Staff Physician
Waukesha Memorial Hospital
Waukesha, Wisconsin
(Chapter 4)

Christopher L. Moore, M.D., R.D.C.S.
Emergency Ultrasound Fellow
Department of Emergency Medicine
Resurrection Medical Center
Chicago, Illinois
(Chapter 5)

Theodore J. Nielsen, R.T., R.D.M.S.
Emergency Ultrasound Director
Windy City Ultrasound, Inc.
Darien, Illinois
(Chapter 3)

Masaaki Ogata, M.D.
Professor of Surgery
Department of Surgery
Kobe Nishi City Hospital
Kobe, Japan
(Chapter 8)

Michael A. Peterson, M.D., R.D.M.S.
Fellowship Director, Emergency Ultrasound
Department of Emergency Medicine
Harbor–UCLA Medical Center
Torrance, California
(Chapters 1 and 17)

David Plummer, M.D.
Attending Staff Physician
Department of Emergency Medicine
Hennepin County Medical Center
Minneapolis, Minnesota
(Chapter 6)

Daniel D. Price, M.D.
Assistant Professor of Emergency Medicine
Department of Emergency Medicine
Highland General Hospital
Oakland, California
(Chapter 17)

Robert F. Reardon, M.D.
Attending Staff Physician
Department of Emergency Medicine
Hennepin County Medical Center
Minneapolis, Minnesota
(Chapter 11)

Geoffrey A. Rose, M.D.
Director, Cardiac Ultrasound Laboratory
Sanger Clinic
Division of Cardiology
Carolinas Medical Center
Charlotte, North Carolina
(Chapter 5)

John S. Rose, M.D.
Assistant Professor of Emergency Medicine
Division of Emergency Medicine
University of California–Davis Medical Center
Sacramento, California
(Chapter 15)

Simon Roy, M.D., R.D.M.S.
Assistant Professor
Department of Emergency Medicine, Ultrasound
    Section
Boston Medical Center
Boston, Massachusetts
(Chapter 7)

Joseph Salomone, M.D.
Residency Director
Department of Emergency Medicine
Truman Medical Center
Kansas City, Missouri
(Chapter 2)

Eric Snoey, M.D.
Associate Clinical Professor of Emergency Medicine
University of California–San Francisco School of
   Medicine
Residency Director
Department of Emergency Medicine
Highland General Hospital
Oakland, California
(Chapter 12)

Stuart Swadron, M.D.
Attending Staff Physician
Department of Emergency Medicine
Los Angeles County–USC Medical Center
Assistant Professor of Emergency Medicine
Keck School of Medicine of the University of
   Southern California
Los Angeles, California
(Chapter 9)

Vivek S. Tayal, M.D.
Director, Emergency Ultrasound
Department of Emergency Medicine
Carolinas Medical Center
Charlotte, North Carolina
(Chapter 5)

John Wiesenfarth, M.D.
Assistant Chief
Department of Emergency Medicine
Kaiser Foundation Hospital
Sacramento, California
(Chapter 2)

FOREWORD

Teaching old dogs new tricks has always been a demanding task. As I began my residency in Emergency Medicine in 1976, David K. Wagner shared with me the challenge that he faced learning to read electrocardiograms after he had completed his residency and been in practice for more than a decade as a pediatric surgeon and subsequently as an emergency physician. I find myself in the same situation as I first learned to read CT-scans and now begin to introduce ultrasonography into my own clinical practice. We are trained in medical school to be continuous learners throughout our career. Indeed, we speak of "practicing" medicine to emphasize that we are continuously enhancing our knowledge base and skills.

Drs. Ma & Mateer have created a textbook that provides a strong foundation for those wishing to develop and expand their knowledge of ultrasonography as a tool for emergency physicians. Although focused on the practitioner who wishes to perform the study as a part of her/his practice, the text also is valuable for the practitioner who has immediate medical sonographic technician backup in their emergency department. Understanding the technical aspects of the studies, including common pitfalls and known limitations will benefit all clinicians.

This new text provides technical and clinical information that will enhance the knowledge base of any clinician seeking to develop or improve her/his understanding of emergency ultrasonography. The application of this knowledge is best coupled with hands-on training and careful quality review of interpretations done by the trainee. Like medicine in general, emergency ultrasonography cannot be learned entirely from reading a text. Regular clinical application of the lessons taught is required to develop expertise.

Undoubtedly ultrasound and other imaging technology will improve over time. The information contained within this text will eventually require updating in light of evolving technological advances. Yet this is the time to become acquainted, if not expert, with this body of knowledge that is becoming a daily part of emergency practice in urban, teaching centers. The text provides a practical, reader-friendly approach to understanding the sonographic techniques and resultant images under a variety of circumstances.

Each clinical chapter has a consistent layout and approach. Appropriate background material is provided before the technical aspects are presented. Common findings and pitfalls are provided in each clinical chapter. Representative cases demonstrating the role of emergency ultrasonography in clinical decision making are provided along with abundant image and anatomic line drawings.

The next generation of emergency physicians will wonder why bedside emergency ultrasonography was not more rapidly introduced into our specialty. Emergency physicians need diagnostic information in real time and not the next day. Delays in the care of one patient adversely affect the care of another patient. There are many answers to why bedside emergency ultrasonography has been slowly embraced — some political, some economic, some logistical, and some related to training. This text goes a long way toward lowering the barriers related to training by providing a text that is worthy as a companion of any training program in emergency ultrasonography.

Jerris R. Hedges, MD, MS, FAAEM
Professor & Chair
Department of Emergency Medicine
Oregon Health & Science University
Portland, Oregon

PREFACE

Emergency ultrasound is a young field that is undergoing a period of explosive growth. Unlike many other specialized areas of medicine, where clear pathways for gaining training, certification, and experience have already been well-established, emergency ultrasound is still relatively new and the methods by which it can be integrated into clinical training and practice have yet to be precisely defined. However, clinicians who practice in the emergency department, the critical care setting, and other acute care settings recognize the value of emergency bedside sonography for improving and expediting patient care.

Ten years ago very few graduate medical programs offered electives or clinical experience with emergency ultrasound; now the practice has gained widespread acceptance. Emergency physicians with advanced skills in bedside sonography are being sought for medical directorships and have been appointed onto academic faculties. Fellowship training programs have been developed. Emergency medicine residency programs have incorporated bedside sonography into their training programs. The scope of clinical practice of emergency medicine includes bedside sonography as a specific procedural skill integral to the practice of emergency medicine.

This textbook was written by and for health care workers who are engaged in the practice of emergency and acute care medicine. We selected topics that represent problems most commonly encountered in these clinical settings to provide an educational and reference tool for a broad readership. Our aim was to address the needs of physicians with varied backgrounds and training. Emergency physicians certainly will find this textbook applicable to their daily practice. Physicians who practice in family medicine, internal medicine, pediatrics, critical care, and general surgery should also find this book to be of value for specific clinical scenarios. Sonographers who are expected to perform ultrasound examinations in the emergency and acute care setting may also benefit from this textbook.

In each chapter, the clinical considerations of the specific medical problem are discussed. The clinical indications for performing an emergency ultrasound examination are then listed and reviewed. After reviewing some of the anatomical considerations that directly impact upon the ultrasound examination, the chapter presents the technique for the focused emergency ultrasound examination along with the normal ultrasound findings. Each chapter emphasizes the key aspects of the *focused* emergency ultrasound examination; this textbook did not attempt to cover every element of the normal comprehensive ultrasound examination. The next two sections present the common and emergent abnormalities of the clinical problem, and review common variants and selected abnormalities. Each chapter includes a discussion of the pitfalls involved with performing the focused ultrasound examination. The chapter concludes by presenting several clinical case studies in which the focused emergency ultrasound examination may play a prominent role in patient care.

A number of experts from a variety of specialties have contributed to this textbook. We would like to express our deep appreciation to the *Emergency Ultrasound* chapter contributors for their commitment and hard work in helping to produce this textbook. We also would like to thank them for helping us collect the nearly 700 images that are included in this textbook. We would like to thank Lori Green and Lori Sens from Gulfcoast Ultrasound for their support of this project and for providing us with numerous ultrasound images from their library. We are indebted to several individuals who assisted us with this project; in particular, we would like to thank Andrea Seils, Susan Noujaim, Martin Wonsiewicz, and Nicky Panton at McGraw-Hill Medical Publishing.

O. John Ma, MD

James R. Mateer, MD

CHAPTER 1

Training and Program Development

Michael A. Peterson and Michael J. Lambert

Establishing a training program in point of care limited ultrasound (PLUS) is an exciting and rewarding experience. After acquiring basic PLUS skills, the impact of ultrasound on the clinical practice of medicine becomes so obvious that many clinicians wonder how they got along without this technology. This chapter outlines the process for developing a PLUS training program and addresses common questions encountered when starting a new program. This chapter was written based on our training experience for emergency medicine residency programs. The principles outlined could be applied to residencies in other specialties as well as to groups of practicing physicians who are interested in developing a PLUS program for emergency and acute care settings.

▶ STEPS TO ESTABLISH A POINT OF CARE ULTRASOUND PROGRAM

The following are a set of steps to establish a high-quality PLUS program. These steps should generally proceed in order, except for the selection of the PLUS lead person, which can be done at any time as long as it is before step 7. Early selection of the PLUS lead person is preferable, however, as several of the steps are time consuming and would benefit by having a designated advocate to champion their completion.

1. Determine type of examinations to be performed.
2. Develop a program plan.
3. Select the PLUS lead person(s).
4. Obtain hospital approval of program plan.
5. Acquire an ultrasound machine.
6. Train the lead person(s).

7. Train the group.
8. Perform problem solving.

▶ DETERMINE TYPE OF EXAMINATIONS TO BE PERFORMED

Intuitively, this step seems like an easy task. However, the applications of PLUS continue to expand along with technologic advances in ultrasound and individual operator expertise. For an emergency PLUS program, dogma suggest that you should start with applications that identify specific life-threatening conditions in which diagnostic ultrasound is the gold standard imaging modality. Pioneers in emergency PLUS refer to these as the "primary" applications (Table 1–1). These particular applications were chosen for two specific reasons. First, identification of most of these particular conditions is extremely time sensitive. The quicker the diagnosis can be confirmed, the sooner definitive treatment can be provided. Emergency physicians and trauma surgeons can appreciate the benefits of PLUS when a trauma patient presents with an isolated penetrating injury to the chest. An echocardiogram is frequently ordered to exclude the most potentially life-threatening condition, a hemopericardium. A trained echocardiographer is requested to perform an ultrasound examination that is then interpreted by a cardiologist. While this can usually be obtained in a reasonable time frame during the day, studies obtained after hours can be significantly delayed. During the interim, if the patient's condition deteriorates, the treating physician may be led down numerous other pathways in an effort to ascertain the etiology. Obviously, the rate-limiting step of this imaging modality can have serious consequences.

► **TABLE 1-1.** PLUS EXAMINATIONS

System	Primary Applications	Additional Examinations and Procedures
Abdominal	Free abdominal fluid Abdominal aortic aneurysm Gallstones Hydronephrosis	Solid organ injuries Bladder volume and aspiration Paracentesis
Obstetrics and gynecology	Early intrauterine pregnancy (to exclude ectopic pregnancy)	Adnexal masses Trauma in pregnancy
Cardiothoracic	Pericardial effusion	Hypotension Cardiac arrest Pleural effusions and thoracentesis Transvenous pacemaker placement
Soft tissue and orthopedic	—	Foreign bodies Abscess localization Fracture reduction
Vascular	—	Deep venous thrombosis Line placement

The second reason these "primary" applications were chosen is that it would be difficult for anyone to argue that a technically proficient ultrasound examination at the bedside would not provide a higher level of care, no matter who provided this service. The real issue is whether or not nonimaging specialist physicians can be properly trained in ultrasound to provide this service. Currently, there is a deficiency in the number of physicians who are capable of providing this level of expertise. However, the number of physicians obtaining these sonographic skills is rapidly expanding, especially in emergency medicine and trauma surgery. No one can argue that diagnostic ultrasound imaging available at the point of care is not a step forward. The debate is over the quality of this service when non-imaging specialists perform and interpret these ultrasound examinations. Many believe that ultrasound is a skill that falls within the scope of practice of clinicians. The implementation of a safe and effective ultrasound credentialing process to ensure quality is where clinician leadership will need to focus its efforts. Although these primary applications are the foundation on which emergency PLUS was built, there are additional urgent indications for PLUS that are applicable to many types of clinical practice.

In general, pelvic ultrasound and trauma ultrasound are excellent PLUS applications for most emergency medicine programs to start their education. These are two applications in which a properly trained emergency physician can expedite the rate-limiting step of ordering an ultrasound examination and make a significant impact on the clinical decision-making.

By virtue of geographic location and individual hospital management, emergency departments throughout the country see very different sets of patient populations. Inner-city hospitals in large metropolitan areas, for example, may have a very active trauma program. Their patient population may also be much younger on average than a suburban or rural hospital. A suburban hospital with numerous surrounding extended-care facilities may see a much older population of patients and have minimal trauma exposure.

When it comes to implementing a PLUS program at an institution, the specific patient population must be considered. If the practice environment sees a predominance of elderly patients and very few trauma patients, it would be wise to tailor a PLUS program to better suit the needs of the individual department. Instead of focusing on all the "primary" applications, the initial focus of the program may center on identifying pericardial effusions, gallstones, or deep vein thromboses. A new PLUS program should strive to identify all of the ultrasound examinations it wants to encompass, both now and in the future. Making this decision early allows the program to seek hospital approval for all these examinations from the very start instead of having to apply for additional approval later. It also allows the program to better define equipment needs during the initial equipment purchase, and avoids subsequent equipment purchases at a time when funding may not be as readily available.

Our advice would be to focus initially on training in one or two ultrasound examinations only, and honing these skills before adding more. This allows everyone time to concentrate their skills in obtaining the necessary windows and landmarks specific to that application. It also provides the trainees time to focus on the technical pitfalls inherent in those particular applications. Likewise, by keeping the entire training group on the same page, the PLUS program's lead person can focus quality improvement efforts on those specific applications. Valuable time can be spent making sure everyone is capturing, recording, and interpreting images in a systematic fashion. Specific case study reviews of these applications can be beneficial to everyone involved. The entire group can learn from the success and mistakes of their peers. After competence is achieved, the next application can be introduced in a similarly systematic fashion. There is no need to rush into all of the applications in a haphazard manner. This systematic approach will ensure a safe, methodical, and effective implementation of PLUS into daily clinical practice. Although PLUS by definition is a truncated examination designed to answer a specific clinical question, the acquisition of these skills nevertheless requires significant education and experience.

▶ DEVELOP A PROGRAM PLAN

The program plan defines all aspects of the PLUS training program. The plan directs the PLUS lead person through all the administrative and teaching aspects of the program and serves as a reference for requirements in training. The most expeditious route for developing a plan is to model one after another group or institution's plan, adapting it for the local clinical environment. Many residency programs are very willing to share their program plans. At a minimum, the program plan should include the following elements.

- Definition of specific privileges.
- Training and credentialing requirements.
- Method of recording results.
- Quality improvement plan.
- Continuing medical education requirements.

Definition of Specific Privileges

This section defines exactly what PLUS examinations will be used for in terms of patient care. For example, a specific privilege may be: "Documentation of free abdominal fluid in trauma patients." This could also be shortened to "Documentation of free abdominal fluid" if there is an additional desire to diagnose ascites. Some institutions allow graduated privileges, meaning that physicians can do more with their PLUS examinations as they gain experience. This approach is beneficial in that it allows implementation of PLUS for patient care with less training time. Earlier implementation helps maintain momentum in the training program as physicians see the benefits of their training sooner. The downside is that graduated privileges create a more complex training program. An example of graduated privileges for evaluating an intrauterine pregnancy is included in Table 1–2.

Privileges and training should be constructed toward the identification of *specific findings* (e.g., presence or absence of gallstones) and not toward the general evaluation of disease processes or anatomic structures (e.g., evaluation for "cardiac disease" or "right upper quadrant abdominal pain"). This limited approach is what makes it possible for PLUS providers to achieve proficiency in their examinations with less training than imaging specialists receive.

Training and Credentialing Requirements

Training
The minimum training requirements for a PLUS program have not been established scientifically. No conclusive studies validate any specific set of training requirements

▶ TABLE 1–2. EXAMPLE OF GRADUATED PRIVILEGES

Level of User	Decision-Making Capabilities
Level 1	Able to accurately diagnose a live intrauterine pregnancy (LIUP) in the pregnant patient. Proficient in correctly locating live pregnancy in the uterus by verifying appropriate landmarks by transabdominal (TAS) technique (bladder, uterus, and vaginal stripe) or endovaginal (EV) technique (bladder and uterus). Accurately records images to support diagnosis. Credentialed to disposition patient with documented LIUP and arranging either follow-up diagnostic study in the department of radiology or with patient's personal physician. If LIUP not clearly identified (*see* criteria), must have gold standard diagnostic study obtained while the patient is in ED.
Level 2	Able to accurately diagnose an intrauterine pregnancy (IUP) and an abnormal intrauterine pregnancy (ABNIUP) in pregnant patient. Proficient in correctly locating IUP or ABNIUP in the uterus by verifying appropriate landmarks. Accurately records images to support diagnosis. May disposition patient with documented IUP or ABNIUP with confirmatory study arranged in the department of radiology or with patient's personal physician. If IUP or ABNIUP not clearly identified (*see* criteria), must have confirmatory diagnostic study obtained while the patient is in ED.
Level 3	Able to accurately diagnose no definitive intrauterine pregnancy (NDIUP) in pregnant patient. Proficient in evaluating adnexal and abdomen for possible extrauterine gestation (EUG), adnexal mass or free fluid in the pelvis. Has obtained Doppler skills necessary to evaluate ovaries for cysts and torsion. Accurately records images to support diagnosis. May disposition patient with documented NDIUP and ovarian cysts for outpatient work-up if stable. Obtains consultation in NDIUP, EUG, or ovarian torsion cases with appropriate OB colleagues. Proficient in instructing patients with ectopic precautions, NDIUP protocols, and arranging for any necessary outpatient labs and imaging.

or demonstrate that one approach to training is superior to another. We know that accuracy rates comparable to imaging specialist examinations have been achieved (e.g., identification of free intraperitoneal fluid or deep venous thrombosis), but the minimal amount of training required to achieve these results has yet to be determined.

Some standards for training in ultrasound have been published. The American College of Radiology (ACR) and the American Institute of Ultrasound in Medicine (AIUM) have established their guidelines.[1,2] The ACR and AIUM guidelines are targeted to learning comprehensive imaging of multiple anatomic regions and organs, a goal that is different than that of PLUS. In 1994, a model curriculum for training in emergency PLUS that required fewer training examinations than either the ACR or the AIUM guidelines, was published.[3] This model curriculum represented the best opinion at the time, but now, these criteria are felt to be excessive by some practitioners.[4,5] Most recently, the American College of Emergency Physicians (ACEP) published an expert consensus on ultrasound training that may become the current standard for emergency medicine.[6]

While these guidelines help structure an ultrasound program in a general sense, more specific training criteria should be defined when constructing a training program. The PLUS lead persons still have a fair degree of latitude in designing their individual programs, but a well-constructed program should at least include minimum requirements for each of the following areas.

- Minimum overall didactic hours.
- Minimum overall didactic content.
- Minimum number of overall ultrasound examinations performed.
- Minimum didactic content pertaining to the specific examination.
- Minimum number of examinations performed to look for the specific finding (either positive or negative).
- Minimum number of examinations positive for the finding.

If in doubt about appropriate training criteria, the PLUS lead person should look to model the program after well-established academic training programs with a track record of producing successful PLUS providers. Table 1–3 provides a comparison of suggested minimum training criteria in PLUS for emergency medicine.

Credentialing

Credentialing applies mainly to hospital-based or clinic-based physicians who wish to perform PLUS examinations on their patients while they are in the hospital. Standard methods of credentialing are crucial to safely

► **TABLE 1-3.** RECOMMENDED MINIMUM TRAINING CRITERIA FOR ULTRASOUND FOR EMERGENCY MEDICINE

	ACR[1]	AIUM[2]	Model Curriculum[3] (1994)	ACEP[51] (2001)	Harbor-UCLA Emergency Medicine Residency Full Privileges‡
Didactic hours/training	3 mo.	3 mo. or 100 h	40 h	16 h	24 h
Minimum didactic content	Instrumentation physics	Instrumentation physics	ND	ND	Instrumentation physics Gallstones/AAA Free Abd. Fluid/Pericard. Ef. IUP
Total exams	500	300	150	25–150†	80‡
Minimum didactic hours for a specific indication	ND	ND	ND	ND	1 h each
Minimum exams for specific indication	ND	ND	ND	25	40
Minimum number of positive exams	ND	ND	ND*	Some	10–25%§

AAA = Abdominal aortic aneurysm; IUP = intrauterine pregnancy; ND = not defined.
*At least 50% should be "clinically indicated."
†25 for a single application, 150 for "general privileges."
‡Limited reporting is allowed with 16 hours didactic, 50 total exams, and a minimum of 10 exams for each of 5 primary applications.
§Depends on exam: AAA, Pericardial Effusion, Free Abdominal Fluid = 10%; Intrauterine pregnancy, Gallstones = 25%.

and effectively implement a successful PLUS program. The cornerstone of the credentialing processes revolves around a required number of technically proficient scans and interpretations, as outlined in the training requirements. Until the training requirements are achieved, the physician is in "training status" and cannot use any information from the PLUS examinations to manage patients. Physicians are also cautioned against discussing any of their results with either patients or consultants during the training period to avoid misunderstandings about the accuracy of the results. After the training requirements are met, physicians are credentialed by the hospital and may begin using examinations for patient care. If a graduated credentialing program is used, the physician may be able to use some findings for patient care, but is considered "in training" for other findings and unable to use those findings for patient care.

Hospitals often break down credentialing into *provisional* and *full* privileges. Provisional privileges are awarded immediately after physicians meet the credentialing criteria, but require the physician be *proctored* for a period of time before full privileges are granted. This proctoring is accomplished differently in various programs. Two examples are: (1) requiring that all studies be backed up by a definitive study until a certain number of examinations are completed and the accuracy of all examinations are verified; or (2) requiring that a defined number of examinations be submitted to the ultrasound lead person for review. Once the proctoring requirement is achieved, the lead person submits a recommendation that privileges be upgraded from provisional to full.

Method of Recording Results

The need to document images is somewhat controversial. There are some PLUS advocates who believe that there is no need to include images in the medical record. They contend that since the PLUS examination is essentially part of the physical examination, the results should be documented in a narrative fashion within the medical record, as is done with any physical examination finding. Other PLUS experts believe that because the majority of physicians do not yet possess the skills to perform an ultrasound examination, the PLUS studies are not easily repeatable by subsequent consulting physicians or specialists who examine the patient. In order to expedite intervention for emergent conditions, the consulting physicians will need recorded documentation for review, thus making it imperative to have images to support specific entities.

Numerous methods are available to document the results of the ultrasound examinations. Two questions that need to be answered are: (1) How will written interpretations be documented; and (2) How will images be documented? The answer to the latter question is especially important, as it will influence the type of ultrasound equipment purchased. Documentation of interpretations can be as simple as writing results on the chart, or as complex as entering them in the hospital information system so they are available to all interested health care providers. One solution is to develop a form for the express purpose of reporting PLUS results. These forms can then be included in the medical record. The advantage of the form is that it can be devised so as to restrict interpretations to those findings that physicians are privileged for, and help physicians avoid making interpretations beyond their level of skill. An example of such a report form is included as Figure 1–1.

Several options exist for the documentation of images. These options include videotape, radiograph film, digital archives, or thermal imaging. If results are to be included in the medical record, thermal imaging is the best option. If images are to be archived separately from the medical record, digital storage or videotaping can be used. Archiving images outside the medical record creates logistic problems of compliance with medical record confidentiality and lack of access to the images by other physicians. Some programs use videotaping for quality assurance and teaching purposes only. Most programs choose not to use radiograph film to archive images.

Quality Improvement Plan

Any department implementing a new PLUS program should place a strong emphasis on quality improvement (QI). No other area of emergency ultrasound training will provide as many teaching opportunities as a well-run QI program. If the resources are lacking initially to overread all of the program's ultrasound images, then finding a trained colleague in other specialties to assist with this endeavor is an option. There are pitfalls common to every application of ultrasound that can serve as a springboard for providing feedback and teaching within the program. This is clearly the most advantageous method of enhancing both the technical and interpretative skills of the sonologists.

The cornerstone of the QI program should be having the program's lead person review the ultrasound examinations. For a very active group of physicians performing PLUS examinations, it will be logistically difficult to review every PLUS study, and so a decision must be made on selecting examinations for review. Examinations can be reviewed on either an *indicated* basis or a *random* basis. Indicated reviews occur when a certain indicator is met, such as a reported discrepancy between the PLUS examination and another definitive study or procedure, or when a case is referred by a colleague because of questions regarding the accuracy of the examination. Random reviews are conducted by randomly selecting a predetermined number, or percentage, of examinations to assess the overall performance of the group.

Problems that are encountered during the QI process should be categorized as to their importance. The following represents one method of this categorization.

LIMITED EMERGENCY ULTRASOUND EXAM
Emergency Department, _____ Medical Center

Date: _____

Provider: _____
(PRINT NAME)

_____
(SIGN)

LEVEL I

Trauma
- ☐ Intra-abdominal Fluid
- ☐ Indeterminate

Gallbladder
- ☐ Gallstones
- ☐ Indeterminate

Cardiac
- ☐ Pericardial Fluid
- ☐ Indeterminate

Pelvic
- ☐ Definite IUP
  (IU Fetal Pole or IU Cardiac Activity)
- ☐ Indeterminate

Cardiac
- ☐ Aneurysm_____cm
- ☐ Indeterminate

(ATTACH IMAGES TO REVERSE SIDE OF MEDICAL RECORD COPY ONLY)

LEVEL II

Trauma
- ☐ **Visualization Adequate**
- ☐ **Visualization Inadequate**
- ☐ Intra-abdominal Fluid
- ☐ No Free Fluid

Gallbladder
- ☐ **Visualization Adequate**
- ☐ **Visualization Inadequate**
- ☐ Gallstones
- ☐ Pericholecystic Fluid
- ☐ None of Above
  CBD _____ mm
  Wall Thickness _____ mm

Gallbladder
- ☐ **Visualization Adequate**
- ☐ **Visualization Inadequate**
- ☐ Pericardial Fluid
- ☐ No Pericardial Fluid

Pelvic
- ☐ **Transabdominal**
- ☐ **Transvaginal**
- ☐ **Visualization Adequate**
- ☐ **Visualization Inadequate**
- ☐ Definite IUP
  (IU Fetal Pole or IU Cardiac Activity)
- ☐ Definite Ectopic
  (Ectopic Fetal Pole or Cardiac Activity)
- ☐ Adnexal Mass
- ☐ Pelvic/Abdominal Fluid
- ☐ None of Above Findings

Aorta
- ☐ **Visualization Adequate**
- ☐ **Visualization Inadequate**
- ☐ Aneurysm_____cm
- ☐ No Aneurysm Detected

Hydronephrosis
- ☐ **Visualization Adequate**
- ☐ **Visualization Inadequate**
- ☐ Hydronephrosis Present R/L
- ☐ No Hydronephrosis

Additional Comments:
(Findings in this section are preliminary and require confirmation when clinically indicated)

_____
_____
_____

All Emergency Ultrasounds are considered "Limited Exams".
Exams do not exclude findings other than those recorded above.
Practitioners should procure comprehensive ultrasound examinations when findings not listed here or findings listed under "additional comments" are of concern.

Figure 1–1. Example of PLUS Report Form.

Level I: Minor

These problems usually consist of some problem with the technical component of the examination (e.g., gain too high) or disagreement on diagnostic criteria (e.g., intrauterine pregnancy documented by presence of double decidual ring sign when this is not one of the training criteria). Level I problems have no direct bearing upon the medical management of the patient. Typically, when this level of disagreement is found, a documented written or electronic copy of the disagreement is sent to the recipient.

Level II: Moderate

These problems consist of discrepancies in interpretation between the sonologist's recorded image(s) and the QI review. In these cases, the undiagnosed or misdiagnosed pathology is nonemergent. For example, the sonologist may record a gallbladder examination in which gallstones were diagnosed. Upon review, the QI review discovers a classic novice pitfall of a hyperechoic duodenal area that is mistaken for gallstones. Typically, when this level of disagreement is found, a chart review is undertaken. Depending upon the follow-up that was provided and the patient's clinical condition at the time of disposition, the action taken can range considerably. In the majority of these types of disagreements, the true diagnosis was established by another means or the patient's symptoms were abated.

Level III: Major

These problems consist of significant discrepancies between the sonologist's recorded image(s) and the QI review. For example, the sonologist records a pelvic ultrasound examination on a pregnant patient as an intrauterine pregnancy. The QI review finds no evidence of an intrauterine pregnancy, but does note free fluid in the pelvis and a 3 × 4 cm adnexal mass. In this case, the chart is immediately pulled and reviewed. Depending upon the follow-up provided or whether a confirmatory study was obtained, the patient is immediately contacted by telephone. The patient is then given follow-up instructions appropriate to the changed diagnosis.

Feedback on reviews, both good and bad, should be provided to sonologists in confidence, along with constructive suggestions for improvement. On occasion, mandated remedial education or training may be appropriate at the discretion of the program's lead person. The lead person is also responsible for recommending to the department chief either limitation, suspension, or termination of PLUS privileges for a sonologist in certain circumstances. Records should be kept on specific sonologist performance so that trends indicating provider problems can be recognized and addressed. Actions taken to address such problems as well as the outcome of such actions should be recorded as well. These records are confidential peer review in nature and should be labeled as such. Results of QI activities should be regularly reported to the appropriate QI organization in the department, hospital, or clinic.

Continuing Medical Education

As with training requirements, there are no well-established guidelines to dictate the amount of continuing medical education (CME) one needs to maintain competency in PLUS. A reasonable number of hours along with continued use of bedside ultrasound should easily maintain skill levels and, preferably, even advance them. "Reasonable" should be determined in light of all the other requirements for continuing education within a specialty. If physicians normally receive 50 hours a year of continuing education in all areas of their specialty, then it would seem overbearing to insist that 20 or even 10 of those hours be specific to ultrasound. Likewise, in a residency program, it does not make sense to require 15 to 20 hours a year of ultrasound didactic education if the entire didactic curriculum is only 200 hours per year. In a poll of 42 emergency department ultrasound directors, the question was asked, "How much CME is needed to keep ultrasound skills up?" Responses varied from 0 to 30 hours, with a median of 8 hours. PLUS lead persons should decide on required levels of CME and should consider all the above factors when making this decision.

▶ SELECT THE LEAD PERSON(S)

The PLUS program's lead person is an individual who has some level of expertise in PLUS and oversees the training program at an institution or clinic. Generally, this person is a member of a group of physicians who are being trained and is either hired into the position, or more commonly, is an existing member of the group who is selected for the position and then trained. In a busy program, this duty is sometimes shared among more than one physician. In some instances, the individual who performs this service is someone from outside the group hired on an hourly basis. Whenever possible, it is advantageous to establish this role within the group because the process of training the other group members is continuous and is much easier to accomplish when the lead person is readily available. The group should acknowledge that the lead person will invest a considerable number of hours in training, often up to 100 hours, and this time should be fairly compensated.

▶ OBTAIN HOSPITAL APPROVAL OF THE PROGRAM

When performing PLUS in a hospital setting, it is strongly recommended that this be done under a hospital-approved program of training and credentialing. Going through such an approval process increases the scrutiny of the program by individuals outside the department and may generate valuable additional input into the program structure. Closer scrutiny by others will also lead to a more careful internal review of the program before presentation to the hospital, invariably leading to a better constructed program and tighter control on the indications of PLUS. Approval also ensures that in the event of a significant PLUS-related problem, it will be more difficult for others outside the department to persuade hospital administration to restrict the PLUS program's activities. As with the overall program design, a hospital proposal can be modeled after a successful one from another institution.

Obtaining hospital approval of a PLUS program should be seen as a political process. There has been some resistance to PLUS programs from imaging specialists.[7–10] Knowing which physician groups side with the proposal and which oppose it before open discussion occurs may enhance the application process. In our experience, those physicians who tend to be most supportive are those who also want to establish PLUS programs. These physicians may include emergency physicians, surgeons, nephrologists, and family physicians, among others. Clinicians who already use ultrasound in their practice also can be allies in this process; these physicians include obstetrician-gynecologists, vascular surgeons, and cardiologists.

The following are helpful to refer to in a proposal.

1. The individual specialty society's policy statement regarding use of PLUS. In emergency medicine, for example, the Society for Academic Emergency Medicine,[11] the American Academy of Emergency Medicine,[12] and the American College of Emergency Physicians[13] have supported PLUS use in the emergency department.
2. The American Medical Association's Policy H-230.960[13] citing that individual specialties have the right to determine how to appropriately use ultrasound in their practice.
3. Determining the percentage of residency programs in the individual specialty, as well as clinicians in the region and nationally, who are using PLUS. Has PLUS become or is it becoming the local standard of care? Is it a resident training requirement? For example, more than two-thirds of U.S. residencies in emergency medicine have training programs in PLUS. Performing and interpreting ultrasound is considered part of the core curriculum in emergency medicine.[15]
4. There are numerous articles attesting to the safety and efficacy of PLUS, especially in comparison to ultrasound examinations performed by imaging specialists.

▶ ACQUIRE AN ULTRASOUND MACHINE

This subject will be covered in detail in Chapter 2, "Ultrasound Equipment." When making the decision on a purchase of an ultrasound machine, the best advice is to try out different ultrasound machines "head to head." This can usually be accomplished at PLUS conferences or specialty society meetings. If other colleagues are using PLUS, determine what they like and dislike about their machines. What equipment did they get that they do not use and what do they wish they had gotten? What kind of service do they get from the manufacturer? The relationship with the manufacturer is almost as important as the machine itself, in that the company representatives assist with scheduled maintenance, urgent repairs, equipment upgrades, and, in many instances, actual training within the program. Besides purchasing a machine, other options include renting, leasing, or borrowing an older machine from a department that is upgrading their equipment.

▶ TRAIN THE LEAD PERSON

Several training options are available for the lead person. Most commonly, this person attends one of the many available PLUS courses given by various specialty societies or commercial entities and then undergoes a period of training in his or her own clinical setting. The fastest way to become facile at PLUS is to sit and practice with an experienced sonographer. The best resource for an experienced sonographer is to look for one certified by the American Registry of Diagnostic Medical Sonographers (ARDMS) within the hospital. It may be possible for the lead person-in-training to sit with a sonographer and perform examinations during the sonographer's normal working hours. This approach has the advantage of minimal cost, but is less time-efficient since the trainee will be required to sit through many examinations that may not be applicable to the interests of that trainee. In addition, there may be some examinations, like the Focused Assessment with Sonography for Trauma examination, that may not be routinely performed by sonographers in the ultrasound suite. A better alternative is to hire a sonographer to individually teach the lead person in their own clinical setting during a time when the trainee is free from clinical duties. Sonographers are often eager for extra work and often charge reasonable hourly rates.

The PLUS lead person may require several months of training before they attain the expertise needed to train others within their group. It is imperative that the lead person be well established before the rest of the group begins training. This is important to help facilitate the group through the "training doldrums," which is when the frustrations of training tend to peak. It should be emphasized that the learning curve is quite steep at the beginning but is actually relatively short in length, so that the minimum level of examination competency can be achieved with a manageable number of ultrasound examinations.

▶ TRAIN THE GROUP

Initial training can be either brief or extensive, depending on the training approach that is taken. One training method is conducted in "parallel," where training occurs for several ultrasound examinations at once. The other method is conducted in "serial," where training occurs with one ultrasound examination at a time, without proceeding to another examination until a certain level of proficiency is achieved. The parallel model works best when individual trainees are able to dedicate a larger portion of their time away from patient care to learn a new set of skills, as is typical in residency training programs. The serial model has the advantage of requiring less time input to get a trainee to a minimum level of competency for one particular examination. Serial training is ideal for community-based practitioners who have less time for training and want to incorporate one set of PLUS skills into their practice as rapidly as possible.

All training programs generally have the following components.

- An initial block of didactic instruction.
- An initial "hands-on" exercise.
- A required number of proctored examinations performed on actual patients.

Initial Didactic Instruction

The initial didactic instruction is where members of the physician group get their "jump start" in training. Initial training may consist of anywhere from several hours of instruction, if training in only one examination type, to several days of instruction, if training in multiple examinations. At a minimum, an introduction to the basic physics of ultrasound is required to understand the capabilities and limitations of the technology. Ultrasound is said to be the "art of determining artifact from reality;" understanding the physics, even at a basic level, is essential for this task. In addition, there should be some specific didactic instruction on the examination(s) being taught. It is feasible for the lead person to develop and perform the initial training block, especially if only one or two examinations are to be covered. If several examinations are being taught, then it may be more practical to have group members attend one of the commercially available introductory ultrasound courses. Planning and giving a large hands-on PLUS instruction block is time consuming and may be better left to the professional course organizers. It is important, however, that the lead person ensure that any outside course meets the training requirements established for their program.

At an ultrasound course, 1 to 2 hours is generally spent on ultrasound physics and equipment instrumentation, and an additional hour or two on each specific examination type. Lectures should include discussions of the specific indications for the examination and review of the anatomy, including normal, normal variant, and abnormal ultrasound findings. Teaching should be "finding-based," concentrating on specific limited findings rather than discussing all diseases related to a specific organ or anatomic area. The major finding for each examination type (e.g., gallstones) as well as other findings (e.g., common bile duct diameter, pericholecystic fluid, gallbladder-wall thickness) should be demonstrated, and the appropriate ways to use these findings for clinical decision making should be discussed. Indications for referral for more comprehensive imaging should be emphasized. A comprehensive listing of suggested content for didactic sessions is listed in the Model Curriculum for Emergency Ultrasound.[3]

Initial Hands-On Exercise

The initial hands-on exercise is usually combined with the initial didactic instruction. During this exercise, image acquisition is practiced on normal models in a nonstressful, non-patient care environment. There should be no more than four to five students and one instructor per ultrasound machine in order to maximize student-scanning time. Topics covered should include basic operation of the ultrasound controls, techniques for maximizing image quality, normal ultrasound anatomy, and systematic approaches to the examination types taught in the didactic sessions. Sessions typically last 1 hour for each examination type. Specific "pelvic" models are employed when transvaginal ultrasound is taught, and chronic ambulatory peritoneal dialysis (CAPD) patients may be employed to demonstrate free intraperitoneal fluid on ultrasound examination. CAPD patients can simulate a positive examination by infusing fluid into their peritoneal cavity at will, and can even vary the amount of fluid to give different appearances. In instances where budgetary or planning constraints exist, these sessions can be run with trainees examining each other. Though pathology will not (usually) be demonstrated using this approach, trainees can effectively learn techniques for good image acquisition and systematic examination.

A newer teaching method is the ultrasound simulator that uses a mannequin and computer to simulate scanning. The advantage of a simulator is that it can be programmed to simulate pathology, thus giving the trainee a more varied and yet standardized training experience. Finding enough patients with actual pathology to examine is one of the biggest challenges during training. Simulator technology may hold great promise for the future of PLUS training.

Proctored Examinations

The goals of proctoring are to help establish basic ultrasound skills, solidify the approach to examinations, verify the quality of images produced, and verify the accuracy of the examinations. Once a physician completes the initial training phase, the real learning curve begins. As the physician begins scanning a variety of patients in his or her own clinical environment, the relative complexity of the skill will become evident. The trainee needs to be mentally prepared for this predictably difficult period so that frustration will not inhibit training. "On-line" proctoring is extremely helpful in assisting the physician through this period. On-line proctoring is having the proctor sit with and guide the trainee through the examinations. The lead person can do on-line proctoring, but this is quite time-consuming. On-line proctoring is best accomplished by a less expensive and usually more experienced ultrasound technician.

Some programs choose to proctor "off-line," meaning that trainees perform examinations independently, and then an experienced individual judges the quality and accuracy of the examinations at a later time. A common method of off-line proctoring is to videotape examinations. This method results in slower training but is usually cheaper than hiring an ultrasound technician for on-line proctoring and saves the lead person from doing the on-line proctoring themselves. At least some proctoring, especially in the early training stages, will have to be "on-line" or the trainee will not possess enough skills to make their independent scanning time productive. A reasonable way to control costs, but provide high-quality training, is to employ a combination of both on-line and off-line proctoring.

Another off-line proctoring option is to keep track of how PLUS results compare with other clinical information, including ultrasound examinations performed by imaging specialists, other imaging studies (such as computed tomography scans), or procedures (such as surgery). This method accomplishes verification of accuracy but does not fulfill the other goals of proctoring. If this method is used, trainees should occasionally undergo on-line proctoring as well. Reviewing static ultrasound images generated by trainees as the sole method to proctor off-line is problematic, especially for negative examinations, since pathology may be visible in one imaging plane but not in another and the inexperienced examiner may simply fail to find and photograph the pathology. Static images that are clearly positive can be used for proctoring in a limited manner since it is more difficult to "create" a false positive image (though not impossible), but it is a less desirable option. Proctoring is the longest phase of training, often taking several months to complete. The biggest challenge for a lead person is to maintain enthusiasm for the training program as physicians begin to climb this steep, but short, learning curve.

▶ PERFORM PROBLEM SOLVING

PLUS lead persons usually experience two major problems with their programs. The first is the difficulty in convincing all members of the group to participate in training. The second deals with problems in maintaining trainee enthusiasm during the long proctoring phase. For emergency physicians, when faced with the difficulty of integrating practice PLUS examinations with patient care during busy emergency department shifts, it is tempting to put off using PLUS. The following are some strategies to help avoid these problems.

1. *Maintain easy access.* The easier it is to use the ultrasound machine, the more it will be used. An ultrasound machine in a "safe" but inconvenient place will not be used. The ultrasound machine should be kept in close proximity to patient rooms and in full view. Not only will this remind physicians to use the machine, it will assist with security of the ultrasound machine since it will be noticeable when it is not there.

2. *Examination efficiency.* PLUS examinations can add 5 to 10 minutes to a patient encounter (though they tend to reduce overall length of stay in the emergency department), which can add up over the course of a shift. If physicians perceive the PLUS examination as a major time drain they will not use it. Bringing the machine to the patient room at the time of first contact if a PLUS examination is anticipated can reduce examination times. The examinations should be kept brief. If it appears clear early in the examination that it will be technically difficult and an accurate result is unlikely, the examination should be terminated instead of wasting time trying to locate elusive structures. There will be other patients to scan and, with experience, the trainee will develop strategies for producing acceptable images on technically difficult patients.

3. *Make it easy to keep track of training examinations.* If trainees are required to bring or keep track of individual logbooks, then the program will likely flounder. Logbooks may be forgotten or lost, which can create frustration on the part of trainees. Many programs keep centralized logbooks in the clinical area into which all trainees record their examinations. A centralized logbook has the advantage of keeping all records in one place and allowing proctors to keep records organized for videotape review sessions. Another approach is to have trainees submit individual 3 × 5 cards documenting each patient examined. This allows examinations to be turned in when completed, reducing the number of examinations lost.

4. *Introduce competition.* Competition is an effective motivating factor if applied appropriately.

Physicians tend to be competitive. Periodically publishing the progress of trainees so that they can see how they compare to their peers can encourage those who might otherwise be ambivalent. At a minimum, it reminds everyone to continue practicing their PLUS skills. Introducing a stepped system of achievement is also beneficial, especially if the first level can be achieved in a reasonably short period of time. The Harbor-UCLA program allows some limited reporting of results after as little as 50 examinations; whereas 80 or more examinations are required for more extensive reporting. Being allowed to proctor less experienced trainees can also reward trainees who have achieved designated levels of achievement.

▶ REGISTRY OF DIAGNOSTIC MEDICAL SONOGRAPHERS

Most ultrasound technicians have been registered by the American Registry of Diagnostic Medical Sonographers and carry the title "RDMS," which stands for "Registered Diagnostic Medical Sonographer." This is a certification that can be achieved after a prescribed period of training or experience and satisfactory performance on a standardized examination. This certification is recognized nationally as the standard of training for sonographers. This certification is available to physicians as well, and many propose it as a logical step in the acquisition of ultrasound skills. Tests are given in several specialty areas including the abdomen, adult echocardiography, and obstetrics and gynecology. These examinations are directed toward comprehensive examination rather than limited examination. In order to be certified, an individual must pass both a physical principles and instrumentation examination as well as at least one specialty area examination.

The advantage of this certification is that it is a credential with which hospitals are likely to be familiar, and may lend weight to the physician seeking credentialing in PLUS. Physicians may qualify to sit for the examination after 1 year of full time clinical practice, which includes ultrasound usage and 12 hours of education specific to the examination area. Notably, the ARDMS certification attests to a practitioner's skills in *performing* examinations but not in *interpreting* them.

▶ ELECTIVE TRAINING

An elective in PLUS is a brief training period, usually on the order of 2 to 4 weeks, where a trainee dedicates his or her time specifically to the learning of PLUS without the distraction of other patient care responsibilities. This can be an outstanding method to accelerate the experi-

ence level of a trainee. Setting objectives is the key to elective design. The elective director should be able to answer the question, "What should the trainee be able to do with PLUS by the end of the elective?" Often, the objective is to perform a certain number of PLUS examinations, or it may be to meet the requirements for a particular privilege level. The goals should be made clear to the trainee at the outset of the elective. Example activities include:

1. Performance of a certain number of examinations under direct supervision or by post hoc review of video or static images.
2. Assigned reading, either from texts or journals.
3. Involvement with administrative aspects of the PLUS training program, including ultrasound machine and supply maintenance, record keeping, and proctoring of other trainees. This is the contribution the trainee makes in return for the teaching time they receive. It is also an essential exercise for anyone considering directing a PLUS program in the future.
4. Involvement with other special projects, including research, teaching, or creating teaching materials, such as an ultrasound teaching file.
5. Testing, both written and practical.

The following is an example set of requirements for a 2-week elective.

1. A pre-elective meeting outlining the objectives of the elective.
2. Four to 6 hours of directly supervised scanning distributed over the elective period.
3. An additional 56 hours of hours of time spent independently scanning.
4. Assigned readings from an ultrasound textbook.
5. A written examination at the end of the elective.
6. Tape review sessions as needed for item 3 above.
7. Special projects amounting to an additional 4 to 8 hours (e.g., submit two cases to the ultrasound teaching file).

Ultrasound is a skill of great interest to the residents in emergency medicine as well as medical students applying for emergency medicine residencies. The enjoyment and satisfaction residents have received while doing the ultrasound elective in our program has made it one of the most popular nonrequired rotations in our department, and at the same time, has greatly increased the overall ultrasound expertise in our emergency department.

▶ FELLOWSHIP TRAINING

To master the skills necessary to integrate this powerful imaging modality into clinical practice, and especially for those considering a position as an ultrasound program director, a fellowship in PLUS should be considered. Fellowships provide a means for intensive ultrasound training beyond that which is currently possible within the curriculum of an existing residency program. There is currently a deficiency of PLUS fellowships available to physicians who desire further training. Many of the current experts in PLUS have acquired the skills on their own. They have invested considerable time and expense learning on the job and at educational courses, visiting professorships, or training with an experienced sonographer willing to mentor them. As increasing numbers of physicians become adept with PLUS, there will be more individuals driven to provide a pathway to share their knowledge with others.

For a fellow to obtain a quality educational experience, residency programs will need a solid commitment from their departments to provide the necessary resources. Several vital elements are needed to foster this learning experience. First, there must be a physician who is qualified to mentor an ultrasound fellow. This person should invariably have an extensive experience in PLUS, along with a passion to teach. They would ideally have research experience and academic involvement in one or more of their specialty's ultrasound committees. Second, the fellowship director's department must fully support their efforts to advance ultrasound education and provide protected academic time to mentor each fellow and train physicians within their own department. Departments should provide financial support for a quality ultrasound system and equipment, and administrative support for research. Third, the patient volume and demographics should be sufficient to provide the fellow with experience in all applications of PLUS.

While the curriculum may vary somewhat, the foundation of each ultrasound fellowship program is fairly similar. They provide each ultrasound fellow with a core content of subject matter that is covered within the 1-year program along with several other educational experiences covered in the following sections.

Core Content

The core content refers to the applications (abdominal, cardiac, pelvic, etc.) and specific organ pathology identifiable by PLUS that is clinically relevant to the fellow's specialty. For an emergency medicine ultrasound fellowship, the "Model Curriculum" developed by the SAEM task force in 1993[3] is an appropriate starting point to design content. Since the time of its publication, however, many other useful applications of PLUS in emergency medicine have emerged (lower extremity doppler, musculoskeletal, etc.).

Quality Improvement

Fellows should be involved in the department's ultrasound QI program. This activity offers a high-educational return for time invested since the mistakes of others become teaching material for the fellow.

Journal Club

Reviewing the literature is an important component of an ultrasound fellowship. Although the structure in which this is accomplished may vary, a working knowledge of the pertinent literature is an integral part of the educational process. Structured journal club meetings may also provide a means by which other members of the department can join in the educational development. Likewise, a review of the literature may also provide an avenue to formulate other research ideas.

Teaching Responsibilities

The ultrasound fellow should also be responsible for educating other physicians within the department. Depending upon the prior experience of the ultrasound fellow, this duty may vary considerably. Once the fellow has developed the skills necessary to supervise others safely and competently, their teaching obligations will be utilized to advance the ultrasound education of other physicians within the department. The fellow should have protected nonclinical time devoted to teaching. He or she also may have other elective teaching opportunities outside of the department, such as at local hospitals, society meetings, or national conferences, in which to hone their skills by lecturing and providing hands-on training.

Future Directors

The goal of most ultrasound fellows is to start or direct a PLUS program after graduating from the fellowship. In the majority of cases, this will involve implementing or enhancing a PLUS program at an existing residency program. Experience gathered through their training should include a road map for this important step. Part of this training should involve the fellow in the political arena in which they must interact. This includes the likes of departmental policies on credentialing, ultrasound system maintenance, billing, QI discrepancies, and intradepartmental policies. They will also need assistance in developing lectures, training courses, and various training aides for their program. The fellowship should also include networking with other leaders in their field who will provide them with an opportunity to share ideas and research projects and shape the future of PLUS.

▶ COST OF A POINT OF CARE ULTRASOUND PROGRAM

One of the most common questions posed by physician groups about PLUS is, "How much will it cost us?" Little has been published about the costs of a PLUS program, but after discussing costs with directors of PLUS programs at over 40 academic emergency medicine centers, several generalizations can be made. Some of the costs are easy

▶ **TABLE 1–4.** COST OF A PLUS PROGRAM§

One-Time Costs	
Ultrasound machine*	$30,000 (median); range $16,000–$100,000
Program development	10–40 h or more. May be much more if lead person prepares and delivers all initial training.
Initial training courses	1–3 days per physician. The cost per physician for commercial courses ranges from $500–$1,000. This cost will be reduced if the lead person does the training.
Proctoring	Cost of on-line proctoring each physician in training (ultrasound technicians often cost from $35–$45 per h). Lead person may perform this duty.
Recurring Costs	
Supplies (paper, gel, etc.)	$1,200 (median); range $300–$1,800/yr
Maintenance agreement†	$1,800 (median); range $700–$8,000/yr
Administration of program	Highly variable, based on program structure
Continuing medical education	8 hours/yr (median recommendation), per physician
Time spent examining‡	10 minutes/examination (median estimate)

*An ultrasound machine should be seen as having about a 5–7 year useful life; a machine should work until the end of that period but technology and options will progress so that replacement of the machine should be planned. It is also possible that once the PLUS program is established, a second ultrasound machine may be purchased as a backup to avoid long downtime periods when the primary machine is out of service.
†Highly recommended.
‡This is included to determine how much income might be lost, especially in a busy emergency department, where time spent scanning is lost income due to less patients being seen. It is possible, though unproven, that PLUS might actually increase the number of patients a physician can care for by narrowing the differential diagnosis sooner and moving patients through the clinical setting more swiftly.
§This information was gathered in the year 2000, so by the time of printing some of the equipment costs will have changed. The costs for training seem to have remained more constant over time.

to define (e.g., equipment and supply costs, price of training courses) and some are not as easy to define (e.g., time spent developing a program plan or performing practice ultrasound examinations.) Costs will be highly institution and group dependent, too. Table 1–4 provides rough estimates that are divided into one-time and recurring costs to give a general idea of what can be expected.

▶ BILLING

The second most common question asked by those who must make the balance sheet work for an office or department is, "Can we bill for this service?" The short answer is "yes." There are physicians and departments who bill successfully for PLUS, though the total number is not known. Their numbers are believed to be small at the time of this writing. This is not to say that billing for PLUS is inherently difficult, but reflects that programs at academic centers generally tend to be less aggressive about billing.

There are CPT codes already in existence that are designed to reimburse PLUS examinations. Some examples are:

76705	Limited Abdomen Examination	(e.g., single organ)
76775	Limited Retroperitoneal Examination	(e.g., kidney)
76815	Limited Obstetric Examination	(e.g., fetal heartbeat)
93979	Limited Aorta Examination	
93971	Limited Doppler Lower Extremity Examination	
93308	Limited 2D Echo Heart Examination	

Physicians performing PLUS should be eligible to bill both the technical portion and the interpretive portion of these codes. Reimbursement ranges are estimated to be from $50 to $150 per examination, depending on the type of examination. Physicians interested in reimbursement are encouraged to discuss the feasibility of billing for PLUS with billing experts.

REFERENCES

1. American College of Radiology. Standard for performing and interpreting diagnostic ultrasound examinations. Resolution 22, American College of Radiology, Reston, VA, 1996.
2. American Institute of Ultrasound in Medicine. Training guidelines for physicians who evaluate and interpret diagnostic ultrasound examinations, official statement, March, 1997. *www.aium.org* (11/13/00).
3. Mateer JR, Plummer D, Heller M, et al. Model curriculum for physician training in emergency ultrasonography. Ann Emerg Med 1994;1:95–102.
4. Lanoix R, Leak LV, Gaeta T, et al. A preliminary evaluation of emergency ultrasound in the setting of an emergency medicine training program. Am J Emerg Med 2000;18:41–45.
5. Witting MD, Euerle BD, Butler KH. A comparison of emergency medicine ultrasound training with the guidelines of

the Society for Academic Emergency Medicine. Ann Emerg Med 1999;34:604–609.

6. ACEP emergency ultrasound guidelines—2001. American College of Emergency Physicians, 2001. *www.acep.org* (8/13/01).

7. Hamper UM. Commentary on Hertzberg BS, Kliewer MA, Bowie JD, Carroll BA, DeLong DH, Gray L, Nelson RC. Physician training requirements in sonography: how many cases are needed for competence? AJR Am J Roentgenol 2000;174(5):1221–7. Society of Radiologists in Ultrasound Newsletter, June 2000.

8. Hertzberg B, Kliewer MA, Bowie JD, et al. Physician training requirements in sonography: how many cases are needed for competence? AJR Am J Roentgenol 2000;174:1221–7.

9. Merritt CR: ER ultrasound services-some points to consider. Society of Radiologists in Ultrasound Newsletter, July 1999.

10. Unknown author: Who can perform ultrasound imaging? Society of Radiologists in Ultrasound Newsletter, March 2000.

11. Society for Academic Emergency Medicine. Ultrasound position statement. *www.saem.org/publicat/ultrasou.htm* (7/23/01).

12. American Academy of Emergency Medicine. Performance of emergency screening ultrasound examinations. Position Statement. February, 1999.

13. American College of Emergency Physicians. Use of ultrasound imaging by emergency physicians. Policy Statement. June, 1997.

14. American Medical Association. Privileging for ultrasound imaging. House of Delegates Policy H-230.960, 2000.

15. Task Force on the Core Content of Emergency Medicine Revision: Core content for emergency medicine. Ann of Emerg Med 1997;29:792–811.

CHAPTER 2

Ultrasound Equipment

William E. Durston, Joseph Salomone, and John Wiesenfarth

Many different ultrasound systems are available for emergency and acute care setting applications. Ultrasound machines come in a wide variety of shapes and sizes, from machines as small and portable as a laptop computer to ones about the size of a washing machine. Ultrasound machines also vary widely in their capabilities and in their price ranges. There are numerous considerations that go into choosing the optimal ultrasound system. In this chapter, the different types of ultrasound systems that are currently available are discussed in the context of their potential applications and limitations in different emergency settings. The chapter is intended to serve as a reference to those who are planning to acquire their first ultrasound system or those who are planning to upgrade or replace an existing system. In addition, this chapter is intended to assist those readers who are currently using ultrasonography in the emergency and acute care setting to fully utilize their current system.

► CONTROLS AND SPECIAL FEATURES

In the emergency setting, the most basic function of ultrasound machine is to offer a two-dimensional, grayscale (B-mode) image of the portion of the body that is being scanned. To accomplish this function, all ultrasound machines have certain basic features and controls. Beyond this basic function, most of the ultrasound machines that are currently available offer a variety of special features that enhance the quality of the B-mode image, provide optional M-mode imaging, and allow the operator to derive quantitative measurements and data from images. Many ultrasound machines also incorporate Doppler technology to display and quantify blood flow. While most

ultrasound machines equipped with general purpose transducers allow the operator to obtain fair images of the heart, some systems suitable for the emergency and acute care setting allow advanced cardiac imaging. In addition, modern ultrasound systems offer a number of options for viewing, printing, storing, and transmitting ultrasound images.

► BASIC FEATURES

Power Supply

Most ultrasound machines suitable for the emergency and acute care setting run off of standard wall current. Small, hand-carried machines may also offer the option of running off of rechargeable lithium batteries. For most applications, battery life ranges from 1.5 to 4 h. Batteries can be recharged in about 4 to 5 h.

Turning an ultrasound machine on and off is not always as intuitive as one might expect. On some machines, the power switch is on the control panel. On other machines, it is on the side of the console. Some machines have a power switch at the base of the console designed to be turned on and off with the operator's foot. Since portable bedside ultrasound machines are turned on and off frequently, it is important that the power switch be conveniently located.

The location and design of the power cord connection is another relevant consideration in choosing an ultrasound machine for the emergency setting. Portable bedside ultrasound machines are typically moved frequently by different personnel. It is not uncommon for the power cord to get run over or to be pulled forcefully when someone forgets to unplug the machine before moving it. For these reasons, it is important that the power cord connection have some type of strain relief mechanism and that there be a convenient arrangement for coiling or retracting the cord out of the way when the machine is being moved.

Electronic Processing: Analog versus Digital

Most currently available ultrasound systems employ a combination of analog and digital technology. With all ultrasound machines, the ultrasound signals are sent and received by the transducer in analog form. Some older machines rely exclusively on analog technology for processing and displaying the received signals. Other machines process the received signals using analog circuitry but convert them to digital format before they are displayed. Another approach used by many currently available machines is to convert the received signals immediately from analog to digital form before they are processed.

A detailed discussion of the relative advantages and disadvantages of analog versus digital processing in ultrasonography is beyond the scope of this chapter. Briefly, though, an advantage of analog processing is that the machine powers up faster, usually in a matter of a few seconds. Analog machines also tend to be less expensive than digital machines. Just as analog media such as vinyl records and cassette tapes are being replaced by digital computerized disks, however, analog ultrasound machines are being replaced by ones that rely primarily on digital processing. Digital ultrasound images can be stored, copied, modified, and transmitted without any degradation in quality. Digital processing also facilitates quantification and manipulation of ultrasound data.

Control Panel

All ultrasound machines have some type of control panel, also referred to as the "user interface." The design and complexity of control panels varies considerably among different machines and manufacturers. The study of the function of the various controls on ultrasound machines has been referred to as "knobology," although in addition to knobs, controls may also consist of buttons, keys, switches, toggles, trackballs, rings, or sliding levers. A single "knob" may have many different functions, depending on the mode in which the machine is operating. For example, a trackball may be used to rapidly move from one field to the next during entry of patient data, to move a cursor to annotate an image, to reduce or expand the area that is being scanned, to position electronic calipers for measuring a structure, or to scroll through saved images. The function of a given control is usually indicated by a label or symbol imprinted on the control panel, although some machines employ "soft menu" screens to facilitate identification of the changeable function of certain controls. On some machines, the functions of selected controls are user programmable. As a general rule, the more expensive and versatile an ultrasound machine is, the more controls are present on the user interface. A large selection of controls may be an asset for experienced sonographers who wish to take full advantage of a machine's capabilities in performing definitive scans for a variety of different indications. For relatively inexperienced clinicians who are using an ultrasound machine occasionally to perform limited, goal-directed studies, a complex control panel may be difficult to master.

Patient Data Entry

Except in the most emergent cases, the first step after turning on the power is to enter identifying information for the patient being scanned. On most machines, this is done by means of an alphanumeric keypad. On the small hand-carried machines, a touchpad may be used instead of a keypad. Some ultrasound machines employ "full stroke" alphanumeric keypads with open keys, whereas others use membrane-covered keypads. In general, the full stroke keypads are easier and faster to use, but more prone to damage, especially from spilled liquids.

The patient identification (ID) screen typically prompts the operator to input the patient name, age, sex, and medical record number; the name or initials of the examiner and the name of the ordering physician. Depending on the type of study being done, the patient ID screen may also prompt the operator to input other information, such as the date of the last menstrual period for an obstetric study. The screen may also allow other comments to be entered, such as the indication for the study. On most machines, the date is entered automatically. Once the patient information has been entered on the patient ID screen, it is automatically displayed as a header during actual scanning of the patient and is included on all saved or printed images. At the end of the study, the operator may return to the patient ID screen to record the results. Some machines offer more detailed report pages, customized for the type of study being done.

Acoustic Output (Power)

The amount of energy leaving the ultrasound transducer is referred to as the acoustic output or power, and relates to the amplitude of the sound waves that are emitted.[1] Increasing acoustic output may, in some cases, improve image quality. On the other hand, increasing acoustic output may also increase the risk of adverse biologic effects, including tissue heating and cavitation. In emergency and acute care setting applications of diagnostic ultrasound, the safety of the acoustic output is of greatest concern in scanning pregnant patients. The default acoustic output setting for all diagnostic ultrasound machines is set at a level that is felt to be safe for human tissue, including the in utero fetus. Some machines allow the operator to change the acoustic output either directly, through an output or power knob, or indirectly, by choosing different preset examination formats (see section on More Advanced Controls and Special Features).

On ultrasound machines that allow the operator to adjust the acoustic output, the output is shown on the display screen. The acoustic output is indicated by a standardized mathematical index, with levels above 1.0 corresponding to more significant risk of adverse biologic effects.[2] Indices are displayed both for potential mechanical and thermal tissue injury. Thermal injury is of particular concern when a stationary acoustic beam is used, as in Doppler or M-mode scanning.

In the case of medical imaging, the old medical adage, "First, do no harm," has been translated into the acronym, "ALARA," which stands for using energy levels that are **a**s **l**ow **a**s **r**easonably **a**chievable.[3] Sonographers in the emergency and acute care setting, and particularly novice sonographers who may be fascinated by the appearance of a live intrauterine pregnancy on ultrasound, should be careful to abide by this principle. Operators of ultrasound machines with adjustable acoustic outputs must be familiar with the output controls and with displays indicating the safety of the output. For additional information on the acoustic output of a given machine, operators should consult the manufacturer's representative or the operation manual supplied with the machine.

Gain Control and Time-Gain Compensation

The gain control increases or decreases the amount of returned echoes displayed on the viewing screen. Increasing the gain has the effect of brightening the display while decreasing it has the effect of darkening it. Changing the gain has no effect on acoustic output. By increasing the gain, though, the operator may be able to decrease the acoustic output necessary to provide an optimal image, in accordance with the ALARA principle.

All ultrasound machines have at least one control for adjusting the overall gain. The gain setting is usually shown on the display screen in units of decibels or as a percentage of maximum gain. In addition, many machines have one or more time-gain compensation (TGC) controls. Echoes returning from deeper tissues (far field) are more attenuated than echoes returning from tissues closer to the transducer (near field) because they must travel through more tissue. If an ultrasound machine did not take this into account, the far field would always appear darker than the near field on two-dimensional grayscale images. To provide more uniform-appearing images, the machine boosts the gain on the signals from the far field. The machine recognizes whether signals are returning from superficial or deep tissue by the time it takes them to return to the transducer. The machine performs TGC in-

ternally, without any action required by the operator. Sometimes, though, the internal TGC processing does not result in optimal images. For example, if the practitioner is trying to examine the uterus and adnexal structures through the bladder, the enhanced transmission of echoes through the bladder may cause the structures deep to it to appear too bright. To overcome this problem, many machines have TGC controls which allow the operator to override the machine's internal TGC processing. The simplest TGC control is a single button that allows the operator to adjust the gain on the near half of the field relative to the far half. More expensive machines usually have multiple TGC controls in the form of a series of sliding levers, lined up one above the other, which allow the operator to adjust the gain at multiple levels quickly and smoothly (Figure 2–1). On some machines, TGC adjustments are displayed on the side of the screen

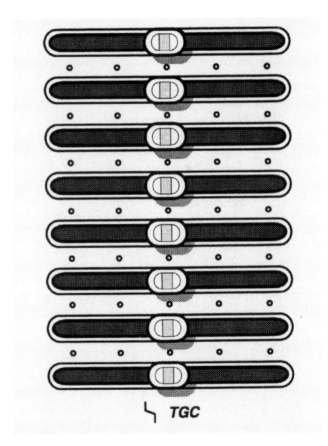

Figure 2–1. Time gain compensation (TGC) controls on the GE Logiq 400 ultrasound machine. Using the eight sliding levers, the operator can quickly and precisely adjust the gain throughout the entire scanning depth. The top lever corresponds to the most superficial tissue layer and the bottom lever to the maximum display depth. Moving a lever to the right in its "slide pot" increases gain; moving the lever to the left decreases gain. *(Reprinted with permission, from Logiq 400 user manual courtesy of General Electric Corporation.)*

as a curved line, with the line on the screen corresponding to an imaginary line drawn through the center of the TGC levers on the control panel.

Depth

Most ultrasound machines allow the operator to adjust the ultrasound scanning depth. If the tissue of interest is just under the skin surface, such as a subcutaneous foreign body, then there is no point in the machine processing signals received from deeper tissues or in displaying these signals on the viewing screen. On the other hand, in a very obese patient, a deep structure such as the abdominal aorta may be off the bottom of the screen if the machine is set to scan at a depth that is optimal for the average patient. By adjusting the imaging depth, the operator can ensure that the tissue or structure of interest is included on the screen, and that extraneous signals from deeper tissues are excluded. The depth of the tissue being scanned is usually displayed on a centimeter scale on the side of the display screen.

Focus and Zoom

Many ultrasound machines allow the operator to adjust the depth at which the ultrasound beam is best focused. Some machines allow the operator to choose multiple concurrent focal depths. Electronically, the focal depth is controlled by minute alterations in the timing of the firing of the crystals in the transducer head. The operator usually controls the focal zone by means of an up/down button on the control panel. Adjusting the focus is most helpful in optimizing images of relatively deep structures. The focal depth is usually displayed as a pointer on the side of the display screen.

On many machines, the width of the scan area can also be adjusted. Ultrasound probes with convex heads produce fan- or sector-shaped images. If the tissue on the outer margins of the image is not of interest, the width of the sector can be narrowed to concentrate more ultrasound beams in a narrower area.

Many machines also offer a "zoom" function that allows the operator to magnify an area of interest. Some machines offer only a single magnification factor. Other machines allow the operator to select from a range of magnifications. The area of interest is usually selected using the trackball, then magnified to full screen size. On some machines, the original image is displayed as a miniature in the corner of the screen, with a frame outlining the portion of the image that has been magnified.

Freeze and Cine Controls

What appears to be a continuous, moving image in two-dimensional scanning is really a series of static images displayed at frame rates so fast that the eye cannot detect flicker between frames. Viewing the motion picture-like images as they are being produced is often referred to as "real-time" ultrasound, as opposed to later viewing of static images. It is generally accepted that more reliable information is obtained during real-time scanning than from viewing static images.[4] Normal structures can be made to appear abnormal, and vice versa, on static images. Viewing images in real time while handling the transducer allows the sonographer to interpret studies in the context of the continual changes in images and artifacts produced by movement of tissue, movement of the transducer, or adjustments on the machine.

Nevertheless, it is important to be able to save selected static images for documentation, review, or quality assurance purposes. All ultrasound machines suitable for emergency and acute care settings have a "freeze" function that allows the operator to lock a static image on the display screen. The freeze button is usually prominently located on the control panel. Some machines also have an optional foot pedal that can be used to freeze images while the operator uses one hand to hold the transducer and the other to make adjustments on the control panel.

Pressing the freeze button at precisely the correct time to save the best static image may occasionally be difficult. For this reason, most machines store a number of frames in a memory bank, which is usually referred to as "cine" (pronounced "sinnie") memory. The number of frames stored in cine memory on different machines varies from as few as 8 to over 1000. In general, a cine memory of 20 frames or more is adequate to catch the desired image. On most machines, the trackball is used to scroll back through cine images. Some machines also offer a cine loop function that replays stored images over and over, either in real time or in slow motion. The cine loop function is particularly useful in echocardiography.

▶ ADVANCED CONTROLS AND SPECIAL FEATURES

Dynamic Range and Grayscale Mapping

Together, dynamic range and grayscale mapping settings help determine how the intensity of the returned echoes is converted into shades of gray on the display screen. All ultrasound machines have built-in default settings for dynamic range and grayscale mapping. Some ultrasound machines allow the operator to adjust these settings to obtain optimal images.

The dynamic range is the range of returning echo intensities that the machine processes in forming a grayscale image. The dynamic range is expressed in decibels. Typical dynamic ranges are from 30 to 78 dB. Higher dynamic range settings tend to give more uniform-appearing images, with more subtle distinctions between tissues of different density. Lower settings give grainier images, with greater contrast between solid and cystic or vascular structures. In general, the best dynamic range is the one that gives a clearest distinction between adjacent tissues of interest.

Within a chosen dynamic range, the ultrasound machine converts different intensities of returning signals into different shades of gray. Some machines employ 64 shades of gray; others use 256. The grayscale map is the correlation between the different returning echo intensities and the shades of gray displayed on the screen. Some machines allow the operator to choose from several different grayscale map curves. By changing the grayscale map, the operator can either emphasize or de-emphasize subtle distinctions in echo intensities at the low, middle, or high end of the dynamic range. Selecting the best grayscale map for a given study is usually a subjective process done through trial and error.

Presettings, Body Position Markers, and Annotation Library

By adjusting settings, such as the acoustic output, dynamic range, grayscale map, scanning depth, focal depth, and gain, the operator can obtain the best possible B-mode image for any given examination. Making these adjustments on every new ultrasound examination, however, would be cumbersome and time consuming. To overcome this problem, many currently available machines have integrated "presets." These are predetermined default settings that are intended to optimize the image for a given type of study. As the name implies, presets allow the user to quickly initialize system settings for a specific examination and assumes a level of capability on the part of the sonographer.

For example, presets on a modern machine might include options for general abdominal, obstetric, gynecologic, vascular, cardiac, renal, urologic, neonatal, musculoskeletal, or small parts scanning. When the operator chooses the type of examination that is going to be done, the machine automatically defaults to the settings that have been predetermined to lead to optimal images for that particular type of study in most patients. Presets also often include an option for the obese or "technically difficult" patient that is likely to start with a higher power output; whereas a preset for obstetric applications would start with a low-power setting. The operator can override the presets if they do not seem optimal for the current patient. On most machines, the operator can also customize the presets. Presets offer the ability to minimize the number of button/switch selections the operator must depress prior to beginning the examination. By implementing the use of presets, operators are afforded an identical starting point to an examination, offering an initial level of consistency among multiple sonographers. Presets become of greater importance as the sophistication of the examination and equipment increases. Systems that offer increased capabilities (e.g., Doppler, etc.) allow a greater number of

scanning parameters to be initialized and manipulated during an examination. It must be remembered, however, that presets allow a standardization of the initial scanning parameters, and manipulating these initial parameters will often be required for specific patients if a quality diagnostic scan, free of misleading data, is to be documented.

Choosing a preset study format may also select a predetermined "library" of terms for use in rapidly annotating images that are to be printed and saved. Annotation libraries usually include both anatomic terms and terms describing transducer position. Choosing terms from the annotation library can save time in typing and can avoid misspellings, as in "Morison's pouch" or "sagittal." On some machines, the operator can customize the content of the annotation library.

In addition to annotating images with words, it is customary to include graphic figures on saved static ultrasound images indicating the position of the transducer relative to the body (Figure 2–2). The body position graphic is usually placed at the lower left-hand corner of the ultrasound image. The position of the transducer relative to the figure is usually controlled with the trackball and a rotation knob. Different machines vary with regard to the numbers and types of body position markers from which the operator may choose. On machines with presets for different types of studies, selecting a given type of study usually brings up a related annotation library and set of body position markers.

Automated Image Enhancement

Even after machine settings have been chosen, some ultrasound machines offer additional controls for enhancement of B-mode images at the push of a single button, similar to features on computer software for automatically enhancing the appearance of scanned images. One such control available on a number of machines is termed "rejection." Turning rejection on filters out low-level echoes usually caused by noise. Rejection may clear up the appearance of cystic and vascular structures, but may also filter out low-level signals from tissues of interest, such as sludge in the gallbladder. Rejection is not to be used as a solution for improper initial TGC and gain settings.

Another control available on some machines is edge enhancement. Edge enhancement emphasizes the grayscale differences between adjacent tissues of different densities, but can also give the appearance of apparent boundaries when none really exist. Some machines offer automatic gain control to give the optimal level of brightness on the image display. One manufacturer offers a control called, "auto tissue optimization (ATO)." In applying ATO (Figure 2–3), the operator indicates the area of greatest interest in the scanned image by framing it within a rectangle. The machine creates an internal histogram of the data within the region of interest and brings that region of interest up to the full 256 shades of gray

Figure 2–2. Body pattern figure with probe orientation marker. *(Reprinted with permission, from Logiq 400 user manual courtesy of General Electric Corporation.)*

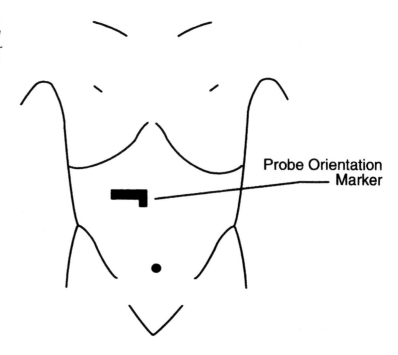

Probe Orientation Marker

available, thereby enhancing the contrast.[5] ATO may be applied during real-time B-mode scanning or after an image has been frozen on the screen.

Tissue Harmonic

Tissue harmonic imaging takes advantage of the fact that as sound waves of a given frequency pass through tissue, harmonics are produced within the tissue at multiples of the initial frequency. For example, if an ultra-sound probe sends out a signal at 2 MHz, harmonics will be produced within the tissue at 4 MHz, 6 MHz, 8 MHz, and so on. In conventional ultrasound scanning, the transducer listens for echoes returning at the same frequency as that at which they were sent out. In tissue harmonic imaging, the transducer listens for sound waves returning at twice the frequency of the pulse that was emitted from the transducer (the second harmonic). The advantage of tissue har-

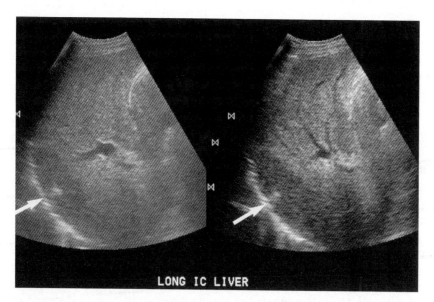

LONG IC LIVER

Figure 2–3. Automated image enhancement. Image on the left was obtained with standard settings. After the image was frozen on the screen, the "automatic tissue optimization" control was selected, resulting in image on right. Arrow points to metastasis in liver. Note the greater contrast between adjacent tissues of slightly different echodensity in the image on the right. *(Image courtesy of General Electric Corporation.)*

monic imaging over conventional scanning is that the harmonic sound waves pass in only one direction, from the tissue to the transducer, before being analyzed. The harmonic sound wave traveling in only one direction is less prone to deflection than the fundamental sound wave emitted from the transducer that must pass through tissue in two directions. Tissue harmonic imaging tends to result in less distortion with greater signal to noise ratio. Artifacts due to side lobes and reverberations are greatly reduced. Subtle distinctions between tissues of slightly different echodensity may be enhanced with tissue harmonics, and acoustic shadowing of calcified structures may be more readily seen (Figure 2–4)[6,7,8]

Three-Dimensional Ultrasound

Three-dimensional viewing is one of the most recent innovations in ultrasonography.[9,10] With currently available ultrasound machines, images must necessarily be presented in two dimensions on the two-dimensional display screen. By shading the images, though, they can be made to appear three-dimensional, a process known as "three-dimensional rendering." Three-dimensional rendering requires that data on the structure of interest actually be acquired in three dimensions instead of the usual two. This is done in one of two methods. In the older method, the operator must manually slide the probe across the patient's skin. The machine analyzes the data from the multiple, two-dimensional B-scans and collates them into a three-dimensional rendering. A newer, more accurate method involves electronic steering of the ultrasound probe. Three-dimensional rendering produces striking images that appear more like anatomic drawings than the usual two-dimensional ultrasound views (Figure 2–5). Whether or not three-dimensional rendering will enhance the accuracy of ultrasonography in the emergency and acute care setting is a question that requires further study.

M Mode

In the motion, or "M mode," tissue movement is depicted along a single narrow ultrasound beam on the vertical axis of the ultrasound screen while time is depicted on the horizontal axis. What the operator sees on the screen is a series of wavy grayscale lines that correspond to movement of the tissue being scanned toward or away from the transducer. In real-time M-mode scanning, the grayscale lines move up and down at the same time as they scroll from right to left. M mode is most often used in cardiac imaging, particularly to depict motion of cardiac valves. Another common use of M mode is to depict fetal cardiac motion. Many modern ultrasound machines allow the operator to switch from B-mode to M-mode scanning, or to display both B-mode and M-mode images simultaneously on a split screen (Figure 2–6).

Color Doppler

Many ultrasound machines now incorporate Doppler technology for the detection and quantification of blood flow. By listening for a frequency shift in the echoes returned from tissue, the machine can detect movement toward or away from the transducer. This frequency shift is converted electronically to color on the screen, with movement toward the transducer typically being depicted as red and movement away from the transducer being depicted as blue. Some machines also offer non-directional Doppler, where flow in any direction is depicted as a single color.

Duplex ultrasound combines high-resolution imaging in real time with simultaneous Doppler capability, providing hemodynamic information with anatomic detail. Duplex scanning has many potential applications in the emergency and acute care setting.[11] One of the most common applications of duplex scanning is to evaluate for

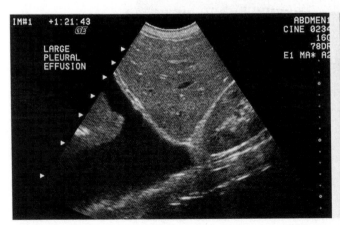
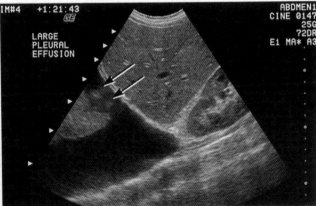

Figure 2–4. Imaging of pleural effusion with and without tissue harmonics. Image on right was obtained through conventional scanning, image on left using tissue harmonics. Note mirror artifact between diaphragm and lung (arrows) with conventional scanning that is not present using tissue harmonics. *(Image courtesy of General Electric Corporation.)*

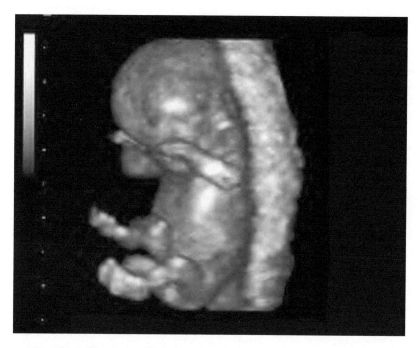

Figure 2–5. Three-dimensional rendering of first trimester fetus. *(Image courtesy of Medison America, Inc.)*

deep vein thrombosis (DVT).[12,13] It has been reported that emergency physicians can perform sonographic venography with acceptable degrees of accuracy after relatively brief training periods.[14–16] Color Doppler may serve as an adjunct during sonographic venography in identifying the arteries and veins and in demonstrating normal augmentation of venous flow after compression of the calf or a Valsalva maneuver. Color Doppler may also facilitate visualization of flow around a partially occluding thrombus (Figure 2–7). Color Doppler is not absolutely nec-

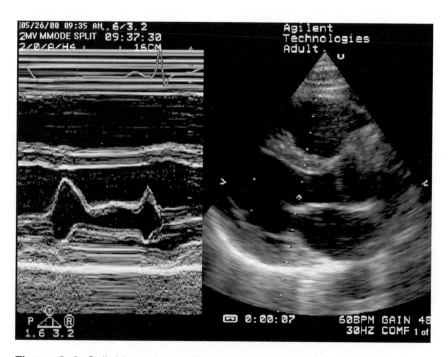

Figure 2–6. Split M-mode and B-mode imaging of the mitral valve. M-mode image on left shows opening and closure of mitral valve over time. Dotted line on B-mode image on the right indicates path of M-mode ultrasound beam. *(Image courtesy of Agilent Technologies.)*

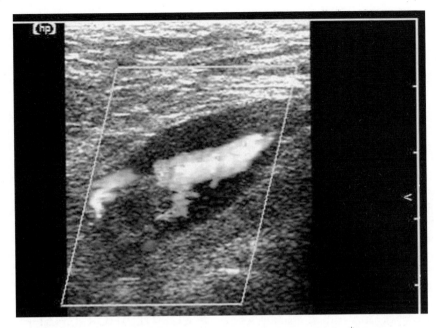

Figure 2–7. Color Doppler (duplex) scanning of partially occluded common femoral vein (greyscale copy). Transducer is oriented longitudinally along course of vein. Flow, indicated by white and light grey, is present in part of the vein. Remainder of vein is filled with clot. *(Image courtesy of Agilent Technologies.)*

essary for sonographic venography, however, as the main criterion for determining the presence or absence of a clot is whether or not the vein is completely compressible on two-dimensional grayscale scanning.

The use of color Doppler by emergency physicians has also been reported in detecting testicular torsion.[17] Relatively inexperienced sonographers may also find color Doppler helpful while scanning the right upper quadrant of the abdomen in helping to distinguish the common bile duct from the adjacent hepatic artery and portal vein. There are many other potential applications of color Doppler in the emergency and acute care setting which, at the time of this writing, have not been reported as being performed by clinicians, but which are well established uses by sonographers in medical imaging. These applications include detection of carotid stenosis in patients with transient ischemic attacks,[18] detection of ovarian torsion,[19,20] evaluation of patients with non-traumatic limb ischemia,[21] evaluation of traumatic vascular injuries,[22] and diagnosing renal[23] and hepatic vein thromboses.[24] Color Doppler has also been reported to show promise in identifying the inflamed appendix,[25] in diagnosing intestinal ischemia,[26] and in evaluating renal trauma.[27]

There are some limitations that come with color Doppler scanning. Movement of tissue due to respirations may be mistaken by the machine as blood flow, in which case, color will appear not only over blood vessels, but over adjacent tissue as well. Some machines allow the operator to adjust the minimum velocity of flow that the machine will detect. Turning up the velocity can reduce respiratory artifact, but will also limit the ability of the machine to detect low-velocity blood flow. Some of the more expensive ultrasound machines have built-in software that helps filter out respiratory artifact.

Another limitation of color Doppler scanning is that when the color Doppler is turned on, there is usually some degradation of the B-mode image. The ultrasound machine can only process a finite amount of information at one time. The time the machine spends in processing the Doppler signal must be taken away from the time spent processing the grayscale image. Most machines compensate by slowing their frame rates during duplex scanning. At frame rates below 25 per second, there is noticeable flicker in the images. More expensive ultrasound machines with faster microprocessors are able to maintain rapid frame rates during duplex scanning.

Quantitative Doppler

In addition to depicting flow qualitatively as red or blue color overlying a two-dimensional grayscale image, many ultrasound machines offer quantification of flow detected in the Doppler mode. A number of factors must be considered to accurately quantify blood flow. These factors include the frequency shift between the emitted and returning echoes, the intensity of the returning echoes, and the angle between the long axis of the transducer beam and the long axis of the vessel or cardiac chamber being studied. Also, flow can be sampled at just one point within a vessel or cardiac chamber or across the entire vessel or chamber. Quantitative Doppler capability is essential to applications such as carotid ultrasound and other arterial studies, in which the velocity of blood flow across a stenotic lesion can be used to estimate the degree of stenosis. Doppler technology is also an integral part of echocardiography. Because of the many factors involved, accurate quantification of blood flow using Doppler technology is technically difficult, and as of the time of this writing, is not commonly performed by physicians at the bedside in the emergency and acute care settings.

The quantitative Doppler mode is typically used in conjunction with B-mode and qualitative color-flow scanning. Simultaneous B-mode, color-flow, and quantitative Doppler scanning is often referred to as "triplex" scanning (Figure 2–8). The screen is split to allow the operator to view the area of interest as a two-dimensional, grayscale image with overlying color on one half of the screen. Using the trackball, the operator can move the Doppler beam to lie over the vessel or other cardiac chamber of interest on this two-dimensional image. The operator can also change the angle of the Doppler beam electronically. A graph of blood flow over time is shown on the other half of the screen. The height of the signals on the vertical axis of the graph corresponds to the velocity of blood flow. Flow is usually also presented as an audible signal from speakers on the ultrasound machine, with the loudness of the signal corresponding to the velocity of flow.

Measurements and Calculations

Most ultrasound machines offer electronic "calipers" for measuring distances or diameters. Examples of simple measurements that are frequently done in the emergency and acute care setting include the diameter of the abdominal aorta, the thickness of the gallbladder wall, the diameter of the common bile duct, the diameter of a gestational sac, or the diameter of an ovarian cyst. Many machines also allow the operator to construct a circle or ellipse for making measurements such as fetal head circumference.

In addition to simple measurements, many modern digital ultrasound machines offer calculation "packages" that automatically convert simple input measurements into clinically important output values. In doing so, the ultrasound machine acts as a computer, using published formulae for performing calculations internally. The operator need not be familiar with the formulae, which are usually included in the operation manual, to obtain the desired values. Examples of typical input measurements and output values are shown in Table 2–1.

▶ ECHOCARDIOGRAPHY

Transthoracic

Most ultrasound systems designed for general emergency and acute care use provide fair images of the heart. Using the typical emergency ultrasound machine and a general purpose transducer, an examiner can usually get good enough views of the heart to evaluate for significant pericardial effusions or grossly impaired contractility.

Some of the earliest reports of ultrasound use by emergency physicians involved echocardiography.[28,29] In the first study to show that echocardiography by emergency physicians was associated with improved survival

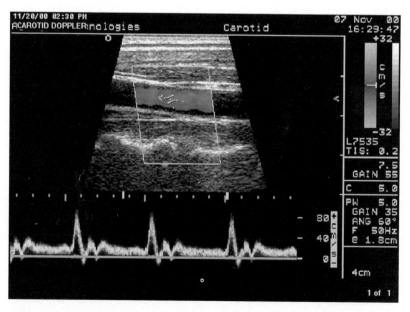

Figure 2–8. Simultaneous B-mode, color Doppler, and spectral Doppler ("triplex") scanning of the carotid artery. *(Image courtesy of Agilent Technologies.)*

► **TABLE 2–1.** EXAMPLES OF INPUT
MEASUREMENTS AND OUTPUT VALUES
FOR CALCULATION PACKAGES ON MODERN
ULTRASOUND MACHINES

Input Measurement(s)	Output Value
1, 2, or 3 distances; 1 or 2 ellipses, or combinations of distances and ellipses	Area or volume
2 lines	Angle
2 distances, 2 ellipses, or 2 tracings	Percent stenosis
Distance between cardiac cycles (in M or PD modes)	Heart rate
Maximum and minimum velocities (in PD mode)	Pressure gradient
Fetal or gestational sac distances (crown rump length, biparietal diameter, sac diameter, etc.)	Gestational age

in penetrating cardiac trauma, the ultrasound machine used in the emergency department was an echocardiogram machine on loan from the hospital's cardiology department.[28] Ultrasound machines designed specifically for performing echocardiography are generally much larger and cost many times more than the typical emergency and acute care machines. Rapid processing and high-frame rates are necessary to obtain good cardiac images, and specialized probes are required to obtain good transthoracic views of the heart through narrow rib interspaces.

Some of the more expensive ultrasound machines designed for emergency and acute care use now offer cardiac imaging capability that approaches the quality of dedicated echocardiography machines. The more advanced systems have the capability of detecting subtle wall motion abnormalities, which have been reported to be one of the most sensitive indicators of myocardial ischemia.[30] Cardiac calculation packages available on some machines also allow estimation of stroke volume, cardiac output, pressure gradients, and valve areas.

Transesophageal

Because the esophagus lies immediately adjacent to the heart and thoracic aorta, transesophageal echocardiography (TEE) allows detailed imaging of cardiac structures and the thoracic aorta. TEE is approximately 95 to 100% sensitive and specific for detecting aortic dissection, and is more accurate than CT scanning or angiography.[31] It is slightly less accurate than MRI scanning[32] but offers the advantage of being able to be performed rapidly at the patient's bedside. TEE has been investigated for use in diagnosing traumatic aortic rupture at the bedside and is considered the primary modality by investigators in France.[33,35,37] Studies also are continuing in the United States to define the appropriate utilization of this modal-

ity for trauma.[34,36] TEE is also highly accurate in detecting valvular lesions and intracardiac thrombi that may be difficult to see on transthoracic echocardiography. The use of TEE is becoming increasingly common in the critical care setting.[38] One disadvantage of TEE is that it is relatively invasive, as compared with transthoracic echocardiography, though patients generally tolerate the procedure well after mild sedation.[39] Another disadvantage is that TEE transducers are presently very expensive, in the range of $35,000. TEE transducers are available for some of the more expensive emergency ultrasound machines. The feasibility and utility of performing TEE in the emergency setting is an area that warrants further study.

► ULTRASOUND TRANSDUCERS

General Considerations

Ultrasound transducers, also referred to as probes, are among the most important and most expensive components of ultrasound systems. They are also the most fragile. As with ultrasound machines themselves, transducers come in a wide variety of shapes, sizes, and price ranges. For most emergency applications, only a few transducers are required. All emergency ultrasound systems should include a general-purpose abdominal probe. Such a transducer is usually all that is necessary to do limited, goal-directed ultrasound examinations for typical indications such as evaluating for gallstones, hemoperitoneum, or pericardial effusion. If the system is going to be used frequently to evaluate patients at risk for ectopic pregnancy, then an endovaginal probe is desirable. To evaluate for DVT or arterial disease, a vascular probe is required. The same probe used for vascular studies may also be used for specialized abdominal studies, such as evaluating for appendicitis. Finally, if the system will be used for detailed echocardiography, a specialized cardiac transducer will be needed. The factors that should be considered in selecting individual transducers for emergency applications are discussed in more detail in the following sections.

Except for the small, hand-carried ultrasound systems, most ultrasound machines allow for more than one transducer to be attached to the machine at one time. Most machines have from two to four transducer ports. On many machines, two ports are potentially "active" and the others are for storage. The operator can switch between transducers in the active ports using the control panel. To switch to a transducer docked in a storage port, it is necessary to disconnect the transducer and physically switch it with a transducer docked in one of the potentially active ports. On some machines, the ports are located on the side of the console; whereas on others, they are located beneath the control panel. Changing transducers docked in ports located beneath the control panel may require one to crouch or kneel down. It is recommended that transducers be changed only when the machine is turned off or in the freeze mode, or when the ports that are being changed have been deselected. Any time a transducer is changed, there is a risk of dropping it or of bending the connector pins. For an emergency setting in which an ultrasound machine will be used for a wide variety of uses, it is desirable to have as many ports as transducers, and as many potentially active ports as possible.

Transducer cords and arrangements for cord storage are of particular concern in the emergency setting. In the ultrasound suites of the medical imaging departments, ultrasound machines are usually conveniently positioned on the patient's right side and are rarely moved. In the emergency and acute care setting, ultrasound machines are typically moved frequently from room to room. In some examination rooms, it might be necessary to place the machine on the patient's left or closer to the head or foot of the gurney than would ordinarily be desirable. It is important that a transducer cord be long enough to reach the patient without putting strain on the cord and its connections to the transducer and the machine. This is particularly an issue in situations in which the transducer connectors are on the right side of the console and the machine must be placed on the left side of the patient. On the other hand, long cords tend to get tangled or in the way, especially when the machine is being moved. Running over a transducer cord or acutely bending it can cause permanent damage. Different machines have different systems for storing transducer cords when the transducer is not in use. These systems generally involve an arm that swings out from the machine and over which the cords are draped. None of these systems is entirely foolproof, and personnel must be cautioned to use great care not to damage transducer cords when moving the machine. Not having to worry about running over transducer cords is one of the advantages of the small, hand-carried ultrasound machines.

The transducer heads are the most fragile part of an ultrasound system. Dropping one on the floor is likely to permanently damage at least some of the crystals in the transducer head. Transducers typically cost from $7,500 to $15,000 a piece, and TEE transducers are even more expensive. Damage to a transducer can be a serious setback for a developing ultrasound program. Some manufacturers offer insurance against transducer breakage. An insurance policy may be particularly advisable for teaching institutions and other departments in which a large number of different personnel will be using the ultrasound machine.

Most ultrasound machines have cradles on the side of the machine in which the transducer heads rest when not in use. Having a secure resting place for the transducer heads is particularly important for machines that are moved frequently and occasionally bumped into. Also, it is important to remind physicians who use the ul-

trasound machine not to leave a transducer lying on the patient's abdomen or beside the patient on the gurney in situations in which the physician must stop scanning to respond to an emergency somewhere else. If the patient moves, the transducer is likely to fall onto the floor.

Transducer Cleaning

For ultrasound transducers that come in contact only with the skin, it is recommended that they be disinfected with a spray cleaner after each use. Spray cleaners designed specifically for ultrasound transducers are available from a number of vendors. Alcohol-containing solutions should be avoided as they lead to drying and cracking of the rubber membranes covering the transducer crystals. For transducers that come in contact with mucous membranes, such as endovaginal and TEE probes, high-level disinfection by soaking in a glutaraldehyde-containing solution for at least 20 min is recommended after each use, even if a probe cover is used over the transducer.[40–42] Glutaraldehyde fumes are potentially toxic to personnel and patients. Special transducer cleaning systems with fume hoods are commercially available and should be used.

Transducer Types

The earliest ultrasound transducers had only a single, stationary piezoelectric crystal in the head that emitted a single ultrasound beam. The returning echo was depicted as a single "A-line" on the ultrasound screen. To produce a two-dimensional image, the operator had to physically move the transducer. A series of A-lines was saved on the screen, one next to the other, as the operator moved the transducer across the skin, creating an image something like unrolling a current day two-dimensional scan. This type of transducer is no longer used, but examples of images produced by this scanning technique may still be found in older textbooks and articles.

The development of transducers with oscillating or rotating crystals in the head revolutionized ultrasonography in the late 1970s.[43] Instead of depending on the operator's hand to sweep the ultrasound beam across the tissue of interest, the crystal is moved in a rapid and precise manner by a tiny motor inside the transducer head. The resultant image is still composed of a series of A-lines side by side, but the crystal is moved so rapidly that what is seen on the screen appears to be a "real-time," two-dimensional image of the tissue being scanned. Mechanical transducers are still available for some machines. Some mechanical transducers have a single crystal in the head, whereas others have several. Many of the mechanical transducers that are currently available produce excellent two-dimensional images. Images produced by mechanical transducers are sector- or pie-shaped, with a narrow apex. The small motor inside the head of a mechanical probe produces a slight vibration that can be felt

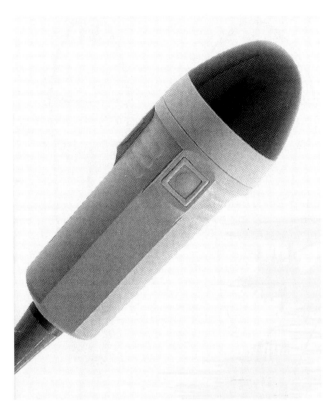

Figure 2–9. Mechanical sector probe. *(Photograph courtesy of Siemens Medical Systems, Inc.)*

by the patient and the operator, though this is not necessarily an unpleasant sensation. The appearance of a typical mechanical transducer head is shown in Figure 2–9.

Mechanical probes with relatively large, moving piezoelectric crystals have been largely replaced by transducers with numerous, much smaller crystals embedded in "arrays" in the head.[44] Such multiple-element transduc-

ers have no moving parts in the head and are, therefore, not susceptible to mechanical failure, though the tiny crystals may be more susceptible to breakage than the larger ones in mechanical probes. Transducers with multiple tiny embedded crystals are technically more difficult to produce than mechanical transducers. They were initially more expensive, though mass production is bringing their cost down. Multiple-element transducers offer an advantage over mechanical transducers in that the ultrasound beams can be steered and focused electronically by altering the sequence of firing of the crystals. The quality of the image produced by multiple-element transducers depends on the number and uniformity of the crystals in the head.

Multiple-element transducers are usually described according to their shape, size, frequency of ultrasound waves emitted, and purpose for which they are intended. Some transducers are designed to be variable frequency, allowing the operator to adjust the frequency of the emitted signals over a range of a few megahertz. For most probes, simultaneous grayscale and Doppler scanning results in a drop in frequency of about one megahertz. Table 2–2 lists those probes most relevant to ultrasound applications in the emergency setting according to probe types, sizes, and frequencies. Probes relevant to emergency ultrasound are discussed as follows.

Convex Probes

Transducers with crystals embedded in a curved, convex array work well for most general emergency and acute care applications, including trauma studies; evaluation of the gallbladder, kidneys, and aorta; and transabdominal scanning of the pelvis. The best compromise between penetration and resolution is usually achieved with a transducer frequency in the range of 3 to 4 MHz. Convex transducers are available with different widths and radiuses

▶ **TABLE 2–2.** ULTRASOUND TRANSDUCERS

Probe Designation*	Principal Uses	Frequency (MHz)	Doppler Frequency†
C364	General abdominal, OB	3.3	2.5
C386	General abdominal, OB	3.5	2.5
C551	Pediatric abdominal, OB	5.0	4.0
E721	Endovaginal, endorectal	6.6	5.0
L546	Deep vascular, small parts, appendicitis	5.2	4.0
L764	Peripheral vascular, small parts, pediatric appendicitis	6.7	5.0
LA39	Small parts	8.7	5.0
S220	Cardiology	2.5	2.2
S317	Cardiology, general abdominal	3.3	2.5
S611	Pediatric cardiology	5.7	4.0

*Letters designate probe type (C = convex array, E = endocavitary, L = linear array, LA = linear annular array, S = sector or phased array). First digit indicates approximate frequency. Last two digits indicate width of probe head in millimeters.
†Frequency of emitted signals during simultaneous B-scan and Doppler (duplex) modes.

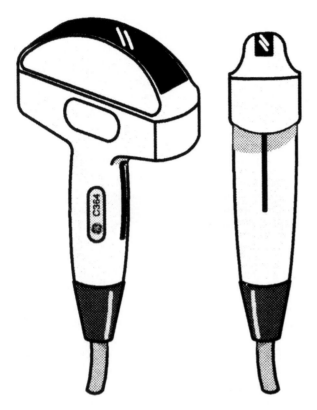

Figure 2–10. Convex transducer, side and oblique views. *(Reprinted from Logiq 400 user manual courtesy of General Electric Corporation.)*

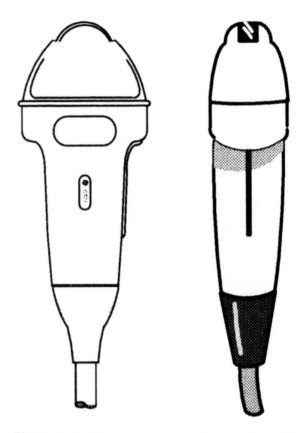

Figure 2–11. Microconvex transducer, side and front views. *(Reprinted from Logiq 400 user manual courtesy of General Electric Corporation.)*

of curvature (Figures 2–10 and 2–11). Transducers with small heads (less than 60 mm) and tight radiuses of curvature are often referred to as "microconvex." Microconvex transducers produce sector- or pie-shaped images with a relatively narrow apex. The small heads help avoid shadowing from rib artifacts when scanning through intercostal spaces. Because the ultrasound beams fan out widely in the far field, though, lateral resolution drops off significantly in deeper tissue. Standard convex transducers with larger heads produce sector-shaped images with wider apices. More crystals can be placed in the heads of larger transducers and there is less fanning of the ultrasound beams as compared to microconvex transducers. Standard convex probes usually produce better images than microconvex probes, therefore, except when scanning through intercostal spaces.

Phased Array Probes

Phased array probes generally have small heads, similar to microconvex transducers, but instead of being curved, the heads are flat (Figure 2–12). The crystals in their heads are arranged in a linear array. By changing the timing in which the crystals are fired, the machine alters the direction of the composite ultrasound beam. For each frame displayed on the screen, the beam is swept once across the tissue, giving a sector-shaped image, much

like that produced by a mechanical or microconvex probe. Phased array probes are also sometimes referred to as sector probes, though mechanical, convex, and microconvex probes all produce sector-shaped images.

Like microconvex probes, phased array transducers can be used for general abdominal scanning and are particularly useful for scanning through intercostal spaces. Because of their flat heads, less pressure is usually required to make complete contact with the skin with phased array probes as compared to convex or microconvex transducers. Phased array transducers are the preferred probes for transthoracic echocardiography. Transducers with frequencies of 2.5 to 3.5 MHz are typically used for general adult echocardiography. Phased array transducers in the range of 5 to 8 MHz are available for pediatric echocardiography. These higher frequency transducers are also advantageous for identifying smaller structures, such as valvular vegetations or intracardiac thrombi, in adults.

Linear Probes

Transducers with crystals embedded in a straight, flat head are generally referred to as linear probes (Figure 2–13). (Convex probes are sometimes referred to as curved linear probes). The ultrasound beams from the crystals in a linear probe are directed straight ahead, parallel to one

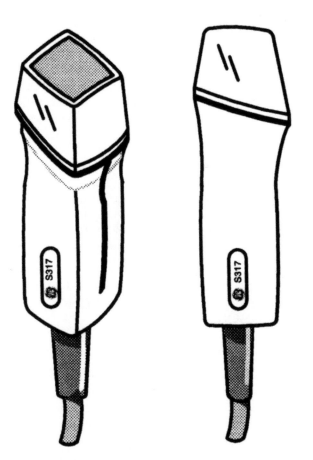
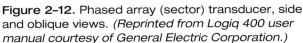

Figure 2–12. Phased array (sector) transducer, side and oblique views. *(Reprinted from Logiq 400 user manual courtesy of General Electric Corporation.)*

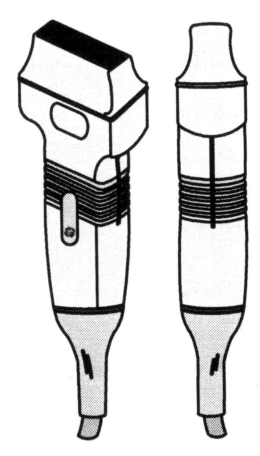

Figure 2–13. Linear transducer, side and oblique views. *(Reprinted from Logiq 400 user manual courtesy of General Electric Corporation.)*

another, leading to a rectangular image rather than a sector-shaped one. The width of the image is the same as the width of the array of crystals in the transducer head. Because of the limited field of view that they provide, linear probes are not good for visualizing large, deep structures. Their parallel beams provide superior resolution for visualizing smaller structures. The most common indication for which linear probes are used is to evaluate for DVT.[14–16] There are also many other potential emergency applications for which the linear probes are the transducers of choice, including evaluating for carotid stenosis[18] and other peripheral vascular disease;[21] examining small parts, such as the thyroid gland[45] and testicles;[17] identifying the inflamed appendix;[46] ruling out foreign bodies in the soft tissue;[47] guiding arthrocentesis[48] and central and peripheral vein cannulation[49,50] and fracture reductions;[51] and evaluating injuries to tendons and ligaments.[52,53]

A variation of the linear array arrangement is the annular array, in which crystals are embedded in a small, flat transducer head in concentric circles rather than in a straight line. This type of transducer emits a high density of ultrasound beams in a small area and produces sector-shaped images. On high-end machines, annular array

probes are used primarily for small parts scanning; however, some manufacturers of portable machines have successfully employed their use for cardiac and general abdominal imaging.

Linear transducers come in a variety of widths and frequencies. For studies in which fine detail is required, such as evaluating for carotid artery disease or small foreign bodies, relatively high-frequency transducers, in the range of 10 MHz, are preferred. For more common emergency applications, such as evaluating for DVT and appendicitis, however, high-frequency probes will not provide adequate penetration in many adult patients. A 5 to 7.5 MHz linear transducer is a good compromise for most emergency applications. A transducer with a wider head (larger than 60 mm) facilitates scanning of the right lower quadrant for appendicitis, but smaller heads (40 to 50 mm wide) are preferred for vascular access and musculoskeletal imaging.

Endocavitary (Endovaginal and Endorectal) Probes

Transducers designed especially for endorectal or endovaginal use are referred to generically as "endocavitary" transducers (Figure 2–14). The use of this type of transducer has also been reported in the oral cavity to rule out peritonsillar abscess.[54] Endorectal transducers are used mainly to look for prostate nodules and accordingly have limited application in the emergency setting. The remainder of this discussion focuses on endovaginal transducers.

An endovaginal transducer is basically a microconvex transducer on a long handle, with the handle designed to facilitate positioning the transducer in the posterior fornix of the vagina. Some endovaginal transducers are designed so that the transducer head points a few degrees away from the long axis of the handle. Slight ventral angulation of the transducer head facilitates scanning an anteverted uterus in the sagittal plane. If the uterus is retroverted, the transducer can be rotated 180°. Similarly, scanning the right adnexa is facilitated by slight angulation of the transducer head to the right. The transducer can be rotated 180° to scan the left adnexa. Some ultrasound systems are designed to allow the operator to steer the ultrasound beam electronically. This feature can significantly reduce patient discomfort during endovaginal scanning.

With endovaginal probes, the transducer head is much closer to the structures of interest than during trans-

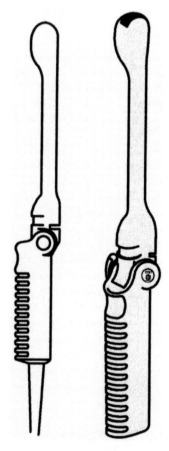

Figure 2–14. Endovaginal transducer, side and oblique views. *(Reprinted from Logiq 400 user manual courtesy of General Electric Corporation.)*

abdominal scanning of the pelvis. As a result, higher frequency transducers with less penetration but greater resolution can be used. Intrauterine pregnancies can usually be positively identified on endovaginal scanning 7 to 10 days earlier than with transabdominal probes.[55] Other findings, such as adnexal masses or small amounts of free fluid in the pelvis, can also usually be seen with greater clarity on endovaginal scanning. Another advantage of endovaginal scanning is that it does not require the patient to have a full bladder. For the usual emergency applications, such as evaluating patients with first trimester bleeding and cramping or non-pregnant patients with pelvic pain, an endovaginal probe with a frequency range of from 5 to 7.5 MHz will provide the best compromise between optimal penetration and resolution.

▶ OPTIONS FOR VIEWING, PRINTING, STORING, AND TRANSMITTING ULTRASOUND IMAGES

Display Monitors

The size and quality of the display monitors vary from machine to machine. The small, hand-carried ultrasound machines typically have small (5 to 8 in. wide) liquid crystal displays that are built into the machine and can be run off of the machine's small internal battery. These displays may be adequate for most general purposes in the emergency and acute care setting, but are difficult to see in poor lighting and do not provide the fine detail of larger monitors. Some hand-carried machines allow the option of being connected to a larger, external display monitor for better image viewing.

Most currently available emergency ultrasound machines have a video display monitor that is positioned on a mechanical arm above the main console. The monitor usually can be tilted or swiveled to provide the optimal viewing angle. Monitors that are 12 to 15 in. wide typically provide excellent images for most emergency applications. Most monitors allow adjustment of brightness and contrast, but are best viewed in dim light. Some emergency ultrasound machines allow conversion from grayscale images on the monitor to shades of orange or blue, which are easier to distinguish in brighter light.

Printing, Storing, and Transmitting Images

Typically during an ultrasound examination, a series of representative static images is taken by the operator to serve as later documentation of the findings of the study, or to allow over-reading of the study by another individual. In the case of ultrasound studies done in medical imaging departments, a sonographer often performs the real-time study and records a provisional interpretation, after which a radiologist reviews the static images and records a final interpretation. In most medical imaging departments, the standard method of recording static images has been to print them on radiographic film. To do so requires a separate matrix camera attached to the ultrasound machine that converts the ultrasound image into radiograph and exposes an radiograph cassette. The camera exposes one section of the radiograph cassette for each static image, so that an radiograph cassette of the size used for a standard chest radiograph can be used to save multiple ultrasound images. After the cassette is exposed, it is developed in a darkroom in the same manner as for standard radiographs, and the final film is read on a radiograph view box. This method of printing ultrasound images onto radiographic film provides high-quality, permanent images, but is relatively cumbersome and expensive. It also has the limitation of not allowing storage of color or moving images.

Thermal Printers

Thermal printers are frequently incorporated as a method for documentation of static (still) images of the ultrasound examination. Thermal printers provide a practical, inexpensive method of printing images from emergency ultrasound machines. Thermal printers are compact and relatively inexpensive. Most currently available emergency ultrasound systems have a slot in the cart designed to accommodate a thermal printer. The typical thermal printer allows the operator to print either portrait or landscape ultrasound images onto a roll of thermal paper, with resultant images from 3.75 to 5 in. wide. Brightness and contrast can be adjusted on the printer to match the printed image to the image on the display monitor. Different grades of thermal paper are available. The dynamic range capabilities of thermal printers and quality of paper has improved a great deal since their inception and when properly adjusted, thermal images provide an acceptable means to view the information as it was displayed on the ultrasound screen. With the higher grades of paper and with optimal printer settings, thermal images approach the clarity of images printed on radiographic film. They offer the advantage over radiographic film of costing only a few cents per image and of taking only a few seconds to print. Also, they do not require a radiograph view box for viewing, and they can be placed in the patient's medical record. Thermal images, however, may degrade over time and the process accelerated if the images are improperly stored. If stored in a dry environment, thermal print image quality remains relatively good for several years. As with radiographic film, thermal prints cannot store color or moving images. Color printers are available that use self-developing photographic film, but these types of prints are considerably more expensive than thermal prints.

Videotape

Most currently available ultrasound machines also offer the option of storing images on a videocassette recorder (VCR) that can be connected to the ultrasound machine. Many ultrasound machine carts have slots for a VCR built into them. Using a VCR, the entire ultrasound study may be stored just as the operator is viewing it in real time, including color Doppler images. The operator can annotate the study verbally by speaking into a microphone that is usually mounted on the display monitor. Numerous studies can be stored on a single VCR cassette, limited only by the length of the videocassette tape and the time taken for each study. Video recording is particularly useful for cardiac and fetal viability examinations or when complete examinations are to be reviewed for quality assurance purposes, especially for progress evaluation of the novice sonographer. Videotape documentation facilitates this process and allows a real-time examination to be documented in part, or as a complete examination and reviewed at a later time. Videotape review is undoubtedly time consuming, but provides an additional assessment of the skill level of the operator during the course of the examination.

Electronic Image Storage and Transmission

Whether ultrasound images are saved on radiographic film, thermal paper, photographic film, or videocassettes, storing and cataloguing sonograms can be cumbersome and can require large storage areas as archives expand. Digital image archiving is often suggested as a documentation solution with many ultrasound systems. Digital storage capabilities vary greatly between each manufacturer and include choices, which may be technology native to the ultrasound system, or peripheral products installed as options. The ability to store digital static (still) images or real-time loops of information will also vary between devices. Many currently available digital ultrasound machines allow electronic storage of ultrasound images on digital data storage media as a more efficient alternative or as an adjunct to the above storage methods. On some analog machines, an optional "frame grabbing" device can be attached to convert analog video signals to digital signals for electronic storage.[56]

Some digital ultrasound machines allow temporary storage of images on the machine's hard drive. The number of images that may be stored may be as few as 16 to as many as several hundred. Images stored on the hard drive can be downloaded at a later time to a computer hard drive or other digital storage devices attached to a computer using standard connector cables and image processing software.

Another option for data storage available on many ultrasound machines is transfer to a computer disk. A computer disk drive may either be built into the ultrasound machine or may be available as an attachable accessory. Some machines use the standard 1.4 megabyte, 3.5-in. floppy computer disks, though the number of images that can be stored on these disks is limited, as a single grayscale ultrasound image may use several hundred kilobytes of memory. Some of the small, portable ultrasound machines use the compact "flash" memory cards of the type used in digital cameras with up to 256 megabytes of memory on a card. Many of the more expensive ultrasound machines allow image storage on magneto-optical (MO) disks that will hold approximately 1200 images on a 640 megabyte disk.

Over the past decade, the National Electrical Manufacturers' Association and various other international organizations involved in medical imaging have collaborated to develop standard formats for digital storage and transmission of medical images. Ultrasound images stored in digital information and communications in medicine (DICOM) format can be transmitted back and forth between remote archives via telephone lines or dedicated digital networks connections.[57] Using this technology, an ultrasound examination performed in the emergency setting can be viewed by a radiologist or other consultant with a compatible workstation in his or her office or at home almost as the study is being done.[58] Instead of storing hard copies of ultrasound images in physical files, digital images can be stored electronically in a picture archiving and communication system (PACS).[59] Patient data and reports can also be stored electronically in a radiology information system (RIS). Along with ultrasound studies, digital imaging studies in other modalities, including magnetic resonance imaging, computerized tomography, nuclear medicine, and digital radiography, can be stored in these filmless archives.[60,61] With a DICOM compatible ultrasound machine, the need to store ultrasound studies as hard copies or even as files on computer disks can be completely eliminated. Ultrasound images taken in the urgent care center, emergency department, trauma center, obstetric unit, or intensive care unit may be stored, if desired, in the same PACS-RIS used for images taken in the radiology department.

▶ ULTRASOUND MACHINE COST

For most departments, cost is a significant consideration in choosing an ultrasound machine. The cost of the ultrasound machine is frequently one of the barriers a department must overcome in starting an ultrasound program. Fortunately, ultrasound machines suitable for emergency use are now available in a wide range of prices, from as low as $10,000 for a small, hand-carried machine to over $150,000 for a machine with all of the special features previously described. The relationship between the cost of an ultrasound machine and the accuracy of studies done in the emergency setting has not been systematically studied. Obviously, the image quality on a $10,000 ultrasound machine will not be the same as the quality on a $150,000 machine. For most limited, goal-directed emergency studies, though, a less expensive machine may be adequate.

The cost of ultrasound transducers contributes significantly to the cost of an ultrasound system. High-quality transducers often cost $10,000 or more. When deciding on which ultrasound system to acquire, it is important to first determine for what type of studies the system is going to be used. When an ultrasound machine is going to be used mainly for the evaluation of trauma, a small portable machine with a single, general-purpose transducer may be adequate. If evaluating for ectopic pregnancy will be a common indication for ultrasound, then an endovaginal transducer will be important. If the ultrasound machine is going to be used for vascular studies or evaluation of appendicitis, a high-frequency linear transducer is essential, and if advanced cardiac imaging is planned, then a cardiac transducer and software package will be required. Depending on the anticipated indications for ultrasound in the emergency setting, it may be desirable to give up some special features, such as color Doppler, in exchange for an extra transducer or better grayscale imaging.

Leasing an ultrasound machine may be a more attractive option than outright purchase for some departments. Leasing overcomes the barrier of the large initial capital outlay. Also, leasing may be the most practical and economical way to upgrade periodically to a new machine as technology advances or as the needs of the department change. It has been demonstrated in the case of ultrasound performed by emergency physicians to evaluate for ectopic pregnancy and cholelithiasis, that leasing one of the more expensive ultrasound machines is cost-effective as compared with the cost of calling in sonographers after regular medical imaging department hours.[62,63]

The details of the warranty, as well as options for an extended warranty and a maintenance agreement, are additional important considerations in the acquisition of an ultrasound machine. Ultrasound machines designed for the emergency and acute care setting are usually fairly resilient, but because they are moved frequently and handled by a variety of personnel, they take more of a beating than most ultrasound machines in medical imaging departments. Most manufacturers offer a 1-year warranty on new ultrasound machines. In some cases, the warranty covers parts only, while in others, it covers parts and labor. Also, damage to ultrasound transducers may or may not be covered in the warranty. Manufacturers also differ with regard to their commitment for the timing of repairs under warranty. Some manufacturers guarantee to provide a replacement machine if the broken one is not repaired within 24 h. For small, hand-carried machines, an insurance policy to cover theft should be considered. Some manufacturers include a theft replacement policy with the purchase of the machine. Finally, the cost of a preventive maintenance program should be considered. Regular preventive maintenance may help detect minor problems before they become major ones. Engineers performing periodic maintenance using standardized testing may also note subtle degradations in image quality that might not be noted by operators in the emergency setting, particularly when there are many different operators who each use the machine occasionally.

Another consideration is what type of technical support is included with the purchase or lease of a machine. Some manufacturers offer full training programs for novice sonographers; whereas others offer technical support on an as needed basis. Using DICOM technology, some manufacturers offer online troubleshooting for ultrasound images transmitted via telephone lines.

Appendix A provides contact information for the United States offices of the major manufacturers of ultrasound machines. Appendix B provides a partial list of the ultrasound machines that are currently available, along with a summary of the features available on each machine and a rough price range. Exact prices are not listed as these may be negotiable and may change over time.

With the wide variety of ultrasound systems currently available, the task of choosing a first ultrasound machine, or of upgrading from an existing machine to a new one, may seem daunting. Because of the competitive market in ultrasound equipment, and the advances in technology that have been made over the past few decades, better systems are becoming available at lower prices. In the end, the decision of which system is best for a given emergency setting involves weighing the numerous factors discussed in this chapter. These factors include not only the capabilities and price of the system, but the level of experience and expertise of the operators and the indications for which the system will be used. In addition to reviewing the information in this chapter, potential purchasers of ultrasound equipment may find it helpful to "test drive" different ultrasound machines themselves. Manufacturers' representatives often display machines at large meetings or at courses on emergency ultrasound. It should be kept in mind, though, that the live models used at exhibits and courses are often chosen on the basis that they have ideal body habitus for ultrasonography. Even the most inexpensive ultrasound systems may produce excellent images on such ideal patients. In some cases, manufacturers' representatives may loan machines for trial use in the patient care setting where a more realistic impression can be gained of the quality of the images that can be obtained on more typical emergency patients.

► ACKNOWLEDGMENT

The editors would like to thank Theodore J. Nielsen, RT, RDMS for his contributions to the hardcopy components section of this chapter.

REFERENCES

1. Plummer D. Principles of emergency ultrasound and echocardiography. Ann Emerg Med 1989;18:1291–97.
2. Standard for real-time display of thermal and mechanical acoustic output indices on diagnostic ultrasound equipment, AIUM/NGMA Standards, Revision 1, UD 3, 1998.
3. Implementation of the principle of as low as reasonably achievable (ALARA) for medical and dental personnel, National Council on Radiation Protection and Measurements (NCRP), Report no. 107, December 31, 1990.
4. Chan V, Hanbridge A, Wilson S, et al. Case for active physician involvement in US practice. Radiology 1996;199:555–560.
5. Kay HH. Auto tissue optimization (ATO) resolves fetal anatomy in the presence of oligohydramnios. 1998 General Electric Systems internal publication 98–5425.
6. Ralls P. Ultrasound tissue harmonics in the diagnosis of liver lesions–"smoking gun" hemangioma. 1998 General Electric internal publication 98–5328.
7. Witte DE, Owen CA. Ultrasound tissue harmonics enhances calcific shadowing. 1998 General Electric internal publication 98–5329.
8. Machin JE, Owen CA. Ultrasound tissue harmonics improves image quality by reducing obscuring artifactual echoes. 1998 General Electric internal publication 98–5326.
9. Campani R, Bottinelli O, Calliada F, et al. The latest in ultrasound: three-dimensional imaging. Part II. Eur J Radiol 1998;27:S183–S187.
10. Estroff JA. Emergency obstetric and gynecologic ultrasound. Radiol Clin North Am 1997;35:921–957.
11. Heller M, Melanson SW. Applications for ultrasonography in the emergency department. Emerg Med Clin North Am 1997;15:735–744.
12. Ellis MH, Manor Y, Witz M. Risk factors and management of patients with upper-limb deep vein thrombosis. Chest 2000;117:43–46.
13. Pearson SD, Polak JL, Cartwright S, et al. A critical pathway to evaluate suspected deep vein thrombosis. Arch Intern Med 1995;155:1773–1778.
14. Frazee BW, Snoey ER, Levitt A. Emergency department compression ultrasound to diagnose proximal deep vein thrombosis. J Emerg Med 2001;20:107–111.
15. Blaivas M, Lambert MJ, Harwood RA, et al. Lower extremity Doppler for deep venous thrombosis–can emergency physicians be accurate and fast? Acad Emerg Med 2000;7:120–126.
16. Jolly BT, Massarin E, Pigman ED. Color Doppler ultrasonography by emergency physicians for the diagnosis of acute deep venous thrombosis. Acad Emerg Med 1997;4:129–123.
17. Blaivas M, Batts M, Lambert M. Ultrasonographic diagnosis of testicular torsion by emergency physicians. Am J Emerg Med 2000;18:198–200.
18. Hennessy MJ, Britton TC. Transient ischaemic attacks: evaluation and management. Int J Clint Pract 2000;54:432–436.
19. Lee EJ, Kwon HC, Joo HJ, et al. Diagnosis of ovarian torsion with color Doppler sonography: depiction of

twisted vascular pedicle. J Ultrasound Med 1998;17:83–89.

20. Kokosa ER. Keller MS, Weber TR. Acute ovarian torsion in children. Am J Surg 2000;180:462–465.

21. Varty K, Nydahl S, Butterworth P, et al. Changes in the management of critical limb ischaemia. Br J Surg 1996;83:953–956.

22. Kuzniec S, Kauffman P, Molnar LJ, et al. Diagnosis of limbs and neck arterial trauma using duplex ultrasonography. Cardiovasc Surg 1998;6:358–366.

23. Chen P, Maklad N, Redwine M. Color and power Doppler imaging of the kidneys. World J Urol 1998;16:41–45.

24. Chawla Y, Kumar S, Dhiman RK, et al. Duplex Doppler sonography in patients with Budd–Chiari syndrome. J Gastroenterol Hepatol 1999;14:904–907.

25. Gutierrez CJ, Mariano MC, Faddis DM, et al. Doppler ultrasound accurately screens patients with appendicitis. Am Surg 1999;65:1015–1017.

26. Danse EM, Laterre PF, Van Beers BE, et al. Early diagnosis of acute intestinal ischaemia: contribution of colour Doppler sonography. Acta Chir Belg 1997;97:173–176.

27. Brown DF, Rosen CL, Wolfe RE. Renal ultrasonography. Emerg Med Clin North Am 1997;15:877–893.

28. Plummer D, Brunette D, Asinger R, Ruiz E. Emergency department echocardiography improves outcome in penetrating cardiac injury. Ann Emerg Med 1992;21:709–712.

29. Hauser AM. The emerging role of echocardiography in the emergency department. Ann Emerg Med 1989;18:1298–1303.

30. Peels CH. Usefulness of two-dimensional echocardiography for immediate detection of myocardial ischemia in the emergency room. Am J Cardiol 1990;65:687.

31. Nienaber CA, von Kodolitsch Y, Nicolas V, et al. The diagnosis of thoracic aortic dissection by non-invasive imaging procedures. N Engl J Med 1993;328:1–9.

32. Nienaber CA, Spielmann RP, von Kodolitsch Y, et al. Diagnosis of thoracic aortic dissection: magnetic resonance imaging versus transesophageal echocardiography. Circulation 1992;85:434–447.

33. Goarin JP, Cluzel P, Gosgnach M, et al. Evaluation of transesophageal echocardiography for diagnosis of traumatic aortic injury. Anesthesiology 2000;93:1373–1377.

34. Feliciano DV, Rozycki GS. Advances in the diagnosis and treatment of thoracic trauma. Surg Clin North Am 1999;79:1417–1429.

35. Berenfeld A, Barraud P, Lusson JR, et al. Traumatic aortic ruptures diagnosed by transesophageal echocardiography. J Am Soc Echocardiogr 1996;9:657–662.

36. Cohn SM, Burns GA, Jaffe C, Milner KA. Exclusion of aortic tear in the unstable trauma patient: the utility of transesophageal echocardiography. J Trauma 1995;39:1087–1090.

37. Vignon P, Gueret P, Vedrinne JM, et al. Role of transesophageal echocardiography in the diagnosis and management of traumatic aortic disruption. Circulation 1995;92:2959–2968.

38. Tousignant C. Transesophageal echocardiographic assessment in trauma and critical care. Can J Surg 1999;42:171–175.

39. Pearson AC, Castello R, Labovitz AJ. Safety and utility of transesophageal echocardiography in the critically ill patient. Am Heart J 1990;119:1083–1089.

40. Storment JM, Monga M, Blanco JD. Ineffectiveness of latex condoms in preventing contamination of the transvaginal ultrasound transducer head. Southern Med J 1997;90:206–208.

41. Milki AA, Fisch JD. Vaginal ultrasound probe cover leakage: implications for patient care. Fertil Steril 1998;69:409–411.

42. Rutala WA. APIC guideline for selection and use of disinfectants. 1994, 1995, and 1996 APIC Guidelines Committee. Association for Professionals in Infection Control and Epidemiology, Inc. Am J Infect Control 1996;24:313–342.

43. Bow CR, McDicken WN, Anderson T, et al. A rotating transducer real-time scanner for ultrasonic examination of the heart and abdomen. Br J Radiol 1979;52:29–33.

44. Kremkay FW. Multiple-element transducers. Radiographics 1993;13:1163–1176.

45. Grant EG, Earll, J, Richardson JD, et al. High-resolution real-time sonography. The study of superficial body parts. Med Clin North Am 1984;68:1609–1629.

46. Puylaert JBCM, Rutgers PH, Lalisang R, et al. A prospective study of ultrasonography in the diagnosis of appendicitis. N Engl J Med 1987;117:666–669.

47. Turner J, Wilde CH, Hughes KC, et al. Ultrasound-guided retrieval of small foreign objects in subcutaneous tissue. Ann Emerg Med 1997;29:731–734.

48. Smith SW. Emergency physician-performed ultrasonography- guided hip arthrocentesis. Acad Emerg Med 1999;6:84–86.

49. Hrics P, Wilber S, Blanda MP, Gallo U. Ultrasound-assisted internal jugular vein catheterization in the ED. Am J Emerg Med 1998;16:401–403.

50. Keyes LE, Frazee BW, Snoey ER, et al. Ultrasound-guided brachial and basilic vein cannulation in emergency department patients with difficult intravenous access. Ann Emerg Med 1999;34:711–714.

51. Durston W, Swartzentruber R. Ultrasound guided reduction of pediatric forearm fractures. Am J Emerg Med 2000;18:72–77.

52. Ahovuo J, Paavolainen P, Homstrom T. Ultrasonography of the tendons of the shoulder. Eur J Radiol 1989;9:17–21.

53. Rockett MS, Waitches G, Sudakoff G, et al. Use of ultrasonography versus magnetic resonance imaging for tendon abnormalities around the ankle. Foot Ankle Intl 1998;19:604–612.

54. Buckley AR, Moss EH, Blokmanis A. Diagnosis of peritonsillar abscess: value of intraoral sonography. Am J Roentgenol 1994;162:961–964.

55. Thorsen MK, Lawson TL, Aiman EJ, et al. Diagnosis of ectopic pregnancy: endovaginal vs. transabdominal sonography. Am J Roentgenol 1990;155:307–310.

56. Stacul F. Ultrasonography and PACS. Eur J Radiol 1998;27:S196–S199.

57. Thomas JD. The DICOM image formatting standard: its role in echocardiography and angiography. Int J Card Imaging Suppl 1998;1:1–6.

58. Martin BD, Levi C, Kelly JL. Enhancing diagnostic ultrasound programs utilizing wide-area image management technology. Int J Circumpolar Health 1998;57:691–693.

59. Andriole KP, Gould RG, Avrin DE, et al. Continuing quality improvement procedures for a clinical PACS. J Digit Imaging 1998;11:111–114.

60. Oberson JC, Welz R, Bovisi L. Development of an electronic radiologist's office in a private institute. Radiographics 2000;20:573–580.

61. Henri CJ, Cox RD, Rubin R, et al. Evolution of a filmless digital imaging and communications in medicine-conformant picture archiving and communications system: design issues and lessons learned over the last 3 years. J Digit Imaging 1999;12:178–180.

62. Durston WE, Carl ML, Guerra WF, et al. Ultrasound availability in the evaluation of ectopic pregnancy in the ED: comparison of quality and cost-effectiveness with different approaches. Am J Emerg Med 2000;18:408–417.

63. Durston W, Carl M, Guerra W, et al. Comparison of quality and cost-effectiveness in the evaluation of symptomatic cholelithiasis with different approaches to ultrasound availability in the emergency department. Am J Emerg Med 2001;19:260–269.

APPENDIX 2–A

Ultrasound Manufacturers with Offices in the U.S.

Acuson, A Siemens Company
1220 Charleston Road
Mountain View, CA 94043
Telephone: 800-422-8766
www.acuson.com

Aloka
10 Fairfield Boulevard
Wallington, CT 06492
Telephone: 800-872-5652
Fax: 203-269-6075
Email: mail@alokah.com

Biosound Esaote, Inc.
8000 Castleway Drive
Indianapolis, IN 46250
Telephone: 800-428-4374
Fax: 317-841-8616
www.biosound.com

GE Medical Systems
P.O. Box 414
Milwaukee, WI 53201
Telephone: 888-202-5528
Fax: 414-544-3384
www.geultrasound.com

Hitachi Medical Corporation of America
Hitachi Medical Systems
660 White Plains Road
Tarrytown, NY 10591-5107
Telephone: 800-852-2080
Fax: 914-524-9716
www.hitachiultrasound.com

Kontron Medical, LLC
31 Industrial Way
Mahwah, NJ 07430
Telephone: 210-825-8414
Fax: 201-825-8516
www.kontronmedical.com

Medison America, Inc.
11075 Knott Avenue
Cypress, CA 90630
Telephone: 800-249-0140
Fax: 714-889-3079
www.medisonusa.com

Philips Medical Systems, N.A.
22100 Bothell Everett Highway
P.O. Box 3003
Bothell, WA 98041-3003
Telephone: 800-526-4963
Fax: 425-485-6080
www.medical.philips.com

Pie Medical
8000 Castleway Drive
Indianapolis, IN 46250-1943
Telephone: 800-927-0708
Fax: 317-698-4743
www.piemedical.com

Shimadzu Medical Systems
20101 South Vermont Avenue
Torrance, CA 90502
Telephone: 800-228-1429
Fax: 310-217-8869
www.shimadzu.com

Siemens Medical Systems, Inc.
Ultrasound Group
P.O. Box 7002
Issaquah, WA 98029
800-367-3569
www.siemensultrasound.com

SonoSite, Inc.
21919 30th Drive SE
Bothell, WA 98021-3904
Telephone: 888-482-9449
Fax: 425-951-1201
www.sonosite.com

Toshiba America Medical Systems, Inc.
2441 Michelle Drive
Tustin, CA 92781
Telephone: 800-421-1968
Fax: 714-734-0362
www.medical.toshiba.com

APPENDIX 2–B

The following table provides examples of the types of ultrasound machines currently available for use in the emergency and acute care setting. The information in the tables was obtained by surveying all the manufacturers in Appendix 2–A. Each company was asked to provide specifications and approximate price ranges for up to three ultrasound machines suitable for use in the emergency department. Information is included in the appendix only for those manufacturers which responded to the survey. Pictures of ultrasound machines were supplied by the respective manufacturers and are reproduced with their permission. The inclusion of certain ultrasound machines in the tables is not intended to represent an endorsement by the authors. The machines listed in the table are sorted first in ascending order by price range and second in alphabetical order by the name of the manufacturer. The key for the price ranges is as follows:

$	$10,000–29,000
$$	$30,000–59,000
$$$	$60,000–89,000
$$$$	≥$90,000

Prices and machine characteristics are subject to change. Also, new models and new features are continually being added, and older models are being phased out. For the latest information on machines available from any given manufacturer, the reader is encouraged to contact the manufacturer's representative directly using the contact information provided in Appendix 2–A.

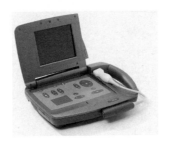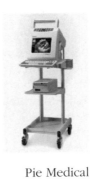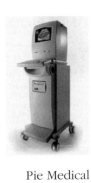

	Philips Medical Systems	Pie Medical	Pie Medical
Company	Philips Medical Systems	Pie Medical	Pie Medical
Model	OptiGo	100 Falco	240 Parus
Dimensions (h, w, d in inc.)	13 × 9 × 3.5	10 × 15 × 14	12 × 16 × 21
Weight (lbs)	7.2	23	33
Battery powered	yes	yes	no
Analog/digital	digital	digital	digital
Frames per sec	up to 55	24	24
Shades of gray	64	256	256
Adjustable acoustic output	no	yes	yes
Levels of TGC control	2	2	2
Adjustable focal depth	no	yes	yes
Zoom	no	yes	yes
Cine memory	60 frames	32 MB	32 MB
Selectable dynamic range	no	yes	yes
Selectable grayscale maps	no	yes	yes
Number of preset protocols	1	100	100
Automated image enhancement	no	yes	yes
Tissue harmonics	no	no	no
Three-D rendering	no	optional	optional
M mode	no	yes	yes
Color Doppler			
Qualitative	yes	no	no
Quantitative	no	no	no
Electronic calipers	yes	yes	yes
Calculation packages			
Volume	no	yes	yes
Obstetric	no	yes	yes
Vascular	no	no	no
Cardiac	no	yes	yes
Number of transducer ports	1	1	2
Active	1	1	2
Storage	0	0	0
Available transducers			
Convex array		3.5–7.5 MHz	3.5–7.5 MHz.
Phased array	25 MHz	no	3.5–7.5 MHz.
Linear array		5–8 MHz	5–8 MHz.
Endovaginal			
Transesophageal echo			
Display monitor width	6.5″	9″	9″
Electronic image storage	256 MB compac flash card	1.44 MB floppy	1.44 MB floppy
DICOM compatible	no	no	no
Price range	$	$	$

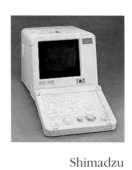 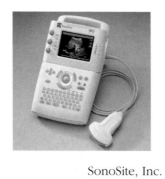 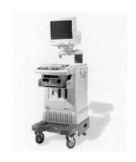

	Shimadzu	SonoSite, Inc.	Philips Medical Systems
Company	Shimadzu	SonoSite, Inc.	Philips Medical Systems
Model	SDU-350 XL	180PLUS	Ultramark 400 C
Dimensions (h, w, d in inches)	11 × 12 × 17	13.3 × 7.6 × 2.5	53 × 20 × 33
Weight (lbs)	29	5.4	232
Battery powered	no	yes	no
Analog/digital	hybrid/digital	digital	digital
Frames per sec	45	up to 100	50
Shades of gray	256	512	256
Adjustable acoustic output	no	no	
Levels of TGC control	8	3	
Adjustable focal depth	26 cm	yes	yes
Zoom	yes	yes	yes
Cine memory	64 frames	120 frames	64 frames
Selectable dynamic range	60 db	yes	yes
Selectable grayscale maps	4	yes	
Number of preset protocols	12	7	
Automated image enhancement	yes	yes	
Tissue harmonics	yes	yes	
Three-D rendering	option	no	
M mode	yes	yes	yes
Color Doppler			
Qualitative	no	yes	yes
Quantitative	na	yes	yes
Electronic calipers	yes	yes	yes
Calculation packages		yes	
Volume	yes	yes	
Obstetric	yes	yes	yes
Vascular	yes	yes	
Cardiac	yes	yes	no
Number of transducer ports			
Active	2	1	
Storage	0	0	
Available transducers			
Convex array	2–8 MHz	2–7 MHz	4–6.5 MHz
Phased array			
Linear array	5–10 MHz	5–10 MHz	7.5 MHz
Endovaginal	4–8 MHz	4–7 MHz	6.5 MHz
Transesophageal echo			
Display monitor width	9″	5″	
Electronic image storage	external floppy disk	120 images internal hard disk	4.3 GB hard disk
DICOM compatible	no	yes	
Price range	$	$	$$

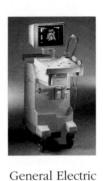 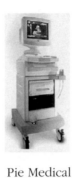 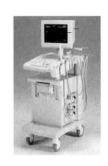

	General Electric	Pie Medical	Shimadzu
Company	General Electric	Pie Medical	Shimadzu
Model	Logiq 200 Pro	Picus	SDU-450 XL
Dimensions (h, w, d in inches)	47 × 16 × 26	15 × 9 × 20	54 × 16 × 23
Weight (lb)	35	33	120
Battery powered	no	No	no
Analog/digital	digital	digital	hybrid/digital
Frames per second	30	Apr-32	155
Shades of gray	256	256	256
Adjustable acoustic output	yes	yes	no
Levels of TGC control	8	8	8
Adjustable focal depth	yes	yes	26 cm
Zoom	yes	yes	yes
Cine memory	64 frames	63 frames	128 frames
Selectable dynamic range	yes	yes	80 db
Selectable grayscale maps	yes	yes	8
Number of preset protocols	8	16	40
Automated image enhancement	yes	yes	yes
Tissue harmonics	no	yes	yes
Three-D rendering	no	optional	optional
M mode	yes	yes	yes
Color Doppler			
Qualitative	no	yes	no
Quantitative	no	yes	no
Electronic calipers	yes	yes	yes
Calculation packages			
Volume	yes	yes	yes
Obstetric	yes	yes	yes
Vascular	no	yes	yes
Cardiac	no	no	yes
Number of transducer ports	2	2	
Active	2	2	2
Storage	0	0	yes
Available transducers			
Convex array	3–7 MHz	2.5–5 MHz.	2–8 MHz.
Phased array			
Linear array	7.5 MHz	5–10 MHz.	12 MHz
Endovaginal	7 MHz		4–8 MHz
Transesophageal echo			
Display monitor width	12″	10″ or 15″	12″
Electronic image storage	540 MB MOD		96 MB image archive card
DICOM compatible	no	yes	no
Price range	$$	$$	$$

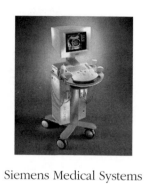 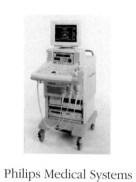 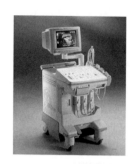

Company	Siemens Medical Systems	Philips Medical Systems	General Electric
Model	SONOLINE Adara	ImagePoint	Logiq 400 Pro
Dimensions (h, w, d in inches)	51 × 19 × 24	40 × 24 × 57	62 × 21 × 37
Weight (lb)	132	308 lbs.	444
Battery powered	no	no	no
Analog/digital	digital	digital	digital
Frames per second	Up to 74	30	30
Shades of gray	256	256	256
Adjustable acoustic output	24dB	no	yes
Levels of TGC control	8	8	8
Adjustable focal depth	yes	yes	yes
Zoom	yes	yes	yes
Cine memory	63 frames	10 seconds	128 frames
Selectable dynamic range	yes	yes	yes
Selectable grayscale maps	yes	yes	yes
Number of preset protocols		50	8
Automated image enhancement	yes	no	yes
Tissue harmonics	no	yes	no
Three-D rendering	yes	no	yes
M mode	yes	yes	yes
Color Doppler			
Qualitative	no	yes	yes
Quantitative	no	yes	yes
Electronic calipers	yes	yes	yes
Calculation packages			
Volume	yes	yes	yes
Obstetric	yes	yes	yes
Vascular	no	yes	yes
Cardiac	yes	yes	no
Number of transducer ports	3	3	3
Active	3	3	2–3
Storage	0	0	0–1
Available transducers			
Convex array	2.5–6.5	2–9 MHz	3–5 MHz
Phased array		2–10 MHz	2–6 MHz
Linear array	5.0–10.0	3–10 MHz	3–12 MHz
Endovaginal	5–7.5 MHz	5–8 MHz	7 MHz
Transesophageal echo		3–8 MHz	
Display monitor width	12″	15″	15″
Electronic image storage		512 MB	600 MB HD, 540 MB MOD
DICOM compatible	yes	yes	yes
Price range	$$	$$$	$$$

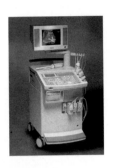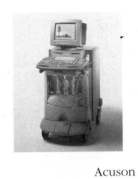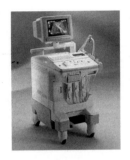

	Siemens Medical Systems	Acuson	General Electric
Company			
Model	SONOLINE Sienna	Sequoia 512	Logiq 500 Pro
Dimensions (h, w, d in inches)	53 × 20 × 34	58 × 26 × 48	62 × 21 × 37
Weight (lb)	287	406	444
Battery powered	no	no	no
Analog/digital	digital	digital	digital
Frames per second	Up to 100	up to 943	30
Shades of gray	256	256	256
Adjustable acoustic output	24dB	yes	yes
Levels of TGC control	8	8	8
Adjustable focal depth	yes	yes	yes
Zoom	yes	yes	yes
Cine memory	63 frames		128 frames
Selectable dynamic range	yes	yes	yes
Selectable grayscale maps	yes	yes	yes
Number of preset protocols	32	50	8
Automated image enhancement	yes	yes	yes
Tissue harmonics	no	yes	yes
Three-D rendering	yes	yes	yes
M mode	yes	yes	yes
Color Doppler			
Qualitative	yes	yes	yes
Quantitative	yes	yes	yes
Electronic calipers	yes	yes	yes
Calculation packages			
Volume	yes	yes	yes
Obstetric	yes	yes	yes
Vascular	yes	yes	yes
Cardiac	no	yes	no
Number of transducer ports	2–4	5	3
Active	2–4	3	3
Storage	0	2	0
Available transducers			
Convex array	2.5–8.0	2–6 MHz	3–5 MHz
Phased array		5–8 MHz	2–6 MHz
Linear array	5.0–12.0	8–15 MHz	3–7 MHz
Endovaginal	5–7.5 MHz	4–8 MHz	7 MHz
Transesophageal echo		yes	yes
Display monitor width	13″	14″	15″
Electronic image storage		1 GB HD, 230 MB MOD	600 MB HD, 540 MB MOD
DICOM compatible	yes	yes	yes
Price range	$$$	$$$$	$$$$

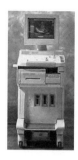 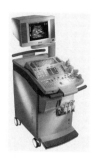

Company	Shimadzu	Siemens Medical Systems
Model	SDU-2200	SONOLINE Omnia
Dimensions (h, w, d in inches)	54 × 17 × 33	57 × 20 × 36
Weight (lb)	330	320
Battery powered	no	no
Analog/digital	digital	digital
Frames per second	120	up to 180
Shades of gray	256	256
Adjustable acoustic output	yes	yes
Levels of TGC control	8	8
Adjustable focal depth	yes	yes
Zoom	yes	yes
Cine memory	128 frames	250 frames
Selectable dynamic range	yes	yes
Selectable grayscale maps	yes	yes
Number of preset protocols	50	32
Automated image enhancement	yes	yes
Tissue harmonics	yes	yes
Three-D rendering	yes	yes
M mode	yes	yes
Color Doppler		
Qualitative	yes	yes
Quantitative	yes	yes
Electronic calipers	yes	yes
Calculation packages		
Volume	yes	yes
Obstetric	yes	yes
Vascular	yes	yes
Cardiac	yes	yes
Number of transducer ports	3	5
Active	3	5
Storage	0	0
Available transducers		
Convex array	2–8 MHz	2.5–8.5
Phased array	2–8 MHz	1.6–6.5
Linear array	2–8 MHz	3.5–12.0
Endovaginal	4–8 MHz	4.2–7.5 MHz
Transesophageal echo	yes	yes
Display monitor width	15″	13″
Electronic image storage	4 GB HD, 9.6 GB DVD	640 MB MOD
DICOM compatible	yes	yes
Price range	$$$$	$$$$

CHAPTER 3
Physics and Instrumentation

Theodore J. Nielsen and Michael J. Lambert

For over 40 years, diagnostic ultrasound has experienced many technologic advances. This provided a pathway for its direct integration into many specialty areas of medicine. With the introduction of smaller, more operator-friendly and less expensive ultrasound systems, an increased number of medical specialties, including emergency medicine, are discovering the benefits of point of care diagnostic ultrasound applications. Patients and physicians have embraced ultrasound as a familiar examination in the diagnostic evaluation. These increased applications, however, introduce a level of potential risk if the operator is not appropriately instructed and guided.

This chapter provides the fundamental platform on which all ultrasound rests its ability to be an effective tool in medical imaging. A basic understanding of ultrasound physics simply must be understood before the operator can enjoy the benefit and reduce the risk of placing the transducer in his or her hand. This chapter is structured to introduce the principles of ultrasound physics and instrumentation that may have more of an immediate effect on understanding and performing emergency ultrasound. To encourage and maintain a standard of excellence, the material that follows is designed to initiate the journey toward more comprehensive information that is available in various other texts and publications.

► UNDERSTANDING SOUND AND ULTRASOUND

History

If we interpret sonar as the inauguration for diagnostic ultrasound, we may draw some comparisons to simplify the concept.

Example: A submarine that possesses sonar capability can control precisely when an acoustic pulse is generated. In addition, it assumes a relative propagation speed as it travels through a specific medium. The amount of elapsed time required for the "echo" to return subsequent to striking an object allows the relative distance to be calculated to the target of interest (Figure 3–1).

Diagnostic ultrasound incorporates a similar concept employing the pulse-echo principle. The transducer provides the source of the sound. The ultrasound system is precisely aware of when the acoustic pulse is generated. This pulse travels at a relatively constant speed until it encounters a reflective surface, at which time a portion of the sound is reflected back toward the source. It is calculated to be traveling through human tissue at body temperature (approx. 1540 m/sec) and the system measures the round-trip time and intensity of the returning "echo." This information may then be represented as a pixel (dot) of information on the display device. The amount of time required for the returning echo determines its relative distance from the transducer. The returning intensity is proportional to the grayscale assignment of the pixel.

Although the pulse-echo principle appears exceedingly simple, there are several pearls to address. Sound waves are actually a series of repeating mechanical pressure waves that propagate through a medium. These pressure waves are measured in hertz (cycles/sec). Typically, audible sound ranges between 16,000 to 20,000 Hz. Ultrasound is technically defined as a "sound" having a frequency in excess of 20,000 Hz. In medicine, ultrasound used for diagnostic purposes incorporates frequencies that generally range between 2 to 15 MHz (megahertz), or 2 to 15 million cycles per sec, well above the range of human hearing. While diagnostic ultrasound frequencies

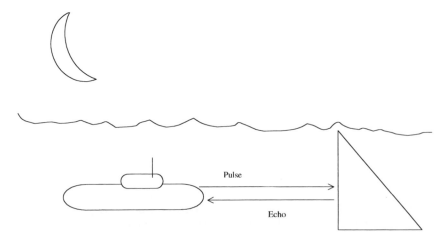

Figure 3–1. Relative distance to/from an object may be determined through a known medium by measuring the round trip time of travel for the returning echo.

extending beyond 15 MHz are available for medical imaging, they are often used for catheter-based technology.

► BASIC DEFINITIONS

A variety of methods may be used to convey an understanding of specific terms. Definitions are often expressed via graphs, charts, and formulas. The text that follows is designed to introduce the reader to the components of an acoustic wave and its terminology (Figure 3–2).

Amplitude

Amplitude is the peak pressure of the wave (height). This may be simply interpreted as the loudness of the wave. A loud sound has a large amplitude. A soft sound has a small amplitude. Although we seldom describe ultrasound images in terms of amplitude, the terminology must be understood as it correlates with the intensity of the returning echo.

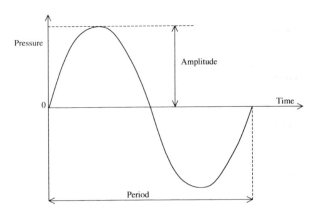

Figure 3–2. Time vs. pressure graph of a sound wave. Amplitude: peak pressure of a wave. Period: time required to complete a single cycle.

Period

Period is the time required to complete a single cycle.

Frequency

Frequency is the number of times per second the wave is repeated. The range of frequencies typically discussed here is between 2 to 15 MHz.

Velocity

Velocity is defined as the speed of the wave. The velocity is dependent upon the material through which the wave is traveling and independent of frequency. Since the speed of ultrasound through a given medium is constant, the closer the molecules are in position to one another, the better the propagation. Therefore, sound travels faster in bone as compared to human soft tissue. When molecules become less dense (gases), the velocity of the sound slows even further. This is not meant to suggest that diagnostic ultrasound may be utilized to visualize structures across this molecular spectrum.

Wavelength

Wavelength (propagation speed/frequency) is the distance the wave travels in a single cycle.

From the very moment the "pulse" is generated inside the transducer we hold in our hand, sound begins to lose energy and progressively weakens, much like the audible note from a piano after striking the key only once. This progressive weakening of the sound as it travels is defined as *attenuation*. Attenuation of the sound is a round-trip effect beginning the instant the pulse is generated inside the transducer, until it returns to the transducer to be registered. There are several factors that contribute to attenuation. These include the medium through which the sound is traveling, the number of interfaces encountered, and the wavelength of the emitted sound.

The type and density of tissue combined with its degree of homogeneity or heterogeneity contributes to the rate of attenuation. It stands to reason that tissue of the same type and density would facilitate the ability to assist in the transmission of the sound rather than inhibit its progression. Conversely, a combination of varying tissues would exhaust energy at an accelerated rate. This is one of the reasons why transabdominal ultrasound scanning of the uterus and ovaries is facilitated by a distended urinary bladder. The fluid inside the bladder provides a pathway of less attenuation and allows an efficient use of the transmitted sound to visualize the posterior anatomy.

Attenuation occurs in several different forms. The first form is *reflection,* or the redirection of part of the sound wave back to its source. This is the foundation on which ultrasound scanning is based. The ultrasound beam should ideally interrogate the anatomy of interest at 90° to maximize the reflection and subsequent visualization of the anatomic structures. Manipulating the transducer so the area of interest is positioned directly under the transducer in the center of the display offers improved visualization and the ability to better appreciate the surrounding anatomical structures (Figure 3–3).

The next definition is *refraction,* or the redirection of part of the sound wave as it crosses a boundary of mediums possessing different propagation speeds.

The third definition is *scattering,* which occurs when the ultrasound beam encounters an interface that is smaller than the sound beam or irregular in shape.

The last concept is *absorption,* which by its name suggests the energy is contained within the tissue. When the acoustic energy is converted to thermal energy, it dissipates as heat within the tissue. This forms the foundation for therapeutic ultrasound that employs a different range of frequencies when compared to diagnostic ultrasound.

Interfaces

When sound crosses a boundary of tissues in contact with one another having a different acoustic impedance, an *interface* is said to occur. *Acoustic impedance* refers to the stiffness or resistance of the tissue to molecular movement and is directly related to tissue density.

Blood cells, water, fat, and muscle all have sufficient differing acoustic impedances to generate a reflection. The greater the density difference between tissues, the stronger the reflection. The intensity of the reflection (how loud the echo is) is determined by how much of a difference exists between the tissues in contact. A small density difference (acoustic impedance) results in a small echo being generated. Conversely, a large difference in density results in a large echo generated with much of the energy lost to reflection. Therefore, little energy remains available to continue for visualization of deeper structures. This premise explains why diagnostic ultrasound cannot "see" through bowel gas or bone, as there is too large a difference in acoustic impedance that exists between these types of interfaces and soft tissue.

Image Resolution

The topic of resolution is often confused with other imaging parameters when discussing diagnostic ultrasound. Resolution refers to the "quality" of the image being produced, which is the ability to differentiate the anatomic

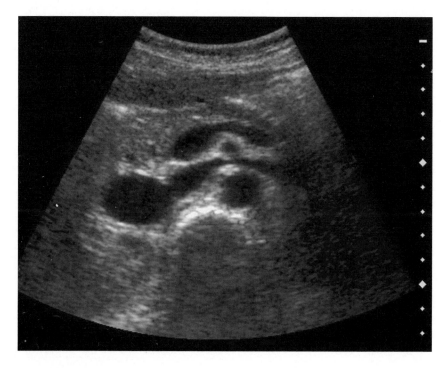

Figure 3–3. Transverse image of the upper abdomen. Maintaining the area of interest in the center of the image allows greater ability to visualize the surrounding anatomy. Vascular structures centered from top include: splenic vein, superior mesenteric artery, left renal vein, aorta, with the inferior vena cava to the left of center.

and pathologic areas of interest with greater detail. Although there are several factors that contribute to the overall image quality, we limit our discussion to the most noteworthy: axial, lateral, and contrast resolution.

Axial Resolution

Axial resolution refers to the system's ability to differentiate two closely spaced echoes that lie in a plane parallel to the direction of propagation of the sound wave (Figure 3–4). The ability to distinguish these echoes in greater number improves our resolution. If we consider the dpi (dots per inch) setting commonly available on a computer printer, the greater dpi setting provides us with greater image resolution and a higher quality image.

There are several factors that contribute to the quality of the axial resolution; however, the rate-limiting step under control by the operator is the ultrasound beam and transducer frequency.

Frequency

There exists an ever-increasing multitude of transducer designs of varying sizes and shapes for seemingly endless applications. While this chapter will not explore the variety of available transducer technologies, there are some general rules that apply to the vast majority we address here.

First, transducer technology is based on the piezo-electric effect. The term piezoelectric is defined as "pressure-electricity" and simply refers to materials that result in the production of a pressure when deformed by an applied voltage. Although quartz is a naturally occurring crystal, the crystal elements incorporated into modern transducers are synthetic. The arrangement and number of crystals within a transducer vary depending upon the manufacturer, transducer design, and its intended application.

Second, transducer frequency usually has a direct effect on image quality and resolution. Generally speaking, if transducer frequency is increased, resolution and image quality improve. However, while resolution may increase, penetration capabilities will decrease. In other words, there will be reduction in the available acoustic energy for penetrating to deeper structures when higher frequencies are selected.

The ultrasound beam is affected, in part, by the frequency emitted by the transducer, with each transducer emitting a "center" frequency during the transmit portion of the cycle. A range of frequencies exists on either side of the center frequency and is known as the *bandwidth*. Many ultrasound systems make use of these bandwidth frequencies during the receive portion of the cycle and thus incorporate broadband transducers. To offer a greater degree of flexibility, additional technology may allow the operator to select one of multiple "center" frequencies available from a single transducer. This selection allows the operator to easily maximize the transmit frequency of the transducer that offers the best resolution for the area of interest. Regardless of which type of transducer

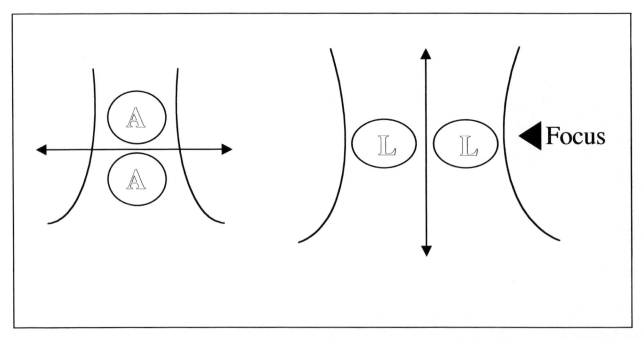

Figure 3–4. Axial resolution (A): ability to differentiate two echoes that lie in a plane parallel to the direction of the sound wave. Lateral resolution (L): ability to differentiate two echoes that are perpendicular to the direction of the ultrasound beam.

technology is utilized, the highest frequency should be used that will penetrate the area of interest and that offers the best resolution. Image resolution is based on many transducer factors including the pulse length of the wave. The pulse length is dependent on specific transducer characteristics set by the manufacturer. This can explain why simply increasing the transmit frequency of a transducer may not consistently result in improved resolution or image quality.

Lateral Resolution

Lateral resolution refers to the ultrasound systems ability to differentiate two closely spaced echoes that are positioned perpendicular to the direction of propagation of the ultrasound beam (see Figure 3–4). Generally, it is agreed upon that lateral resolution will be inferior to axial resolution. While transducer frequency aids in improving lateral resolution, it is the ultrasound beam width that contributes to this side-to-side resolution. When we examine the surface of a transducer, we must remember the width of an average beam emitting from a transducer is approximately 1 to 1.5 mm at a focal depth. For transducers incorporating an internal focusing capability, however, a user selectable adjustment is often available. This adjustment allows the operator to adjust the width of the ultrasound beam relative to depth within the image. If this "focal zone" is positioned on the screen adjacent to the area of interest on the ultrasound image, then the ultrasound beam will in theory be the narrowest at this point allowing for improved lateral resolution. In addition, multiple focal zones can be selected on a single ultrasound image in an attempt to maximize the resolution at specific depths. Since this action requires additional processing time, a slower frame rate will occur and the image will appear to have less of a real-time appearance. Single focal zone capabilities are generally sufficient for most abdominal and cardiac examinations, while multiple focal zones are often of greater value when examining superficial structures when transducer movement is at a minimum and additional signal processing time is of less concern.

Contrast Resolution

Referring to the previous section on Interfaces and Acoustic Impedance, we learned that the greater the density difference between tissues, the stronger the reflection. The amount of reflection (how loud the echo is) is determined by how much of a difference exists between the tissues in contact with one another. A small difference results in a small echo being generated. One should remember that the returning echoes consist of varying strengths or amplitudes. Contrast resolution refers to the ultrasound system's ability to assign a grayscale value to returning echoes of varying amplitudes. Many diagnostic ultrasound systems allow an assignment of 256 shades of gray, which facilitates the ability to discriminate between the subtleties that exist between tissues. Often times, a higher contrast (less shades of gray) may be more pleasing to the human eye but may in fact contain less diagnostic information. This dynamic range of information (measured in decibels or db) is often a programmable feature on ultrasound systems and may be examination specific. Abdominal examinations often display a greater dynamic range when compared to cardiac examinations when extended grayscale information may be of less value. The optimum setting allows a clear differentiation between the area of interest and the surrounding anatomy.

Transducers

The chapter discussing equipment explores the variety of available transducer technologies. It is of importance to note that specific designs and shapes may be employed to assist in gaining access to a particular imaging "window." The surface area of a transducer in contact with the patient is referred to as the "footprint" of the probe. Large footprint transducers may be suitable for general abdominal imaging; however, small footprint transducers facilitate intercostal access. Whichever design is selected, one should note that axial and lateral resolution, along with focal and depth capabilities, will also change. A transducer that allows easier access may, in fact, not provide as high a resolution simply due to the laws of physics. This is entirely acceptable if the desired echo information can be obtained.

Consider two convex transducers with varying degrees of curvature (Figure 3–5A and B).

Scan lines of information are emitted from the transducer at right angles to the surface of the probe offering a geometrically steered array. Notice that the lines of information are positioned farther apart deep in the field on the tightly curved array simply due to the design of the transducer. This contributes (in part) to the more rapid deterioration of the quality of the returning echoes positioned posteriorly and laterally within the image. The smaller footprint transducer (while inferior in image quality when compared to the larger curved array) facilitates intercostal access to the desired scanning window.

Display Device

The final contributing factor to the quality or resolution of the image lies in the ability to display the information. High-definition monitors, flat screen panels, and computer screens all possess characteristics that affect the ability to satisfactorily view the returning acoustic information with varying degrees of resolution. A variety of screen sizes combined with the angle of the viewing screen also affect the display of the returning echo information. Fixed position monitors can compromise the operator's ability to

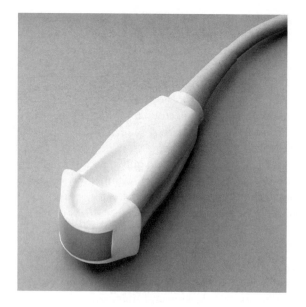

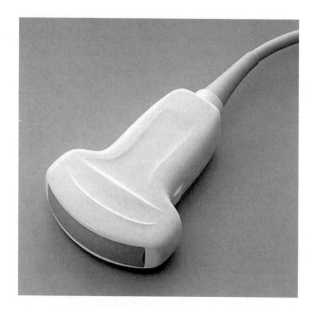

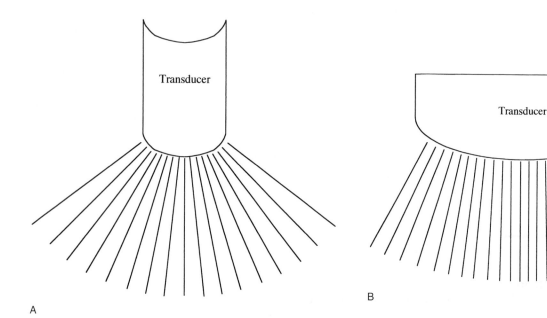

A

B

Figure 3–5. Small curvature transducers (A) generally facilitate intercostals access. However, the lines of information are positioned farther apart in the far field on the tightly curved array. This may result in the lateral resolution declining more rapidly when compared to a transducer with a larger curvature (B).

view the screen comfortably, especially when standing, whereas screens with an adjustable viewing angle can be positioned to suit the operator. There may not be one clear solution that fits everyone so it is worth noting that a variety of display technologies exist and the end-user must make a decision as to the viewing requirements of the application.

▶ MODES

A variety of imaging modalities are incorporated into diagnostic ultrasound. Historically, *A mode* or "amplitude" provided one of the first looks into the human body using sound. A mode ultrasound incorporated an oscilloscope display for returning amplitude information and a tradi-

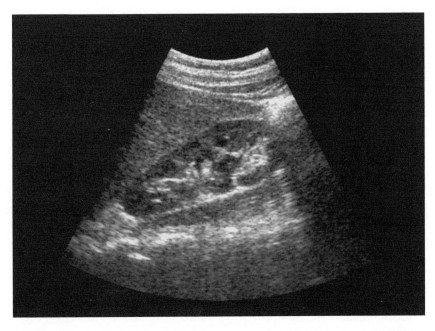

Figure 3–6. Grayscale sonography allows visualization of subtle differences within the renal architecture.

tional picture, as we know it, did not exist. The peak amplitude information on the vertical axis provided information regarding the strength or "loudness" of the wave, while the horizontal axis provided reflector distance information from the transducer.

Fortunately, *B mode* or "brightness" converted these amplitude waveforms into an image allowing better correlation with anatomic structures. Early B mode images consisted of a bi-stable display generally depicting dots of

information on a contrasting background. Grayscale scanners progressed from eight shades of gray to the advanced systems of today that may display up to 256 shades of grayscale information. These shades of gray allow subtle differences within tissues to be visualized (Figure 3–6).

Often used for cardiology examinations, *M mode,* or "motion," permits a simultaneous display of the two-dimensional B mode image and a characteristic waveform (Figure 3–7). This waveform depicts the motion or deflec-

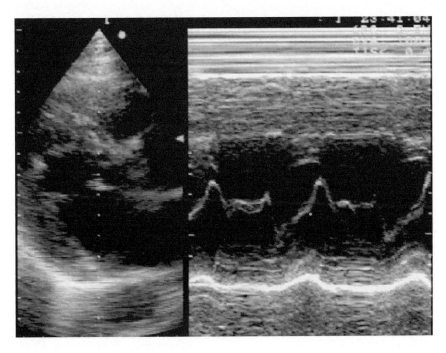

Figure 3–7. Split screen B mode / M mode image of the mitral valve.

tion of the tissue relative to the transducer on the vertical axis and represents time on the horizontal axis. M mode technology can be of value in the emergency and acute care setting during pregnancy examinations and permits measurement and documentation of fetal cardiac activity.

D mode, or "Doppler," is presented in a few different forms. Doppler technology relies on the interpretation the "frequency shift" that exists between the transmitted and received Doppler signal, while the anatomy (blood within the vessel) is moving as it is imaged.

Let us consider a railroad engineer on a moving train as an example. As the train whistle is engaged, the pedestrian at the crossing will experience an increase in the pitch (Doppler shift) of the whistle as the train approaches and a decrease in the pitch as the train continues to move away. The train engineer, however, does not experience this shift in sound since he or she is traveling with the sound, and an audible shift in frequency does not occur. Doppler ultrasound technology makes use of this "frequency shift" and the angle of interrogation of a vessel is a prominent factor in the quality and accuracy of the Doppler signal.

Spectral Doppler provides a characteristic waveform (Figure 3–8) and allows a quantitative assessment for blood flow analysis consisting of continuous or pulsed wave technologies. Continuous wave Doppler (often incorporated for interrogation of higher velocities) samples an area or line of information positioned within the ultrasound image extending along a vertical axis from the transducer. Pulsed wave Doppler allows the user to position a sample area along the vertically positioned Doppler line. The operator adjusts this sample "gate" by selecting its size and relative position (depth) within the image from the point the Doppler information is to be obtained.

The introduction of color Doppler in the early 1980s allowed a visual representation of the directional properties of flow and often facilitated the placement of the sample gate for spectral evaluation. Directional information of flow with respect to the transducer provides the operator with a visual representation of the moving blood cells (Figure 3–9). Velocity range selections, filters, and other numerous adjustments contribute to the color Doppler display and require a working knowledge of Doppler physics.

Power Doppler utilizes a slightly different component of the returning signal and often displays a greater sensitivity for evaluation of reduced flow components, as it may be slightly less angle-dependent than spectral or conventional color Doppler technologies. Power Doppler capabilities are suggested to be of increased value when low flow states (e.g., testicular or ovarian torsion) are suspected (Figure 3–10).

Each form of Doppler consists of benefits and limitations; however, regardless of which Doppler technology is employed, its operation appears deceptively simple. A complete understanding of Doppler physics and velocity components is beyond the scope of this chapter and it is strongly recommended the reader pursue additional edu-

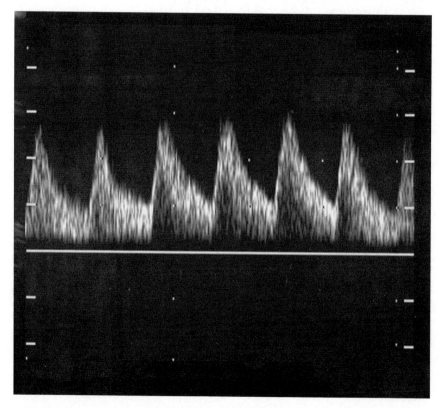

Figure 3–8. Spectral Doppler waveform.

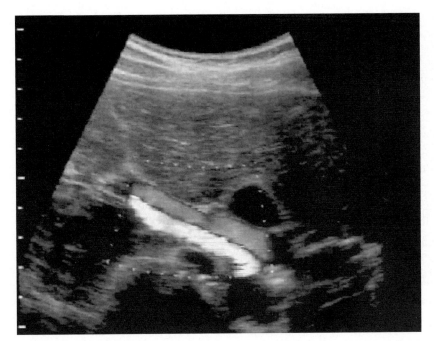

Figure 3–9. Color-flow Doppler provides directional information. In this grayscale copy, the right renal artery flow is represented by light gray and the right renal vein by medium gray within the sample area.

cational pathways for learning this valuable addition to ultrasound imaging prior to incorporating it into the imaging examination.

▶ TWO-DIMENSIONAL IMAGING

Echogenicity

Medical terminology offers a "standard language" when discussing specific items. Diagnostic ultrasound also incorporates terminology used to identify and describe the

ultrasound image. The descriptive terms brighter, whiter, blacker, darker, and so forth, are subject to a variety of interpretations. These descriptive terms are more effectively replaced by the term *echogenicity.*

Echogenicity refers to the amplitude display of the returning echoes. If a structure presents as *hyperechoic,* it is said to be more echogenic (of increased amplitude) than the surrounding anatomy. Conversely, *hypoechoic* structures appear less echogenic (of decreased amplitude). *Isoechoic* information has the same echogenicity as the surrounding structures. Finally, *anechoic* refers to

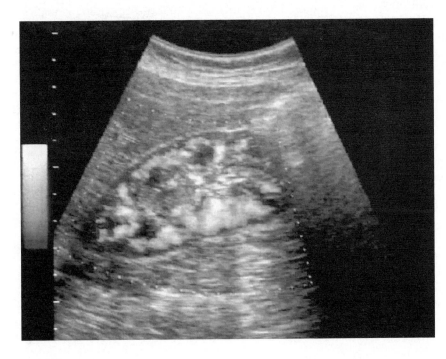

Figure 3–10. Power Doppler. Coronal view of the right kidney (grayscale copy). Light gray areas within the cortex represent detected blood flow.

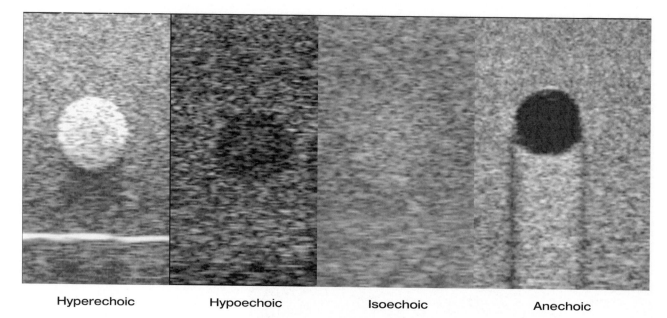

| Hyperechoic | Hypoechoic | Isoechoic | Anechoic |

Figure 3–11. Comparative echogenicity demonstrated with an ultrasound phantom.

the absence of echoes. Typically, fluid-filled structures appear anechoic (Figure 3–11).

▶ SCANNING PLANES AND TRANSDUCER ORIENTATION

One of the fundamental differences between diagnostic ultrasound and other imaging modalities lies not only in the speed of image acquisition and display, but in the ability to quickly alter the scanning plane of the transducer. Allowing the transducer to become an extension of the hand allows the operator the flexibility to interrogate anatomic structures three dimensionally (with two dimensions displayed at any one time) by rotating the transducer 90° to the original plane of interrogation. Some technology actually splits the viewing screen and allows three-dimensional real-time display under certain circumstances.

Traditional scanning planes include *longitudinal*, or *sagittal*, whereby the transducer is oriented along the long axis of the patient's body (Figure 3–12A).

Rotating the transducer 90° places the transducer in a *transverse*, or *axial*, orientation, providing a cross-sectional display of the anatomical information similar to viewing a computed tomography (CT) image (Figure 3–12B). A combination of planes results in an *oblique* transducer orientation (Figure 3–12C).

Positioning the transducer laterally from the longitudinal plane results in a *coronal*-scanning plane (Figure 3–12D). This position acoustically "slices" the anatomy in an anterior to posterior scanning plane, noting that it is in fact a thin slice of sound being emitted from the transducer (see lateral resolution). This scanning plane will become of greater importance for the successful completion of the focused assessment with sonography for trauma (FAST) examination.

Which Way Is Up?

As with the standard in terminology, a similar criterion exists when discussing the anatomic display of ultrasound imaging. While monitor or display information will change depending upon the type of examination performed (e.g., endovaginal, cardiac, etc.). This discussion is limited to display orientation for transabdominal imaging.

Many transducers offer an identification mark that is placed on the exterior assembly. Since no standard exists with respect to the size or type of identification mark, some manufacturers may utilize a depression located on one side of the transducer, while others may offer a different solution (Figure 3–13). This identification mark is required to be oriented with a corresponding identification mark located on the display device. By maintaining a level of consistency between with these indicators, it offers two distinct benefits. First, a standard display of information may be presented on the image screen and the documentation device maintaining correct orientation. Second, an expectation should exist on the part of the operator that when the transducer is moved in a particular direction on the patient, a specific portion of the display (anatomy) will enter/exit the field of view. In addition to the cephalic to caudal and right to left information displayed, the areas that are closest to the transducer (anterior) will appear more toward the top of the image, while posterior anatomy will be positioned farther away from the transducer.

▶ INSTRUMENTATION

Several key controls exist that require a thorough understanding if an acceptable ultrasound image is to be obtained and valuable information is not to be omitted.

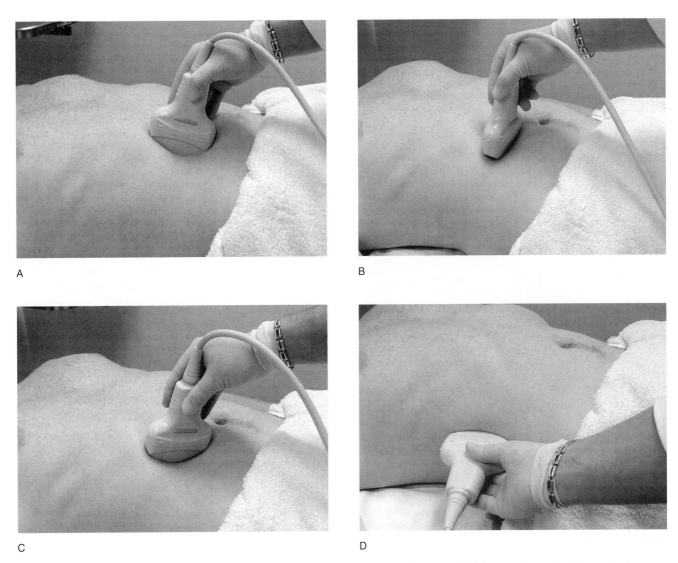

A

B

C

D

Figure 3–12. (A) Sagittal/Longitudinal plane. (B) Transverse/Axial plane. (C) Oblique plane. (D) Coronal plane.

Time Gain Compensation

Two receiver controls exist that allow the operator to manually adjust the intensity (brightness or amplitude display) of the returning echoes. The first control is labeled TGC or time gain compensation. We must remember that attenuation affects much of the ability of the ultrasound wave to propagate through the tissue at intensity equal to its original value. Since attenuation is a fact of ultrasound scanning, controls must exist that permit the operator to amplify these returning echoes at a desired depth. TGC allows the operator to "compensate" the "gain" (intensity) of the returning echoes due to the additional "time" required for the echoes to return to the transducer from structures that were positioned more posteriorly. Consider the human liver as an acoustic example. The normal human liver is a rather homogeneous structure. In other words, the echogenic-

ity displayed in the anterior portion of the liver should in fact be identical to that of the posterior echoes. However, due to the factor of attenuation, there remains considerably less acoustic energy available to display these posterior echoes at the same intensity as those positioned more anteriorly. TGC provides the operator the ability to amplify returning echoes at a given depth so as to display the intensity (brightness) of ALL of the returning echoes equally, regardless of their relative distance from the transducer. While TGC is a widely accepted term for this control, some manufacturers may reduce the number of controls and replace the traditional "slide pots" (potentiometers) with knobs or buttons labeled "Near" and "Far." While the controls are called something different, they are basically TGC controls. If the screen is artificially divided into two halves horizontally, the upper half would be interpreted as the "near" and the lower half as the "far." The principle,

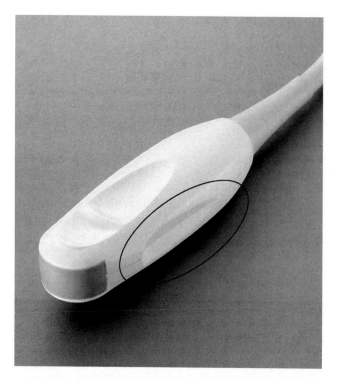

Figure 3–13. The transducer orientation indicator for this probe is encircled. The type of indicator varies among manufacturers.

however, remains the same. The controls are to be manipulated so as to achieve a "balance" of image intensity from the top of the screen to the bottom.

Gain

The gain control offers an additional parameter for adjusting the intensity of the returning echoes. While the TGC control allows amplification of the returning echoes relative to depth, the gain control amplifies all of the returning echoes equally, regardless of where they occur. Often measured in decibels (db) or a numerical value, this control increases or decreases the overall intensity (brightness) of the returning echoes. While the physical manipulation of the TGC and gain is relatively simple, it is imperative to combine their adjustment with the knowledge of echogenic anatomy. In other words, understanding the expected sonographic appearance of anatomy greatly contributes to the ability of the sonographer to create a quality diagnostic image.

Depth, Range, Magnification, and Zoom

The function of depth is to adjust the field of view on the display device, which allows more or less depth to be displayed. This results in an overall change in size of the displayed image. Allowing more depth to be displayed results in a sonographic image that appears smaller on the

screen. Conversely, allowing less depth to be displayed results in an increase in magnification of the image and is useful when targeting a specific area of visualization. The operator, however, must be keenly aware of the anatomy in question. An image display depth that is too shallow may result in the anatomic area of interest being omitted from the field of view.

The "zoom" function is very similar to the depth/range control, with some distinct differences. Often times, the zoom function permits the operator to select an area of interest on the display device and increase the magnification of this region. While the level of magnification may be an adjustable or a fixed value, it allows the operator to target a specific area of interest for display. This function is often performed during a real-time scan, as the echo information is actually acquired on a larger scale. The ability to zoom a "frozen" image does exist on some products. This ability may be compared to enlarging a 35-mm slide with some expected loss of resolution within the image.

Acoustic Power

The power selection refers to the transmit or output power (amplitude) employed to pulse the transducer in all modes of ultrasound. Often indicated as a percentage or numerical value, its on-screen display is present on those products that allow an adjustment of its value. A percentage of systems allow this parameter to be adjusted, while others have "fixed" this transmit value within the system. Acoustic power adjustments are often excluded in ultrasound examinations. Other operators may include it in their routine scanning, particularly in early obstetrical evaluations (see Biologic Effects section).

Adjustment of acoustic power may be warranted during ultrasound examinations. Often times, a lower acoustic power setting (transmit control) is desired if the returning echo information may be achieved by increasing the TGC and gain settings (receiver controls), especially during first trimester pregnancy examinations. Conversely, increasing the acoustic power may be warranted when the returning echo information does not provide a sufficient diagnostic display through adjustment of the remaining controls. Increasing acoustic power however, increases the potential risk of biologic effects. Risk factors are displayed as mechanical indices (MI) and thermal indices (TI) on the display screen. While other operator controlled parameters may also contribute in calculating the MI and TI, increasing the acoustic power and the resultant MI and TI values provide the operator with information to assist in determining whether the increase in acoustic power and the echo information obtained outweigh any potential increase in risk. Ultrasound equipment operators should be familiar with the acoustic power, MI, and TI information located in the operator's manual or from the manufacturer. Encouraging a prudent use of diagnostic ultrasound, the ideal scanning environment includes a transmit power selection that is of sufficient value to allow adequate visualization of the desired anatomy through manipulation of the remaining controls.

Measurement and Analysis

The measurement and analysis packages will vary between ultrasound systems. Ultrasound systems typically offer multiple "sets" of electronic calipers allowing various measurements to be performed on a single ultrasound image (Figure 3–14). The calipers automatically adjust their value for the change in depth, range, or magnification.

In addition to basic measurements, an extensive array of application-specific analysis packages is available, which allow assignment of the measurement data (e.g., obstetrical reports). It is important to remember that there is a vast selection of gestational parameters available for measurement and as many authors from which to choose. It is possible the "default" gestational charts in a particular ultrasound product may not necessarily parallel the choice of the user and alternate gestational parameters or authors may need to be selected. Each department may evaluate the need and selection of analysis packages; however, basic measurements remain the primary need in the emergency environment.

▶ IMAGE ARTIFACTS

The importance of understanding image artifacts and their formation is paramount. Unrecognized artifacts are frequently the source of misleading information. The ability to recognize and interpret echo information not only includes the anatomic reflections we expect to visualize, but also includes the formation of echoes that appear as a result of image phenomenon. For the simplicity of this chapter, artifacts will be defined as any echo information that does not correspond to the anatomic information as it is positioned and reflected from within the patient. The origin of these artifactual echoes may occur from within the patient, as a result of changes in the acoustic wave or from an external source. Some of the frequent image artifacts encountered are explored.

Shadowing

Acoustic shadowing is one of the most common and frequently encountered imaging artifacts in diagnostic ultrasound. Shadowing may occur for several different reasons, including anatomic or pathologic or changes undergone by the ultrasound beam.

Acoustic shadowing frequently occurs when the sound encounters a highly reflective (high attenuation) surface, much like the example of when a beam of light emitting from a flashlight is aimed directly at a mirror. The reflected energy is returned to the transducer with little acoustic energy available to continue traveling to

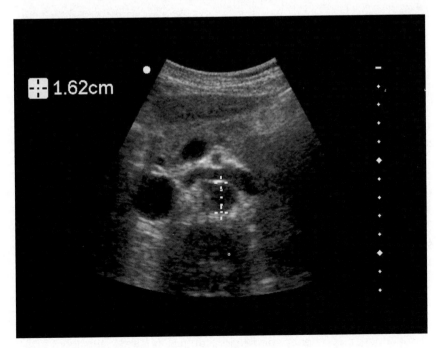

Figure 3–14. Measurement of the anterior to posterior diameter of the transverse aorta using the electronic calipers.

deeper structures. Gallstones, renal stones, ribs, or tissue calcifications are some of the reasons a shadow may exist. Figure 3–15A demonstrates a gallbladder with no contents visualized within its lumen. When the scanning plane is changed slightly, the ultrasound beam now crosses the boundary of the gallstone, reflecting the acoustic energy at its surface, and an acoustic shadow presents (Figure 3–15B).

Acoustic Enhancement

As sound crosses a boundary where less signal attenuation occurs, acoustic enhancement of the beam is often

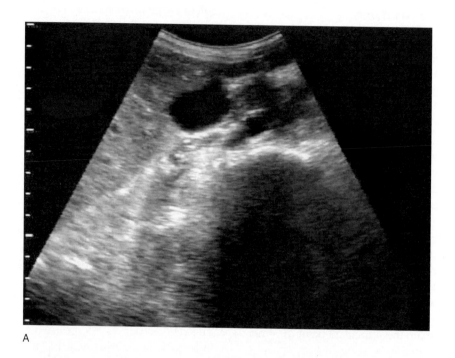

A

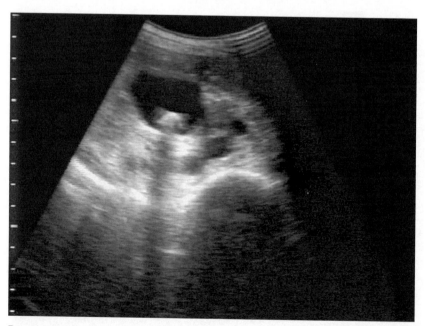

B

Figure 3–15. (A) Transverse view of the gallbladder. (B) Slight changes in transducer placement or angulation can demonstrate significant changes in the image display. In this view, a gallstone with posterior shadowing is revealed.

the result. The effects of acoustic enhancement are quite simply the opposite of high-attenuating objects. Ultrasound is based on the principle of energy transmitted and reflected (attenuation) with part of the energy continuing to encounter additional reflectors.

As sound encounters ultrasound friendly objects (e.g., simple cysts, distended normal gallbladder, urinary bladder, some types of solid tissue, etc.), less attenuation of the signal occurs, which results in a greater amount of acoustic energy available to continue its journey along the same angle of travel. This increase in acoustic energy results in a similar increase in echogenicity (hyperechoic) immediately posterior to the area where less attenuation of the signal occurred. This type of imaging artifact is commonly used to confirm the presence of areas suspected to be fluid-filled in etiology and is also referred to as "increased acoustic transmission" (Figure 3–16).

Refraction

Shadows may also occur due to changes in the ultrasound beam. We are familiar with the childhood example of refraction using light and a pencil in a glass of water that results in a visible distortion of the pencil. In ultrasound, a change in the sound beam direction results when there is an oblique incidence of the sound beam as it crosses a boundary of tissue with different propagation speeds. Note the bilateral shadows that present parallel to the sound beam and tangentially to the wall of the structure being examined as the sound crosses from a boundary of tissue to an anechoic fluid-filled structure. As the sound crosses this boundary, a change in the beam direction occurs and an acoustic shadow results (Figure 3–17). When an acoustic shadow presents, it is wise to identify the path so we may appreciate its origin.

Gas

The presence of bowel gas is possibly the first identifiable artifact abdominal sonographers encounter on their first day. Referring back to the discussion of Acoustic Impedance, we remember the large differences in density that exists between gas and soft tissue. Diagnostic ultrasound is not equipped to handle these large differences and much of the acoustic energy is scattered with little or no appreciable diagnostic information visualized. Slight transducer pressure or a change in patient and/or transducer positioning may minimize the obstacle; however, often times, experience will dictate when additional views may not prove of benefit (Figure 3–18).

Reverberation

When sound "bounces" between two highly reflective objects, reverberation artifacts appear as recurrent bright arcs displayed at equidistant intervals from the transducer. Commonly, this artifact will appear at the anterior aspect of the distended urinary bladder or near the layers of the

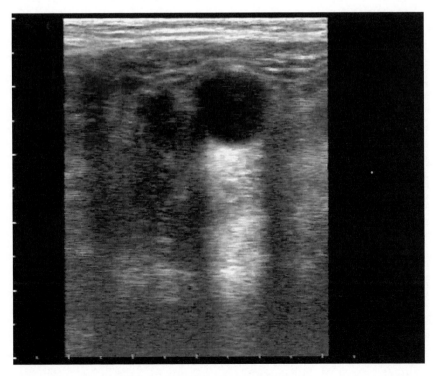

Figure 3–16. Acoustic enhancement. Note increase in echogenicity posterior to the anechoic area.

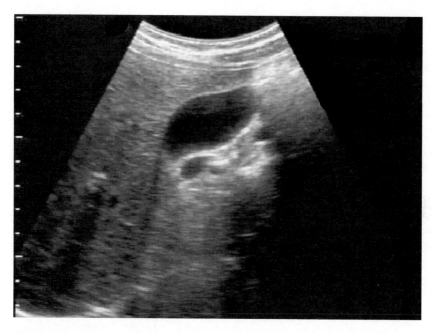

Figure 3–17. Longitudinal view of the gallbladder. Note the edge artifact producing a narrow shadow extending posteriorly from the wall of the gallbladder.

abdominal wall and become more of a nuisance when interrogating structures that are positioned in close proximity. Figure 3–19 demonstrates an anterior gallbladder with multiple reverberation artifacts identified adjacent to the anterior wall. Changes in transducer positioning, patient positioning, or transducer transmit frequency, may reduce their appearance; however, their presence is not likely to be confused with a pathologic condition.

Mirroring

Mirror artifacts are displayed as objects that appear on both sides of a strong reflector. These artifacts can be confusing in appearance and occur due to changes in the reflected beam. Ultrasound assumes that sound is traveling in a straight line and the distance (or depth) of the reflector is proportional to the travel time necessary to make the

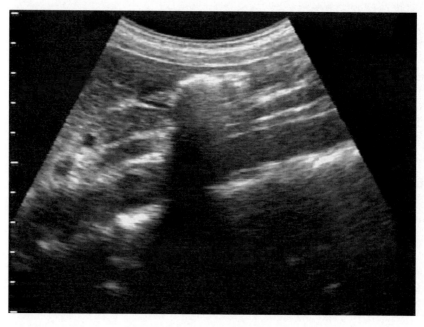

Figure 3–18. Longitudinal aorta is partially obscured by overlying bowel gas.

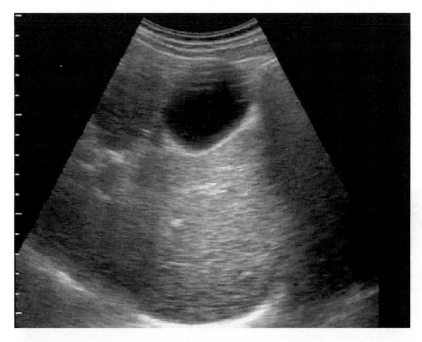

Figure 3–19. Reverberation artifacts are noted in the anterior aspect of the gallbladder.

return trip. When the ultrasound beam undergoes multiple reflections as it returns, an incorrect interpretation of the signal timing ensues and results in a duplication of structures. The more posterior echo information is the "false" echo. Mirror artifacts are common around the diaphragm and may depict hepatic structures appearing on both sides of the diaphragm. Changes in transducer or pa-

tient positioning should alleviate any real threat to misdiagnosis (Figure 3–20).

Motion Artifacts

Motion artifacts can be traced to a variety of sources. Transducer movement, patient respirations, and transmitted

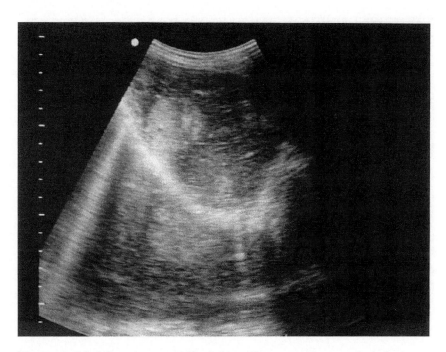

Figure 3–20. Mirror image artifact. Liver tissue and hyperechoic liver lesions are duplicated above the diaphragm.

pulses from cardiac activity may all contribute to blurring of the image as the "freeze" button has been depressed. Frequently, this fuzzy image may be improved through a function called "cine memory" that allows the operator to view a number of frames that preceded the frozen image. The exact number of available image frames will vary by ultrasound product and other parameters set forth by the manufacturer. In fact, often it is less than 1 second of information remaining in memory. This may not sound like an abundance of time; however, at 20 to 30 frames/sec, a frame of information free of motion artifact is generally available. Cine memory is particularly helpful when Doppler is performed since the area demonstrating the specific frame of interest may be identified (Figure 3–21A and B).

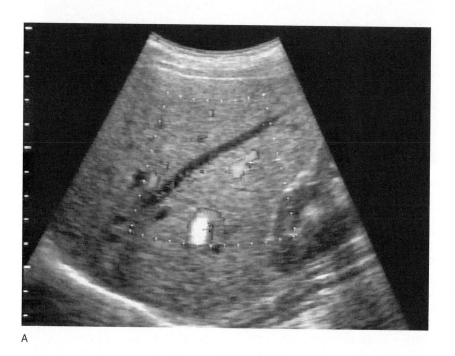

A

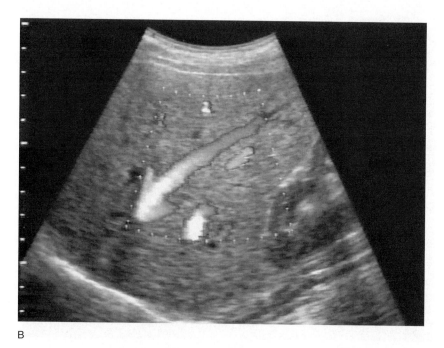

B

Figure 3–21. Two separate frames recalled from cine memory. Frame B demonstrates more color flow information than Frame A.

Side Lobes

It is easy to envision one ultrasound beam being emitted from the probe along a plane parallel to the central axis of the transducer. In reality, ultrasound beams of lower intensity, called "side lobes," may originate at angles to the primary beam and are generally of little consequence. Highly reflective interfaces return echoes via this pathway of side lobes and present as false information. This false information may be introduced as an oblique line of acoustic reflection. Changes in the scanning angle often confirm these returning echoes as side lobes (Figure 3–22).

Noise

Electronic noise can obscure the primary echo information as it is displayed. We may recall the familiar "lines" of information that interrupt our viewing of a television program when an electric tool is activated nearby or an airplane passes overhead. Electronic noise occurs when these signals disturb the primary signal of information. Sources of electronic noise vary and include electronic devices in the trauma bay, other devices that are supplied by the same electrical service, and radio frequency signals traveling through the air. Shielding these devices is often difficult and understanding noise as an occasional artifact in imaging is necessary.

Technique

Referring back to the Instrumentation section, incorrect TGC and gain settings can create confusing image patterns (Figure 3–23 A, B, and C). Note that in Figure 3–23D, excessive gain settings create an image pattern where the subtleties between the liver and right kidney have disappeared, creating a uniformly hyperechoic image and obscuring the ability to appreciate echogenicity. There is no substitute for experience and understanding of the echogenicity relating to specific anatomy.

▶ QUALITY ASSURANCE

Quality assurance is a topic often interpreted as the "quality" of the ultrasound examination that is solely dependent upon the skill level of the operator. While the operator is in direct control over the views obtained and system settings to perform a quality examination, the consistency with which the ultrasound system produces quality examinations over time cannot be overlooked.

Diagnostic ultrasound phantoms exist in part to allow a reproducible standard to be documented to ensure that the ultrasound system and its components are operating at the performance level defined by the product manufacturer. Ultrasound system and transducer performance can change over time. Multipurpose ultrasound phantoms allow evaluation of transducer parameters, measurement calibration, focal zone, axial and lateral resolution, sensitivity, functional resolution, and grayscale displays (Figure 3–24). Specialty phantoms are available to examine transducer beam profile and slice thickness in

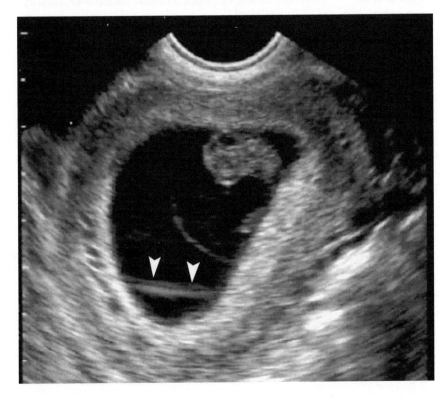

Figure 3–22. Endovaginal image reveals intrauterine gestation with embryonic pole and thin amniotic membrane. Side lobe artifact is demonstrated within the gestational sac (Arrowheads).

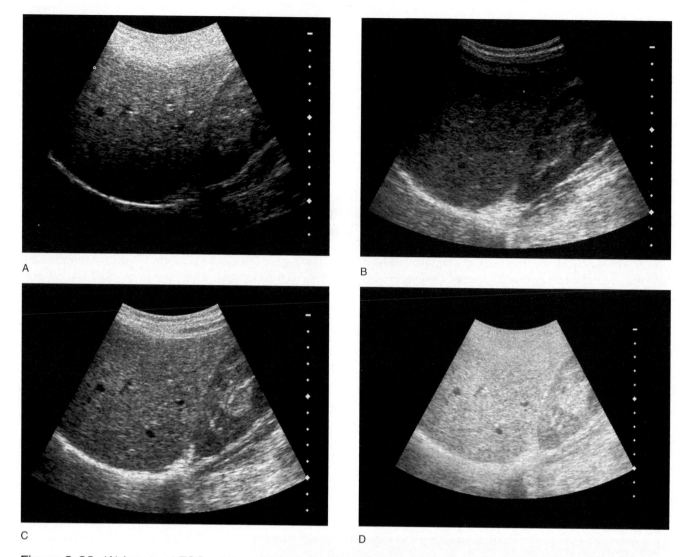

Figure 3–23. (A) Incorrect TGC settings. Maladjusted far field/posterior TGC setting does not permit visualization of posterior structures. (B) Incorrect TGC settings. Maladjusted near field/anterior TGC setting does not permit visualization of structures positioned closer to the transducer. (C) Correct TGC and gain settings. By balancing the display of echogenic information, one can appreciate the subtleties which occur among tissues. (D) Excessive gain settings reduce the ability to differentiate subtleties among various tissues.

addition to Doppler phantoms. Scheduled performance evaluations should be incorporated at regular intervals to ensure the ultrasound system and documentation devices are operating at peak performance.

▶ BIOLOGIC EFFECTS

Risk factors do exist in diagnostic ultrasound and their effects over time have yet to be discovered, especially as new diagnostic ultrasound technology continues to develop and be implemented. The American Institute of Ultrasound in Medicine (AIUM) has adopted an acronym termed ALARA: As Low As Reasonably Achievable. The term reminds the sonographer that the amount of

time for an examination, along with equipment settings, contributes to prudent use of diagnostic ultrasound. The receiver controls (i.e., TGC, gain, etc.) need to be optimized prior to increasing acoustic power capabilities in an attempt to secure or improve the desired image (Appendix A).

▶ CONCLUSION

A basic understanding of ultrasound physics must be understood before the operator can enjoy the benefit of bedside sonography and reduce any of its potential risks. Prudent use of diagnostic ultrasound remains at the forefront of discussion, and to dismiss any potential

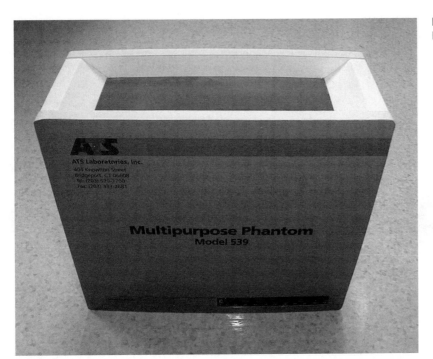

Figure 3-24. ATS Multipurpose Phantom Model 539.

biologic effect as a trivial matter would result in an injustice to patient care. By implementing emergency ultrasound, there remains a responsibility to the patient community that diagnostic ultrasound examinations include our understanding and implementation of physics and instrumentation. This is the first step in assuring that a high-quality examination is performed while minimizing any potential risk to the patient or operator.

REFERENCES

1. Gill K. Abdominal ultrasound: a practitioner's guide. Philadelphia: Saunders, 2000.
2. Goodsit MM, Carson JY, Witt TG, et al. Real time B-mode ultrasound quality control test procedures. Report of AAPM ultrasound task group no. 1. Am Assoc Phys Med 1998;27;23–25.
3. Kurtz AB, Middleton AB. Ultrasound: the requisites. Philadelphia: Saunders, 1996.
4. Kremkau FW. Diagnostic ultrasound: principles and instruments, 6th ed. Philadelphia: Saunders, 2002.
5. Lin GS, Milburn DT, Briggs S. Power Doppler how it works, its clinical benefits and recent technological advances. JDMS 1998;14:45–48.
6. Nilsson A Ingemar Loren I, Nirhov N, et al. Power doppler sonography: alternative to computed tomograph in abdominal trauma patients. JUM 1999;18:129–132.
7. Rumack CM, Charboneau JW, Wilson SR. Diagnostic ultrasound, 2nd ed. Philadelphia: Saunders, 1998.
8. Stephen E. Felkel S. Ultrasound safety mechanical and thermal indices: a primer. JDMS 1999;15:98–100.
9. Tempkin BB. Ultrasound scanning: principles and protocols, 2nd ed. Philadelphia: Saunders, 1998.

▶ APPENDIX A

Further reading includes the AIUM publications listed below on ultrasound safety and are available by contacting AIUM.

American Institute of Ultrasound in Medicine
www.aium.org
800-638-5352
14750 Sweitzer Lane
Suite 100
Laurel, MD 20707

Ultrasound Safety Publications

Bioeffects and Safety of Diagnostic Ultrasound

Evaluation of Research Reports: Bioeffects Literature Reviews (1962–1982).

Evaluation of Research Reports: Bioeffects Literature Reviews (1985–1991).

Evaluation of Research Reports: Bioeffects Literature Reviews (1992–1998).

How to Interpret the Ultrasound Output Display Standard for Higher Acoustic Output Diagnostic Ultrasound Devices (technical bulletin).

Mechanical Bioeffects from Diagnostic Ultrasound: Consensus Statements.

Medical Ultrasound Safety

What You Should Know About the Safety of Your Ultrasound Examination (patient pamphlet).

CHAPTER 4

Trauma

O. John Ma and James R. Mateer

Over the past 20 years, trauma surgeons in Europe and Japan have demonstrated the proficient use of ultrasonography in evaluating blunt trauma patients.[1–9] During the 1990s, emergency physicians and trauma surgeons in the United States have prospectively evaluated the applications of ultrasonography in trauma and have presented results comparable to other investigators worldwide.[10–18]

The focused assessment with sonography for trauma (FAST) examination is a bedside screening tool to aid clinicians in identifying free intrathoracic or intraperitoneal fluid. The underlying premise behind the use of the FAST examination is that clinically significant injuries will be associated with the presence of free fluid accumulating in dependent areas. The FAST examination was developed as a limited ultrasound examination, focusing primarily on the detection of free fluid, and was not designed to universally identify all sonographically detectable pathology.

► CLINICAL CONSIDERATIONS

The rapid and accurate diagnosis of injuries sustained by trauma patients can be difficult, especially when they are associated with other distracting injuries or altered mental status from head injury or drug or alcohol use. In the United States, the three generally accepted diagnostic techniques for evaluating abdominal trauma patients are diagnostic peritoneal lavage, computed tomography (CT) of the abdomen, and ultrasonography. Each of these diagnostic modalities has their own advantages and disadvantages.

Diagnostic peritoneal lavage remains an excellent screening test for evaluating abdominal trauma. The advantages of diagnostic peritoneal lavage include its sensitivity, availability, relative speed with which it can be performed, and low complication rate. Disadvantages, however, include the potential for iatrogenic injury, its misapplication for evaluation of retroperitoneal injuries, and its lack of specificity.

Computed tomography of the abdomen has a greater specificity than diagnostic peritoneal lavage, thus making it the initial diagnostic test of choice at many trauma centers. Oral and IV contrast material should be given to provide optimal resolution. Advantages of CT scan include its ability to precisely locate intra-abdominal lesions preoperatively, to evaluate the retroperitoneum, to identify injuries that may be managed nonoperatively, and its noninvasiveness. The disadvantages of CT scanning are its expense, time required to perform the study, need to transport the trauma patient to the radiology suite, and the need for contrast materials.

Ultrasonography offers several advantages over diagnostic peritoneal lavage and the abdominal CT scan. Numerous studies have demonstrated that the FAST examination, like diagnostic peritoneal lavage, is an accurate screening tool for abdominal trauma.[1–19] Advantages of the FAST examination are that it is accurate, rapid, noninvasive, repeatable, portable, and involves no contrast material or radiation exposure to the patient. There is limited risk for patients who are pregnant, coagulopathic, or have had previous abdominal surgery. The average time to perform a complete FAST examination of the thoracic and abdominal cavities is 2.1[20] to 4.0 min.[12] One major advantage of the FAST examination is the ability to also evaluate for free pericardial and pleural fluid. Disadvantages include the inability to determine the exact etiology of the free intraperitoneal fluid and the operator-dependent nature of the examination. Other disadvantages of the FAST examination are the difficulty in interpreting the views in patients who are obese or have subcutaneous air or excessive bowel gas and the inability to distinguish intraperitoneal hemorrhage from ascites. The FAST examination also cannot evaluate the retroperitoneum as well as CT scanning.

In light of the evolving nonoperative approach to certain types of solid-organ injuries, a positive diagnostic peritoneal lavage by itself is becoming less of an indication for immediate exploratory laparotomy than the amount of hemorrhage and the clinical condition of the patient. Since the FAST examination can reliably detect small amounts of free intraperitoneal fluid and can be used to estimate the rate of hemorrhage through serial examinations, ultrasonography is replacing diagnostic peritoneal lavage for most current indications.

▶ CLINICAL INDICATIONS

The clinical indications for performing the FAST examination are:

- Acute blunt or penetrating torso trauma
- Trauma in pregnancy
- Pediatric trauma
- Subacute torso trauma

ACUTE BLUNT OR PENETRATING TORSO TRAUMA

At level 1 trauma centers, the primary utilization of the FAST examination has been for the rapid detection of free intraperitoneal fluid in patients who have sustained significant blunt torso trauma. More recently, trauma programs have begun to incorporate the FAST examination into the primary patient assessment for detecting the presence, amount, and location of intracavitary hemorrhage in general.

With blunt trauma, the FAST examination is particularly useful for patients who: (1) are too hemodynamically unstable to leave the emergency department for CT scanning; (2) have a physical examination that is unreliable secondary to drug intoxication, distracting injury, or central nervous system injury; or (3) have unexplained hypotension and an equivocal physical examination.

With penetrating trauma patients, the FAST examination should be performed when it is not certain that immediate surgery is indicated. In patients with multiple wounds, the FAST examination can be used to quantify and locate the source of internal hemorrhage. When the trajectory of a penetrating wound is uncertain, the FAST examination may quickly identify the course by the presence of free fluid within the compartments involved. This is particularly helpful when the entry location is the precordium, lower chest, or epigastrium. The FAST examination can, therefore, be used to prioritize such life-saving interventions as pericardiocentesis, pericardiotomy, thoracostomy, thoracotomy, laparotomy, or sternotomy. The FAST examination is useful in evaluating patients who have sustained stab wounds to the abdomen where local wound exploration indicates that the superficial muscle fascia has been violated. Also, the FAST examination may be useful in confirming a negative physical examination when tangential or lower chest wounds are involved.

In non-level 1 trauma centers, emergency physicians and surgeons often lack the immediate availability of CT scans and formal two-dimensional echocardiograms. The availability of bedside ultrasonography and physicians trained to perform the FAST examination in these settings will significantly improve patient evaluation, initial treatment, consultation, and the timely transport of patients to trauma centers when indicated. When the FAST examination demonstrates intracavitary fluid in these settings, surgeons and operating room personnel can be consulted immediately and/or transport to a level 1 trauma center can be initiated. When the diagnostic imaging personnel and surgeons are out of the hospital, and the severity of the patient's injuries are not clinically evident, a positive FAST examination could save up to an hour or more of time to definitive surgical treatment.

Although the FAST examination is used most commonly to detect free intraperitoneal fluid, it may also aid in the rapid identification of free pericardial or pleural fluid, and in the evaluation of the fetus in the pregnant trauma patient. In addition, the FAST examination has been evaluated in the management of pediatric trauma patients and can be utilized in patients who present with subacute trauma but with a significant mechanism of injury or concerning physical examination.

Detection of Free Intraperitoneal Fluid

By the latter half of the 1990s, for patients who had sustained blunt or penetrating abdominal trauma, the FAST examination's utility for detecting free intraperitoneal fluid had been almost universally recognized. While computed tomography remained the gold standard for detecting specific intraabdominal pathology, the FAST examination had gained acceptance as a rapid screening tool for identifying free intraperitoneal fluid.

During the 1980s, surgeons in Germany developed bedside utilization of ultrasonography for evaluation of trauma patients. Although excellent results were reported in early studies, with the sensitivity ranging from 84 to 100% and the specificity from 88 to 100%, these findings went largely unnoticed in the United States, in part, because the articles were not initially translated into English.[2–7]

In the 1990s, a number of prospective studies (with study sizes greater than 100 patients) had been reported on this issue in the English literature.[1,8-19] The majority of these studies focused on the FAST examination for the evaluation of free intraperitoneal fluid in blunt abdominal trauma patients only. These studies reported the sensitivity and the specificity to range from 69 to 90% and 95 to 100%, respectively.

Tiling and co-workers were the first investigators to suggest that the FAST examination could provide comprehensive evaluation for significant areas of hemorrhage, including pericardial, pleural, intraperitoneal, and retroperitoneal. Their prospective study of 808 blunt trauma patients found a sensitivity of 89% and a specificity of 99% for free intraperitoneal fluid. Their clinical algorithm incorporates the FAST examination during the initial patient evaluation (Figure 4–1).[1]

In one of the first North American trauma ultrasound studies, Rozycki and colleagues demonstrated the FAST examination to have an overall sensitivity of 79% and specificity of 95.6%. They concluded that appropriately trained surgeons could rapidly and accurately perform and interpret FAST examinations and that ultrasonography was a rapid, sensitive, and specific diagnostic modality for detecting intraperitoneal fluid and pericardial effusion.[10] In another study, they successfully used ultrasonography as the primary adjuvant modality to detect hemoperitoneum and pericardial effusion in injured patients. In the FAST examinations of 371 patients, they had an 81.5% sensitivity and 99.7% specificity. The researcher stated that ultrasonography should be the primary adjuvant instrument for the evaluation of injured patients because it was rapid, accurate, and potentially cost-effective.[11] They

also devised a suggested algorithm for the use of ultrasonography in evaluating patients with blunt abdominal trauma (Figure 4–2).

In 1995, Ma and Mateer prospectively demonstrated that the FAST examination could serve as a sensitive, specific, and accurate diagnostic tool in the detection of free intraperitoneal and thoracic fluid in patients who had sustained major blunt or penetrating trauma. Overall, the FAST examination had a sensitivity of 90%, specificity of 99%, and accuracy of 99%. In evaluating the subgroup of blunt trauma patients, which consisted of 165 out of the 245 patients, the FAST examination was 90% sensitive, 99% specific, and 99% accurate. In evaluating the subgroup of penetrating trauma victims, which consisted of 80 out of the 245 patients, the FAST examination was 91% sensitive, 100% specific, and 99% accurate.[12] Since emergency physicians performed all the FAST examinations, it became the first prospective study to support that appropriately trained emergency physicians could accurately perform and interpret FAST examinations. The results reiterated that a FAST examination of the entire torso could successfully provide early and valuable information for the presence of free fluid in both the peritoneal and thoracic cavities. Additionally, the FAST examination was found to be equally sensitive, specific, and accurate for both blunt and penetrating torso trauma. Penetrating trauma patients could benefit from the rapid and accurate information yielded by ultrasonography. The identification and localization of significant hemorrhage in penetrating trauma patients would allow physicians "to prioritize resources for resuscitation and evaluation."[10]

Most studies have utilized a multiple view FAST examination for evaluation of trauma patients. Some investigators have employed a single view technique, examining only Morison's pouch for free intraperitoneal fluid.[21-23] In one study, all patients were placed in the Trendelenburg position and the perihepatic (Morison's pouch) was the single area examined. The results of this technique was reported to be 81.8% sensitive, 93.9% specific, and 90.9% accurate.[21]

The single view (perihepatic) imaging technique was compared against the multiple view technique of the FAST examination for the identification of free intraperitoneal fluid in patients who had sustained major blunt or penetrating torso trauma. For detecting free intraperitoneal fluid, when comparing the multiple view FAST examination of the abdomen to the gold standard, the multiple view FAST examination technique had a sensitivity of 87%, a specificity of 99%, and an accuracy of 98%. When comparing the perihepatic single view of the abdomen to the gold standard, the single view FAST examination technique had a sensitivity of 51%, a specificity of 100%, and an accuracy of 93%.[13] Based on this and other studies, the more sensitive and accurate FAST examination method for detecting free intraperitoneal fluid was determined to be the multiple views technique.[13]

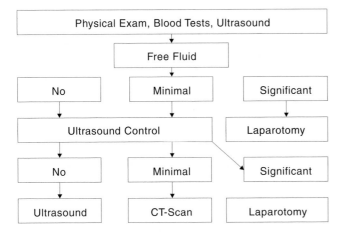

Figure 4–1. Tiling's algorithm for managing blunt abdominal trauma. *(Reprinted with permission from Tiling T, Bouillon B, Schmid A, et al. Ultrasound in blunt abdomino-thoracic trauma. In: Border JR, Allgoewer M, Hansen ST, et al, eds. Blunt multiple trauma: comprehensive pathophysiology and care. New York: Marcel Dekker, 1990;415–433.)*

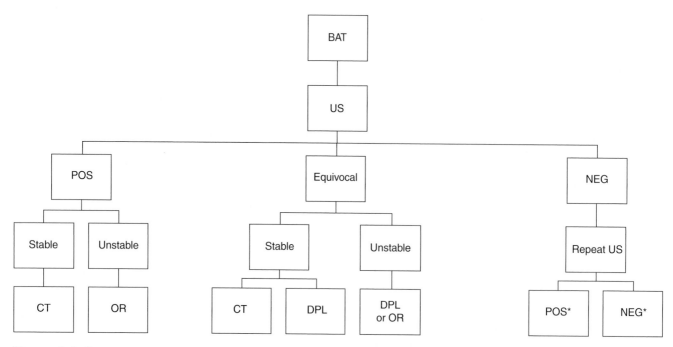

Figure 4–2. Suggested algorithm for the use of ultrasonography in the evaluation of the patient with blunt abdominal trauma. *(Reprinted with permission from Rozycki GS, Shackford SR. Ultrasound: what every trauma surgeon should know. J Trauma 1996;40:2.)*

Clinical pathways and protocols have been derived from the use of the FAST examination. An ultrasound-based key clinical pathway has been shown to reduce the number of diagnostic peritoneal lavage procedures and CT scans required to evaluate blunt abdominal trauma without increased risk to the patient. Using the key clinical pathway, diagnostic peritoneal lavage procedures were reduced from 17 to 4%, and CT scans reduced from 56 to 26%. The injury severity score increased from 11.6 to 21.5 for diagnostic peritoneal lavage patients and from 4.6 to 8.3 for CT scan patients. FAST examinations were used exclusively in 65% of the patients. This ultrasound-based key clinical pathway was found to result in significant reductions in the utilization of diagnostic peritoneal lavage and CT scanning in the evaluation of blunt abdominal trauma without increased risk to the patient (Figure 4–3). The investigators estimated cost savings of $450,000 per year using this key clinical pathway.[24] The issue of cost savings of the FAST examination has also been addressed in another study. For blunt trauma patients, the FAST examination was found to be more efficient and cost effective compared to CT scanning or diagnostic peritoneal lavage. There was a significantly shorter time to disposition at approximately one-third the cost in the ultrasonography group.[25] An ultrasound-based scoring system has been developed to quantify the amount of intraperitoneal blood in blunt abdominal trauma patients and to assess the need for therapeutic exploratory laparotomy. Scores ranged from 0 to 8. The system assigned two points for significant fluid collections and one

point for minor fluid collections. A score of 3 correlated with 1000 mL of fluid. In the study, of those patients who had a score of 3 or more, 24 of 25 patients (96%) required therapeutic laparotomy. Of those who had a score of less than 3, therapeutic laparotomy was required in only 9 of 24 patients (38%). The FAST examination was found to be a useful adjunct in helping to make clinical decisions during the resuscitation period.[26] In another study evaluating the role of the FAST examination in determining the need for therapeutic laparotomy, none of the patients with negative FAST examination results died or sustained identifiable mortality as a consequence of their negative scans.[27]

Detection of Pericardial Fluid

In the hypotensive patient who has sustained penetrating trauma to the torso, the echocardiographic portion of the FAST examination may prove to be the most beneficial aspect. Echocardiography remains the gold standard diagnostic procedure for detecting pericardial effusions. The classic physical examination findings of acute cardiac tamponade—distended neck veins, hypotension, and muffled heart tones—are present in less than 40% of patients with surgically proven cardiac tamponade.[28] Timely emergency department procedures and expeditious transport of the patient to the operating room can be accomplished by ultrasound diagnosis of hemopericardium.

In 1992, Plummer and co-investigators evaluated the effect of bedside echocardiography performed by emer-

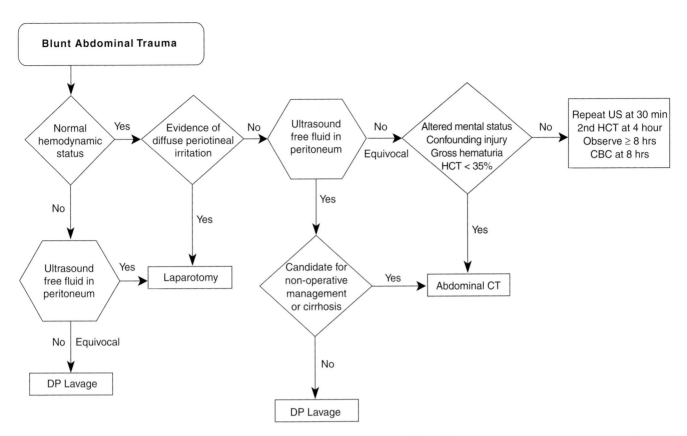

Figure 4-3. Key clinical pathway for the evaluation of blunt abdominal trauma. *(Reprinted with permission from Branney SW, Moore EE, Cantrill S, et al. Ultrasound-based key clinical pathway reduces the use of hospital resources for the evaluation of blunt abdominal trauma. J Trauma 1997;42:1086–1090.)*

gency physicians on the outcome of 49 patients with penetrating cardiac injuries over a 10-year period. Compared to a retrospective control group, the use of bedside echocardiography significantly reduced the time of diagnosis and disposition to the operating room from 42.4 ± 21.7 min to 15.5 ± 11.4 min. The actual survival rate improved from 57.1 to 100%.[29]

The accuracy of emergency ultrasound has been evaluated after it was introduced into five level I trauma centers for the diagnosis of acute hemopericardium. Surgeons or cardiologists (four centers) and technicians (one center) performed pericardial ultrasound examinations on patients with penetrating truncal wounds. By protocol, patients with positive examinations underwent immediate operation. In 261 patients, pericardial ultrasound examinations were found to have a sensitivity of 100%, specificity of 96.9%, and accuracy of 97.3%. The mean time from ultrasound to operation was 12.1 ± 5 min. This further demonstrated that ultrasound should be the initial modality for the evaluation of patients with penetrating precordial wounds because it is accurate and rapid.[30]

Over the years, numerous studies have examined the role of echocardiography in blunt cardiac trauma. The utility and role of ultrasound, particularly with the diagnosis of cardiac contusion, remain unclear (see Chapter 5 for a comprehensive review of this topic).

Detection of Pleural Fluid

Since patients who have sustained major trauma routinely present to the emergency department immobilized on a long-spine board, clinicians may have difficulty identifying bilateral hemothoraces or a small unilateral hemothorax on the initial supine chest radiograph. The FAST examination can detect hemothorax before the completion of a chest radiograph. Results can be used as additional information when the chest radiograph is equivocal.

Of the six anatomic areas scanned by the FAST examination, only two are required to identify the presence of free pleural fluid in the two pleural cavities. Thus, tube thoracostomy for trauma patients may be expedited with use of ultrasonography.

Ma and Mateer demonstrated that the FAST examination could serve as a sensitive, specific, and accurate diagnostic tool in detecting hemothorax in major trauma patients. When comparing the FAST examination and the chest radiograph to the criterion standard definitions, both diagnostic tests had an equal sensitivity (96.2%), specificity (100%), and accuracy (99.6%) for detecting pleural fluid. They concluded that ultrasonography was comparable to the chest radiograph for identifying hemothorax.[31]

Ultrasonography can detect smaller quantities of pleural fluid than the chest radiograph. It is estimated that an upright chest radiograph can accurately detect a minimum of 50 to 100 mL of pleural fluid.[32] A supine chest radiograph can detect a minimum of 175 mL of pleural fluid.[33] By contrast, it is estimated that ultrasonography can detect a minimum of 20 mL of pleural fluid.[9]

This should not suggest that ultrasonography can replace the chest radiograph during the initial evaluation of trauma patients. The chest radiograph holds several indispensable advantages over ultrasonography since it can identify pneumothorax, mediastinal injuries, and bony injuries. Although the FAST examination cannot replace the chest radiograph, it can complement chest radiograph findings by rapidly identifying hemothorax in the supine patient. By utilizing the FAST examination to initially identify hemothorax, the standard chest radiograph of the trauma patient can be performed after tube thoracostomy, thereby sparing the patient an additional chest radiograph. Also, ultrasonography can help to differentiate between pleural fluid and pleural thickening or pulmonary contusion when the supine chest radiograph is equivocal.

TRAUMA IN PREGNANCY

Trauma continues to be one of the leading causes of nonobstetrical mortality in pregnant patients.[34] Moreover, it contributes to fetal death more frequently than maternal death.[35–39] Ultrasonography can be a valuable adjunct for rapid diagnosis of traumatic injuries, both for the mother and fetus.[40–42]

The pregnant trauma patient presents unique diagnostic and management issues for the emergency physician and trauma surgeon. Maternal shock carries a high fetal mortality rate.[38] Although there are two lives at stake, proper assessment and stabilization of the mother will provide the best opportunity for fetal stability. Therefore, rapid assessment of the pregnant trauma patient is essential for early identification of life-threatening injuries. The FAST examination clearly may play a role in the timely assessment of pregnant trauma patients.

In this setting, ultrasonography offers several advantages over abdominal CT scan and diagnostic peritoneal lavage. The FAST examination can aid in the timely identification of pregnant trauma patients who need exploratory laparotomy immediately, and can help avoid delays in management while other diagnostic tests are obtained. The FAST examination can be performed at the bedside and involves no contrast material or radiation exposure to the mother or fetus. Sonography can rapidly assess the pregnant trauma patient for hemoperitoneum and intrathoracic hemorrhage, and can assess the fetus for fetal heart tones, activity, and approximate gestational age. While ultrasonography is useful for identifying fetal heart tones and fetal movement, it is not as accurate in diagnosing uterine rupture or placental abruption, and it may be more technically difficult for advanced third trimester pregnancy.[43]

The identification of free intraperitoneal fluid can be related to hemorrhage from solid organ injuries or amniotic fluid from uterine rupture or both. Ultrasonography should not be considered a reliable method for the specific identification of uterine rupture. The presence of an intrauterine organized hematoma and/or oligohydramnios, however, may suggest this diagnosis. Finally, although ultrasonography can be utilized to confirm immediate fetal viability, it cannot be used to rule out fetal placental injury. While ultrasonography is used as an adjunct for diagnosis of placental abruption, it is not sufficiently sensitive to exclude this diagnosis.[43] Continuous cardiotocographic monitoring, which has been demonstrated to accurately detect significant placental abruption, should be utilized as early as possible for all pregnant patients with significant blunt trauma.[44] (Please see Chapter 12 for further reading.)

PEDIATRIC TRAUMA

The precise role of the FAST examination in evaluating pediatric trauma patients has not been as well defined as in adults. The utilization of bedside ultrasonography in a pediatric trauma center setting was pioneered in Montreal, Quebec in the late 1970s. Their accuracy for detecting splenic and hepatic injuries approached 90% with experience. Bedside ultrasonography has become their initial diagnostic procedure of choice unless multiple organs are involved (particularly head trauma), in which case, CT scanning is initially utilized.[45] Later reports from the medical center (1993) confirmed the continued utilization of the FAST examination. In children, the bedside FAST examination holds several advantages. It obviates the need for sedation prior to CT scan. The thin abdominal wall of children enhances the resolution of the ultrasound image. Also, CT scanning can be more difficult to interpret in children due to the relative lack of intraperitoneal fat stripes.[46]

Subsequent studies, primarily performed by radiologists, have not been as optimistic with their results for pediatric trauma. Two studies demonstrated that 31 to 37% of children with solid organ injuries do not have associated hemoperitoneum.[47,48] This finding potentially would limit the utility of the FAST examination in this setting since the underlying premise of the technique is to detect free fluid. Other studies have shown the sensitivity of the FAST examination in children to range from 30 to 80% and the specificity to range from 95 to 100%.[49–51] For these initial studies in children, the FAST examination's sensitivity appears to fall short of the results found in adult trauma patients and this may be due to the unique pathophysiology of pediatric trauma patients. As further clinical studies are performed, investigators should consider the opinion of Luks and colleagues: "The use of ultrasound in the primary evaluation of blunt abdominal trauma does not require it to surpass other modalities in diagnostic accuracy, as long as it identifies all potentially life-threatening conditions."

Although ultrasound alone was not always diagnostic, there were no false positive or false negative results when used in conjunction with a clinical protocol.[46] Since the vast majority of solid organ injuries are managed nonoperatively in the pediatric population, the important applicability of serial examinations with ultrasonography may be further demonstrated in the future.

SUBACUTE TRAUMA

Patients occasionally present one or more days after the traumatic event with complaints of chest or abdominal pain. The issues of evolving hemothorax, hemoperitoneum, or subcapsular organ hemorrhage should be considered. When solid organ injuries are strongly considered, CT scanning is the preferred diagnostic method. When the index of suspicion is lower, bedside ultrasonography can be utilized to confirm the absence of unexpected abnormalities. A common scenario is a patient with suspected left-sided rib injuries who has left upper quadrant abdominal tenderness on examination. With subacute trauma, a splenic injury is likely to have evolved to the point where it could be detected by ultrasonography. The confirmation of a normal perisplenic ultrasound examination (without hemoperitoneum or subcapsular hemorrhage) would validate the clinician's suspicion of an isolated ribcage injury. In this case, an unexpected abnormal ultrasound examination would significantly alter the patient's treatment and disposition.

► ANATOMIC CONSIDERATIONS

The shape of the peritoneal cavity provides three dependent areas when a patient is in the supine position. These areas are divided by the spine longitudinally and the pelvic brim transversely. The site of accumulation of intraperitoneal fluid is dependent on the position of the patient and the source of bleeding.[13] Free intraperitoneal fluid has the propensity to collect in dependent intraperitoneal compartments formed by peritoneal reflections and mesenteric attachments (Figure 4–4A–E).

The main compartment of the peritoneal cavity is the greater sac, which is divided into the supramesocolic and inframesocolic compartments. These two compartments are connected by the paracolic gutters. The right paracolic gutter connects Morison's pouch with the pelvis. Morison's pouch is the potential space between the liver and the right kidney. The left paracolic gutter is shallower than the right and its course to the splenorenal recess is blocked by the phrenicocolic ligament. Thus, free fluid will tend to flow via the right paracolic gutter since there is less resistance. In the supine patient, the most dependent area of the supramesocolic compartment is Morison's pouch. Overall, however, the rectovesical pouch is the most dependent area of the supine male and the pouch of Douglas is the most dependent area of the supine female.[52]

In the supine patient, free intraperitoneal fluid in the right upper quadrant will tend to accumulate in Morison's pouch first before overflowing down the right paracolic gutter to the pelvis. In contrast, free intraperitoneal fluid in the left upper quadrant will tend to accumulate in the left subphrenic space first, and not the splenorenal recess, which is the potential space between the spleen and left kidney. Free fluid overflowing from the left subphrenic space will travel into the splenorenal recess and then down the left paracolic gutter into the pelvis. Free fluid from the lesser peritoneal sac will travel across the epiploic foramen to Morison's pouch. Free intraperitoneal fluid in the pelvis will tend to accumulate in the rectovesical pouch in the supine male and the pouch of Douglas in the supine female (Figure 4–5).[52]

Positioning of the patient during the FAST examination may allow redistribution of free fluid in some cases but it may require patient angles of 30° to 45° (decubitus or Trendelenburg) for fluid to flow completely over the spine or pelvic brim. In addition, intraperitoneal hemorrhage often results in a combination of liquid and clotted blood. The organized hemorrhage may not redistribute to another compartment with patient repositioning.

If an initial abbreviated FAST examination is required, the data from one study suggest that for supine patients, an isolated pelvic view may provide a slightly greater yield (68% sensitivity) than does an isolated view of Morison's pouch (59% sensitivity) in the identification of free intraperitoneal fluid.[13]

The quantity of free intraperitoneal fluid that can accurately be detected on ultrasound has been reported to be as little as 100 mL.[8] Tiling considered a small anechoic stripe in Morison's pouch to represent about 250 mL of fluid and a 0.5 cm anechoic stripe to correspond to more than 500 mL of fluid within the peritoneum.[1]

► TECHNIQUE AND NORMAL ULTRASOUND FINDINGS

The FAST examination consists of multiple ultrasound views of the abdomen and lower thorax. The standard examination is performed with the patient in the supine position. Figure 4–6 demonstrates the six areas of the FAST examination protocol. A sweeping motion of a standard 3.5 MHz probe should be used for each view to maximize the information obtained. The scan planes are longitudinal (sagittal), transverse, and coronal.

The sensitivity of the FAST examination can be influenced by a number of factors, which include the

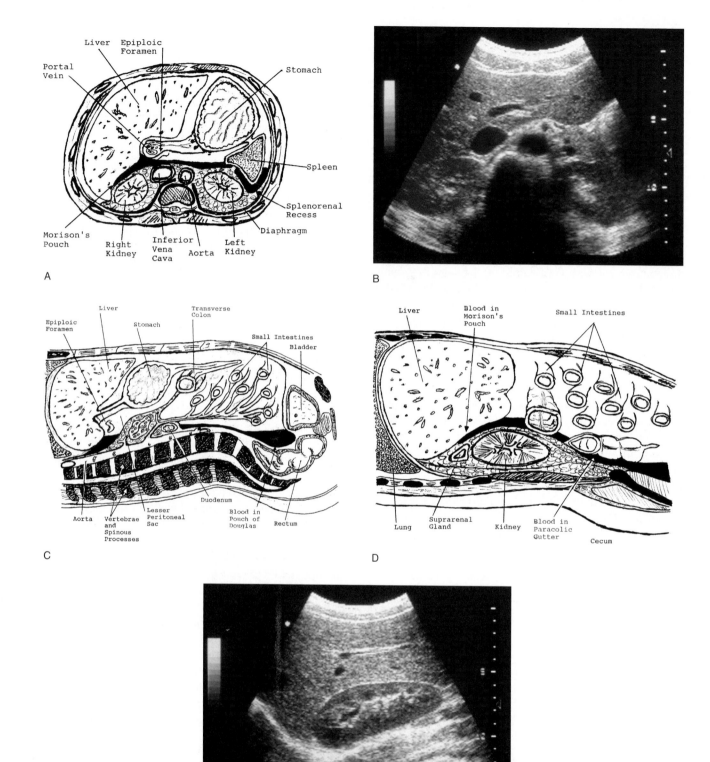

Figure 4–4. Transverse illustration of the upper abdomen, which demonstrates the dependent compartments where free intraperitoneal fluid may collect (A). A transverse ultrasound view of the normal upper abdomen is depicted for comparison (B). Longitudinal illustration of the midline (C) and right paramedian abdomen (D) that demonstrate the dependent compartments where free intraperitoneal fluid may collect. A longitudinal ultrasound view of the normal right upper abdomen is depicted for comparison (E). *(Courtesy of Lori Sens and Lori Green, Gulfcoast Ultrasound; B, E; Mark Hoffmann, MD, A,C,D.)*

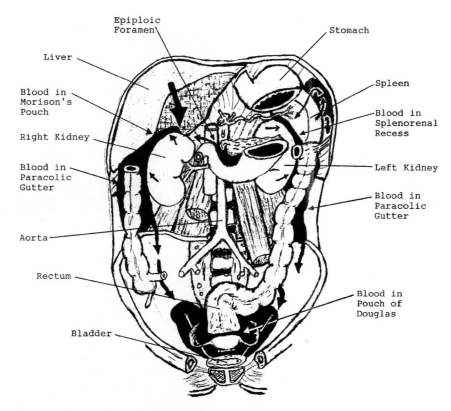

Figure 4–5. Movement patterns of free intraperitoneal fluid within the abdominal cavity. *(Courtesy of Mark Hoffmann, MD.)*

experience of the sonographer, type of equipment, timing of the FAST examination during the resuscitation, performance of serial examinations, the number of anatomic areas examined, and the position of the patient.

First, the subxiphoid four-chamber view of the heart (Figure 4–6, area 1) should be used to examine for free pericardial fluid. For this pericardial view, the ultrasound probe is placed in the subxiphoid area and angled toward the patient's left shoulder. A coronal section of the heart should provide an adequate four-chamber view of the heart. From this view, global cardiac function and chamber size can be inspected briefly. The normal pericardium is seen as a hyperechoic (white) line surrounding the heart and, by using an anterior to posterior sweeping motion, the pericardium can be fully evaluated. (Figure 4–7).

Next, the right intercostal oblique and right coronal views (see Figure 4–6, areas 2 and 3, respectively) should be used to examine for: right pleural effusion, free fluid in Morison's pouch, and free fluid in the right paracolic gutter. From these views, the right diaphragm, the right lobe of the liver, and the right kidney also should be inspected briefly. For these perihepatic views, the ultrasound probe is placed in the mid-axillary line between the eighth and 11th and ribs with an oblique scanning plane. The probe indicator should be pointing toward the right posterior axilla at the proper angle to keep the image plane between the ribs. The liver, right kidney, and Morison's pouch

should be readily identified (Figure 4–8A). The angle of the probe can be directed more cephalad to examine for pleural fluid superior to the right diaphragm. The right diaphragm appears as a hyperechoic structure (Figure 4–8B); pleural fluid can be identified as an anechoic stripe superior to the diaphragm. The right pararenal retroperitoneum and paracolic gutter are viewed by rotating the transducer to the coronal imaging plane (probe indicator towards the axilla) and positioning the probe caudally below the 11th rib in the mid- to posterior axillary line (Figure 4–9).

The left intercostal oblique and left coronal views (see Figure 4–6, areas 4 and 5, respectively) should be used to examine for: left pleural effusion, free fluid in the subphrenic space and splenorenal recess, and free fluid in the left paracolic gutter. From these views, the left diaphragm, the spleen, and the left kidney also should be inspected briefly. For these perisplenic views, the ultrasound probe is placed at the left posterior axillary line between the eighth and 11th ribs with an oblique scanning plane. The probe indicator should be pointing toward the left posterior axilla. If the left kidney is identified first, the probe should be directed slightly more cephalad to locate the spleen (Figure 4–10). The angle of the probe can then be directed more cephalad to examine for pleural fluid superior to the left diaphragm. The left diaphragm appears as a hyperechoic structure; pleural fluid can be identified as an anechoic stripe superior to the diaphragm. The

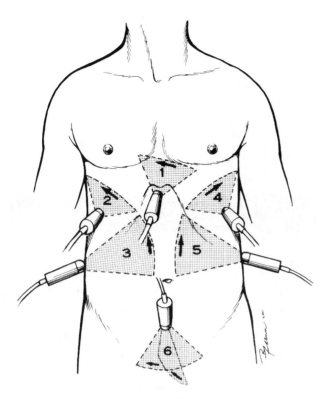

Figure 4–6. Ultrasound probe positions for the focused assessment with sonography for trauma (FAST) examination. *(Reprinted with permission from Ma OJ, Mateer JR, Ogata M, et al. Prospective analysis of a rapid trauma ultrasound examination performed by emergency physicians. J Trauma 1995;38:879-885.)*

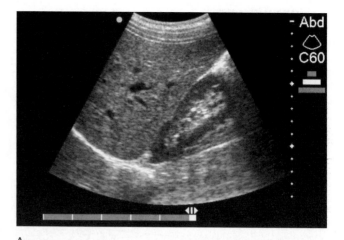

A

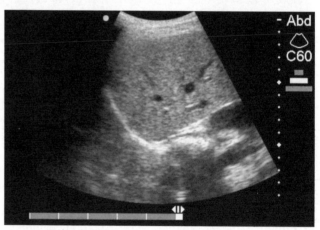

B

Figure 4–8. (A) Right intercostal oblique view. The liver, right kidney, and Morison's pouch are readily identified. (B) Right intercostal oblique view. The right diaphragm appears as a hyperechoic structure.

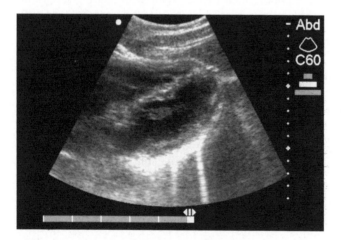

Figure 4–7. Subxiphoid four-chamber view of the heart. The normal pericardium is seen as a hyper-echoic (white) line surrounding the heart.

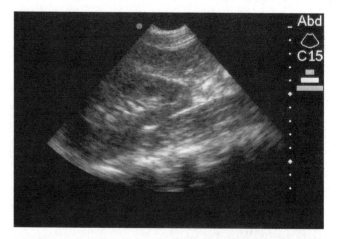

Figure 4–9. Right coronal view. The right pararenal retroperitoneum and paracolic gutter areas are identified above the psoas muscle in this view.

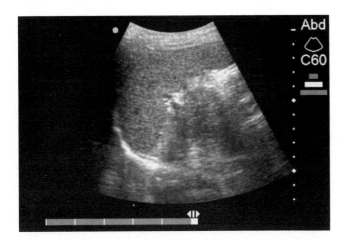

Figure 4–10. Left intercostal oblique view. A longitudinal view of the spleen, a portion of the diaphragm, and surrounding areas are visualized.

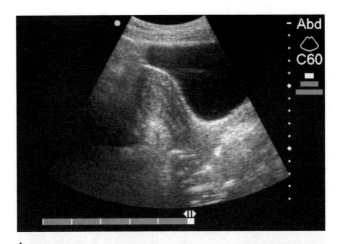

A

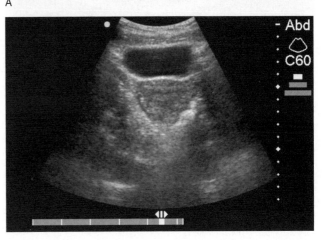

B

Figure 4–12. Pelvic views (A, longitudinal and B, transverse). Ideally, these views should be obtained prior to placement of a Foley catheter. In addition to potential fluid spaces, the bladder, the prostate or uterus, and the lateral walls of the pelvis can also be inspected briefly.

left pararenal retroperitoneum and paracolic gutter are viewed by rotating the transducer to the coronal imaging plane (probe indicator toward the axilla) and positioning the probe caudally below the 11th rib in the mid- to posterior axillary line. The left kidney is often more difficult to visualize than the right kidney because it is positioned higher in the abdomen and can be obscured by overlying gas in the stomach and colon (Figure 4–11).

Finally, the pelvic (longitudinal and transverse) views (see Figure 4–6, area 6) should be used to examine for free fluid in the anterior pelvis or cul-de-sac (pouch of Douglas). Ideally, these views should be obtained prior to placement of a Foley catheter. From these views, the bladder, the prostate or uterus, and the lateral walls of the pelvis also should be inspected briefly (Figure 4–12A,B). For these pelvic views, the ultrasound probe should be placed 2-cm superior to the symphysis pubis along the midline of the abdomen with the scanning plane oriented longitudinally and the probe aimed caudally into the pelvis. The probe indicator should be pointing toward the patient's head. The probe is then rotated 90° counter-clockwise to obtain transverse images of the pelvis. Fluid in the bladder appears as a well-circumscribed and contained fluid collection that appears anechoic. In women, the uterus will be seen posterior to the bladder.

▶ COMMON AND EMERGENT ABNORMALITIES

On ultrasound images, free fluid appears anechoic (black) or hypoechoic (if the blood is clotted) and, since it is not contained within a viscus, will have sharp edges as opposed to rounded edges.

1. *Hemopericardium.* Free pericardial fluid is identified as an anechoic stripe surrounding the heart

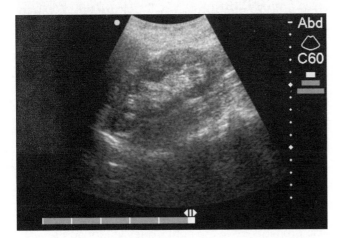

Figure 4–11. Left coronal view. The left pararenal, paracolic gutter areas, and kidney are examined in this view.

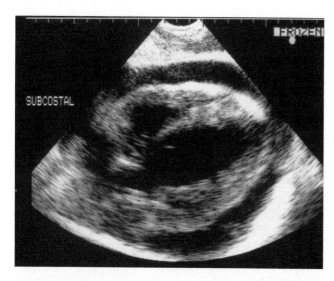

Figure 4–13. Hemopericardium. Free pericardial fluid is identified as an anechoic surrounding the heart within the parietal and visceral layers of the bright hyperechoic pericardial sac.

within the parietal and visceral layers of the bright hyperechoic pericardial sac (Figure 4–13).

2. *Free pleural fluid.* The right or left diaphragm appears as a bright hyperechoic structure; free pleural fluid can be identified as an anechoic stripe superior to the diaphragm (Figure 4–14).

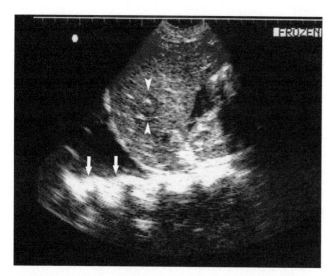

Figure 4–14. Free pleural fluid. The right diaphragm appears as a bright hyperechoic structure. Free pleural fluid can be identified as an anechoic space superior to the diaphragm. The pleural fluid allows visualization of the lateral chest wall (arrows), which cannot be visualized when the air filled lung is normally present. The patient also has a circular defect in the liver (arrowheads) from a bullet wound, and fluid in Morison's pouch.

3. *Hemoperitoneum.* Morison's pouch is a common site for blood to accumulate when any solid intra-abdominal organ has been injured (Figure 4–15A). Free fluid appears as an anechoic stripe in Morison's pouch (Figure 4–15B) or the right paracolic gutter (adjacent to the lower pole of the right kidney) (Figure 4–16A). Retroperitoneal fluid appears as a hypoechoic stripe adjacent to the psoas muscle (Figure 4–16B).

4. In the perisplenic region, free fluid appearance and location are similar to the description for the perihepatic area. Free intraperitoneal fluid appears as an anechoic stripe in the subdiaphragmatic

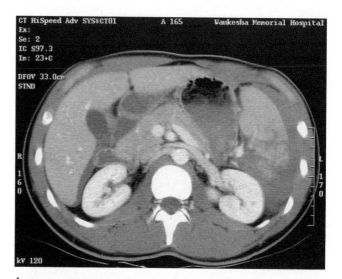

A

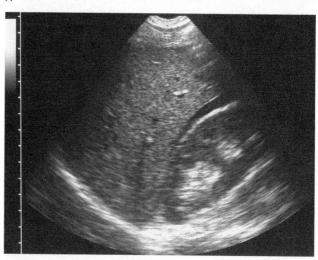

B

Figure 4–15. Hemoperitoneum. The abdominal contrast CT (A) demonstrates a fractured spleen with surrounding hematoma but a small stripe of fluid is also present above the right kidney in Morison's pouch. A right intercostal oblique ultrasound view from the same patient reveals a thin stripe of fluid in Morison's pouch (B).

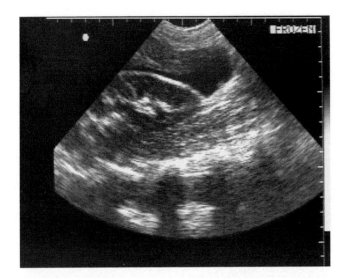

A

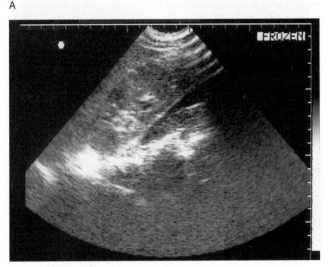

B

Figure 4–16. (A) A right coronal view demonstrates fluid in the paracolic gutter (adjacent to the lower pole of the right kidney). (B) Retroperitoneal fluid. A coronal view of the right kidney reveals fluid accumulation overlying the psoas muscle stripe and medial to the kidney.

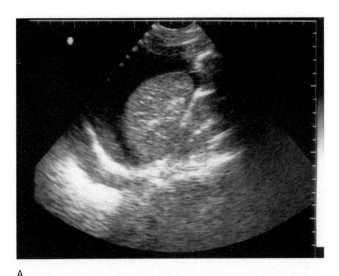

A

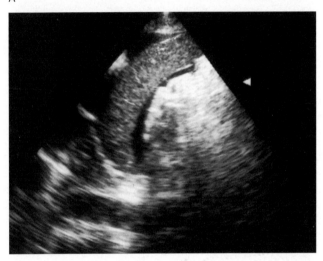

B

Figure 4–17. (A) Left intercostal oblique view reveals the spleen surrounded by hypoechoic fluid in the sub-diaphragmatic space. A small amount of clotted blood is also noted adjacent to the bright curvilinear diaphragm. (B) A coronal view of the spleen shows free intraperitoneal fluid as an anechoic stripe in the splenorenal recess. The tubular fluid filled object at the bottom of the image is the aorta. *(Courtesy of Lori Sens, Gulfcoast Ultrasound, B.)*

space (Figure 4–17A), splenorenal recess (Figure 4–17B), or the left paracolic gutter. Since the splenorenal recess is not the most common site for free intraperitoneal fluid to accumulate in the left upper quadrant, it is essential to visualize the left diaphragm and left subphrenic space.

5. Since the pelvis is the most dependent area of the peritoneal cavity, free intraperitoneal fluid often accumulates in this area (Figure 4–18A, B). Liquid blood or ascites floats above the bowels and will be located adjacent to the bladder and anterior peritoneum (Figure 4–18C). Blood clots in the pelvis are located in the cul-de-sac and may distort the contour of the bladder (Figure 4–19A,B).

▶ COMMON VARIANTS AND SELECTED ABNORMALITIES

When performing the FAST examination, it is essential to recognize common normal variants that can mimic positive findings. When examining the perihepatic views, fluid in the gallbladder, duodenum, hepatic flexure of the colon, or inferior vena cava (IVC) may be erroneously identified as free intraperitoneal fluid (Figure 4–20A). When examining the perisplenic views, fluid in the stomach or splenic flexure of the colon or blood within the

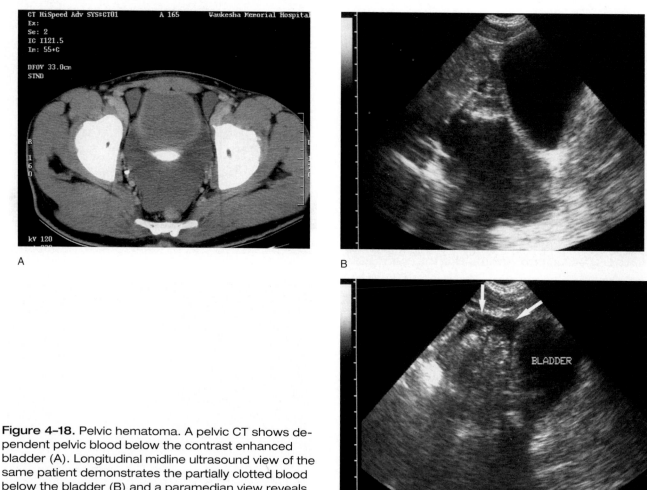

Figure 4–18. Pelvic hematoma. A pelvic CT shows dependent pelvic blood below the contrast enhanced bladder (A). Longitudinal midline ultrasound view of the same patient demonstrates the partially clotted blood below the bladder (B) and a paramedian view reveals liquid density blood floating above the bowels and located adjacent to the bladder and anterior peritoneum (arrows) (C).

vena cava or portal veins may be erroneously identified as free intraperitoneal fluid (Figure 4–20B). When examining the pelvic views, fluid within a collapsed bladder or an ovarian cyst may be incorrectly identified as free intraperitoneal fluid. In the male patient, the seminal vesicles may be incorrectly identified as free intraperitoneal fluid. Also, premenopausal women occasionally may have a small baseline amount of free fluid in the pouch of Douglas.[53]

Occasionally, when performing the FAST examination, the clinician may directly detect injury in a solid organ, which is usually the spleen or liver. While this is not the specific goal of the FAST examination, it is helpful to understand some of the sonographic features of solid organ injury. When the patient is stable and serial follow-up examinations (control examinations) are being performed, the clinician has more time to evaluate for possible obvious solid organ injuries. Acute solid organ lacerations may appear as fragmented areas of increased or decreased echogenicity. Contained intraparenchymal or subcapsular hemorrhages can appear initially as isoechoic or slightly hyperechoic, which can make them difficult to reliably detect (Figure 4–21A–C). The examiner must pay close attention to contour and organ tissue irregularities to observe these injuries (Figure 4–22A,B). CT is more sensitive for acute organ injuries and should be ordered when these are suspected (see Figure 4–15A). Over time, contained hemorrhage will become hypoechoic, with the area lacking sharp margins. A subcapsular hemorrhage may appear as a crescent-shaped hypoechoic stripe surrounding the organ (Figure 4–23).

Intraperitoneal fat is usually hyperechoic but, in some cases, is relatively hypoechoic. When the fat is present in the perinephric areas, it can be mistaken for intraperitoneal fluid or hematoma. Intraperitoneal fat (as opposed to hematoma) will be a consistent density throughout and will not move with respirations. Intra-

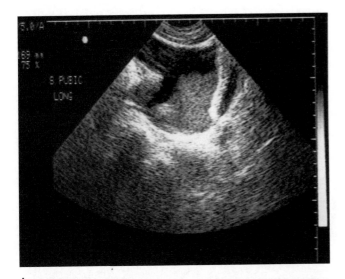

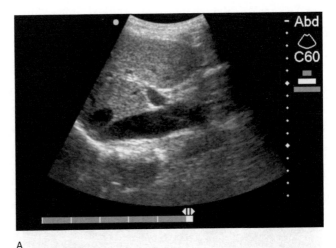

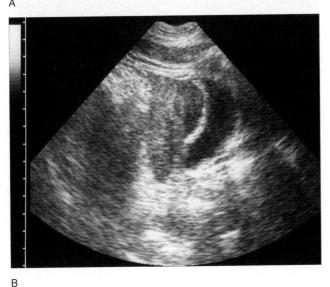

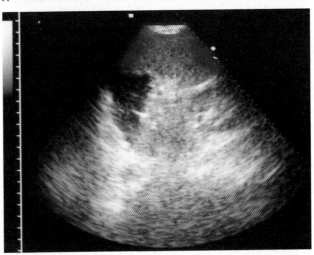

Figure 4–19. Longitudinal pelvic views demonstrate a collapsed bladder and dependent clotted blood in the cul-de-sac with liquid blood above (A). Blood clots in the pelvis may distort the contour of the bladder. The uterus-like object, in the center of the image in this male patient, is actually hematoma (B).

Figure 4–20. Fluid pitfalls. Oblique view of the liver shows fluid below, which is contained within the IVC (A). When examining the perisplenic views, fluid in the stomach (or other bowels) may be erroneously identified as free intraperitoneal fluid (B).

peritoneal hematoma contains gray-level echoes but will be accompanied by hypoechoic fluid areas as well.

A pericardial fat pad can be hypoechoic or contain gray-level echoes. The pericardial fat pad is almost always located anterior to the right ventricle and is not present posterior to the left ventricle (Figure 4–24). Pericardial fluid or hemorrhage will be located in both the anterior and posterior pericardial spaces. A small amount of fluid (less than 5 mm) may be present within the dependent pericardium, but is usually considered to be physiologic when it is visualized during systole only.

▶ PITFALLS

1. *Contraindication.* The only absolute contraindication to performing the FAST examination is when immediate operative management is clearly indicated, in which case the FAST examination could delay patient transport to the operating room.
2. *Over-reliance on the FAST examination.* A clinical pitfall is the over-reliance of an initial negative FAST examination in caring for the trauma patient. There is still no substitute for sound clinical judgment. Each FAST examination is a single data point in the overall clinical picture of the trauma patient. When mandated by the mechanism of injury or an evolving physical examination,

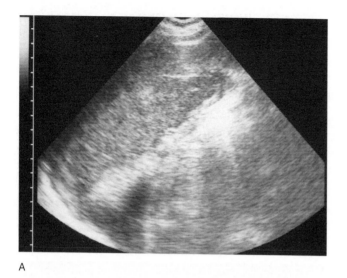

A

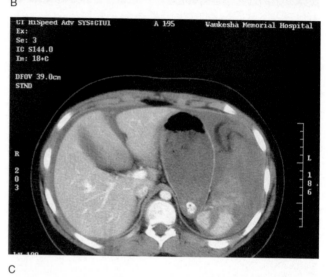

B

C

Figure 4–21. Intercostal oblique views of the spleen. The initial view (A) showed only a questionable area of isoechoic tissue between the spleen tip and the ultrasound probe. The spleen does not have obvious injuries. A slightly different view of the spleen (B) reveals a 1.5- 2-cm echogenic stripe (arrowheads) around the spleen (contained hematoma) and an irregular echo pattern from the splenic tissue (the hemispleen closest to the diaphragm is hyperechoic). (C) CT of the same patient shows a large intraparenchymal and perisplenic hematoma with contrast enhanced spleen fragments posteriorly.

serial FAST examinations or an abdominal CT scan should be performed on the patient. Serial FAST examinations are a common practice in Germany and are gaining acceptance in the United States.[54] They are used to determine if new intraperitoneal fluid has developed or if existing intraperitoneal fluid is expanding.

3. *Limitations of the FAST examination.* Limitations include difficulty in imaging patients who are morbidly obese or have massive subcutaneous emphysema. Also, in a patient at risk for ascites, it may be difficult to determine whether the free intraperitoneal fluid is ascites or blood. To help distinguish between the two, general ultrasound findings that point to ascites secondary to chronic liver disease include: nodular cirrhosis of the liver (Figure 4–25A), generalized thickening of the gallbladder wall (Figure 4–25B), enlargement of the

caudate lobe, enlargement of the spleen (Figure 4–25C), or engorgement of the portal venous system. The clinician could also clarify the issue by performing an ultrasound-directed needle paracentesis of the fluid to distinguish ascites from hemoperitoneum. Another limitation is that ultrasound is not as reliable as CT scanning in distinguishing and grading precise solid organ injury.

4. *Limitations associated with pregnancy.* There are limitations of the FAST examination in pregnant trauma patients that should be noted. Evaluating the pouch of Douglas for hemoperitoneum in the presence of a gravid uterus requires careful consideration. The distortion of usual landmarks and the difficulty with differentiating between intrauterine versus extrauterine fluid can make this a challenging examination for the inexperienced sonologist. Also, the dependent portions of the peri-

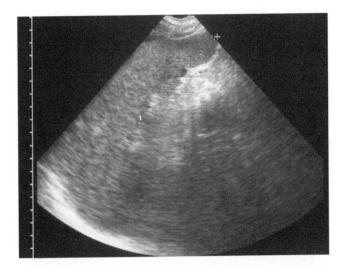

A

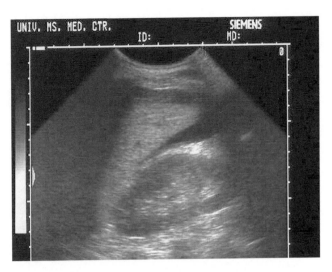

Figure 4–23. Subcapsular hemorrhage. This intercostal oblique view of the liver appears to have free fluid in Morison's pouch and a hypoechoic stripe between the probe and liver tissue. There was no other evidence for free fluid on ultrasound. The patient's CT revealed a contained subcapsular hematoma of the liver and no free fluid *(Courtesy of Verena Valley, MD)*.

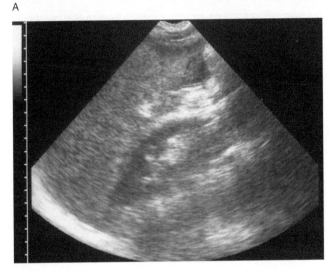

B

Figure 4–22. Initial oblique view of the spleen (A) showed enlargement (long axis is 17 cm) and a contour irregularity (narrow inferior tip). A slightly different view of the same patient revealed clots and liquid blood near the spleen tip (B). Compare these ultrasound findings with the CT findings from the same patient in Figure 15A. The splenic fractures were not readily apparent on the ultrasound views.

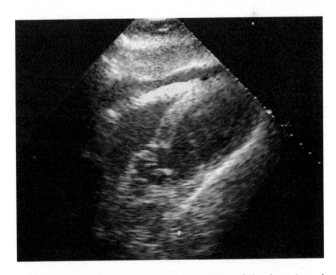

Figure 4–24. Subcostal long axis view of the heart and pericardium. A pericardial fat pad can be hypoechoic or contain grey level echoes. The pericardial fat pad is almost always located anterior to the right ventricle and is not present posterior to the left ventricle.

toneal cavity may become further distorted with advanced third trimester pregnancy, making the diagnosis of free intraperitoneal fluid versus intrauterine fluid more difficult.[42] Also, as previously discussed, the FAST examination alone cannot exclude uterine rupture or placental abruption.

5. *Technical difficulties with the FAST examination.* Most clinicians have little difficulty locating Morison's pouch but have greater difficulty locating the splenorenal recess and left pleural space. One common technical error is not placing the ultrasound probe posterior or superior enough.

The probe often must be placed in the posterior axillary line at the eighth to ninth intercostal space to visualize these structures. With some patients, visualizing the pericardium can be difficult. Placing the probe as close to the xiphoid as possible and depressing the probe toward the spine can facilitate the subcostal cardiac view. Even so, the patient may have to take a deep breath or the

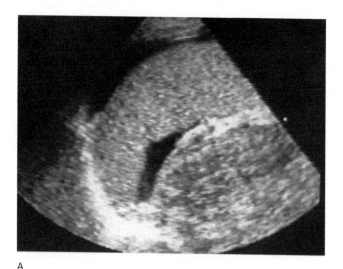

A

B

Figure 4–25. (A) Cirrhosis of the liver. This oblique view of the right lobe demonstrates the findings of contracted size, increased echogenicity, and irregular texture of the liver. There is surrounding echo-free ascites. *(Courtesy of Simon Roy MD.)* (B) An oblique right upper quadrant view of the abdomen shows a contracted liver, massive ascites, and generalized thickening of the gallbladder wall. This gallbladder finding is common with chronic liver disease and ascites. (C) Long axis view of the spleen measures more than 17 cm. *(Courtesy of Lori Sens, Gulfcoast Ultrasound.)*

C

depth of the image adjusted to visualize the entire pericardium. If subcostal views are ineffective, then parasternal views should be attempted. Breathing or ventilation can interfere with the examination (from lung or rib artifact) or enhance the examination when it brings organs closer to the ultrasound probe (diaphragm, heart, liver, spleen, or kidneys). Fluid in a partially emptied bladder can be mistaken for free intraperitoneal fluid. This scenario can be clarified with complete catheter emptying of the bladder or by retrograde bladder filling and repeat examination.

6. *Injuries undetected by ultrasound.* Certain injuries may not be detected initially by the FAST examination. These include perforation of a viscus, bowel wall contusion, pancreatic trauma, or renal pedicle injury. Newer ultrasound imaging techniques, such as power color Doppler, may be used to evaluate renal tissue perfusion in patients with suspected renal pedicle injury. The entire

diaphragm also cannot be visualized using ultrasonography.

▶ CASE STUDIES

Case 1

Patient Presentation

A 48-year-old man presented to the emergency department after he slid into a telephone pole when his motorcycle skidded on a patch of ice. He was wearing a helmet but lost consciousness at the scene of the crash. The patient complained of abdominal pain but denied any chest pain, shortness of breath, headache, or nausea and vomiting. He admitted to drinking "at least a dozen" beers earlier in the evening.

On physical examination, his blood pressure was 88/48 mm Hg; pulse, 122 beats per minute; respirations, 18 per minute; and temperature, 37°C. He was arousable but drowsy and slurring his words. He had a strong odor of alcohol on his breath. His head, neck, pulmonary, and cardiovascular examinations were unremarkable. The abdominal examination was soft, diffusely tender, and without peritoneal signs. His extremities revealed diffuse deep abrasions but without bony injury. His neurologic examination was unremarkable except for his depressed mental status.

Management Course

After being infused 2 L of intravenous crystalloid fluid, the patient's blood pressure was 92/60 mm Hg and his pulse was 116 beats per minute. A supine chest radiograph was normal. Urinalysis revealed gross hematuria. His serum ethanol level was 342 mg/dL. A FAST examination of the abdomen performed by the emergency physician revealed a large quantity of free intraperitoneal fluid in Morison's pouch (Figure 4–26), the right paracolic gutter, and in the pelvic cul-de-sac. The decision to perform an abdominal CT scan or diagnostic peritoneal lavage was deferred by the attending trauma surgeon. Instead, a head CT scan was performed in 10 min, which was negative for intracranial pathology. The patient was then taken directly to the operating room for an exploratory laparotomy, which revealed large liver and right kidney lacerations and 1.5 L of hemoperitoneum.

Commentary

Case 1 was an example of a patient presenting to the emergency department hypotensive after sustaining blunt abdominal trauma. His profound alcohol intoxication and possible closed head injury complicated his examination and evaluation. Since the patient was too hemodynamically unstable to leave the trauma room, the FAST examination was an ideal diagnostic study to evaluate the patient. The FAST examination revealed gross free intraperitoneal fluid. The information provided by the FAST examination in this case negated the need for an abdominal CT scan or diagnostic peritoneal lavage. Instead, time was saved by the expeditious use of a head CT scan to evaluate for intracranial pathology followed by the direct transport of the patient to the operating suite.

Case 2

Patient Presentation

An 18-year-old woman presented to the emergency department after sustaining a gunshot wound to her right flank. She complained only of abdominal pain. She denied any other complaints and reported no other injuries. The patient believed that she was about 4 months pregnant and had not received any prenatal care. She denied any significant past medical history.

On physical examination, her blood pressure was 128/78 mm Hg; pulse, 94 beats per minute; respirations, 18 per minute; and temperature, 37°C. She was comfortable and appeared in no acute distress. Her pulmonary and cardiovascular examinations were normal. The abdominal examination was soft, nontender, and without peritoneal signs. A gravid uterus, 3-cm below the umbilicus, was noted. The rectal examination revealed normal sphincter tone and guaiac negative brown stool. A small entrance wound was noted in the right flank region, approximately 40-cm below the right scapula, and the exit wound was found on the right lateral abdominal wall, at the level of the umbilicus.

Management Course

The patient remained hemodynamically stable in the emergency department. An upright chest radiograph was normal. Her urinalysis showed no red blood cells. As arrangements were being made by the trauma surgeon to take the patient to the operating room for an exploratory laparotomy, a FAST examination of the abdomen performed by the emergency physician revealed: no evidence of hemoperitoneum, fetal heart tones present at 140 beats per minute, the fetus moving actively within the uterus, and a fetal gestational age of 15.5 weeks by biparietal diameter (Figure 4–27). The obstetrics consultant agreed with the emergency physician's clinical and ultrasonographic findings. Because of the patient's unremarkable abdominal examination and the normal FAST examination, the trauma surgeon opted to defer exploratory laparotomy in favor of admission and observation of the patient. After admission, a CT scan of the patient's abdomen confirmed the absence of intraabdominal pathology. The patient was observed for 2 days and serial

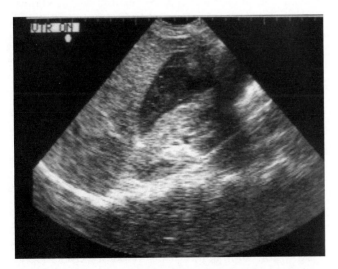

Figure 4–26. A large quantity of free intraperitoneal fluid is present in Morison's pouch. The fluid is mildly echogenic due to clotting of the blood.

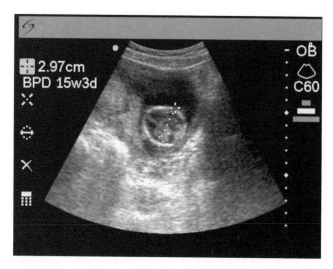

Figure 4–27. Suprapubic longitudinal view of the uterus and a transverse view of the fetal head demonstrate a gestational age of 15.5 weeks by biparietal diameter.

abdominal examinations remained unremarkable. She was discharged with the diagnosis of an extraperitoneal gunshot wound to the abdomen. The patient went on to deliver a healthy, 2655-g baby girl.

Commentary

Case 2 was an example of penetrating trauma to the abdomen in a pregnant patient. Based on the mechanism of injury, the trauma surgeon initially believed that the patient needed exploratory laparotomy to investigate for possible intraperitoneal or retroperitoneal injury. The FAST examination demonstrated no evidence of intra-abdominal fluid and an active, viable fetus. Based on this information, the surgeon opted to obtain further imaging studies and observe the patient instead of performing exploratory laparotomy. The information provided by the FAST examination in this case negated the need for a non-therapeutic laparotomy and any associated morbidity to the mother or fetus.

Case 3

Patient Presentation

A 19-year-old man presented to the emergency department after sustaining a single stab wound to his lower chest, just below the sternum. The weapon, according to the patient, was an 8-in. kitchen knife. He was complaining of diffuse abdominal pain but denied any shortness of breath, chest pain, or neurologic changes.

According to the paramedics, the patient had complained of abdominal pain at the scene and had one episode of emesis of clear fluid that was "mixed with blood." He had an out-of-hospital blood pressure of 90/60 mm Hg and had received 1 L of lactated Ringer's prior to his arrival in the emergency department.

On physical examination, his blood pressure was 82/58 mm Hg; pulse, 132 beats per minute; respirations, 32 per minute; temperature 37.2°C. He was a well-developed, thin man who was extremely anxious. The patient's head and neck examination were unremarkable. No jugular venous distention was noted. On his chest wall, there was a single stab wound immediately below the xiphoid process. No active bleeding from the wound site was noted and no subcutaneous crepitus was palpated. His lungs were clear, and there were equal breath sounds bilaterally. On cardiovascular examination, the patient was tachycardic with a regular rhythm and a normal S_1 and S_2. There were no murmurs, gallops, or rubs appreciated. His abdomen was soft but had moderate tenderness to palpation in the midepigastric region. No guarding or rebound tenderness was appreciated. On rectal examination, he had normal sphincter tone and guaiac negative brown stool. His extremity and neurologic examinations were normal.

Management Course

The patient's cardiac monitor revealed sinus tachycardia at 128 beats per minute. His upright anteroposterior chest radiograph was normal. Nasogastric tube lavage was negative for bright red blood or coffee-ground contents. Urinalysis was negative for red blood cells. After resuscitation with 2 L of lactated Ringer's, the patient's blood pressure was 102/64 mm Hg and pulse 110.

As preparations were being made to explore the wound in the trauma room, the patient acutely became lethargic and his blood pressure dropped to 64/40 mm Hg. Jugular venous distention was noted in the neck. A FAST examination revealed no evidence of hemoperitoneum but did demonstrate a significant pericardial effusion inhibiting cardiac wall activity (Figure 4–28). Pericardiocentesis aspirated 35 cc of blood from within the pericardium. The patient's mental status improved and his blood pressure increased to 96/54. The patient was emergently transported to the operating room for a thoracotomy that revealed an epicardial vessel had been lacerated.

Commentary

Case 3 was an example of a patient who sustained a stab wound to the midepigastric area. Upon initial presentation, it was unclear if the patient had sustained a thoracic or abdominal injury or both. Since it can evaluate both the thorax and abdomen, the FAST examination was an ideal diagnostic study to evaluate the patient. The FAST examination excluded the presence of hemoperitoneum but demonstrated free pericardial fluid that was inhibiting cardiac wall activity and, subsequently, the patient's hemodynamic status. The information provided by the FAST examination in this case supported the decision to perform an emergent pericardiocentesis as a temporizing measure and to transport the patient to the operating room for a definitive procedure.

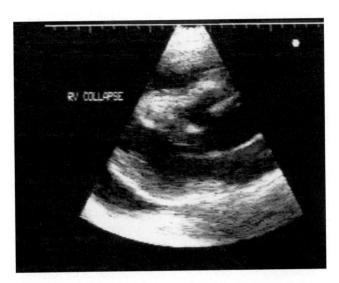

Figure 4-28. Pericardial tamponade. A parasternal long axis view of the heart reveals a pericardial effusion located in both the anterior and posterior portion of the pericardial cavity. The right ventricle is partially collapsed indicating tamponade.

REFERENCES

1. Tiling T, Bouillon B, Schmid A, et al. Ultrasound in blunt abdomino-thoracic trauma. In: Border JR, Allgoewer M, Hansen ST, et al, eds: Blunt multiple trauma: comprehensive pathophysiology and care. New York: Marcel Dekker, 1990:415–433.

2. Halbfass HJ, Wimmer B, Hauenstein K, et al. Ultrasonic diagnosis of blunt abdominal injuries. Fortschr Med 1981;99:1681.

3. Aufschnaiter M, Kofler H. Sonographic acute diagnosis in polytrauma. Aktuel Traumatol 1983;13:55.

4. Hoffman R, Pohlemann T, Wippermann B, et al. Management of blunt abdominal trauma using sonography. Unfallchirurg 1989;92:471.

5. Seifert M, Petereit U, Ortmann G. Sonographs of the diagnostic multi-system trauma patients. Zentrlbl Chir 1989;114:1012.

6. Kohlberger VEJ, Strittmatter B, Waninger J. Ultrasound diagnostic technique after abdominal trauma. Fortschr Med 1989;107:244.

7. Wening JV. Evaluation of ultrasound, lavage and computed tomography in blunt abdominal trauma. Surg Endosc 1989;3:152.

8. Kimura A, Otsuka T. Emergency center ultrasonography in the evaluation of hemoperitoneum: a prospective study. J Trauma 1991;31:20–23.

9. Rothlin MA, Naf R, Amgwerd M, et al. Ultrasound in blunt abdominal and thoracic trauma. J Trauma 1993;34:488–495.

10. Rozycki GS, Ochsner MG, Jaffin JH, et al. Prospective evaluation of surgeons' use of ultrasound in the evaluation of the trauma patient. J Trauma 1993;34:516–527.

11. Rozycki GS, Ochsner MG, Schmidt JA, et al. A prospective study of surgeon-performed ultrasound as the primary adjunct modality for injured patient assessment. J Trauma 1995;39:492–500.

12. Ma OJ, Mateer JR, Ogata M, Kefer MP, et al. Prospective analysis of a rapid trauma ultrasound examination performed by emergency physicians. J Trauma 1995;38:879–885.

13. Ma OJ, Kefer MP, Mateer JR, et al. Evaluation of hemoperitoneum using a single vs. multiple-view ultrasonographic examination. Acad Emerg Med 1995;2:581–586.

14. Hoffman R, Nerlich M, Muggia-Sullam M, et al. Blunt abdominal trauma in cases of multiple trauma evaluated by ultrasonography: a prospective analysis of 291 patients. J Trauma 1992;32:452–458.

15. Tso P, Rodriquez A, Cooper C, et al. Sonography in blunt abdominal trauma: a preliminary progress report. J Trauma 1992;33:39–44.

16. Lentz KA, McKenney MG, Nunez DB, et al. Evaluating blunt abdominal trauma: role for ultrasonography. J Ultrasound Med 1996;15:447–451.

17. McElveen TS, Collin GR. The role of ultrasonography in blunt abdominal trauma: a prospective study. Am Surg 1997;63:18188.

18. Rozycki GS, Ochsner MG, Feliciano DV, et al. Early detection of hemoperitoneum by ultrasound examination of the right upper quadrant: a multicenter study. J Trauma 1998;45:878–883.

19. Bode PJ, Edwards MJ, Kruit MC, et al. Sonography in a clinical algorithm for early evaluation of 1671 patients with blunt abdominal trauma. AJR Am J Roentgenol 1999;172:905–911.

20. Thomas B, Falcone RE, Vasquez D, et al. Ultrasound evaluation of blunt abdominal trauma: program implementation, initial experience, and learning curve. J Trauma 1997;42:38–388.

21. Jehle D, Guarina J, Karamanoukian H. Emergency department ultrasound in the evaluation of blunt abdominal trauma. Am J Emerg Med 1993;11:342–346.

22. Hilty WE, Wolfe RE, Moore EE, et al. Sensitivity and specificity of ultrasound in the detection of intraperitoneal fluid. Ann Emerg Med 1993;22:921.

23. Branney SW, Wolfe RE, Moore EE, et al. Quantitative sensitivity of ultrasound in detecting free intraperitoneal fluid. J Trauma 1995;39:375–380.

24. Branney SW, Moore EE, Cantrill S, et al. Ultrasound-based key clinical pathway reduces the use of hospital resources for the evaluation of blunt abdominal trauma. J Trauma 1997;42:1086–1090.

25. Arrillaga A, Graham R, York JW, et al. Increased efficiency and cost-effectiveness in the evaluation of the blunt abdominal trauma patient with the use of ultrasound. Am Surg 1999;65:31–35.

26. Huang MS, Liu M, Wu JK, et al. Ultrasonography for the evaluation of hemoperitoneum during resuscitation: a simple scoring system. J Trauma 1994;36:173–177.

27. Porter RS, Nester BA, Dalsey WC, et al. Use of ultrasound to determine the need for laparotomy in trauma patients. Ann Emerg Med 1997;29:323–330.

28. Carrel R, Shaffer M, Franaszek J. Emergency diagnosis, resuscitation and treatment of acute penetrating cardiac trauma. Ann Emerg Med 1982;11:50–517.

29. Plummer D, Brunette D, Asinger R, et al. Emergency department echocardiography improves outcome in penetrating cardiac injury. Ann Emerg Med 1992;21:709–712.

30. Rozycki GS, Feliciano DV, Ochsner MG, et al. The role of ultrasound in patients with possible penetrating cardiac wounds: a prospective multicenter study. J Trauma 1999;46:543–551.

31. Ma OJ, Mateer JR. Trauma ultrasound examination versus chest radiography in the detection of hemothorax. Ann Emerg Med 1997;29:312–316.

32. Rubens MB. The pleura: collapse and consolidation. In Sutton D, ed. A textbook of radiology imaging. 4th ed. Edinburgh: Churchill Livingstone, 1987:393.

33. Juhl JH. Diseases of the pleura, mediastinum, and diaphragm. In Juhl JH, Crummy AB, eds. Essentials of radiologic imaging. 6th ed. Philadelphia: JB Lippincott, 1993:1026.

34. Varner MW. Maternal mortality in Iowa from 1952 to 1986. Surg Gynecol Obstet 1989;168:555–562.

35. Lane PL. Traumatic fetal deaths. J Emerg Med 1989;7:433–435.

36. Agran PF, Dunkle DE, Winn DG, et al. Fetal death in motor vehicle accidents. Ann Emerg Med 1987;16:1355–1358.

37. Pepperell RJ, Rubinstein E, MacIsaac LA. Motor-car accidents during pregnancy. Med J Aust 1997;1:203–205.

38. Stafford PA, Biddinger PW, Zumwalt RE. Lethal intrauterine fetal trauma. Am J Obstet Gynecol 1988;159:459–459.

39. Crosby WM, Costiloe JP. Safety of lap-belt restraint for pregnant victims of automobile collisions. N Engl J Med 1971;284:632–636.

40. Pearlman MD, Tintinalli JE, Lorenz RP. Blunt trauma during pregnancy. N Engl J Med 1990;323:1609–1613.

41. Sherer DM, Schenker JG. Accidental injury during pregnancy. Obstet Gynecol Surg 1989;44:330–338.

42. Drost, TF, Rosemury AS, Sherman HF, et al. Major trauma in pregnant women: maternal/fetal outcome. J Trauma 1990;30:574–578.

43. Ma OJ, Mateer JR, DeBehnke DJ. Use of ultrasonography for the evaluation of pregnant trauma patients. J Trauma 1996;40:665–668.

44. Pearlman MD, Tintinalli JE, Lorenz RP. A prospective controlled study of outcome after trauma during pregnancy. Am J Obstet Gynecol 1990;162:1502–1510.

45. Filiatrault D, Longpre D, Patriquin H, et al. Investigation of childhood blunt abdominal trauma: a practical approach using ultrasound as the initial diagnostic modality. Pediatr Radiol 1987;17:373–379.

46. Luks FI, Lemire A, St-Vil D, et al. Blunt abdominal trauma in children: the practical value of ultrasonography. J Trauma 1993;34:607–610.

47. Taylor GA, Sivit CJ. Posttraumatic peritoneal fluid: is it a reliable indicator of intraabdominal injury in children? J Pediatr Surg 1995;30:1644–1648.

48. Coley BD, Mutabagani KH, Martin LC, et al. Focused abdominal sonography for trauma (FAST) in children with blunt abdominal trauma. J Trauma 2000;48:902–906.

49. Thourani VH, Pettitt BJ, Schmidt JA, et al. Validation of surgeon-performed emergency abdominal ultrasonography in pediatric trauma patients. J Pediatr Surg 1998;33:322–328.

50. Patel JC, Tepas JJ. The efficacy of focused abdominal sonography for trauma as a screening tool in the assessment of injured children. J Pediatr Surg 1999;34:4–47.

51. Mutabagani KH, Coley BD, Zumberge N, et al. Preliminary experience with focused abdominal sonography for trauma (FAST) in children: is it useful? J Pediatr Surg 1999;34:48–54.

52. Meyers MA. The spread and localization of acute intraperitoneal effusion. Radiology 1970;94:547–554.

53. McKenney KL, Nunez DB, McKenney MG, et al. Ultrasound for blunt abdominal trauma: is it free fluid? Emerg Radiol 1998;5:203–209.

54. Henderson SO, Sung J, Mandavia D. Serial abdominal ultrasound in the setting of trauma. J Emerg Med 2000;18:79–81.

CHAPTER 5

Cardiac

Vivek S. Tayal, Christopher L. Moore, and Geoffrey A. Rose

The emergent use of cardiac ultrasound provides clinicians in the emergency setting with a remarkable window into the most critical of all organs for resuscitation. By visualizing the heart, the clinician receives important information about both cardiac structure and function.[1] Abnormal physiologic states can be determined and followed by the acoustic window into the heart. The current use of bedside echocardiography in the emergent situation is the ideal 21st century representation of the "stethoscope of the future."

Echocardiography can be the most challenging and the most satisfying application of emergency ultrasound.[2] This specific organ is not only surrounded by impediments to ultrasound, but it is moving in multiple planes. Whereas grayscale transthoracic two-dimensional echocardiography is the predominant mode presently applied by emergency and acute care physicians, other modes, such as M mode and Doppler, and approaches such as transesophageal, are complementary to present examinations.

The cardiac applications of emergency ultrasound include its use in cardiac arrest, hypotension of unclear etiology, trauma to the heart and great vessels, acute chest pain, and procedural applications.[1,2] The list of applications of emergent echocardiography is growing as more physicians learn and apply the modality in innovative ways.

► CLINICAL CONSIDERATIONS

Evaluation of cardiac emergencies at the bedside has traditionally been dependent on many indirect tests, including the physical examination, pulse oximetry, electrocardiogram (ECG), and plain chest radiograph. Each of these tests adds to the complete clinical picture, but often

lacks specificity in certain emergency pathophysiologic states such as cardiac tamponade, hypotension, chest pain, and aortic dissection. Direct visualization of the cardiac structures, however, can immediately provide the clinician information about functional and structural processes only inferred by the clinical examination.

The physical examination of the cardiovascular system, estimated to provide an overall clinical accuracy of 20%, includes inspection, palpation, percussion, and auscultation.[3] These aspects of the clinical evaluation, while important and required, often lack sensitivity and specificity for diagnosis of life-threatening conditions. Pulse oximetry reveals the saturation of hemoglobin through capillary blood in the skin or appendage. Effective in normal and some hemodynamically compromised states, pulse oximetry can be compromised by low blood flow states, especially in cardiac arrest. Electrocardiography detects conduction of electrical signals through the cardiac conducting system, chamber enlargement, ischemic syndromes, metabolic abnormalities, and inflammatory syndromes. Although the ECG is specific at times for various ischemic syndromes, it lacks specificity for other acute cardiac emergencies, such as aortic dissection, cardiac tamponade, or pulmonary embolism. Plain chest radiography can reveal general cardiac silhouette size as well as pulmonary findings, reflecting indirectly on the various functions of the two sides of the heart. Its findings also are fairly non-specific.

Other alternative diagnostic tests to echocardiography include computed tomography (CT) and magnetic resonance imaging (MRI). CT imaging of the heart would require dynamic CT to capture significant intracardiac anatomic abnormalities or fluid collections. For imaging the great vessels of the chest, advantages of CT are that it is widely available and rapid. Other advantages include its non-invasive nature and its accuracy, as the sensitivity and specificity for detecting aortic dissection approach 100%. Disadvantages of CT include the need to transfer a patient out of the emergency department and into the medical imaging suite, the administration of contrast material, and the need for patient cooperation.[4–7] MRI is also highly sensitive and specific for detecting aortic and cardiac structural disease. Its accuracy is 100% in most studies. MRI is non-invasive and provides more complete anatomic data than CT scanning. MRI, however, also requires a patient to be moved outside of the resuscitation arena. It requires a longer examination period and is not as readily available as CT. Also, the constraints of a high magnetic field must be factored in.[4–7]

Arteriography, though excellent for coronary anatomic and valvular function, may not detect pericardial effusion or right-sided cardiac disease without a right-heart catheterization. Difficulties with arterial catheterization include availability of catheterization laboratory, personnel, and contrast agent issues. Invasive methods, such as thoracoscopy, pericardial window, and thoracotomy, may provide direct visualization of the heart through operative maneuvers. The morbidity and mortality of a thoracic procedure, even with cardiac bypass shunting, is not insignificant.[4–7]

Transthoracic echocardiography compares favorably for the evaluation of cardiac emergencies, especially in a busy and noisy emergency or acute care setting.[8,9] Echocardiography can add to the clinical evaluation by confirming high central venous pressure, detecting valvular abnormalities, and confirming enlargement of the heart.[1] Echocardiography clearly can indicate cardiac mechanical activity beyond the ability of palpation or Doppler peripheral arterial pulse acquisition in the low-flow patient. It can identify pericardial fluid collections that have not impacted cardiac hemodynamic status. Echocardiography can measure cardiac pressure gradients in chambers and across valves. Indirectly, echocardiography indicates the etiology of altered hemodynamics. In the future, echocardiography may be able to detect specific coronary lesions and myocardium at risk.

Transesophageal echocardiography (TEE) can be used as an alternative or complementary diagnostic tool to transthoracic echocardiography. Although transthoracic echocardiography does not require sedation or airway protection, TEE is a more invasive procedure that may necessitate those maneuvers. Nevertheless, although not yet widely used by emergency or acute care physicians, TEE has the capability of obtaining excellent resolution of intracardiac abnormalities with little artifact or ultrasound window difficulty. TEE is portable and can be performed at the bedside and during ongoing cardiopulmonary resuscitation without interruption of chest procedures. Other advantages include that it is reproducible, rapid, and accurate. Disadvantages of TEE are that it is very operator dependent, may not be well tolerated by some patients, and may expose patients to vomiting and aspiration. Limitations of TEE are that it may not visualize the extension of aortic dissection into supra-aortic arteries. It can be difficult to assess a small distal portion of the ascending aorta and branches of the aortic arch behind the respiratory tract.[4–7] Table 5–1 compares transthoracic echocardiography to various other diagnostic testing and evaluation methods.

▶ CLINICAL INDICATIONS

The clinical indications for performing a limited echocardiography examination in the emergency setting include:

- Cardiac arrest states
- Trauma to the heart and great vessels
- Acute hypotension
- Acute chest pain
- Guidance for procedures

▶ **TABLE 5–1.** EMERGENT TRANSTHORACIC ECHOCARDIOGRAPHY CONTRASTED WITH OTHER DIAGNOSTIC TESTS

Criteria	TTE	Clinical Examination	CVP	PA Line
Ease of use	+++	+++	+	+
Diagnostic cardiac accuracy	+++	+	+	++
Lack of invasiveness	+++	+++	+	+
Limitations	Aortic anatomy, coronary anatomy, pulmonary anatomy, valvular vegetation	Pulmonary embolism, myocardial ischemia	LVEDP not measured	Invasive pressures only measured
Strengths	Repeatable, noninvasive, bedside intracardiac anatomy	Valvular, lack of invasiveness	Availability, right heart pressures	Blood sampling, LVEDP accurate measurement

0 = None; + = Minimal; ++ = Moderate; +++ = Large.
CT = computed tomography; CVP = central venous pressure; ECG = electrocardiogram; LVEDP = left ventricular end diastolic pressure; MRI = magnetic resonance imaging; PA = pulmonary artery; TTE = transthoracic echocardiography.

CARDIAC ARREST STATES

Cardiopulmonary Resuscitation

Echocardiographic visualization of the heart during cardiopulmonary resuscitation (CPR) is difficult due to chest compressions being performed. Use of transthoracic echo during pulse checks, however, may reveal abnormalities, such as pericardial effusion or detection of myocardial activity, without the artifact of manual CPR. TEE can provide visualization of the heart without cessation of mechanical chest compressions; however, there is no literature that advocates its use during CPR.

Pulseless Electric Activity

In the emergency setting, the palpation or auscultation of peripheral pulses can be difficult to assess in cardiac arrest or hypotensive patients. While asystole, ventricular fibrillation, and ventricular tachycardia are usually evident on cardiac monitoring, the diagnosis of pulseless electric activity (PEA) depends on the determination of a pulse, either centrally or peripherally. PEA, formerly called electromechanical dissociation, is electrical activity on a cardiac monitor without a palpable pulse. Segments of the population with this condition may actually have myocardial activity that is indeterminable by means other than ultrasound. In previous eras, this was called pseudoelectromechanical dissociation.[10–12] Ultrasound not only can determine cardiac activity, but it also may also diagnose a pericardial effusion, dilated ventricular chamber, or small tachycardic heart reflective of etiologies of PEA.[8,13,14] Echocardiography can diagnose specific etiologies of PEA, such as pericardial tamponade, hypovolemia, massive pulmonary embolism, cardiac rupture, and massive myocardial infarction. Treatment can then be directed at the suspected cause.

Asystole

When the presenting arrest rhythm is asystole, absence of echocardiographic activity during the resuscitation can provide important information about the patient's ultimate prognosis and aid in the determination of cessation of efforts. Studies of patients in asystole have shown that the absence of cardiac contractions in conjunction with clinical judgment and end-tidal CO_2 readings generally prognosticate poor outcome.[15] One study of 136 patients showed that the 71 patients with asystole on the emergency department monitor were not resuscitated regardless of initial rhythm.[15] Both real-time and M-mode tracing can help determine the presence of cardiac activity. Cardiac activity can be seen in one or more of the heart structures, but only ventricular contraction should alert the clinician that a pseudo-PEA state is occurring. Agonal or morbid ultrasonographic findings that are possible during electrical asystole include slow valvular contractions, slow atrial contraction, and a dilated, minimally contracting left ventricle.[10]

Ventricular Fibrillation

Ventricular fibrillation is typically a diagnosis made by reviewing the cardiac monitor; however, ventricular fibrillation masquerading as asystole has been diagnosed by emergent echocardiography.[16,17] Fine ventricular fibrillation can be seen on ultrasound as a quivering of the ventricles.[15] Supraventricular motion is variable, as regular left atrial contractions may continue during untreated ventricular fibrillation.[18]

TRAUMA TO THE HEART AND GREAT VESSELS

Traumatic injury to the heart is usually categorized into two categories: penetrating trauma to the pericardium and cardiac structures and blunt cardiac contusion. Penetrating

	ECG	Chest Radiograph	Arteriography	CT
	+++	+++	+	++
	++	++	+++	++
	+++	+++	+	++
	Lack of anatomical findings, nonspecificity for valvular lesions and aortic disease	Chamber size, hemodynamics, location of disease	Dye load, catheterization laboratory availability, valvular anatomy, right and left heart—different procedures	Breath hold, intracardiac anatomy, pressure readings
	Availability	Pulmonary disease, availability	Coronary anatomy, chamber pressure, aortic disease	Other thoracic and abdominal anatomy, aortic disease

injury to the heart is an indication for the use of emergent echocardiography (Algorithm 5–1).[12] The diagnosis of pericardial effusion by cardiac ultrasound was first made in the 1960s.[19] Timely emergency department procedures and expeditious transport of the patient to the operating room can be accomplished by ultrasound diagnosis of hemopericardium. In 1992, Plummer and coworkers demonstrated a reduction in time to diagnosis and overall patient mortality by the use of echocardiography in the emergency department for penetrating injuries to the heart.[9] Rozycki and colleagues also found echocardiography to be effective and accurate in the hands of surgeons evaluating patients with penetrating chest injuries.[20] The pericardium should be visualized during the focused assessment with sonography for trauma (FAST) examination.

Blunt injury to the heart, usually associated with deceleration injuries and sternal trauma, is commonly labeled as "cardiac contusion." The most common clinical features associated with a significant myocardial contusion are tachycardia out of proportion to blood loss, arrhythmias (especially premature ventricular contractions and atrial fibrillation), and conduction defects. The chest radiograph is most useful for detecting associated injuries. Radionuclide angiography can be used to evaluate the wall motion of the right and left ventricles. Cardiac enzymes have been proven to be of little benefit in diagnosing this injury. Echocardiography can assess the functional aspect of this injury. Echocardiographic findings of significant cardiac contusion include dyskinesia of the right ventricle, a small pericardial effusion, and variable left ventricular function (Algorithm 5–2). Cardiac contusion remains a part of the differential diagnosis in the blunt trauma patient with significant chest pain, sternal injury, electrocardiographic changes, or hypotension of unknown etiology.

Traumatic rupture of the aorta is usually diagnosed by mechanism of injury, a widened mediastinum on upright chest radiograph, and clinical judgment. While aortography traditionally has been considered the gold standard, its resource and time intensiveness has made it a second-line diagnostic procedure. Helical CT of the chest, MRI, and TEE are all very sensitive and specific for diagnosing aortic rupture, with accuracy rates reported as high as 100%.[21–23] In this scenario, a view of the distal descending aorta is critical for making the diagnosis. Since TEE is portable, experienced physicians in the emergency department, operating room, or intensive care unit can perform it.

ACUTE HYPOTENSION

This use of echocardiography for diagnosing undifferentiated hypotension is the most promising use of echocardiography in the emergency setting. By visualizing the heart in hypotensive, near-arrest or cardiac arrest states,

the emergency physician can gain clinical insight into the problem, initiate appropriate maneuvers for resuscitation, and monitor the resuscitation.[10,12,17,18]

Pericardial effusion with cardiac tamponade is an immediately reversible cause for acute hypotension. Patients who present with unexplained shortness of breath or who are at risk for pericardial effusion are excellent candidates to undergo emergent echocardiography.[8,24,25] Emergency physicians and others clinicians have been able to use limited echocardiography to make the diagnosis of pericardial effusion in the setting of penetrating trauma, blunt trauma, hypotension, shortness of breath, and cardiac arrest.[26]

Pericardial effusion can be well tolerated or present with life-threatening signs. The collagen fibers of the pericardium usually are taut, so that rapid development of as little as 50 mL of fluid may affect hemodynamics while the pericardial cavity can adapt to the slow accumulation of up to several hundred mL of fluid without tamponade. Cardiac tamponade is, therefore, not dependent on the amount of fluid within the pericardial sac but the pressure within it.[27,28] Cardiac tamponade may be defined clinically or echocardiographically. True cardiac tamponade is defined as the presence of pericardial effusion causing circulatory collapse (as indicated by blood pressure and perfusion status). Echocardiographic tamponade, which accompanies clinical cardiac tamponade (but may precede it), shows diastolic collapse of the right heart and is often referred to as impending tamponade. Cardiac tamponade can result from either fluid, solid, or gas in the pericardial sac, causing elevated pericardial pressure and preventing adequate right ventricular flow. This results in decreased left ventricular flow and cardiac output. As pericardial pressure rises, extramural right heart pressure rises, and filling of the right side of the heart is ultimately impaired. The filling of the right ventricle during diastole shows "collapse." The usual left ventricular relaxation during diastole toward the right ventricle is "flattened" by the rising pressure of the right ventricle. Cardiac output is slowly reduced unless there is release of the tamponade (Figure 5–1). Cardiac tamponade, the state of cardiac impairment caused by an accumulation of pressure within the pericardial sac, is a critical aspect of undifferentiated hypotension, dyspnea of unknown origin, precordial trauma, and chest pain states.[27,28]

The diagnosis of cardiac tamponade cannot exist without a pericardial effusion. It should be noted, however, that in patients who have recently undergone cardiac surgery, pericardial effusions may be loculated but nevertheless exert a significant hemodynamic effect. Beck's triad and pulsus paradoxus have limitations. Beck's triad may be found in less than 30% of patients with cardiac tamponade. It is a late finding in trauma patients with known cardiac effusion.[29] Pulsus paradoxus has multiple other etiologies, including emphysema, pulmonary embolus, right ventricular infarction, restrictive cardiomyopathy, extreme obesity, and ascites.[27] Pulsus paradoxus

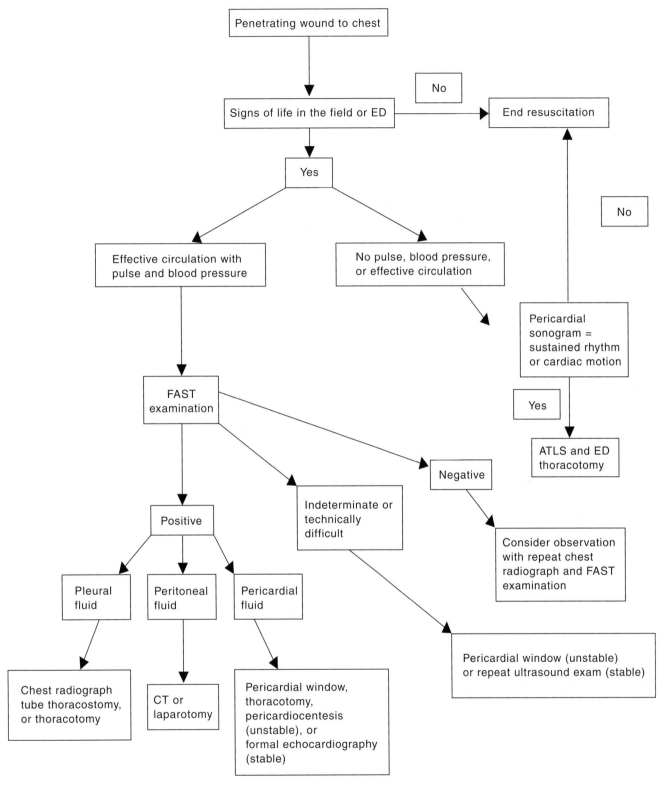

Algorithm 5–1. Penetrating cardiac trauma.

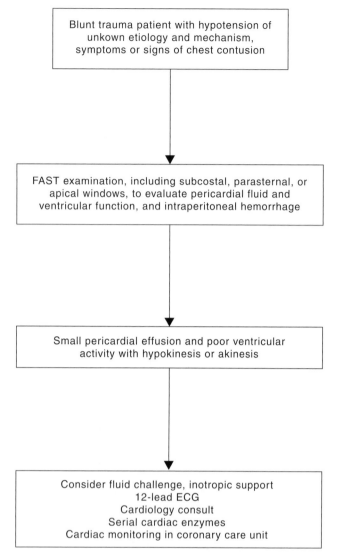

```
┌─────────────────────────────────────┐
│  Blunt trauma patient with hypotension of │
│     unkown etiology and mechanism,        │
│  symptoms or signs of chest contusion     │
└─────────────────────────────────────┘
                    │
                    ▼
┌─────────────────────────────────────┐
│  FAST examination, including subcostal,   │
│  parasternal, or apical windows, to       │
│  evaluate pericardial fluid and           │
│  ventricular function, and intraperitoneal│
│  hemorrhage                               │
└─────────────────────────────────────┘
                    │
                    ▼
┌─────────────────────────────────────┐
│  Small pericardial effusion and poor      │
│  ventricular activity with hypokinesis or │
│  akinesis                                 │
└─────────────────────────────────────┘
                    │
                    ▼
┌─────────────────────────────────────┐
│  Consider fluid challenge, inotropic      │
│  support                                  │
│  12-lead ECG                              │
│  Cardiology consult                       │
│  Serial cardiac enzymes                   │
│  Cardiac monitoring in coronary care unit │
└─────────────────────────────────────┘
```

Algorithm 5–2. Blunt cardiac trauma.

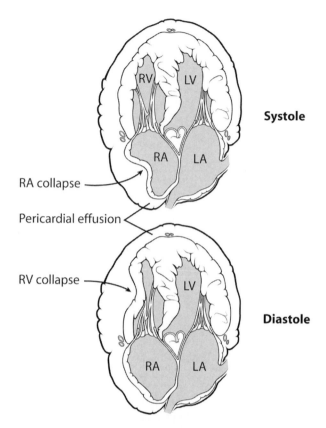

Figure 5–1. Physiology of cardiac tamponade.

may be absent in patients with left ventricular dysfunction, decreased intravascular volume, aortic stenosis, and atrial septal defect. The exclusion of pericardial effusion by echocardiography can then allow the clinician to focus the resuscitation of the patient in shock or respiratory distress on other clinical entities.

In addition to excluding cardiac tamponade, assessment of left ventricular function may help determine volume status. Visualization of a small, hyperkinetic left ventricle suggests hypovolemia, whereas a dilated, hypokinetic left ventricle suggests a primary cardiac cause.[30–32] One study demonstrated that transthoracic echocardiography provided information that was similar to a pulmonary artery catheter in 86% of patients. This information can guide the clinician's mode of resuscitation.[33]

The degree of decrease of the ejection fraction, seen on echocardiography, has been shown to predict mortality in congestive heart failure and myocardial infarction,

and can be used to guide pharmacologic therapy in these situations.[34,35] Paradoxically, increased ejection fraction has also been associated with increased mortality in septic shock.[36] Worsening septic shock causes a decreased systemic vascular resistance, and an increased ejection fraction can be a marker for this more advanced state.

ACUTE CHEST PAIN

When a patient presents with acute chest pain in the emergency setting, echocardiography can assist with differentiating between some of the life-threatening etiologies of chest pain. Myocardial ischemia, pulmonary embolism, and aortic dissection are in the differential diagnosis of acute chest pain and each possesses distinct echocardiographic features. In addition, echocardiography may help distinguish pericarditis from the more serious disease entities in the differential diagnosis of chest pain.

Myocardial Ischemia

The diagnosis of the various cardiac ischemia states can be made by echocardiographic findings of wall motion abnormalities. Though requiring more technical skill, emergency physicians have accurately identified gross left ventricular dysfunction on echocardiography.[37] Myocardial function is immediately affected by ischemia, and can precede ECG changes. New regional wall motion abnormalities, however, often cannot be differentiated from old wall motion changes without reviewing prior echocardiograms.

Studies have demonstrated that the recognition of regional wall motion abnormalities during echocardiography in acute chest pain patients is a sensitive predictor for Q-wave myocardial infarction.[38,39] The limitations of echocardiography for chest pain patients seem to lie with the non-Q-wave myocardial infarction where some patients may have "normal regional wall motion." Sensitivity for acute myocardial infarction generally is high, but specificity remains moderate due to old wall motion abnormalities.[38,39]

Conversely, the ability of resting echocardiography to exclude cardiac ischemia seems limited. Studies have demonstrated that resting echocardiography in acute chest pain patients was not sufficiently sensitive for the detection or exclusion of cardiac ischemia.[40,41] In the emergency department, however, the combination of resting echocardiography and cardiac enzyme serum markers can be a promising combination for the stratification of patients at risk for complications within the hospital and on discharge.[42] The identification of echocardiographic abnormalities can expedite admission for stable patients who are being evaluated in an emergency department chest pain observation unit.

Echocardiography plays an important role in the continuing noninvasive evaluation of patients with known myocardial infarction, including evaluation of its complications, such as left ventricular systolic dysfunction, development of ventricular septal defects, left ventricular rupture, and mitral regurgitation.[43] More chronic complications, such as pericarditis, pericardial effusion, left ventricular aneurysm, and left ventricular thrombus, can also be evaluated by echocardiography.

Pulmonary Embolism

Pulmonary embolism is usually not evident on echocardiography until a substantial portion of the pulmonary arterial bed is occluded. Massive pulmonary embolism can produce a dilated, stiff right ventricle, rivaling the size of the usually larger left ventricle. Though suggestive, a dilated right ventricle in the hemodynamically compromised patient should prompt further testing with TEE, CT of the chest, pulmonary arteriogram, or MRI to evaluate for pulmonary embolism. Echocardiography has not yet proven sufficient accuracy for diagnosis of pulmonary embolism by itself, but may help to expedite intervention for patients with a moderate to high probability of pulmonary embolism. Studies evaluating the utility of right ventricular dilatation, abnormal septal motion, and tricuspid regurgitation, alone and in various combinations, have found sensitivities ranging between 50 and 93% and specificities

ranging between 81 and 98%.[44–50] TEE can be helpful in the diagnosis of pulmonary embolism, especially if there is a large central clot.[51–53] Sensitivities for TEE have been reported to be 80 to 84% for a central clot, with specificities as high as 100%,[51] although false positive cases have been recorded.[50–52] TEE can be particularly useful in the hemodynamically compromised patient who is too unstable to leave the emergency department.

In patients with known pulmonary embolus, evidence of right heart strain by echocardiography can provide prognostic indicators. Presence of right ventricular strain by echocardiography has been found to be significantly related to in-hospital, 3-month, and 1-year mortality rates.[53–55] One of the larger studies to look at the use of thrombolytic therapy versus heparin therapy involved the use of right heart strain on echocardiography to define a "major pulmonary embolism."[56] The researchers included 719 patients with "major" pulmonary embolus, of which 169 received thrombolytic therapy. The 30-day mortality rate in the thrombolytic group was 4.7% compared to 11.1% in the group that received heparin alone. This data have been used as evidence that right heart strain on echocardiography in this clinical setting supports the use of thrombolytic therapy.[57] However, the study has been criticized for not being randomized, with the heparin group being slightly older and with more co-existing cardiac problems.

Aortic Dissection

Aortic dissection occurs when the intima is violated, allowing blood to enter the media and dissect between the intimal and adventitial layers. Common sites for tear include the ascending aorta and the region of the ligamentum arteriosum. Aortic dissection can be classified by two systems. The DeBakey classification categorizes aortic dissection as: type I, which involve the ascending aorta, the aortic arch, and the descending aorta; type II, which involves only the ascending aorta; and type III, which involves only the descending aorta. The Stanford classification categorizes aortic dissection as: type A, which involves the ascending aorta; and type B, which involves only the descending aorta.[4–7]

Aortic dissection and intramural hematoma can be detected by transthoracic echocardiography on parasternal long, parasternal short, and suprasternal views. A linear echogenic flap, indicative of aortic dissection, can be seen across the aortic lumen anywhere along its length. The ascending aorta can be seen on the parasternal views. The descending aorta is usually only seen in cross-section on parasternal views. The aortic arch can be visualized on the suprasternal view in a segment of the population.[4–7]

TEE provides much better resolution and visualization of aortic dissection than transthoracic echocardiography. Spiral CT, TEE, and MRI have been demonstrated to have comparable sensitivity, and specificity, with accuracy rates approaching 100%.[4-7] Sommer and co-workers found that all three modalities approach 100% sensitivity; the specificities for spiral CT, TEE, and MRI were 100%, 94%, and 94%, respectively.[58]

Important issues to address with aortic dissection include: (1) presence of pericardial involvement as a sign of imminent mortality without surgical intervention; (2) presence of ascending aorta involvement without pericardial involvement; (3) evidence of isolated descending aorta involvement; (4) location of the entry site; and (5) evidence of involvement of major branch vessels.[4-7]

GUIDANCE FOR PROCEDURES

Pericardiocentesis

Pericardiocentesis is the aspiration of fluid from the pericardial sac. Typically, it is performed in a blind fashion after palpation of landmarks in the subxiphoid region. Complications of pericardiocentesis include lacerations of cardiac chambers or structures, pneumothorax, pneumopericardium, and liver laceration. Echocardiography has been proven to help guide pericardiocentesis in a subxiphoid, parasternal, or apical approach, depending on the location of maximum fluid.[59,60] The ultrasound probe can be placed at a site away from the needle entrance site. Sterile saline injections from the (agitated) syringe into the pericardial sac, as viewed on real-time ultrasound, can provide guidance as to the correct placement of the needle in the pericardial sac.[59,60]

Detection of Pacing Capture

In transcutaneous and transvenous pacing, the detection of pacer capture can be difficult in the patient with other rhythmic muscular contractions.[61,62] Visualization of ventricular contraction by echocardiography subsequent to the pacing spike indicates that capture has occurred. The proper placement of the pacing wire within the right ventricle can also be detected by ultrasound.[62]

▶ ANATOMIC CONSIDERATIONS

Heart

The heart is a hollow muscular organ, placed between the lungs and enclosed within the pericardium. It is divided by a septum into two halves, right and left, each half being further subdivided into two cavities, the atrium and the ventricle (Figure 5–2). Blood flows from the right atrium into the right ventricle through the tricuspid valve. From the right ventricle, unoxygenated blood is carried to the lungs through the pulmonary artery. Blood flows from the left atrium into the left ventricle through the mitral valve. From the left ventricle, oxygenated blood is distrib-

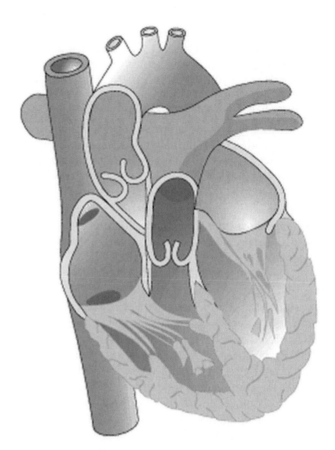

Figure 5–2. Cardiac circulation.

uted to the body through the aorta. The outflow tract through the aortic valve into the proximal aorta starts anteriorly and revolves posteriorly into the posterior mediastinum next to the esophagus. The aorta is divided into the ascending aorta, the aortic arch, and the descending aorta. The ascending aorta is approximately 5 cm in length; the only branches of the ascending aorta are the coronary arteries. The aortic arch has three branches: the innominate artery, the left common carotid artery, and the left subclavian artery.

The pericardium is composed of two layers, the parietal and visceral layers, which normally oppose each other without any significant fluid accumulation. The pericardium attaches to the superior left atrium and envelops the proximal aspects of the great vessels (Figure 5–3).

Thoracic Cavity

The thoracic cavity provides both windows and impediments to the accurate sonographic view of the heart (Figure 5–4). The heart has very few sonographic windows since ribs, the sternum, and the lungs surround it (Figure 5–5). Common windows include the parasternal, apical, subcostal, and suprasternal views. The left parasternal interspace allows for small sonographic windows into the mediastinum. The superior aspect of the abdomen also allows for soft tissue windows via the left lobe

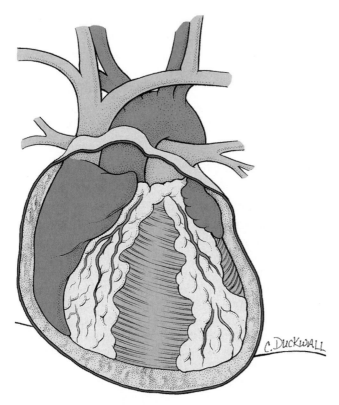

Figure 5–3. Pericardium.

of the liver. The heart can shift closer to the chest wall in the left decubitus position.

Cardiac Axes

The heart has a long axis from the right shoulder to the left hip. The transverse view, or short axis of the heart, is rotated 90° from the long axis of the heart (left shoulder to right hip) (Figure 5–6). The apical view, or four-chamber axis, is a coronal image of the heart from its apex to its base. The apex of the heart is usually located at the nipple line in the anterior axillary line. The base of the heart lies in an axis, anterior to posterior, from the parasternal right second intercostal space to the posterior thorax next to the esophagus.

▶ TECHNIQUE AND NORMAL ULTRASOUND FINDINGS

Transthoracic Echocardiography

For cardiac transthoracic echocardiographic studies, either a curved linear array probe or a phased array sector probe with median frequencies of 3.5 MHz (2.5 to 5.0 MHz) should be used. Table 5–2 lists the advantages and disadvantages of using curved linear array probes and phased array sector probes in the emergency department.

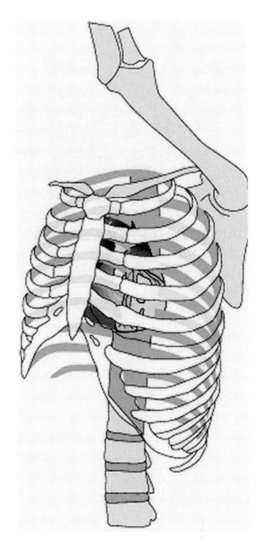

Figure 5–4. Chest cage.

The settings on the ultrasound machine may need to be adjusted to allow for a lower dynamic range (more black and white), lower depth, preprocessing curves to adjust gray scale and edge enhancement, and a more equal time gain compensation. These setting changes are accomplished easily on most machines by selecting the cardiac preset on machine start up. The machine and probe should be positioned to the patient's left in echocardiography. In the emergency and acute care setting, however, the sonologist often needs to be flexible with regard to available space for location of the machine and approach to the patient. The arrow (right/left indicator) on the monitor is usually oriented to the right side of the image which is the opposite of abdominal or pelvic imaging, and is done automatically via presets or manually by toggling the flip image (horizontal) button. The probe indicator, therefore, is oriented to the patient's left for transverse images. Table 5–3 provides a comparison of imaging techniques for the heart when using an echocardiography preset versus an abdominal/pelvic preset. Regardless of the

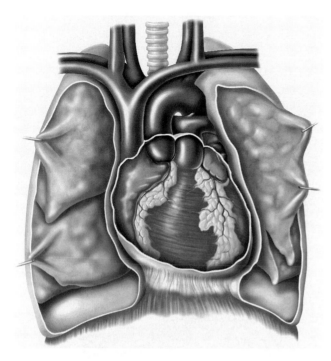

Figure 5–5. Surrounding structures.

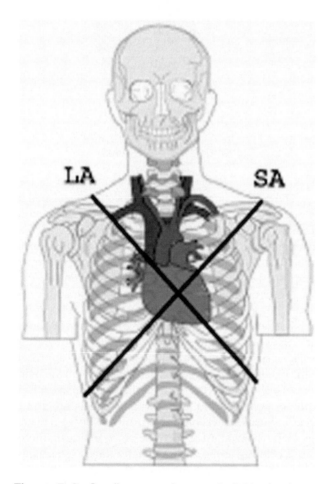

Figure 5–6. Cardiac axes. Long axis (LA), short axis (SA).

▶ **TABLE 5–2.** COMPARISON OF CURVED LINEAR ARRAY WITH PHASED ARRAY TRANSDUCERS

Transducer Type	Curved Linear Array	Flat Phased Array
Image on monitor	Sector	Sector
Moving structures capture	Poor	Good
Small window capability	Generally worse	Excellent
Grayscale differentiation of echogenic structures	Good	Poor

machine setup, what is most important is to orient the images in a standard fashion on the monitor. This facilitates recognition of the cardiac chambers for the sonologist and for any others who may review the images.

Most patients requiring emergent echocardiography will be in the supine position during resuscitation. If the situation is less emergent and the patient is cooperative, superior images may be obtained from placing the patient in a left lateral decubitus position, with their left hand under their head. Skills that need to be obtained to enhance viewing all of the cardiac windows include transducer movement, rotation, tilting, and angling (Figure 5–7). Once these skills are obtained, clinicians will be able to visualize significant echocardiographic findings or use alternate windows to gain images.

Transesophageal Echocardiography

Usually performed at the bedside, regardless of the patient's hemodynamic status, TEE requires more preparation. If the patient's airway is not completely stable, the patient should be intubated to protect the airway. Suction should be at the bedside and the patient should be on a cardiac monitor. Patients should undergo conscious sedation in the typical fashion. Unless there is a question of a spinal injury, the TEE examination should be performed with the sedated patient in the left lateral decubitus position.

Biplanar and multiplanar probes are used. Biplanar TEE can rotate in the transverse and long axes of the esophagus. Multiplanar TEE can rotate from a transverse position through intermediate positions to the reversed transverse position. All aspects of the heart, ascending aorta (except for the superior aspect where the right mainstem bronchus crosses the aorta), mid to distal aortic arch, and descending aorta can be imaged adequately with TEE. Transesophageal images are dependent on the relative positions of the cardiac structures and esophagus in each position.

TYPICAL CARDIAC WINDOWS

Probe orientation is based on echocardiography preset as previously described.

► **TABLE 5–3.** TRANSTHORACIC TRANSDUCER ORIENTATION ON THE SUPINE PATIENT

Ultrasound Preset	Echocardiography	Abdomen and Pelvis
Machine and probe location	To the patient's left	To the patient's right
Monitor indicator	Right side of the screen	Left side of the screen
Subcostal	Probe marker directed to the patient's left flank	Probe marker directed to the patient's right flank
Apical four-chamber	Probe marker directed to the left shoulder Probe aimed to right shoulder	Probe marker directed to the right hip Probe aimed to left shoulder
Parasternal long	Probe marker directed to the patient's right shoulder (10 o'clock)	Probe marker directed to the patient's left hip (4 o'clock)
Parasternal short	Probe marker directed to the patient's left shoulder (2 o'clock)	Probe marker directed to the patient's right hip (8 o'clock)

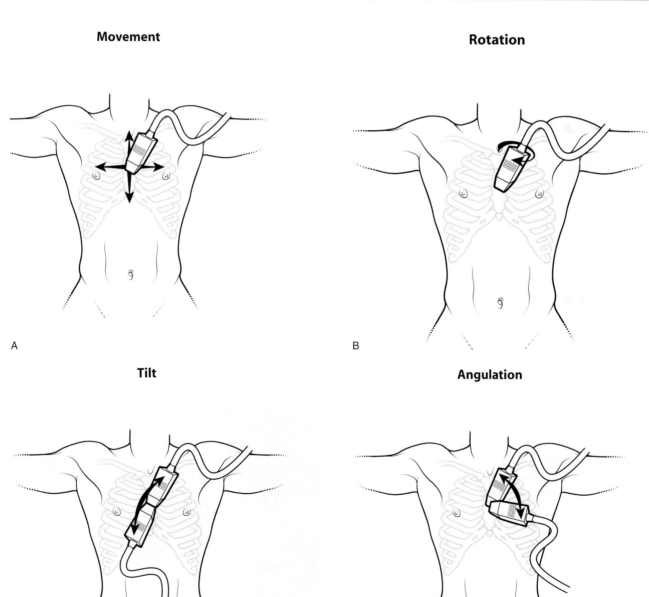

Figure 5–7. Transducer skills.

Subcostal Four-Chamber View

The subcostal view is the most useful view for emergency ultrasound. It usually does not interfere in resuscitative measures such as thoracostomy, CPR, subclavian line insertion, or intubation. It is easily learned, repeated, and performed as part of both the cardiac and trauma ultrasound evaluations.

The subcostal view should be performed at the subxiphoid position of the abdomen (Figure 5–8). The probe should be held at a 15° angle to the chest wall and aimed toward the left shoulder. The probe marker should be aimed toward the patient's left hip. The transducer should be angled up or down depending on the depth of the chest cavity to obtain images of the beating heart. The depth should then be adjusted to visualize the atria at the bottom of the monitor screen. Tips on gaining this image include using an appropriate amount of ultrasound gel, using a shallow angle to the chest wall, moving the transducer to the right to use the left lobe of the liver as a window, and moving off the xiphoid and over to the lower intercostal spaces to image the barrel-chested patient with a larger anterior to posterior diameter.

The subcostal four-chamber view should be seen as primarily a diagonal view of the ventricles, atria, pericardium, and the left lobe of the liver (Figures 5–9 and 5–10). If the transducer is angled at a more acute angle toward the abdomen, the left lobe of the liver, inferior vena cava, and the hepatic veins should be visualized.

While the subcostal four-chamber long axis view is primarily used in emergency ultrasound for the detection of pericardial effusion and cardiac activity, the interatrial and interventricular septum may also be viewed. Also, this may be the only view obtainable in the patient with emphysema due to the large amount of lung volume pushing mediastinal structures inferiorly.

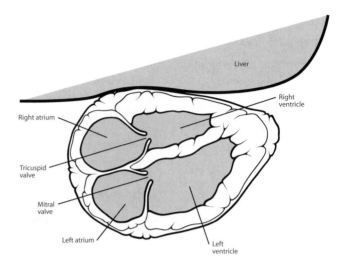

Figure 5–9. Subcostal four-chamber diagram.

Subcostal Short Axis View

The subcostal short axis view should be performed by rotating the ultrasound probe 90° clockwise from the four-chamber view and aiming it towards the patient's left arm. This view should resemble the parasternal short axis view and provide the "doughnut" view of the left ventricle (Figures 5–11 and 5–12).

Subcostal Long Axis View

The subcostal long axis view, which is widely used for trauma patients, uses a sagittal body axis with the probe marker aimed toward the patient's feet (Figures 5–13 and 5–14). A sagittal section of the body views the heart, the left lobe of the liver, the inferior vena cava,

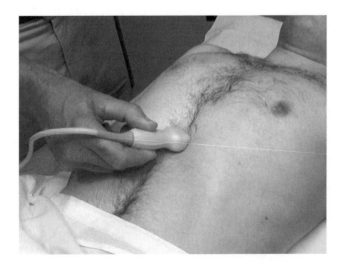

Figure 5–8. Probe position for subcostal four-chamber view.

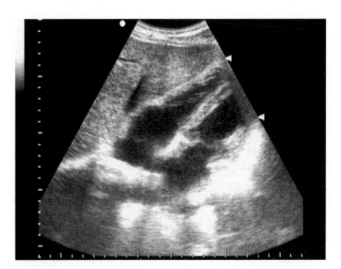

Figure 5–10. Subcostal four-chamber normal ultrasound.

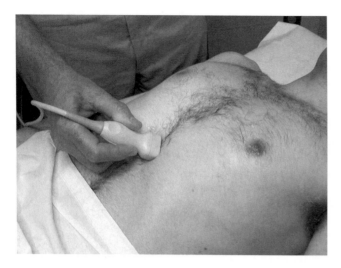

Figure 5–11. Probe position for subcostal short axis view.

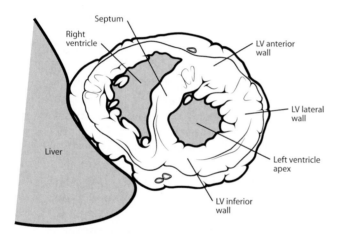

Figure 5–12. Subcostal short axis (SAX).

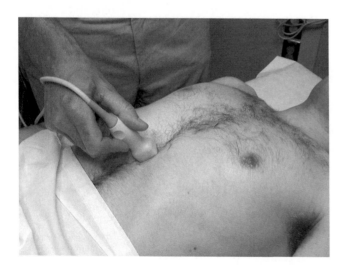

Figure 5–13. Probe position for subcostal long axis (LAX) view.

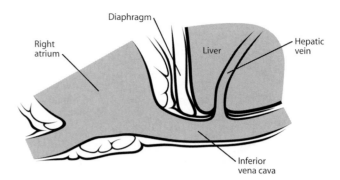

Figure 5–14. Subcostal long axis diagram.

and hepatic veins. This view has the advantage of visualizing an anterior pericardial effusion, cardiac activity, and elevated right heart pressures, as manifested by a dilated and stiff inferior vena cava and hepatic vein. Disadvantages of this view are the lack of visualization of cardiac chamber size and activity and posterior cardiac effusions.

Parasternal Long Axis View

The parasternal long axis view can be best obtained by accepting the long axis of the heart to be roughly from the right shoulder to the left hip (Figures 5–15, 5–16, and 5–17). The transducer should be placed perpendicular to the third or fourth intercostal space immediately to the left of the sternum with the probe indicator directed toward the right shoulder. The following structures can be visualized from anterior to posterior on the monitor: right ventricular free wall, right ventricular cavity, interventricular septum, left ventricular cavity, and the posterior left ventricle. On the basal side of the image (right side of the screen), the aortic valve with its

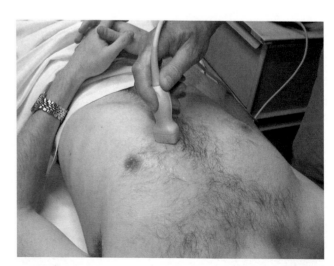

Figure 5–15. Probe position for parasternal long axis (PSL) view.

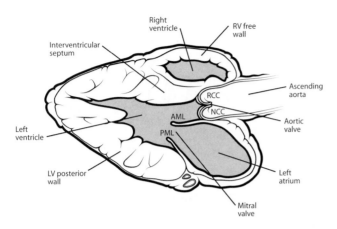

Figure 5–16. Parasternal long axis diagram.

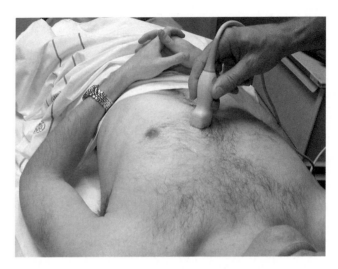

Figure 5–18. Probe position for parasternal short axis (PSS) view.

inflow and outflow tracts, the mitral valve with its inflow and outflow tracts, the left atrium, the posterior pericardium, and possibly the descending aorta should be seen (see Figure 5–17). The probe should be rotated to obtain the best axis to view these structures. Angling and tilting may be needed, but less so than for the short axis view. A reduction in size of the image may be needed to focus on certain structures or enlargement of the field of view to see below the left ventricle and left atrium.

Parasternal Short Axis View

The parasternal short axis view of the heart stretches from the left shoulder to the right hip, and should be obtained in the left third or fourth intercostal space next to the sternum. If the parasternal long axis view has already been obtained, the parasternal short axis view should be obtained by maintaining the window gained

for the long axis view and then rotating the probe marker 90° clockwise toward the left shoulder. This provides the "doughnut" view of the heart, especially the left ventricle (Figures 5–18, 5–19, and 5–20). Once this window is obtained, the transducer position should be maintained tightly on the chest wall, and the transducer should be tilted down toward the apex (Figures 5–21 and 5–22) or up toward the base of the heart (Figures 5–23 and 5–24). These various short axis views should allow visualization of the left ventricle from the apex though the papillary muscle, mitral valve (see Figure 5–19), and up to the left atrium. A superior short axis view visualizes the right atrium, tricuspid valve, right ventricle, and pulmonary valve draping over the aortic valve ("Mer-

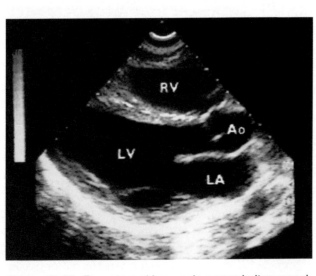

Figure 5–17. Parasternal long axis normal ultrasound.

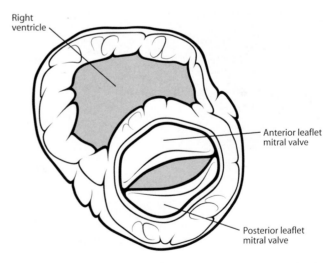

Figure 5–19. Parasternal short axis diagram at mitral valve.

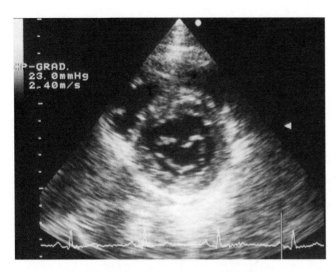

Figure 5–20. Parasternal short axis normal ultrasound at mitral valve.

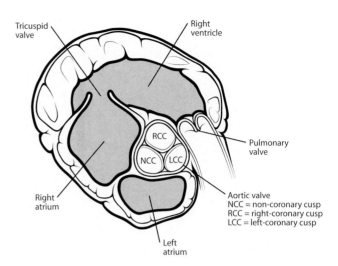

Figure 5–23. Parasternal short axis diagram at aortic valve.

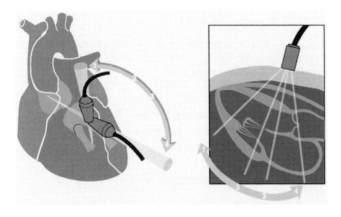

Figure 5–21. Parasternal probe movement for short axis views.

cedes Benz sign") in cross-section in the middle of the view (see Figure 5–23 and 5–25).

Apical Four-Chamber View

The apical four-chamber view is a coronal view of the heart that views all four chambers in a slice. Alterations of this view include the apical two-chamber view, the apical three-chamber view, and the apical five-chamber view. Regardless of the number of chambers, the view is best observed by obtaining the window at the apex of the heart, usually where the nipple line is located. Alteration

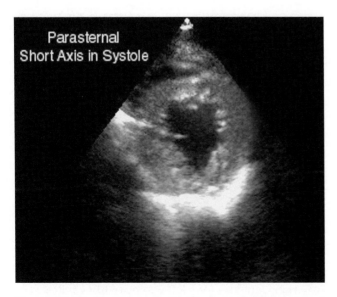

Figure 5–22. Parasternal short axis normal ultrasound at apex.

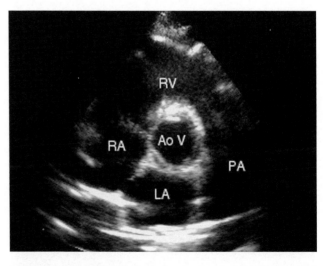

Figure 5–24. Parasternal short axis normal ultrasound at aortic valve. RV = right ventricular outflow tract, RA = right atrium, LA = left atrium, PA = pulmonary artery, Ao V = aortic valve.

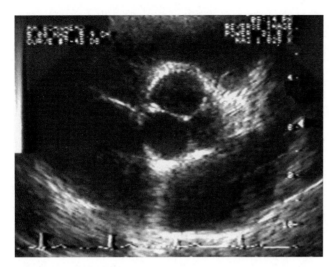

Figure 5–25. Mercedes Benz sign. Parasternal short axis at aortic valve demonstrates closure of all 3 cusps. *(Courtesy of Lori Sens and Lori Green, Gulfcoast Ultrasound.)*

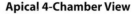

Apical 4-Chamber View

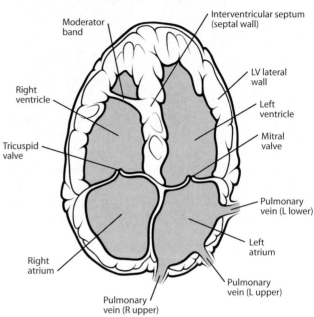

Figure 5–27. Apical four-chamber diagram. Note that the right ventricle is depicted larger than normal size for illustrative purposes.

of this position may be needed to adjust for breast tissue, emphysema, chest deformities, and other anatomic changes. Whenever possible, the patient should be rotated toward the left side to reduce lung artifact. The transducer should be placed roughly at this position in the fifth intercostal space aimed toward the right shoulder with the marker directed towards the left (Figures 5–26, 5–27, and 5–28). Some rotation may be needed to allow for all four chambers to be viewed. A rounded, foreshortened heart is usually artifactual, and the transducer should be aimed in a more anterior direction. On this view, the right ventricle with its lateral wall, the interventricular septum (septal wall), the left ventricle with the lateral wall, the two atria, the interatrial septum, and the pulmonary veins should be visualized. This view is advantageous for as-

sessing right ventricular function and the left ventricle for function and presence of blood clots. Interatrial abnormalities, such as myxoma, may be well visualized.

Apical Two-Chamber View

For the apical two-chamber view, the ultrasound probe should be placed in the same location as for the apical four-chamber view but the transducer should be rotated

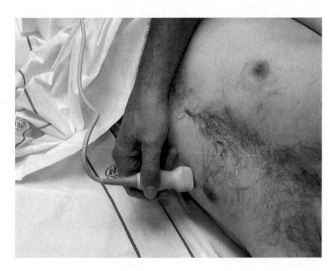

Figure 5–26. Probe position for apical four-chamber view.

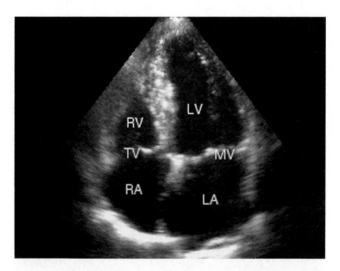

Figure 5–28. Apical four-chamber normal ultrasound. RV = right ventricle, LV = left ventricle, MV = mitral valve, LA = left atrium, RA = right atrium, TV = tricuspid valve.

90° counterclockwise until the marker is directed towards the head of the patient (Figures 5–29, 5–30, and 5–31). This view evaluates anterior and inferior walls, thus complementing the apical four-chamber view of the left ventricle for wall motion and function.

Suprasternal View

The suprasternal view provides a glimpse of the aortic arch with its three main branches: the brachiocephalic artery, the left carotid artery, and the left subclavian artery. The ultrasound probe should be placed in the sternal notch with the transducer marker pointed to the left and aimed as far anteriorly as possible (Figures 5–32, 5–33, and 5–34). While it is difficult to obtain in many patients, this view may provide a confirmation of aortic aneurysm or dissection. Aortic aneurysm or dissection can be detected in the patient with an optimal window. The right pulmonary artery in cross section can be viewed below the aortic arch. If the transducer is rotated 90° to visualize the aortic arch in cross section, the left pulmonary artery may be seen. Occasionally, the superior vena cava may be viewed lateral to the ascending aorta. The left atrium lies inferior to the pulmonary arteries and, in an optimal window, all four pulmonary veins can be viewed.

Transesophageal Windows

Although TEE is not routinely utilized at this time by emergency or acute care physicians, the normal examination is included as a source of high-resolution cardiac images that are free from artifacts commonly associated with the transthoracic method. In this section, the windows indicate the position of the probe, and not the axis of the heart. Therefore, in transverse or longitudinal planes, the four-chamber, short axis, or long axis views of the heart can be seen.

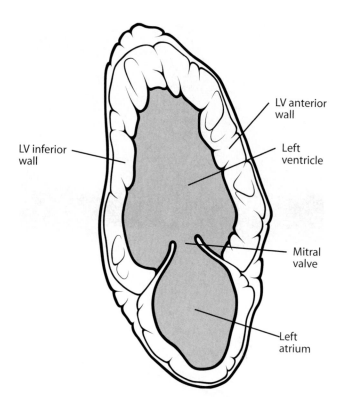

Figure 5–30. Apical two-chamber diagram.

TEE Transverse Great Vessel

Immediately after the trachea, the main pulmonary artery and its division can be viewed. Past this level, the aortic valve, left atrium, and right atrium can be seen. The sinuses of Valsalva can be seen with origins of the main coronary arteries coming off the left and right coronary cusps of the aortic valve, respectively. At this level, other structures that can be seen include the interatrial septum, left atrial appendages, and pulmonary veins (Figures 5–35 through 5–40).

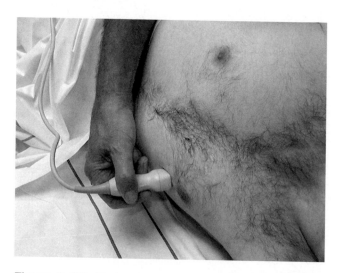

Figure 5–29. Probe position for apical two-chamber view.

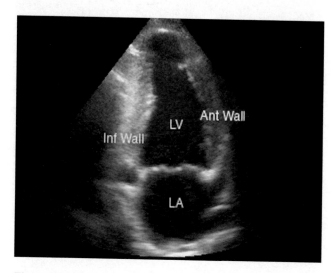

Figure 5–31. Apical two-chamber normal ultrasound.

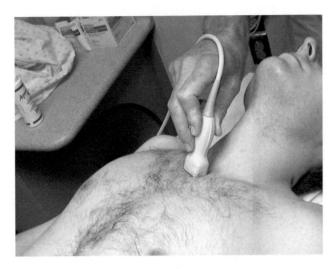

Figure 5–32. Probe position for suprasternal view.

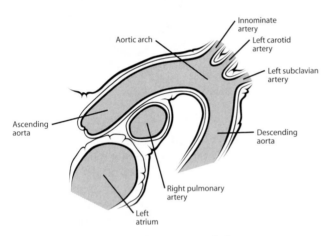

Figure 5–33. Suprasternal diagram.

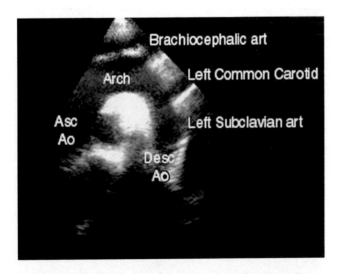

Figure 5–34. Suprasternal normal ultrasound.

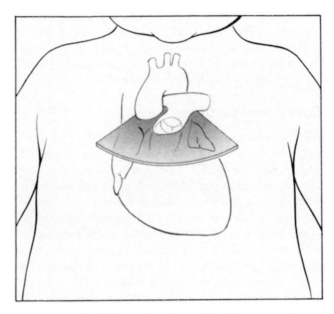

Figure 5–35. TEE aortic valve and pulmonary artery transverse technique.

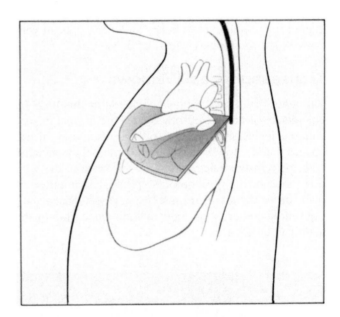

Figure 5–36. TEE aortic valve and pulmonary artery transverse technique (lateral view).

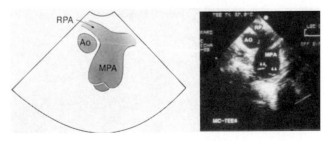

Figure 5–37. TEE aortic valve and pulmonary artery transverse ultrasound view with diagram.

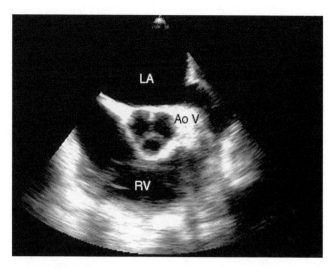

Figure 5–38. TEE transverse aortic valve.

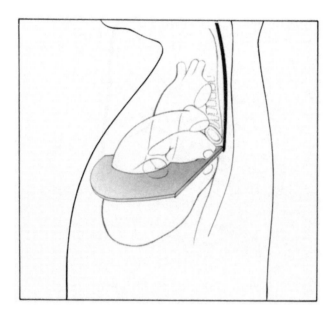

Figure 5–40. TEE left atrium and aortic valve transverse technique (lateral view).

TEE Transverse Mitral Valve

Once the transducer is at the level of the left atrium, the mitral valve and all four cardiac chambers (albeit somewhat foreshortened) can be viewed (Figures 5–41 through 5–44).

TEE Longitudinal Left Atrium and Left Ventricle

Looking through the left atrium, the left atrium, mitral valve, and left ventricle can be viewed (Figures 5–45, 5–46, and 5–47).

TEE Longitudinal Aortic Valve and Ascending Aorta

The probe should be oriented anteriorly to obtain a view of the aortic valve, ascending aorta, and left ven-

tricular outflow tract. Views for aortic dissection may be obtained in this area as the aortic root is well visualized (Figure 5–48).

TEE Transgastric

By angling the probe superiorly, a long and short axis view of the left ventricle can be obtained. The circular view, however, is flipped 180° from the TEE short axis view of the left ventricle. Thus, the wall closest to the transducer is the posterior wall, and the wall furthest away is the anterior wall (Figures 5–49 and 5–50).

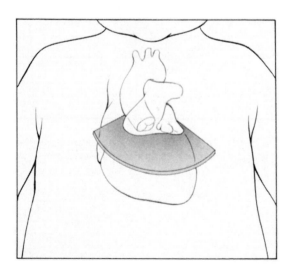

Figure 5–39. TEE left atrium and aortic valve transverse technique.

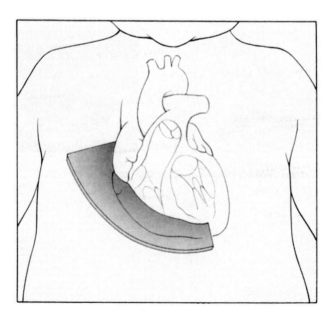

Figure 5–41. TEE four-chamber transverse technique.

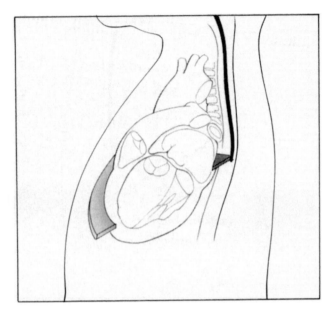

Figure 5-42. TEE four-chamber transverse technique (lateral view).

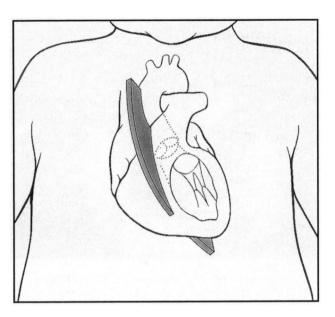

Figure 5-45. TEE aortic valve, left ventricle, and mitral valve longitudinal technique.

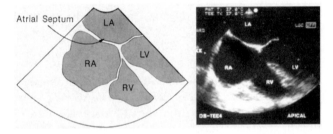

Figure 5-43. TEE four-chamber transverse ultrasound view.

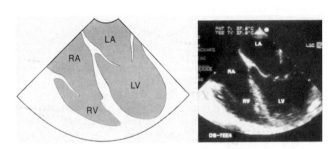

Figure 5-44. TEE four-chamber transverse ultrasound view.

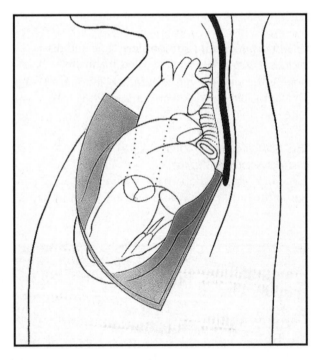

Figure 5-46. TEE aortic valve, left ventricle, and mitral valve longitudinal technique (lateral view).

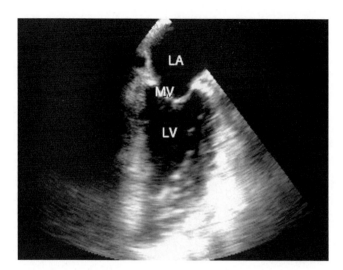

Figure 5–47. TEE left atrium, mitral valve, and left ventricle normal longitudinal ultrasound view.

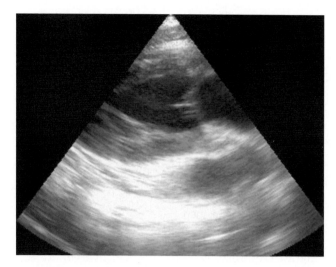

Figure 5–49. TEE left atrium and left ventricle long axis transgastric technique.

Two-Dimensional Measurement

Chamber dimensions and sizes should be measured at right angles to the long axis of the respective chamber. Measurement of the chamber sizes, wall thickness, and the left ventricular function may be helpful. By measuring the left ventricular dimensions in systole and diastole, the ejection fraction can be calculated manually or by using the ultrasound machine calculation package. Critical to the two-dimensional measurement is the ability to visualize the endocardium and a cine memory to scroll to the correct point in the cardiac cycle for measurement. Table 5–4 lists linear dimensions of normal cardiac structures.

Left Ventricular Function Measurement

Left ventricular function is frequently expressed as ejection fraction. Three common methods exist for the mea-

surement of ejection fraction: contrast ventriculography, radionuclide cineangiography, and echocardiography.[63] Currently, echocardiography is the most common method for measuring ejection fraction due to cost, ease of use, and availability.[64]

Several methods exist for the echocardiographic measurement of ejection fraction. These range from observation and fairly simple M-mode measurements to complicated biplane calculations.[65] Many ultrasound software packages have the ability to estimate volume and calculate ejection fraction. This is typically done by border tracing and measurement of cavity length in an apical four-chamber and apical two-chamber view.

Although it may be satisfying to actually calculate a value for ejection fraction, it has been shown that visual estimation of ejection fraction is as good or better

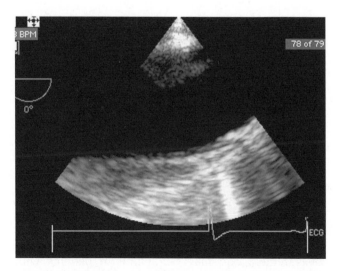

Figure 5–48. TEE ascending aorta normal longitudinal ultrasound view.

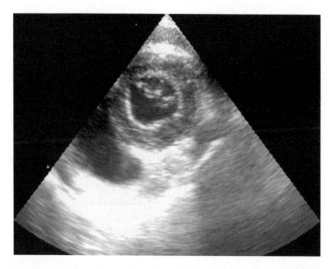

Figure 5–50. TEE left ventricle short axis transgastric technique.

▶ **TABLE 5–4.** NORMAL FINDINGS ON 2-D ECHOCARDIOGRAPHY

	Range	Range Indexed to BSA	Upper Limit of Normal
Aorta			
Annulus diameter	1.4–2.6 cm	1.3 ± 0.1 cm/m^2	<1.6 cm/m^2
Diameter at leaflet tips	2.2–3.6 cm	1.7 ± 0.2 cm/m^2	<2.1 cm/m^2
Ascending aorta diameter	2.1–3.4 cm	1.5 ± 0.2 cm/m^2	
Arch diameter	2.0–3.6 cm		
Short axis diastole	3.5–6.0 cm	2.3–3.1 cm/m^2	
Left ventricle			
Short axis systole	2.1–4.0 cm	1.4–2.1 cm/m^2	
Long axis diastole	6.3–10.3 cm	4.1–5.7 cm/m^2	
Long axis systole	4.6–8.4 cm		
End diastolic volume, men	96–157 ml	67 ± 9 mL	
End diastolic volume, women	59–138 ml	61 ± 13 mL	
End systolic volume, men	33–68 ml	27 ± 5 mL	
End systolic volume, women	18–65 ml	26 ± 7 mL	
Ejection fraction, men	0.59 ± 0.06		
Ejection fraction, women	0.59 ± 0.07		
LV wall thickness (end diastole)	0.6–1.1 cm		Men ≤ 1.2 cm Women ≤ 1.1 cm
LV mass, men	<294 g	109 ± 20 g/m^2	≤150 g/m^2
LV mass, women	<194 g	89 ± 15 g/m^2	≤120 g/m^2
Left atrium			
Long axis AP diameter	2.3–4.5 cm	1.6–2.4 cm/m^2	
Apical four-chamber Medial–lateral diameter	2.5–4.5 cm	1.6–2.4 cm/m^2	
Apical four-chamber Superior–inferior diameter	3.4–6.1 cm	2.5–3.5 cm/m^2	
Mitral annulus			
End diastole	2.7 ± 0.4 cm		
End systole	2.9 ± 0.3 cm		
Wall thickness	0.2–0.5 cm	0.2 ± 0.05 cm/m^2	
Right ventricle			
Minor dimension	2.2–4.4 cm	1.0–2.8 cm/m^2	
Length diastole	5.5–9.5 cm	3.8–5.3 cm/m^2	
Length systole	4.2–8.1 cm		
Pulmonary artery			
Annulus diameter	1.0–2.2 cm		
Main pulmonary artery	0.9–2.9 cm		
Inferior vena cava			
At right atrial junction Diameter	1.2–2.3 cm		

AP = anterior to posterior; BSA = body surface area; LV = left ventricle.
Source: Adapted from Otto CM, Pearlman AS. Normal cardiac anatomy in textbook of clinical echocardiography. Philadelphia, Saunders, 1995; p. 35.

than calculated ejection fraction and is much easier to perform.[65–67] This is the most frequent method in clinical use today. With training and practice, noncardiologists may be able to estimate ejection fraction with reasonable accuracy.[37] It is important to note that both estimated and calculated ejection fractions are more accurate when the ventricle is regularly shaped and contracts in a symmetric fashion. Wall motion abnormalities and other variations in shape may significantly confound the echocardiographic measurement of ejection fraction.[34]

Central Venous Pressure
Right atrial pressures can be estimated by viewing the respiratory change in the diameter of the inferior vena cava. Table 5–5 shows common measurements of inferior vena cava diameter and change with respiration used to estimate the right atrial pressure. This amounts to a non-invasive central venous pressure measurement and may be helpful in patients with hypotension and uncertain volume status. It is also possible to estimate the end-systolic pulmonary artery

► **TABLE 5-5.** INFERIOR VENA CAVA (IVC) ESTIMATES OF RIGHT ATRIAL (RA) PRESSURE

IVC Size (cm)	Respiratory Change	RA Pressure (cm)
< 1.5	Total collapse	0–5
1.5–2.5	> 50% collapse	5–10
1.5–2.5	< 50% collapse	11–15
> 2.5	< 50% collapse	16–20
> 2.5	No change	> 20

pressure (approximates the wedge pressure) by measuring the flow velocity of the tricuspid regurgitant jet, and applying it to a formula or calculation package. The specifics of this measurement are beyond the scope of the text.

M Mode

M mode (motion mode) allows for one-dimensional tracing of structures over time. M mode can record motion of structures faster than human vision and record subtle changes. Measurements of valve diameter, wall motion, wall thickness, and stroke volume are possible. There are several uses of M-mode tracing but the most common in emergency ultrasound is the tracing through the left ventricle for measurement of left ventricular size and function and to confirm the presence of a pericardial effusion.

M Mode Left Ventricle

This is usually performed perpendicular to the long axis of the left ventricle in the parasternal long or short axis at the level of the tips of the mitral valve leaflets. This tracing cuts through the right ventricle, interventricular septum, left ventricle anterior wall, left ventricle posterior wall, and posterior pericardium. The end systolic diameter (ESD) is measured at the small dimensions or at the end of the T wave on a simultaneous ECG tracing (Figure 5–51). A

second measurement during end diastole is taken just prior to ventricular thickening and contraction or at the start of the QRS interval on simultaneous ECG tracing. The distance between the posterior left ventricular wall and the posterior parietal pericardium can be quantified if there is fluid present.

M Mode Mitral Valve and Left Ventricular Dysfunction

An M-mode tracing at the mitral valve level shows the right ventricular free wall, interventricular septum, the mitral valve leaflets, the posterior left ventricular wall, and the pericardium. The mitral valve leaflets open and close as single lines joining together (Figure 5–52). The early diastolic motion of the anterior leaflet is termed the E point. The distance between this E point and the left ventricular septal wall is measured as the E-point septal separation (EPSS). A large EPSS in the absence of mitral stenosis reflects left ventricular systolic dysfunction, left ventricular dilatation, and aortic regurgitation.

Doppler Measurements

The use of the Doppler principle in ultrasound depends on the measurement of frequency shifts from moving red blood cells within cardiac structures. The velocity of the red blood cells depends on the transducer frequency, the speed of red blood cells in vessels, and the angle between the beam and the direction of flow. The sampling beam should be positioned as parallel to flow as possible.

Laminar flow is flow as one would imagine inside a tube, with a leading edge of fast flow and slow flow along the walls. Pressure differences drive blood across the vessel or in the heart. With turbulent flow, blood is moving in all directions but is moving forward. At stenoses,

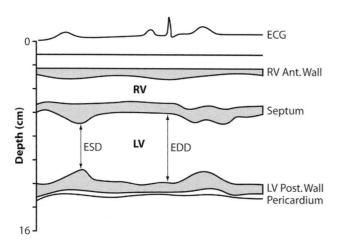

Figure 5-51. M mode of left ventricle.

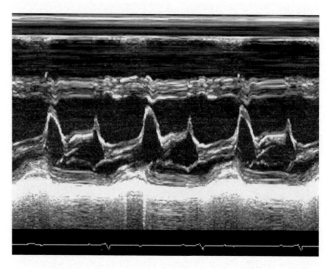

Figure 5-52. M mode mitral valve level.

▶ **TABLE 5–6.** SPECTRAL DOPPLER SAMPLING SITES

Doppler Measurement	Sample Location	Normal Velocity (m/s)
Right atrial pressure	Subcostal in central hepatic vein SSN	Systole = 0.32–0.69 Diastole = 0.06–0.45
Right ventricular pressure	Right ventricular inflow tract Apical four-chamber	0.3–0.7
Pulmonary artery pressure	Right ventricular outflow tract Parasternal short or subcostal short axis beyond pulmonary valve leaflets	0.5–1.3
Left atrial pressure	Apical four-chamber	Systole 0.56 Diastole 0.44
Left ventricular end diastolic pressure	Apical four-chamber Parasternal long	E (early filling)velocity 0.67–1.3 A (atrial contraction) velocity 0.2–0.7
Left ventricular outflow	Apical five-chamber	0.7–1.1
Ascending aorta	Left ventricle apex SSN	1.0–1.7

SSN = suprasternal notch.

the flow is faster than at wider areas because the volume of blood moving across the stenosis must be the same as in other areas of the heart. Doppler measurements are taken in different windows to measure flows from different chambers and vessels. Table 5–6 shows these velocity sampling sites.

Color Doppler Flow

Color Doppler flow is a representation of flow, usually as red or blue, in regards to the direction from the transducer (Figure 5–53). Conventionally, red flow is toward the transducer and blue flow is away from the transducer. It should be noted that the colors red and blue do not necessarily signify arterial or venous flow or vessels. In addition, degrees of velocity are mapped as shades of red and blue. Variance or turbulence may be mapped as green or yellow.

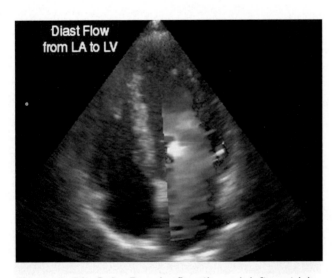

Figure 5–53. Color Doppler flow through left ventricle, apical four-chamber view (grayscale).

▶ COMMON AND EMERGENT ABNORMALITIES

Cardiac Tamponade

Cardiac tamponade is not dependent on the amount of fluid in the pericardial sac but on the rate of fluid accumulation within the pericardial sac (Figure 5–54).[27] Emergent echocardiography findings of cardiac tamponade include a pericardial effusion, right atrial collapse during systole, right ventricular diastolic collapse (see Figure 5–1 and 5–55), lack of respiratory variation in the inferior vena cava and hepatic veins, and a swinging heart.[27] Left atrial or left ventricular collapse can occur in localized left-sided compressions or in severe pulmonary hypertension.

Pericardial Effusion

Pericardial effusion is characterized by an anechoic fluid collection between the parietal pericardium and the vis-

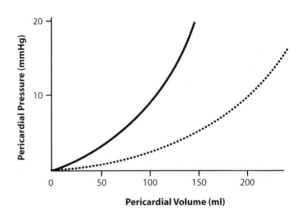

Figure 5–54. Pericardial P/V curve with acute (solid line) versus chronic effusion (dotted line).

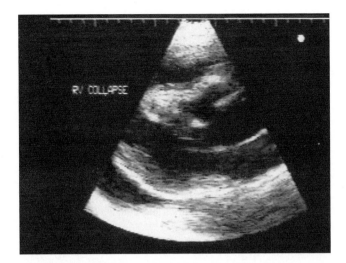

Figure 5–55. Cardiac tamponade. PSL view with diastolic collapse of right ventricle. *(Courtesy of James Mateer, MD.)*

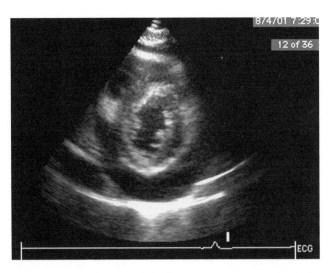

Figure 5–57. Pericardial effusion (parasternal short axis).

ceral pericardium (Figures 5–56 through 5–60). For all practical purposes, the visceral pericardium is not visualized by transthoracic echocardiography. However, the combined interface of the parietal and visceral pericardium is echogenic.

On transthoracic echocardiography, pericardial effusions can be judged as small or large. Small pericardial effusions are seen as an anechoic space less than 1 cm thick and are often localized, usually between the posterior pericardium and left ventricular epicardium. Large effusions are seen as an anechoic space greater than 1 to 2 cm thick, and usually surround the heart completely. In patients with larger effusions, the heart may swing freely within the pericardial sac (Figure 5–61).

Pericardial volumes of up to 50 cc may be normal; however, pathologic fluid collections, if slow in pro-

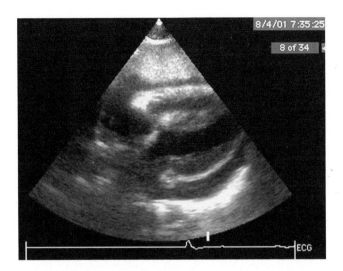

Figure 5–58. Pericardial effusion (subcostal).

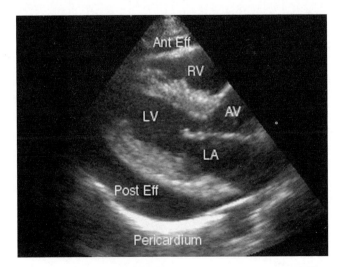

Figure 5–56. Pericardial effusion (parasternal long axis).

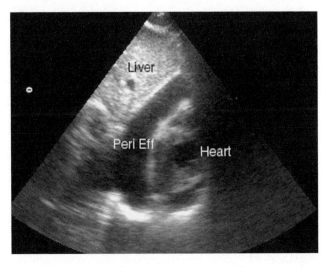

Figure 5–59. Pericardial effusion (subcostal long axis).

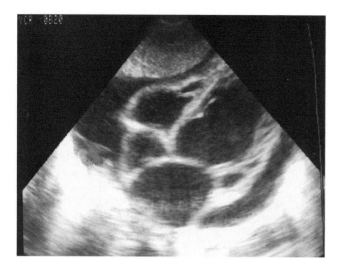

Figure 5–60. Chronic pericardial effusion (subcostal four-chamber).

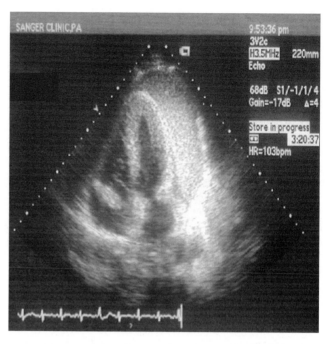

Figure 5–62. Exudative pericardial effusion.

gression, can accumulate hundreds of cubic centimeters. Pericardial fluid is usually anechoic, but exudative effusions, such as pus, malignant effusions, and blood mixed with fibrin material, can be echogenic (Figures 5–62 and 5–63). Pericardial fluid collections can be complicated by gas-collecting infections or by gas-causing tamponade (pneumopericardium).

Myocardial Ischemia

Abnormal wall motion and abnormal ventricular emptying or relaxation characterizes left ventricular dysfunction (Figure 5–64). Wall motion is graded as hypokinesis (reduced ventricular wall thickening and motion), akinesis (absent wall thickening and motion), and dyskinesia (paradoxical motion of the wall, that is, outward movement of the wall during systole).[38,68] Wall

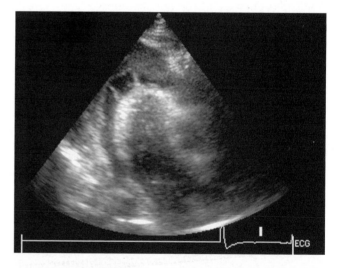

Figure 5–63. Pericardial effusion with fibrin.

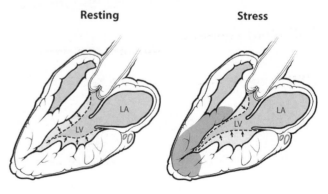

Figure 5–64. Wall motion abnormality.

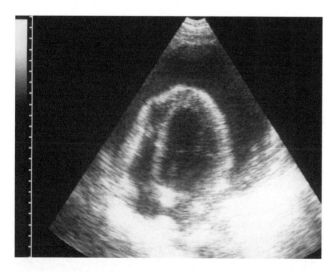

Figure 5–61. Large effusion, apical view. *(Courtesy of James Mateer, MD.)*

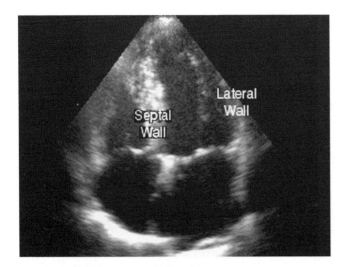

Figure 5–65. Left ventricle walls in apical four-chamber view (labeled).

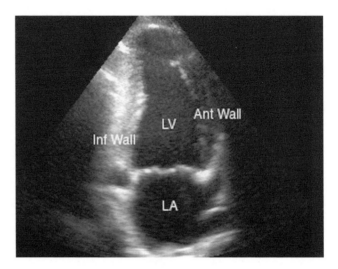

Figure 5–67. Left ventricle walls in apical two-chamber view (labeled).

motion can be characterized by gross ventricular wall dysfunction or segmental wall motion defects that usually follow the distribution of coronary blood perfusion (Figures 5–65, 5–66, and 5–67).

Echocardiography can detect ischemic changes with diastolic dysfunction, increased left ventricular diastolic filling, decreased left ventricular diastolic compliance, and reduced left ventricular diastolic compliance. As the ischemia transforms to transmural infarction, there is impaired systolic thickening, reduction in endocardial motion, and dyssynchronous contraction of myocardial segment. Left ventricular chamber size increases with reduction in systolic ejection fraction (Figure 5–68). Acute findings of left ventricular dysfunction are indicated by wall motion abnormalities, usually regional in the distribution of a coronary artery or its branch (Figure 5–69).

Chronic findings of left ventricular dysfunction, leading to a dilated cardiomyopathy, include a dilated left ventricle, global wall motion abnormalities, and immobile aortic root. The left atrium may be dilated and there may be thrombus at the apex.

Right ventricular dysfunction or dilatation may be the only sign of severe pulmonary disease, pericardial disease, or right-sided ischemia. The right ventricle is a thin and narrow chamber that is generally half the size of the left ventricle. While a dilated right ventricle may be seen in any view, the four-chamber apical or the parasternal long views may be particularly useful.

Pulmonary Embolism

Hemodynamically significant pulmonary embolism produces cardiovascular changes that may be evident by

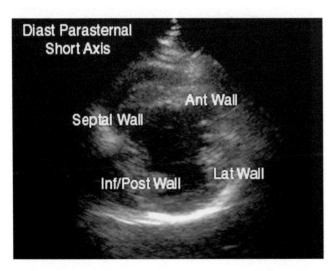

Figure 5–66. Left ventricle walls in parasternal short axis view (labeled).

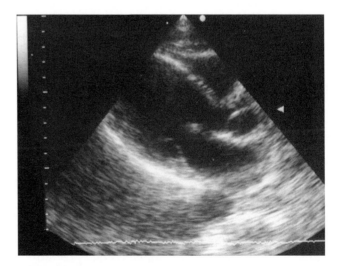

Figure 5–68. Dilated left ventricle in parasternal long axis view.

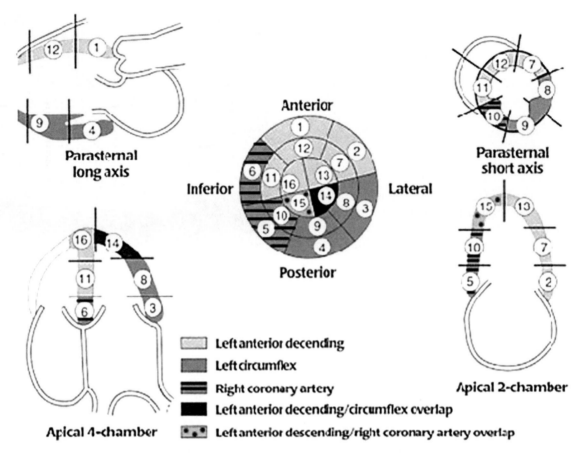

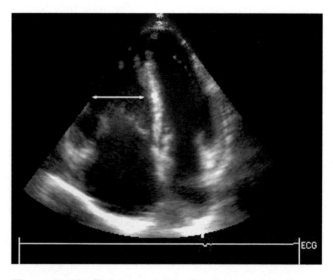

Figure 5-69. Left ventricle wall segments.

echocardiography. While direct visualization of a blood clot may be seen either in the right heart or the pulmonary arteries (by TEE approach), most echocardiographically visible changes are indirect indexes of right heart strain caused by pumping against a fixed blood clot in the lung. These changes include right ventricular dilatation, right ventricular hypokinesis, tricuspid regurgitation, and abnormal septal motion.

The normal right ventricular end diastolic diameter is 21 ± 1 mm in a parasternal long axis view. Abnormal values for this view have been documented as measurements greater than 25 to 30 mm (Figure 5-70). Normal right ventricle to left ventricle ratio, usually obtained in an apical four-chamber view, is less than 0.5. Abnormal ratios are cited from greater than 0.5 up to greater than 1.

Tricuspid regurgitation can occur when pulmonary artery pressures exceed right ventricular end diastolic (right atrial) pressures. Measurement of tricuspid regurgitation requires spectral Doppler velocity measurement and is usually obtained on the apical four-chamber view. While many healthy persons have a trivial degree of tricuspid regurgitation, up to 90% of patients with pulmonary embolism will have measurable tricuspid regurgitation.[69] Normal pulmonary artery systolic pressure is approximately 25 mm Hg in a healthy person, corresponding to a regurgitant jet of less than 2 m/s. Over 3 m/s

would correspond to a pulmonary artery pressure of 46 mm Hg. Studies using cut-off values for diagnosis of pulmonary embolism typically cite over 2.5 to 2.7 m/s as being elevated.

In addition to right heart strain, a blood clot in the lung may cause decreased venous return to the left heart.

Figure 5-70. Right ventricle enlargement. Apical four-chamber transverse diameter exceeds 2.5 cm.

This may result in decreased left ventricular end diastolic diameter as well as "paradoxical septal motion." The normal interventricular septum relaxes outward (toward the right ventricle) in diastole. With increased right end diastolic pressures and decreased left-sided pressures, abnormal motion of the septum in diastole can be visualized. While this septal deviation toward the left ventricle (also described as "septal flattening") may also be observed in systole, its presence is more pronounced in diastole and is especially prominent in the acute phase of massive pulmonary embolus.[70]

All of the indirect indicators of right heart strain may occur in other conditions aside from pulmonary embolus. These conditions include right ventricular infarct, emphysema, and primary pulmonary hypertension. It is worthwhile to note that the acutely strained right heart rarely has the muscle mass to elevate pulmonary artery pressure into the extremely high range. Values well over 40 mm Hg should suggest a chronic elevation.[69] An increase in muscle mass on measurement of the right ventricular free wall may also indicate a more chronic etiology for right ventricular strain as opposed to a thin, acutely dilated right ventricle. The normal right ventricular free wall is 2.4 ± 0.5 mm, and is generally considered hypertrophied at measurements of 5 mm and greater.[71]

Ascending Aortic Dissection

Aortic dissection is characterized by an echogenic, linear, mobile flap within the aortic lumen (Figure 5–71). Aortic dissection may be difficult to detect without TEE, and a negative transthoracic echocardiography examination does not exclude the diagnosis. On transthoracic echocardiography, the parasternal long axis view may be the only view to adequately view a flap for the first 2 cm of the ascending aorta, while the descending aorta also may be seen on the parasternal long axis view behind the left atrium. The arch of the aorta may be seen on the transthoracic echocardiography suprasternal view in a minority of patients. In addition to the linear flap,

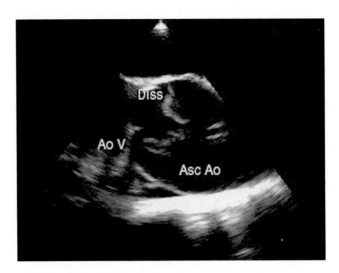

Figure 5–72. TEE longitudinal view of an aortic dissection.

aortic dissection is characterized on echocardiography as having two lumens, true and false, with different flow patterns (Figures 5–72, 5–73, and 5–74).[72,73]

Complications of aortic dissection include occlusion of any portion of the aorta or branch vessel creating ischemia or infarction of end organs.[4–7] Aortic regurgitation, coronary artery occlusion, and pericardial effusion .aortic dissection. Dissection that involves the aortic arch may manifest in acute stroke or upper extremity ischemic presentations. Dissection that starts or continues down the descending aorta may manifest in ischemia to the spinal cord, renal arteries, or lower extremities.

Traumatic Aortic Rupture

The traumatic rupture of the descending aorta usually occurs at the isthmic level of the descending aorta distal to

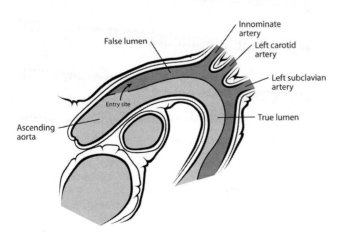

Figure 5–71. Type A aortic dissection.

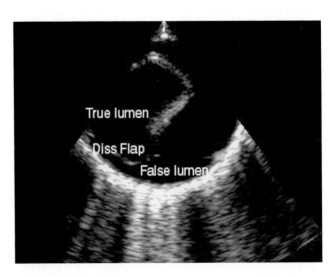

Figure 5–73. TEE transverse view of an aortic dissection with flap.

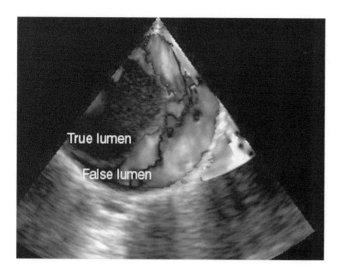

Figure 5–74. TEE aortic dissection, color Doppler with T & F lumens (grayscale).

the left subclavian artery near the ligamentum arteriosum.[73] Tears also can occur at the origin of the brachiocephalic arteries, above the diaphragm, and in the descending aorta. These branch vessel injuries may represent a limitation of TEE, as the take off and proximal extent of these vessels may not reliably be seen by TEE.

An intimal tear may be visualized with careful TEE scanning at the distal arch level. Tears may appear as small intimal flaps, a blood clot localized to the intima or the media, pseudoaneurysm, mediastinal hemorrhage, or abnormal contour of the aortic lumen. Doppler findings include similar blood flow velocities on both sides of the medial flap or a mosaic of colors surrounding the disrupted wall.

Asystole

Asystole is seen as a lack of ventricular contraction on echocardiography. Contractions of the mitral valve or atria may continue as the end of an irreversible pathologic process.[18] Pooling of blood may be seen and clots of echogenicity may form. As asystole continues, there are progressive decreased left ventricular diastolic and systolic volumes associated with rising left ventricular pressures. Ventricular wall thickness progressively increases until the heart becomes motionless.[14]

Cardiopulmonary Resuscitation

Echocardiography observed during CPR reveals left ventricular deformation and mitral valve closure during compression (systole). Mitral valve opening, aortic regurgitation, and anterior translation can be seen during the relaxation phase of CPR.[14]

► COMMON VARIANTS AND SELECTED ABNORMALITIES

Ascending Aortic Aneurysm

Dilation of the ascending aorta over 1.5 times the normal segment can reflect an aneurysmal change (Figure 5–75) aneurysm of the ascending aorta involves all layers of the vessel wall. A false aneurysm, or pseudoaneurysm, involves a penetration of the intima and media layers only. Most thoracic aneurysms are fusiform but may be saccular. Concomitant aortic dissection may occur as well.

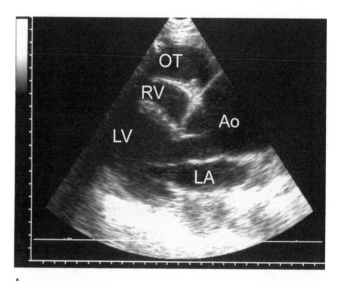

A

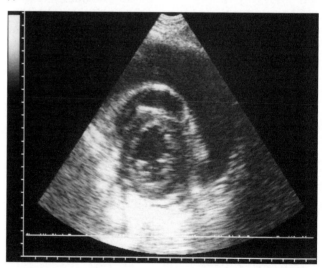

B

Figure 5–75. (A) Aortic aneurism. Parasternal long axis view shows a 6-cm. aneurism in the ascending aorta. (B) The anterior fluid is not a pericardial effusion but instead is contained within the dilated RVOT (seen best on parasternal short axis view). Ao = Aorta, LA = left atrium, LV = left ventricle, RV = right ventricle, OT = RV outflow tract. *(Courtesy of James Mateer, MD.)*

On echocardiography, the aorta is usually measured at several locations: aortic annulus, aortic leaflet tip, ascending aorta, aortic arch, and descending aorta. The length and levels of dilatation should be noted. As with the abdominal aorta, if the thoracic aorta is measured to have a diameter of 5 to 6 cm, then the patient should be referred to a cardiothoracic surgery consultant.

The role of transthoracic echocardiography is limited as the aortic arch and descending aorta cannot be fully visualized due to the depth of the aorta in many views. There is also difficulty in viewing the endothelium and poor windows due to intervening bone and air. TEE, CT, and MRI are similar in accuracy for the detection and evaluation of aortic aneurysm.

Thrombus

While a thrombus may be detected in any cardiac chamber, slow-moving chambers or lower pressures chambers are at greater risk for developing a thrombus. A thrombus can be hyperechoic, isoechoic, and even hypoechoic in appearance (Figures 5–76 and 5–77). It is usually laminated, with the layers paralleling the chamber wall. A thrombus is usually homogeneous with irregular borders, and may fill in the apices of the ventricles or attach themselves to the chamber wall or valves of the atria. Near field or time gain compensation may have to be adjusted to visualize suspected areas. A thrombus may make differentiating the pericardial layers difficult.

High-frequency transducers that utilize cardiac scanning windows close to the cardiac chamber in question provide the best imaging. While transesophageal transducers are needed for thrombus detection in atria, transthoracic scanning is adequate for thrombus detection in the ventricles. If color Doppler is available, the swirling vortices of flow may indicate the presence of a thrombus.

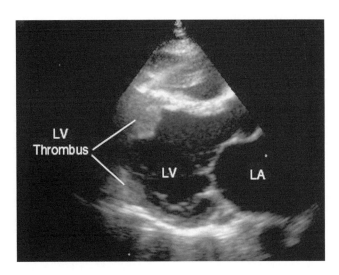

Figure 5–77. Left ventricular thrombus.

Normal structures, such as the left atrial appendages, right atrial Chiari network, and right ventricular moderator bands, must be distinguished from thrombus.

Vegetations

Findings of irregularities on valvular surfaces should prompt further investigation and consultation for more definitive diagnosis (Figures 5–78 and 5–79). Vegetations can be echogenic or isoechoic and have an irregular appearance. Vegetations may be seen on any valve leaflet or part of the apparatus. Laminated or pedunculated attachments to the leaflet of the valve should prompt suspicion. In

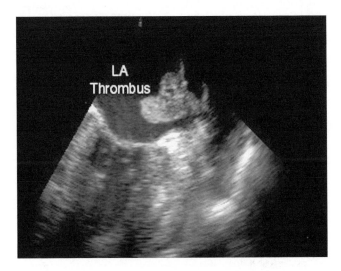

Figure 5–76. TEE left atrial thrombus.

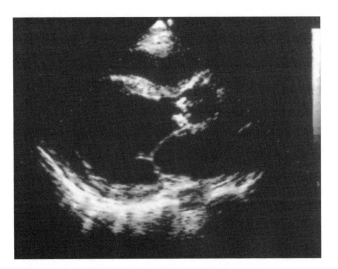

Figure 5–78. Endocarditis. Parasternal long axis view reveals echogenic mobile vegetations on the aortic valve leaflets. *(Courtesy of Lori Sens and Lori Green, Gulfcoast Ultrasound.)*

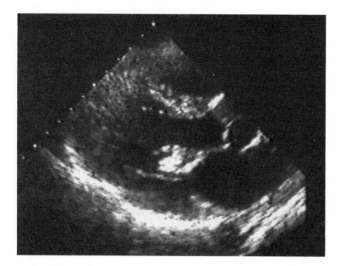

Figure 5–79. Endocarditis. Parasternal long axis view with echogenic mobile vegetations on the mitral valve leaflets. *(Courtesy of Lori Sens and Lori Green, Gulfcoast Ultrasound.)*

general, they do not restrict valvular motion. Some valve leaflets may not coapt together correctly. Typical appearance of normal valves includes smooth echogenic leaflets. All suspected cases should be referred for transesophageal imaging and formal cardiology consultation.

Valvular Abnormalities

Valvular dysfunction and structural abnormalities have not traditionally been a focal part of the emergent echocardiography examination. However, these abnormalities may present as an incidental finding and should be recognized for appropriate referral. Most hemodynamically significant valvular abnormalities will eventually cause cardiac chamber enlargement and/or hypertrophy and this may lead the sonologist to the diagnosis (Figures 5–80 and 5–81).

In the setting of acute myocardial infarction, the sudden holosystolic murmur from mitral regurgitation associated with a papillary muscle rupture can be recognized by the gross prolapse or dysfunction of the mitral valve leaflets (Figures 5–82 and 5–83). Additionally, with Doppler capability, a large ventricular septal defect may be seen with color flow imaging.

Tricuspid and pulmonary valve abnormalities usually are not of emergent significance, unless large masses or clots are obstructing them. The mitral valve in acute ischemic events or traumatic events may provide a clue to injury. Aortic valve involvement may be associated with ascending aortic abnormalities.

Myxoma

Myxomas, which are uncommon benign fibrous tumors, are usually attached to a septal wall. Myxomas are usu-

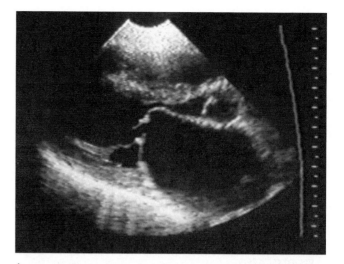

A

B

Figure 5–80. Mitral stenosis. Parasternal long axis view (A) shows the typical features: left atrium enlargement, ballooning of the valve, and a "hockey stick" appearance of the anterior leaflet. Apical four-chamber example (B) of this condition. *(Courtesy of Lori Sens and Lori Green, Gulfcoast Ultrasound.)*

ally echogenic, globular, and smooth. They are pedunculated with a stalk on one wall. They are usually seen attached to an atrial wall, most often the left atrium (Figures 5–84 and 5–85).

▶ PITFALLS

1. *Contraindications.* No contraindications exist for transthoracic echocardiography unless its use is interfering with life-saving procedures and treatments. Contraindications for TEE include coagulopathy and esophageal strictures, masses, and varices (Table 5–7).

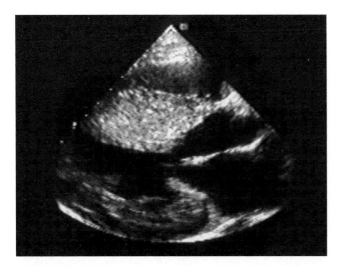

Figure 5–81. Assymetric septal hypertrophy. A thickened, echogenic left ventricle septum is noted in a parasternal long axis view in a patient with this condition (also known as IHSS). *(Courtesy of Lori Sens and Lori Green, Gulfcoast Ultrasound.)*

2. *Inability to obtain adequate views.* Some patients cannot be imaged well by transthoracic echocardiography. These include patients with subcutaneous emphysema, pneumopericardium, large anterior to posterior girth, and chest wall deformities. Suggestions for improving image acquisition include maintaining transducer contact with the chest wall, use of an adequate amount of conduction gel, use of adjacent cardiac windows, and angling, rotating, and tilting the transducer, as necessary. The patient may be turned in the left lateral decubitus position to bring the heart closer to the anterior chest wall.

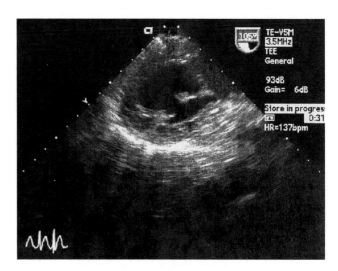

Figure 5–83. Ruptured papillary muscle. TEE view shows both ends of the disrupted papillary muscle.

a. The subcostal window is a mainstay of the emergency cardiac ultrasound examination during resuscitation of a critically ill patient. Suggestions for improving image acquisition for this view include ensuring that the transducer is at a shallow angle to the plane of the body (15° in general) and moving the transducer to the patient's right in the subxiphoid space instead of the more intuitive left side. This helps to avoid the air-filled stomach and uses the left lobe of the liver as a soft tissue window. Also, asking the patient to take a deep inspiration or, if the patient is intubated, providing a large tidal volume, will help push the heart towards the subxiphoid space.

b. The parasternal view is limited by retrosternal air or altered anatomy. Moving the transducer

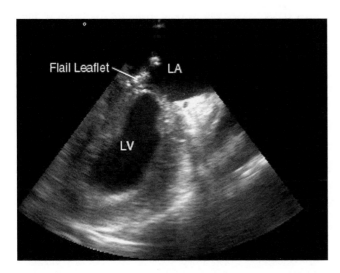

Figure 5–82. Flail leaflet. The anterior mitral leaflet is prolapsing into the left atrium on TEE long axis view.

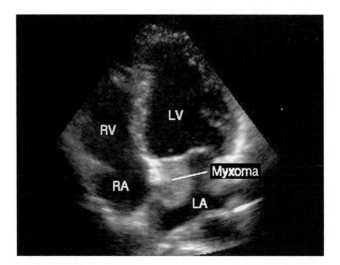

Figure 5–84. Left atrium myxoma shown on apical four-chamber view.

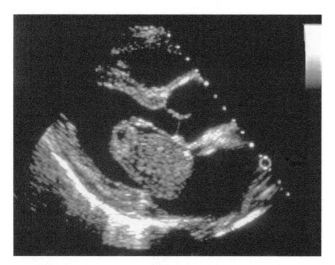

Figure 5–85. Left atrium myxoma shown on a Parasternal long axis view. The mass was mobile and prolapsing into the left ventricle on the real-time examination. *(Courtesy of Lori Sens and Lori Green, Gulfcoast Ultrasound.)*

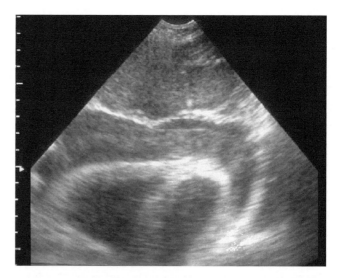

Figure 5–86. Hemopericardium. Echogenic clotted blood with a thin stripe of liquid blood above is shown in this subcostal view.

to the left, and then up and down along the anterior to posterior axis may help with obtaining a better view.

   c. The apical view may be improved by changing the angle and aiming the transducer towards the head or right elbow instead of the right shoulder.

3. *Reversed orientation.* Proper imaging requires knowledge of the orientation of the transducer. Reverse orientation may lead the sonographer to mistake ventricular hypertrophy for normal and vice versa. For example, a dilated right ventricle is an important clue for massive pulmonary embolus, but may be falsely identified as normal if a normal left ventricle is viewed on the reversed side of the monitor screen.

4. *Fluid versus blood clot or fat.* Fluid (pericardial fluid, pus, or defibrinated blood) will appear as anechoic. However, a blood clot may be echogenic initially (Figure 5–86). The borders of clot

usually have a thin anechoic stripe. Viewing other windows may assist with identifying free fluid in other aspects of the pericardium. Fat is commonly located in the anterior precordial space. In some patients, this appears hypoechoic and can be mistaken for fluid or hematoma. Clues to identification are mildly echogenic septations characteristic of fat and the lack of any dependent pooling of fluid within the posterior pericardial space (see Figure 4–24 in Trauma).

5. *Gain issues.* Gain should be adjusted to allow the posterior aspect of the heart to have the highest time gain compensation. Cardiac cavities should be anechoic and cardiac structures should be echogenic.

6. *Depth.* Depth should be adjusted to visualize posterior to the cardiac structure in question. The focus, if adjustable, should be placed at the structure of interest. Too much magnification can alter proper interpretation and too shallow depth can minimize pathologic findings.

▶ **TABLE 5–7.** PATIENT SELECTION FOR TRANSESOPHAGEAL ECHOCARDIOGRAPHY

Absolute Contraindications	Relative Contraindications
Esophageal stricture or stenosis	Respiratory failure (without definitive airway management)
Esophagitis	Upper airway abnormalities
Esophageal–gastric varices	Full stomach
Esophageal masses	Prior esophageal surgery
Esophageal diverticulum	Radiation therapy
Perforated viscus	
Gastric volvulus	
Gastrointestinal bleeding	
Combative or unwilling patient	

7. *Dynamic range.* Many machines used for emergency ultrasound applications are preset for abdominal applications; this includes the dynamic range setting. In cardiac ultrasound, the image is more black and white. The dynamic range should be lower than that in abdominal or pelvic imaging.

► CASE STUDIES

Case 1

Patient Presentation

A 33-year-old woman presented to the emergency department complaining of dizziness, which she described as a lightheaded feeling. This was associated with a 2-day history of malaise and mild dyspnea, but she denied any vaginal bleeding, melena, chest pain, headache, extremity pain, vomiting, or pelvic pain. She had given birth to a healthy son 4 weeks earlier but denied any problems with the pregnancy or delivery.

On physical examination, her blood pressure was 90/60 mm Hg, heart rate 116 beats per minute, respiratory rate 26 per/min, and temperature 99.0°F. She was in mild distress. She had no jugular venous distention. Her lungs were clear. Cardiovascular examination revealed tachycardia without murmurs or gallops. Abdominal and pelvic examinations were unremarkable. Her rectal examination revealed guaiac-negative stool. Her lower extremities revealed bilateral obese legs with no cords or erythema.

Management Course

An ECG revealed sinus tachycardia with no ischemic changes. Her chest radiograph was normal. Her hemoglobin was 14.0 g/dL and her blood sugar was 78. A urine pregnancy test was negative and urinalysis was normal. The patient continued to have a blood pressure that hovered around 85/60 mm Hg.

Due to the unexplained hypotension, a bedside echocardiogram was performed that showed a dilated right ventricle (Figure 5–87). A pericardial effusion was not present and the global left ventricular function was good. A spiral CT of the chest was ordered to evaluate for pulmonary embolus. The spiral CT was positive for a massive pulmonary embolus in both main pulmonary branches. Thrombolytic therapy was unsuccessful so the patient underwent thrombectomy on cardiac bypass. The patient was discharged in good condition after 2 weeks.

Commentary

Case 1 centered on the findings of unexplained hypotension in a previously healthy woman. The bedside echocardiographic examination revealed gross abnormalities of

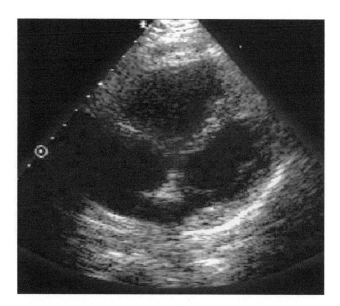

Figure 5–87. Case 1. subcostal four-chamber view shows a dilated right ventricle (chamber closest to the probe).

the right ventricle and suggested further investigation for the dilated right ventricle in a young woman. Hypotension may present with clear clinical etiologies; however, if there is no apparent cause, emergent echocardiography may provide some guidance for further evaluation.

Case 2

Patient Presentation

A 65-year-old man presented to the emergency department with a 6-h history of left-sided chest pain radiating to his left arm and mid-back. He described the pain as pressure-like and acute in onset. This episode occurred at rest. He denied any associated dyspnea, nausea, vomiting, diaphoresis, or abdominal pain. His past medical history was significant for hypertension and hypercholesterolemia. He smoked 2 packs of cigarettes per day. He could not remember the names of his medications.

On physical examination, his blood pressure was 195/110 mm Hg, heart rate 56 beats per minute, respiratory rate 18 per/min, and temperature 98°F. He appeared anxious and was in moderate distress. He demonstrated no jugular venous distention. His lungs were clear. His cardiovascular examination revealed regular rate and rhythm with no murmurs. He had equal pulses in all extremities. His abdominal and rectal examinations were normal.

Management Course

The ECG demonstrated 1 mm of ST segment elevation in the lateral leads with reciprocal changes in the inferior leads. A chest radiograph revealed a tortuous aortic silhouette, borderline widened mediastinum, and cardiomegaly. The patient was administered an aspirin tablet

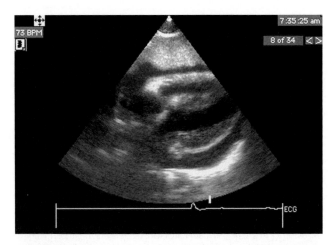

Figure 5–88. Case 2. Subcostal view reveals pericardial effusion.

and started on a nitroglycerin drip. While the nurses were preparing heparin and thrombolytic therapy, a bedside echocardiographic examination was performed because of the suspicious chest radiograph findings. This revealed a pericardial effusion on the subcostal view (Figure 5–88). The descending aorta had an echogenic linear flap on the left parasternal long view. A suprasternal view was nondiagnostic. The order for anticoagulation and thrombolysis was discontinued. The cardiologist on call was consulted and agreed with the echocardiography findings. His TEE examination demonstrated a type A aortic dissection involving the left coronary artery (Figure 5–89). The patient was transported directly to the operating room for a repair of the aortic dissection. He had an uneventful postoperative course.

Commentary

Case 2 was an example of a patient presenting to the emergency department with symptoms and an ECG sug-

gestive of an acute myocardial infarction. On bedside echocardiography, however, the patient was found to have an acute, type A aortic dissection. In this case, the emergency physician had a high index of suspicion for a concomitant aortic dissection because of the patient's history and chest radiograph findings. His access to bedside ultrasound allowed him to assess for findings consistent with other diagnoses in the differential diagnosis and avoid thrombolysis for this condition.

Case 3

Patient Presentation

A 55-year-old woman was found without a pulse on a walkway in the park. Bystander CPR was initiated immediately and a fire department automated external defibrillator shocked the patient three times after their arrival. The patient converted into a PEA rhythm. The patient was intubated and administered endotracheal epinephrine and atropine. The patient was transported to the hospital without a pulse in this PEA rhythm.

Management Course

In the emergency department, the patient was found to be in a PEA rhythm. Bilateral breath sounds were present. Routine advanced cardiac life support measures were continued. A bedside echocardiographic examination revealed ventricular activity with a dilated left ventricle and no pericardial effusion (Figure 5–90). A 2-L crystalloid fluid bolus was administered along with a dopamine IV drip. The patient regained a palpable pulse. Her blood pressure was measured at 72/48 mm Hg and an ECG revealed a large anterior wall myocardial infarction. A harsh holosystolic murmur at the left sternal border was auscultated. A TEE examination by the cardiologist consultant demonstrated a ruptured papillary muscle with prolapse of the anterior leaflet of the mitral valve (see Figure 5–83). The patient was transported to the cardiac

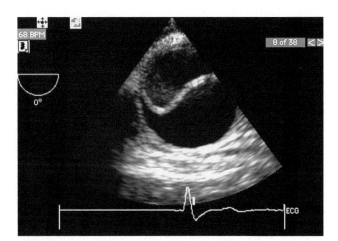

Figure 5–89. Case 2. Aorta on TEE short axis view shows the intimal flap.

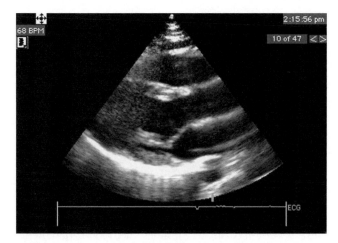

Figure 5–90. Case 3. Parasternal long axis view shows a dilated left ventricle.

catheterization laboratory where a two-vessel proximal coronary artery occlusion was discovered (99% left anterior descending artery and 95% right coronary artery). Mitral regurgitation was seen. The patient was transported to the operating room for coronary artery bypass grafting and mitral valve repair.

Commentary

Case 3 was an example of a patient presenting to the emergency department in cardiac arrest with a PEA rhythm. While no peripheral pulse was palpated, cardiac activity was seen on bedside echocardiography. The patient was treated for undifferentiated hypotension until peripheral pulses were palpated. An anterior myocardial infarction was diagnosed on the ECG. The echocardiography also revealed rupture of a papillary muscle, which was consistent with the physical examination findings of a holosystolic murmur. In this case, emergency echocardiography played a vital diagnostic role during the resuscitation of cardiac arrest.

► ACKNOWLEDGMENT

The authors would like to thank Anne Olson, Medical Illustrator at Carolinas Medical Center, for her contributions to this chapter.

REFERENCES

1. Hauser AM. The emerging role of echocardiography in the emergency department. Ann Emerg Med 1989; 18:1298–1303.
2. Oh JK, Meloy TD, Seward JB. Echocardiography in the emergency room. Echocardiography 1995;12:163–171.
3. Mangione S, Nieman L. Cardiac auscultatory skills of internal medicine and family practice trainees. A comparison of diagnostic proficiency. JAMA 1997;278:76–79.
4. Flachskampf FA, Daniel WG. Aortic dissection. Cardiol Clin 2000;18:807–817.
5. Dmowski AT, Carey MT. Aortic dissection. Am J Emerg Med 1999;17:372–378.
6. Pretre R, Segesser LK. Aortic dissection. Lancet 1997;349:1461–1464.
7. Desanctis RW, Doroghazi RM, Austen WG, et al. Aortic dissection. N Engl J Med 1987;317:1060–1065.
8. Plummer D. Principles of emergency ultrasound and echocardiography. Ann Emerg Med 1989;18:1291–1297.
9. Plummer D, Brunnette D, Asinger R, Ruiz E. Emergency department echocardiography improves outcome in penetrating cardiac injury. Ann Emerg Med 1992; 21:709–712.
10. Rose J, Bair A, Mandavia D, Kinser D. The UHP ultrasound protocol: a novel ultrasound approach to the empiric evaluation of the undifferentiated hypotensive patient. Am J Emerg Med 2001;19:299–302.
11. Blaivas M, Fox J. Outcome in cardiac arrest patients found to have cardiac standstill on the bedside emergency department echocardiogram. Acad Emerg Med 2001;8:616–621.
12. Mayron R, Gaudio FE, Plummer D, et al. Echocardiography performed by emergency physicians: impact on diagnosis and therapy. Ann Emerg Med 1988;17:150–154.
13. Salen P, O'Connor R, Passarello B, et al. Can cardiac sonography and capnography be used independently and in combination to predict resuscitation outcomes? Acad Emerg Med 2001;8:610–615.
14. Klouche K, Weil MH, Sun S, Tang W, et al. Echo–doppler observations during cardiac arrest and cardiopulmonary resuscitation. Crit Care Med 2000;28:212–213.
15. Calinas-Correia J, Phair I. Is there a pulse? Resuscitation 1999;1:201–202.
16. Amaya SC, Langsam A. Ultrasound detection of ventricular fibrillation disguised as asystole. Ann Emerg Med 1999;33:344–346.
17. Hendrickson R, Dean A, Costantino T. A novel use of ultrasound in pulseless electrical activity: the diagnosis of an acute abdominal aortic rupture. J Emerg Med 2001;21:141–144.
18. Bocka JJ, Overton DT, Hauser A. Electromechanical dissociation in human beings: an echocardiographic evaluation. Ann Emerg Med 1998;17:450–452.
19. Feigenbaum H, Waldhausen JA, Hyde LP. Ultrasound diagnosis of pericardial effusion. JAMA 1965;191:157.
20. Rozycki GS, Feliciano DV, Ochsner MG, et al. The role of ultrasound in patients with possible penetrating cardiac wounds: a prospective multicenter study. J Trauma 1999;46:543–51.
21. Pretre R, Chilcott M. Blunt trauma to the heart and great vessels. NEJM 1997;336:626–630.
22. Olsovsky MR, Wechsler AS, Topaz O. Cardiac trauma: diagnosis, management, and current therapy. Angiology 1997;48:423–427.
23. Rosenthal MA, Ellis JI. Cardiac and mediastinal trauma. Emerg Med Clinics N Am 1995;13:887–892.
24. Blaivas M, Lambert MJ. Incidence of pericardial effusion in patients presenting to the emergency department with unexplained dyspnea. Acad Emerg Med 2000;7:492.
25. Mandavia D, Hoffner R, Mahaney K, Henderson S. Bedside echocardiography by emergency physicians. Ann Emerg Med 2001;38:377–382.
26. Kimura BJ, Pezeshki B, Frack SA, DeMaria AN. Feasibility of "limited" echo imaging: characterization of incidental findings. J Am Soc Echocard 1998;11:746–750.
27. Tsang TSM, Oh JK, Seward JB. Diagnosis and management of cardiac tamponade in the era of echocardiography. Clin Card 1999;22:446–452.
28. Sagrista-Sauleda J, Angel J, Permanyer-Miralda G, Soler-Soler J. Long-term follow-up of idiopathic chronic pericardial effusion. N Engl J Med 1999;341:2054–2059.
29. Guberman BA, Fowler NO, Engel PJ, Gueron M, et al. Cardiac tamponade in medical patients. Circulation 1981;64:633–640.
30. Chenzbraun A, Pinto FJ, Schnittger I. Transesophageal echocardiography in the intensive care unit: impact on diagnosis and decision-making. Clin Card 1994;17:438–444.
31. Glance LG, Keefe DL, Carlon GC. Transesophageal echocardiography for assessing the cause of hypotension. Crit Care Med 1991;19:1213–1214.

32. Sanfilippo AJ, Weyman AE. The role of echocardiography in managing critically ill patients. J Crit Illness 1988;3:27–44.

33. Kaul S, Stratienko AA, Pollock SJ, et al. Value of two-dimensional echocardiography for determining the basis of hemodynamic compromise in critically ill patients: a prospective study. J Am Soc Echocard 1994;7:598–606.

34. Cheitlin M, Alpert JS. ACC/AHA guidelines for the clinical application of echocardiography. Circulation 1997; 95:1686–1744.

35. Rihal C, Nishimura RA, Hatle L, et al. Systolic and diastolic dysfunction in patients with clinical diagnosis of dilated cardiomyopathy. Circulation 1994;90:89–92.

36. Kumar A, Haery C, Parillo J. Myocardial dysfunction in septic shock. Crit Care Clin 2000;16:251–287.

37. Moore CL, Rose G, Taval V, et al. Determination of left ventricular function by emergency physician echocardiography of hypotensive patients. Acad Emerg Med 2001;8:266.

38. Horowitz RS, Morganroth J, Parrotto C. Immediate diagnosis of acute myocardial infarction by two-dimensional echocardiography. Circulation 1982;65:323–329.

39. Sabia P, Afrookteh A, Towuchstone DA, et al. Value of regional wall motion abnormality in the emergency room diagnosis of acute myocardial infarction. Circulation 1991;84:I85–I92.

40. Levitt MA, Promes SB, Bullock S, et al. Combined cardiac marker approach with adjunct two-dimensional echocardiography to diagnose acute myocardial infarction in the emergency department. Ann Emerg Med 1996;27:1–7.

41. Muttreja M. Clinical use of ischemic markers and echocardiography in the emergency department. Echocardiography 1999;16:187–192.

42. Mohler EM, Ryan T, Douglas SS. Clinical utility of troponin t levels and echocardiography in the emergency department. Am Heart J 1998;135:253–260.

43. Reardon MJ, Carr CL, Diamond A, et al. Ischemic left ventricular free wall rupture: prediction, diagnosis, and treatment. Ann Thorac Surg 1997;64:1509–1513.

44. Grifoni S, Olivivotto I, Pieralli F, et al. Utility of an integrated clinical, echocardiographic, and venous ultrasonographic approach for triage of patients with suspected pulmonary embolism. Am J Cardiol 1998;82:1230–1235.

45. Kasper W, Meinerz T, Henkel B, et al. Echocardiographic findings in patients with proved pulmonary embolism. Am Heart J 1986;112:1284–1290.

46. Nazeyrollas P, Metz D, Chapoutot L, et al. Diagnostic accuracy of echocardiography-doppler in acute pulmonary embolism. Int J Cardiol 1995;47:273–280.

47. Nazeyrollas P, Metz D, Jolly D, Mailler B. Use of transthoracic Doppler echocardiography combined with clinical and electrocardiographic data to predict acute pulmonary embolism. Eur Heart J 1996;17:779–786.

48. Perrier A, Tamm C, Unger P-F, et al. Diagnostic accuracy of Doppler-echocardiography in unselected patients with suspected pulmonary embolism. Int J Cardiol 1998; 65:101–109.

49. Rudoni R, Jackson RE, Godfrey G, et al. Use of two-dimensional echocardiography for the diagnosis of pulmonary embolism. J Emerg Med 2001;16:5–8.

50. Steiner P, Lund G, Debatin JF, et al. Acute pulmonary embolism: value of transthoracic and transesophageal echocardiography in comparison with helical CT. Am J Radiol 1996;167:931–936.

51. Cerel A, Burger AJ. The diagnosis of a pulmonary artery thrombus by transesophageal echocardiography. Chest 1993;103:128–131.

52. Richaud M, Drobinski G, Montalescot G, et al. Diagnosis of pulmonary embolism by transesophageal echocardiography. Eur Heart J 1992;13:1000–1001.

53. Ritoo D, Sutherland G, Samuel L, et al. Role of transesophageal echocardiography. Chest 1993;103:103–105.

54. Kasper W, Konstantinides S, Geibel A, et al. Prognostic significance of right ventricular afterload stress detected via echocardiography in patients with clinically suspected proven pulmonary embolism. Heart 1997;77:346–349.

55. Ribiero A, Lindmarker P, Johlin-Dannflet A, et al. Echocardiography Doppler in pulmonary embolism: right ventricular dysfunction as a predictor of mortality rate. Am Heart J 1997;134:45–47.

56. Konstantinides S, Geibel A, Olschewski M, et al. Association between thrombolytic treatment and the prognosis of hemodynamically stable patients with major pulmonary embolism. Circulation 1997;96:882–888.

57. Goldhaber S. Pulmonary embolism thrombolysis: broadening the paradigm for its administration. Circulation 1997;96:716–718.

58. Sommer T, Fehske W, Holzknecht N. Aortic dissection: a comparative study of diagnosis with spiral CT, multiplanar transesophageal echocardiography and MR imaging. Radiology 1996;199:347–352.

59. Maggiolini S, Bozzano A, Russo P, et al. Echocardiography-guided pericardiocentesis with probe-mounted needle: report of 53 cases. J Am Soc Echo 2001;14:821–824.

60. Tsang TSM, El-Najdawi EK, Seward JB, et al. Percutaneous echocardiographically guided pericardiocentesis in pediatric patients: evaluation of safety and efficacy. J Am Soc Echo 1998;11:1072–1077.

61. Ettin D, Cook T. Using ultrasound to determine external pacer capture. J Emerg Med 1999;17:1007–1008.

62. Macedo W, Sturmann K, Kim JM, Kang J. Ultrasonographic guidance of transvenous pacemaker insertion in the emergency department: a report of three cases. J Emerg Med 1999;17:491–496.

63. Rumberger JA, Behrenback T, Bell MR, et al. Determination of ventricular ejection fraction: a comparison of available imaging methods. Mayo Clin Proc 1997;72:860–870.

64. Jensen-Urstad K, Bouvier F, Hojer J, et al. Comparison of different echocardiographic methods with radionuclide imaging for measuring left ventricular ejection fraction during acute myocardial infarction treated by thrombolytic therapy. Am J Cardiol 1998;81:538–544.

65. Mueller X, Stauffer J, Jaussi A, et al. Subjective visual echocardiographic estimate of left ventricular ejection fraction as an alternative to conventional echocardiographic methods: comparison with contrast angiography. Clin Cardiol 1991;14:898–907.

66. Amico A, Lichtenberg GS, Resiner SA, et al. Superiority of visual versus computerized echocardiographic estimation of radionuclide left ventricular ejection fraction. Am Heart J 1989;118:1259–1265.

67. Stamm R, Carabello B, Mayers D, Martin R. Two-dimensional echocardiographic measurement of left

ventricular ejection fraction: prospective analysis of what constitutes an adequate determination. Am Heart J 1982;104:136–144.

68. Oh JK, Miller FA, Shub C, et al. Evaluation of acute chest pain syndromes by two-dimensional echocardiography: its potential application in the selection of patients for acute reperfusion therapy. Mayo Clin Proc 1987;62:59–66.

69. Come PC. Echocardiographic recognition of pulmonary arterial disease determination of its cause. Am J Med 1988;84:384–394.

70. Jardin F, Dubourg O, Gueret P, et al. Quantitative two-dimensional echocardiography in massive pulmonary embolism: emphasis on ventricular interdependence and leftward septal displacement. J Am Col Cardiol 1987;10:1201–1206.

71. Stein P, Dalen J, Goldhaber S, et al. Opinions regarding the diagnosis and management of thromboembolic disease. Chest 1996;109:233–237.

72. Vignon P, Gueret P, Vedrinne JM, et al. Role of transesophageal echocardiography in the diagnosis and management of traumatic aortic disruption. Circulation 1995;92:2959–2968.

73. Vignon P, Lang RM. Use of transesophageal echocardiography for the assessment of traumatic aortic injuries. Echocardiography 1999;16:207–219.

CHAPTER 6

Abdominal Aortic Aneurysm

David Plummer

Abnormalities of the abdominal aorta present catastrophically and with regularity to the emergency department. Patients presenting with a rupturing abdominal aortic aneurysm (AAA) may pose a diagnostic challenge to physicians. These patients may have no medical history of AAA to guide the physician. Signs and symptoms may be immediately life-threatening or deceptively nonspecific. Failure to diagnose and treat in a timely manner is most often fatal. There is no mystery why it remains the thirteenth leading cause of death in the United States despite improvements in outcome of almost every other type of cardiovascular disease.[1] Emergency and acute care physicians need to develop improved clinical strategies for rapidly diagnosing a ruptured AAA and expediting their disposition to the operating room. Few patients have as much to benefit from immediate limited bedside ultrasound as those who present with a ruptured AAA.

► CLINICAL CONSIDERATIONS

Few conditions in emergency medicine present as catastrophically as a ruptured AAA. Of the rapidly fatal disease entities that emergency and acute care physicians encounter, AAA remains one of the most misunderstood conditions.[2] These patients present a particular challenge because they require immediate diagnosis and treatment to survive. At the same time, these patients may have poor overall health, may be poor historians, are critically ill, and often have no history of AAA. The diagnosis does not reveal itself with sufficient predictive value by historical features or physical examination. Formal imaging confirmation requires time and resources, and the delay may prove fatal. Even when convinced of the diagnosis, the emergency physician must compel others to engage

in immediate surgery. Time to diagnosis and disposition has been cited as an independent predictor of survival.[2]

Multiple factors, including hypertension, smoking, age, atherosclerotic vascular disease, and genetics, interplay to cause progressive changes in the aorta's intimal and medial layer resulting in a gradual dilatation of the external diameter of the abdominal aorta. This dilatation is considered aneurysmal when the external diameter becomes 1.5 times that of normal. Therefore, adult males over 55 years of age are considered to have aneurysms when the aortic diameter reaches 3.0 cm or greater.[3] Many authors consider more liberal definitions of AAA, such as loss of the normal distal tapering of the aorta. However, patients in these earlier phases of AAA formation are at extremely low risk for rupture. The debate over these latter definitions remains academic for the physicians who face catastrophic aortic rupture almost exclusively in patients with AAA greater than 5 cm in size.

The factors predisposing to aneurysm formation make it more prevalent in the aging population. The incidence of AAA is 11% in men over 65 years of age.[4] The overall prevalence of AAA at autopsy is 1.8 to 6.6%. The average age of patients presenting with AAA is 75 years. AAA rarely presents in young adults and infants.[5] AAA is more common in men than in women with a male-to-female ratio of approximately 7:1.[5] Rupture of an AAA is the cause of death in 1.2% of males and 0.6% of females in the U.S. Over the past three decades, there has been more than a 300% increase in overall, as well as age-specific, prevalence of AAA. Because of the increasing prevalence of AAA due to an aging population, most believe that physicians will encounter an increasing number of patients arriving alive to the emergency department suffering from a ruptured AAA.

The natural history of AAA is to enlarge and rupture, resulting in death. Aneurysms enlarge at an average rate of 0.4 cm per year, with a high individual variability. The single most important factor associated with rupture is maximal cross-sectional aneurysm diameter. Although rupture under 4 cm has been described, and diagnosed in the emergency department by bedside ultrasound, this occurrence is very rare.[6] The threshold appears to occur at greater than 5.0 cm in size as these patients have a 22% risk of rupture within 2 years. The risk of rupture is estimated at 1 to 3% per year for aneurysms 4 to 5 cm, 6–11% per year for aneurysms 5 to 7 cm, and 20% per year for aneurysms greater than 7 cm. The most frequent site of aortic rupture is the left retroperitoneum (87%).[7] Retroperitoneal ruptures are usually posterior and may be contained by the psoas muscle and adjacent periaortic and perivertebral tissue. This type of rupture may occur without significant blood loss initially and the patient may be hemodynamically stable on presentation. These patients may have periaortic fluid and hematoma that is difficult to visualize by ultrasound. Rarely, an AAA may rupture into the inferior vena cava to produce an acute massive arteriovenous fistula or into the duodenum with upper gastrointestinal bleeding.[8]

Prior to rupture, most AAAs are asymptomatic. Slowly expanding aneurysms can erode adjacent structures and can be associated with vague abdominal and back discomfort. Acutely expanding aneurysms can produce severe, deep back pain or abdominal pain radiating to the back even before rupture. The expanding unruptured mass can cause a femoral neuropathy from compression of the femoral nerve against the iliopsoas muscle resulting in hip and thigh pain, quadriceps muscle weakness, and positive psoas sign. Intramural clot is a source of peripheral emboli and 5% of abdominal aneurysms present with embolization to the lower extremity. Unfortunately, because of the nonspecific signs and symptoms associated with unruptured AAA, these patients may not be diagnosed in a timely manner.[9]

Patients presenting with a ruptured AAA pose a difficult clinical problem. Often, patients have no medical history of AAA to guide the physician. Patients can experience pain in the abdomen, back, flank, or buttocks. The pain is acute, severe, and constant, and it may radiate to the chest, thigh, inguinal area, or scrotum. When back pain is present, it is most often not affected by movement. Occasionally, patients can have chest pain induced by retroperitoneal blood and this may be accompanied by nausea and vomiting. The symptom complex can result from extrinsic compression of adjacent structures. Compression may result in ureteral obstruction or vertebral erosion. The duration of symptoms before presentation is highly variable. Patients with ruptured AAA occasionally have symptoms for several days or even weeks before seeking medical attention.[10,11] A long duration of symptoms, therefore, does not exclude the diagnosis of ruptured AAA.

Unexplained syncope, hypotension, hypovolemia, or cardiovascular collapse is the most common presenting sign of ruptured AAA. Clinical shock is present between 35 and 70% of patients but tachycardia is present in only 50%. Patients who experience shock or syncope may demonstrate transient improvement in symptoms with intravenous (IV) fluids, but this will be followed by hemodynamic deterioration if diagnosis and treatment are delayed.[12,13]

The physical examination is notoriously unreliable for diagnosing ruptured AAA.[14] The familiar triad of abdominal/back pain, a pulsatile abdominal mass, and hypotension (recognized as pathognomonic of ruptured AAA) is seen in less than one-third of cases.[15] Because of the difficulty in distinguishing the abdominal aorta from surrounding structures by palpation, the size of an aneurysm may be misjudged. Hypovolemia and hypotension preclude a good pressure wave formation during cardiac systole, which diminishes the pulsatile component of the AAA. Perfusion distal to a ruptured AAA is usually well maintained through a patent, albeit ruptured, lumen; most patients have normal femoral pulses. Asymmetry or absence of femoral pulses is more commonly associated with aortic dissection. Extension of an aortic aneurysm into the iliac arteries or the presence of isolated iliac aneurysms cannot be appreciated on physical examination. Bruits arising from associated narrowed arteries may be heard but are also uncommon. Ecchymoses of the anterior abdominal wall, flank, thigh, inguinal area, scrotum, penis, perineum, or perianal area can all occur as a result of intraabdominal hemorrhage, but are distinctly uncommon. These non-specific physical findings and atypical pain profile subject patients with ruptured abdominal aortic aneurysm to a high rate of initial misdiagnosis. The most common errors include diagnosing the patient with nephrolithiasis, diverticulitis, intestinal ischemia, pancreatitis, appendicitis, perforated viscus, bowel obstruction, musculoskeletal back pain, gastrointestinal bleed, or acute myocardial infarction.

Clinicians have diagnostic imaging options for evaluating patients suspected of having a ruptured AAA. The lateral cross table lumbar spine radiograph may display an enlarged aortic profile, but is insensitive and non-specific. Computed tomography (CT) is the most precise test for imaging AAA. CT scanning with timed intravenous contrast infusion provides good images of the aorta, aortic lumen, and branch vessels. CT scanning is much more sensitive than ultrasound in detecting the location and extent of retroperitoneal hemorrhage. Rarely, the CT scan is falsely positive for rupture with an intact aneurysm. CT scanning provides more information than ultrasound about other retroperitoneal or intraperitoneal disorders and may reveal diagnoses such as pancreatitis, diverticulitis, or mesenteric ischemia. CT scanning, however, requires radiology technicians, radiologists, and significant time to perform. It also requires that the patient be moved to the radiology suite, which is often logistically difficult to perform. An IV contrast load is required for CT scanning and is harmful to hypovolemic and hemodynamically compromised patients. As a result, the patient must be stable to perform CT scanning.

Arteriography has been the historical procedure of choice for diagnosing ruptured AAA. Arteriography provides reliable information on artery lumen caliber and branch vessel disease. However, because most aneurysms contain a variable amount of thrombus lining the aneurysm wall, assessment of the size of the aneurysm by arteriography is unreliable. In addition, arteriography is expensive, invasive, and suffers the other pitfalls ascribed to CT scanning. Therefore, the patient must be stable to undergo arteriography. Magnetic resonance imaging (MRI) is also very accurate for diagnosing ruptured AAA, but patients must be stable to undergo MRI. The precise role of MRI in the evaluation of AAA continues to be investigated.

Bedside ultrasound has been reported to be 100% sensitive for the presence of an AAA.[16] Although the quality of the examination can be influenced by the expertise of the examiner, nearly 100% accuracy can be obtained even with brief training.[17] There is not much inter-observer variability, even in inexperienced hands.[18] Ultrasonography is inadequate to demonstrate the presence of extraluminal, retroperitoneal blood associated with rupture, which is found with a sensitivity approaching 4%.[19] However, in the appropriate clinical setting, the demonstration of a large AAA can be considered ruptured until proven otherwise. Therefore, these patients should undergo immediate bedside screening ultrasound on arrival.[20,21]

▶ CLINICAL INDICATIONS

The clinical indication for performing an emergency bedside ultrasound examination of the abdominal aorta is:

- Possible ruptured AAA

Abdominal Aortic Aneurysm

Patients older than 50 years of age presenting with unexplained syncope, hypotension, hypovolemia, weakness, cardiovascular collapse, abdominal pain, back pain, or flank pain require consideration of ruptured AAA. Patients who present with arterial emboli, femoral neuropathy, quadriceps pain, or retroperitoneal inflammation should also be considered. Younger patients (50 years old or less) are several times more likely to present with symptomatic AAA disease at the time of initial diagnosis.[22] Symptoms may persist for hours to days prior to presentation.

▶ ANATOMIC CONSIDERATIONS

The abdominal aorta begins where the descending aorta enters the abdomen through the aortic orifice of the diaphragm. Its maximum external diameter is normally 2.0 cm (2.1 cm for males over 55 years and 1.8 cm for females over 55 years) and tapers to approximately 1.5 cm at the distal aspect where it bifurcates. The first large branch of the abdominal aorta is the celiac trunk (Figure 6–1). The celiac trunk arises from the anterior wall of the abdominal aorta approximately 1 to 2 cm below the level of the diaphragm and gives off the following branches: splenic artery, the common hepatic artery, and left gastric artery. The splenic artery is the largest of the three arteries from the celiac trunk. It passes to the left along the superior border of the pancreas. The next aortic branch is the superior mesenteric artery (SMA), which arises from the anterior wall of the aorta approximately 2 cm from the celiac trunk. The renal arteries come off the lateral wall of the aorta just distal to the SMA, while the inferior mesenteric artery arises from the anterior wall just proximal to the bifurcation. The renal arteries and inferior mesenteric artery are often difficult to visualize. In a stable patient, the issue of renal artery involvement may be important for the surgeon. This can be estimated by noting the relative positions of the more commonly visualized structures. The SMA branches off the aorta approximately 2 cm above the renal arteries. The left renal vein is usually positioned directly anterior or slightly superior to the left renal artery. The common iliac arteries arise at the bifurcation approximately at the level of the umbilicus or the level of the fourth lumbar vertebra.

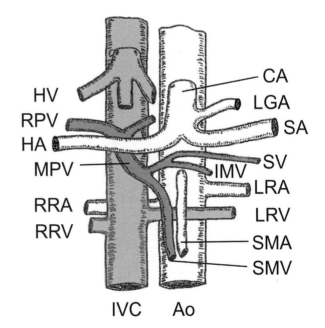

Figure 6–1. Branches of the abdominal aorta, IVC and portal veins. Ao = aorta; CA = celiac artery; HA = common hepatic artery; HV = hepatic vein; IMV = inferior mesenteric vein; IVC = inferior vena cava; LGA = left gastric artery; LRA = left renal artery; LRV = left renal vein; MPV = main portal vein; RPV = right portal vein; RRA = right renal artery; RRV = right renal vein; SA = splenic artery; SMA = superior mesenteric artery; SMV = superior mesenteric vein; SV = splenic vein.

▶ TECHNIQUE AND NORMAL ULTRASOUND FINDINGS

A curved array 2.5 to 3.5 MHz transducer should be used to examine the aorta. This allows the best balance of resolution and penetration in most adults. A lower frequency probe should be selected for greater penetration if required by a patient with a large body habitus. Standard two-dimensional grayscale imaging is adequate; additional features such as color Doppler and power Doppler are not required. A maximal depth (20 to 24 cm) should be selected along with maximum output with appropriate time gain compensation settings. Upon visualizing the aorta, the examiner should reduce depth and output.

Initially, with the patient supine, sonic conducting gel should be applied to the subxiphoid area and extended to the umbilicus in the patient's midline. The transducer should be placed in the patient's midline at the xiphoid process. Often, the examiner will have just completed a quick inspection of the heart from a subxiphoid window and the transducer will be correctly positioned on this external landmark. This position also corresponds to the first window employed in the focused assessment with sonography for trauma (FAST) examination (Figure 6–2).

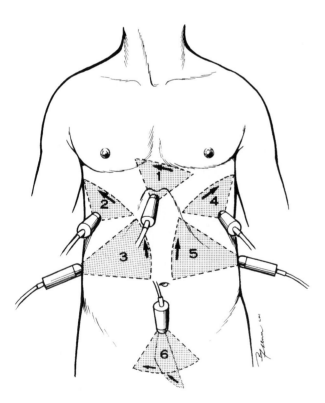

Figure 6–2. Ultrasound probe positions for the focused assessment with sonography for trauma (FAST) examination. *(Reprinted with permission from Ma OJ, Mateer JR, Ogata M, et al. Prospective analysis of a rapid trauma ultrasound examination performed by emergency physicians. J Trauma 1995;38:879–885.)*

From the subxiphoid region, the transducer angle should be swept inferiorly, positioning the plane of the transducer perpendicular to the patient in the transverse plane (Figure 6–3). The transducer position should be oriented so that the right side of the patient appears on the left side of the monitor, as viewed by the physician. The structures closest to the transducer—the skin, subcutaneous tissue, and the left lobe of the liver—should be positioned near the top of the display. The liver acts as an acoustic window to view deeper structures. The first landmark to seek is the anterior portion of the bony vertebral body. This structure presents as a densely hyperechoic, concave down, and shadow-casting arch (Figure 6–4). Two vascular anechoic structures present themselves immediately anterior to the vertebral body. Because they are closer to the transducer, they are displayed nearer the top of the screen. The aorta is on the patient's left and the inferior vena cava on the patient's right. In addition, the aorta can be differentiated from the inferior vena cava by its thicker, white walls and by its pulsatile motion as opposed to the undulating motion of the inferior vena cava. The aorta is not compressible with gentle transducer pressure, whereas the inferior vena cava is compressible. The normal aortic lumen is anechoic, whereas a circumferential thrombus is typically moderately echogenic.

Anterior to posterior (AP) diameter from outer wall to outer wall in transverse section provides the most accurate measurement of the external diameter of the abdominal aorta. The resulting image in patients with a rupture is usually immediately positive for a large AAA. With an average external diameter of over 7.5 cm and a range of up to 14 cm, an AAA is often clear immediately on initial probe application. This AP dimension is the most reliable orientation for assessing maximum diameter and avoids the "cylinder tangent" error associated with the longitudinal view and described below. If a careful measurement is required, then the freeze-frame should be used along with

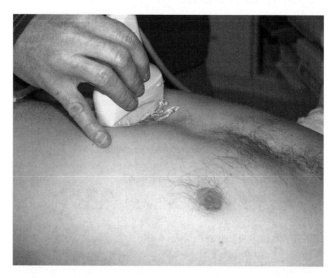

Figure 6–3. Initial transducer position for rapid imaging of the abdominal aorta.

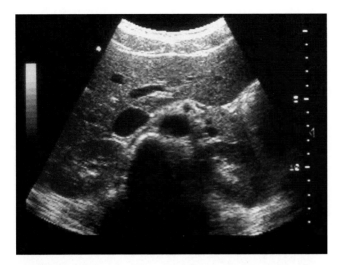

Figure 6–4. Transverse view of the upper abdomen. By using a large convex probe in a thin patient, the relative positions of the anatomic landmarks can be visualized. The liver serves as an acoustic window to the structures below. The aorta and IVC are immediately above the spine (Large, dark shadow at the bottom of the image). Both kidneys are seen adjacent to the spine. *(Courtesy of Lori Sens and Lori Green, Gulfcoast Ultrasound.)*

the caliper measurement software. If at any point during the examination an AAA is clearly demonstrated and rupture is suspected, then a surgeon should be consulted immediately. Further examination for the presence and extent of any free intraabdominal fluid can be performed via the windows described in the FAST examination.

When time allows, the examination should be completed by visualizing the entire length of the abdominal aorta. Keeping the transducer perpendicular to the patient in the transverse plane, the transducer should be moved from xiphoid to umbilicus. Bowel gas in the unprepared patient that interposes between the transducer and the aorta will obliterate the image. Bowel gas can be displaced to the right and left with gentle pressure applied through the transducer in an anterior to posterior direction. Landmark structures that ensure an adequate segment of the aorta has been imaged include the celiac trunk (Figure 6–5A), SMA (Figure 6–5B), and the bifurcation of the aorta (Figure 6–5C). Arising from the aorta anteriorly, the celiac trunk and the SMA can be visualized in the epigastrium. In this transverse plane, the celiac trunk, left gastric artery, SMA, and common hepatic artery form a characteristic appearance. Careful inspection reveals the splenic vein visualized anterior to the SMA, and the left renal vein can

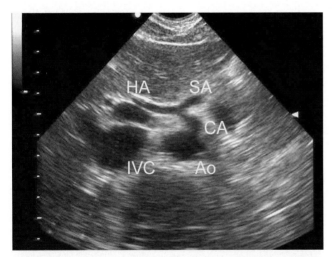

A

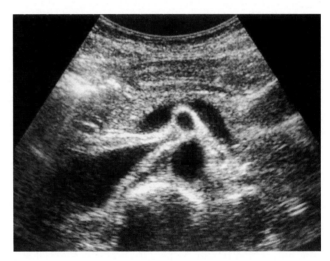

B

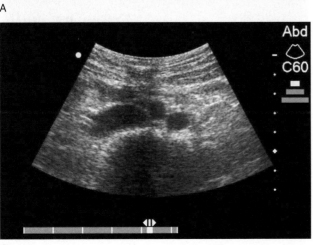

C

Figure 6–5. Transverse views of the abdominal aorta. (A) Level of the celiac artery. Ao = aorta; CA = celiac artery; HA = common hepatic artery; IVC = inferior vena cava; SA = splenic artery. (B) Level of the superior mesenteric artery (SMA). Because the SMA is surrounded by fat, it is usually outlined by a thick brightly echogenic wall. The aorta is immediately below the SMA and the splenic vein is wrapped around and above the SMA. *(Courtesy of Masaaki Ogata, MD.)* (C) Bifurcation level. Vascular structures from the left side of the image to the right include the IVC, right common iliac artery and left common iliac artery. *(Courtesy of James Mateer, MD.)*

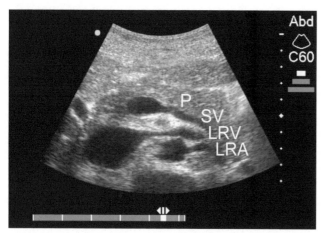

Figure 6–6. Transverse view of the upper abdominal aorta and surrounding vessels. LRA = left renal artery; LRV = left renal vein; P = pancreas; SV = splenic vein. The left renal vein usually courses from the IVC to the kidney by passing between the SMA and aorta. The left renal artery may be visualized in a thin patient without overlying gas. *(Courtesy of James Mateer, MD.)*

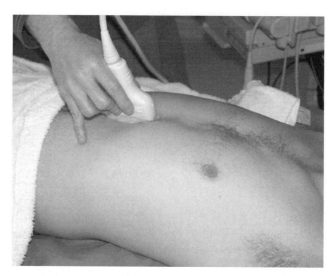

Figure 6–7. Transducer position for longitudinal views of the aorta.

be seen interposed between the aorta and the SMA (Figure 6–6). The pancreas can be visualized just distal to the origin of the SMA in transverse section, anterior to the splenic vein. Calcified plaques may be appreciated along the wall of the aorta and may produce shadowing; shadows will also result from the lateral cystic shadow (edge artifact). The aortic bifurcation is visualized at the L4 level, near the umbilicus externally. Adequate visualization of this entire length of abdominal aorta is required to exclude AAA. Should its diameter be adequately visualized and appear normal over this length, then this excludes a ruptured AAA with an essentially 100% negative predictive value.

To visualize the aorta in long axis, or sagittal plane, the examiner should return to the starting point at the subxiphoid area. First, the aorta should be visualized in short axis and centered in the sector. The transducer should be rotated on its long axis while maintaining the aorta in the center of the sector (Figure 6–7). While rotating, the aorta will appear to elongate until 90° of rotation is reached. At this point, the beam plane will be in the sagittal plane, and the aorta will be visualized in the long axis (Figure 6–8). Proper image orientation requires the patient's head at the left of the screen and the feet at the right. This will yield an aortic image coursing on the screen from left lower to right upper; as the aorta becomes more superficial it progresses distally. Proper visualization will include the celiac trunk and the SMA. The SMA arises from the aorta anteriorly and lies immediately anterior to the longitudinal aorta. The advantage of the long axis view is that it is more intuitive to interpret than the transverse view.

If helpful, the inferior vena cava can be intentionally visualized using the same windows. The examiner should return to subxiphoid area with the transducer in short axis orientation. The inferior vena cava will appear on the patient's right of the aorta and anterior to the shadow-casting vertebral body. The transducer should be rotated 90° to visualize the inferior vena cava in long axis, again with the deeper, proximal portion on the examiner's left on the monitor (Figure 6–9). The right renal artery may be seen posterior to the inferior vena cava.

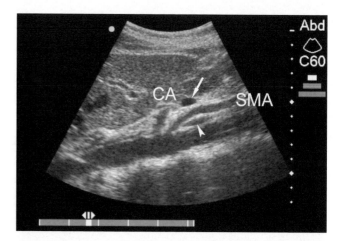

Figure 6–8. Longitudinal view of the abdominal aorta. The celiac artery (CA) is the first vessel to branch off the aorta. The superior mesenteric artery (SMA) is immediately below the celiac artery and courses parallel to the aorta. The splenic/portal vein (arrow) and the left renal vein (Arrowhead) can be seen in short axis immediately above and below the SMA. *(Courtesy of James Mateer, MD.)*

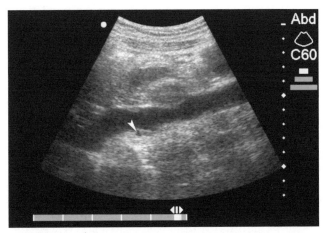

Figure 6–9. Longitudinal view of the inferior vena cava (IVC). The position of the right renal artery is indicated (arrowhead) as it courses behind the IVC. *(Courtesy of James Mateer, MD.)*

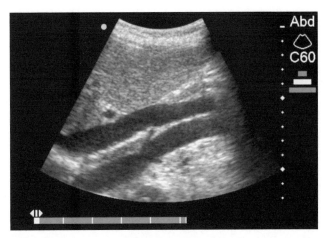

Figure 6–11. Coronal view of the aorta. The IVC is above the aorta in this right coronal view. Both renal arteries are seen branching off the aorta at a 45° angle (forming an arrowhead appearance in the mid aorta). The renal arteries are not routinely visualized in this view. *(Courtesy of James Mateer, MD.)*

Obesity and bowel gas diminish the chances of a quality examination. The physician can utilize other techniques to partially compensate for this. First, the patient can be rolled into a left lateral decubitus position (Figure 6–10). This will allow bowel contents and pannus to fall to the patients left and not be interposed between the transducer and the aorta. Second, the transducer can be placed in the right anterior axillary line and, using the hepatic acoustic window, the aorta can be imaged in the coronal plane. The examination should be initiated with the image display at maximum depth. This will yield an image with the inferior vena cava toward the top of the screen and the aorta lying deeper (Figure 6–11).

▶ COMMON AND EMERGENT ABNORMALITIES

1. *Abdominal aortic aneurysm.* The primary abnormality that the physician seeks is aneurysmal enlargement of the abdominal aorta. This is most commonly visualized in the transverse view as an aorta greater than 3.0 cm in diameter (Figure 6–12). Aneurysmal dilation is usually fusiform, resulting in a uniform symmetric concentric enlargement of the circumference (Figure 6–13). Localized out-pouching of a segment of the aortic wall results

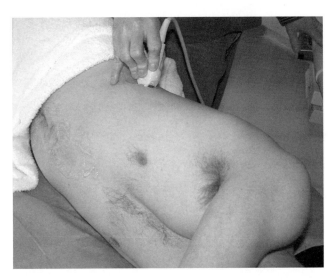

Figure 6–10. Transducer position for coronal views of the aorta.

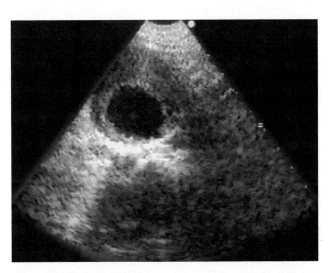

Figure 6–12. Transverse view of an AAA. This fusiform aneurism demonstrates a thickened wall secondary to mural thrombus.

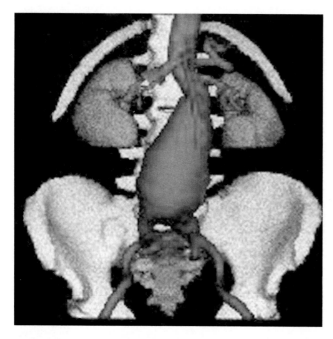

Figure 6–13. Fusiform aneurysm. Aneurysmal dilation is usually fusiform, resulting in a uniform symmetric, concentric enlargement of the circumference.

in saccular aneurysm formation which is much less common (Figure 6–14). Aneurysmal dilatation is most often confined to the infrarenal aorta and usually terminates proximal to the bifurcation. Contiguous thoracoabdominal aneurysms occur in a minority of cases (2%) and involve the thoracic aorta in addition to the abdominal aorta, including the segment involving the celiac, supe-

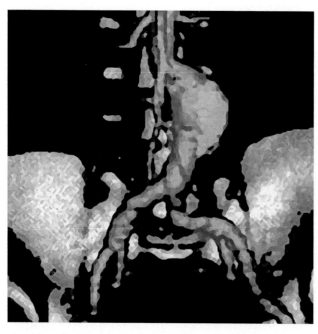

Figure 6–14. Localized out-pouching of a segment of the aortic wall results in saccular aneurysm formation.

rior mesenteric, and renal arteries. The iliac arteries are involved in 40% of patients with AAA, and occasionally, iliac artery aneurysms occur in an isolated fashion (Figure 6–15).

2. *Circumferential thrombus.* With increasing diameter, the laminar flow rate decreases at the periphery, resulting in blood stagnation and thrombus formation. This circumferential thrombus is well visualized by ultrasound (see Figure 6–12). Thrombus exists in ruptured as well as intact AAA. It is not an indication of rupture or dissection, and is not a false lumen.

3. *Hemoperitoneum.* Rupture into the peritoneal cavity can present with acute hemoperitoneum (Figure 6–16) that may be visualized with the right intercostal oblique window of the FAST examination (see Figure 6–2) or other windows.

► COMMON VARIANTS AND SELECTED ABNORMALITIES

1. *Tortuosity of the aorta.* Variations of the position and size of vessels are common. The aorta often becomes tortuous with age. This can cause diffi-

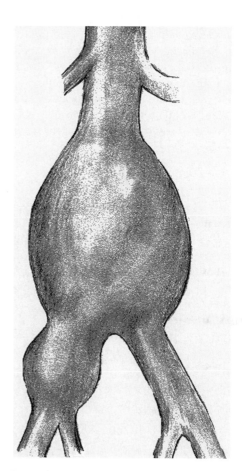

Figure 6–15. Iliac artery aneurism. A fusiform AAA with extension into the right common iliac artery is illustrated.

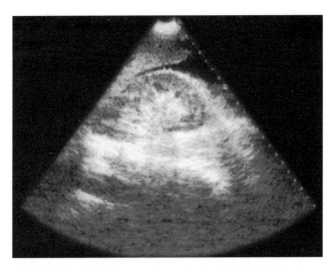

Figure 6–16. Coronal view of the right kidney area demonstrates free intraperitoneal fluid.

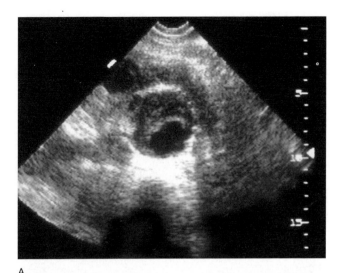

A

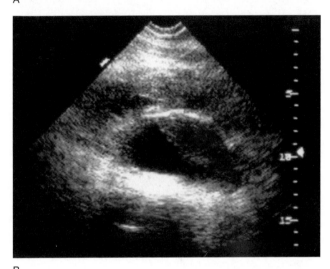

B

Figure 6–18. Contained rupture of an AAA. (A) Transverse view reveals an AAA with mural thrombus. Wrapping around the anterior aorta is a hypoechoic mixed density area (from contained hemorrhage and hematoma). (B) Longitudinal view of the same patient. *(Courtesy of James Mateer, MD.)*

culty with following the course of the vessel and finding the correct plane for transverse and longitudinal views (Figure 6–17).

2. *Contained aortic rupture.* A contained rupture of an AAA is not commonly diagnosed with ultrasound. When present, it may be seen as a hypoechoic mixed density area (from contained hemorrhage and hematoma) surrounding the aorta (Figure 6–18).

3. *Hydronephrosis.* A large AAA can cause secondary complications by compressing surrounding structures. Compression of the left ureter can lead to hydronephrosis and eventually to a perinephric urinoma from calyceal rupture (Figure 6–19).

4. *Acute abdominal aortic dissection.* This disease entity may be confused with ruptured AAA and can occur with or without a coexisting aneurysm. Only 2 to 4% of patients with an aortic dissection experience it in the abdominal aorta. The presenting symptoms are similar to those seen in ruptured AAA.[23]

5. *Aortovenous fistula.* Formation of an aortovenous fistula occurs when an AAA ruptures into an adjacent vein; the left renal vein or the inferior vena cava is involved most often. Because these aneurysms are usually large (11-13 cm on average), a pulsatile mass can often be palpated on examination.[24] The presenting symptoms are similar to those seen in AAA rupture. An ultrasound examination demonstrating a large AAA, along with a

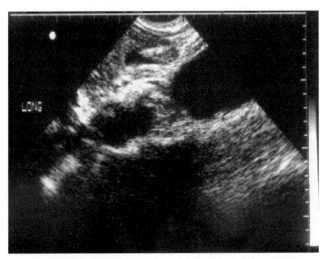

Figure 6–17. Longitudinal view of an AAA. The normal distal tapering of the aorta is reversed. The echogenic area within the aorta is not a clot, but is the sidewall of the vessel due to tortuosity. *(Courtesy of James Mateer, MD.)*

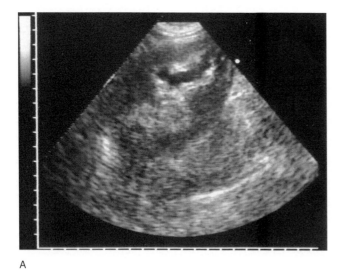

A

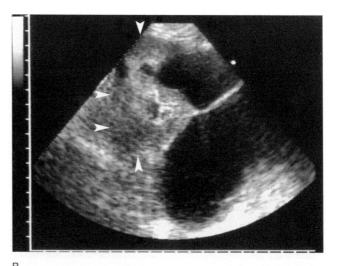

B

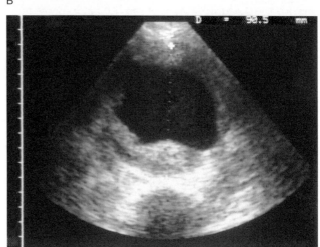

C

Figure 6–19. Hydronephrosis from AAA. (A) An anterior coronal view of the inferior pole of the left kidney reveals mild hydronephrosis. (B) A posterior coronal view of the lower flank (angled superiorly) in the same patient shows a septated fluid collection that communicates with the collecting system of the kidney. The renal borders are outlined (Arrowheads). The contained fluid collection is a perinephric urinoma secondary to ureteral compression with calyceal rupture from a large (9.5 cm) AAA (C). *(Courtesy of James Mateer, MD.)*

CT scan documenting a retroaortic left renal vein and an IVP showing absence of left renal filling, may help confirm the diagnosis.

▶ PITFALLS

1. *Contraindication.* The only absolute contraindication to performing this examination is if it delays clearly indicated, immediate surgical intervention.
2. *Over-reliance on examination.* The finding of an enlarged aorta alone is not sufficient to diagnose rupture of the abdominal aorta. There are no reliable ultrasound findings of retroperitoneal hematoma associated with the most common form of AAA rupture. The finding of AAA accompanied by other clinical manifestations, such as acute hemodynamic compromise, strongly suggest the diagnosis of rupture. When hemodynamically stable,

contained rupture may be diagnosed by definitive imaging prior to intervention.
3. *Errors in imaging.* Two common errors in imaging should be avoided. First, the physician must take care not to inadvertently sweep the plane of the beam into a right parasagittal plane, which may result in a long axis view of the inferior vena cava (Figure 6–20). The inferior vena cava here is thin walled, easily compressed, and can be mistaken for the abdominal aorta. The examiner can avoid this error by visualizing the celiac trunk and SMA, ensuring proper orientation over the aorta (Figure 6–21). The second possible error can result from the cylinder tangent effect. In unprepared patients, limited window accessibility may result in a situation in which the plane of the beam enters the cylinder of the aorta at a tangent. In this event, the ultrasound machine will display an incorrect AP diameter (Figure 6–22). This is not an artifact error but an opera-

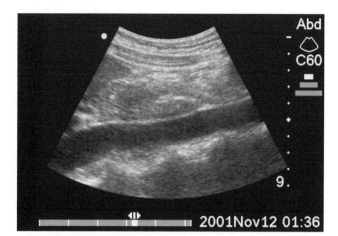

Figure 6–20. Long axis view of the IVC. Note the thinner walls compared to the aorta, and the lack of branching vessels. *(Courtesy of James Mateer, MD.)*

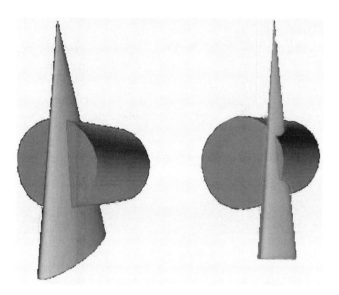

Figure 6–22. The cylinder tangent effect. A longitudinal beam slice through the center of the vessel will show the maximum diameter. An off center slice will show a reduced diameter.

tor error and should be kept in mind if assessing AP diameter by sagittal views only.

4. *Patient factors limiting imaging.* Obesity and bowel gas always render ultrasound imaging more difficult. Failure to determine the involvement of the major branches of the aorta makes operative planning more difficult for the surgeon.

5. *Failure to consider the diagnosis.* When elderly patients present with the common complaints of back pain or flank pain, the diagnosis of AAA must be considered. A common misdiagnosis for AAA is renal colic. Since AAA can present with hydronephrosis (see Figure 6–19), the aorta should also be imaged in older patients undergoing ultrasound examination for renal colic.

▶ CASE STUDIES

Case 1

Patient Presentation

A 65-year-old man presented to the emergency department after a witnessed syncopal episode. Upon awaking in the morning, the patient complained of feeling weak and constipated. His wife witnessed him go into the bathroom and suffer a sudden collapse. The patient had a history of well-controlled hypertension.

On physical examination, the patient was awake, alert and oriented. His blood pressure was 100/50 mm Hg; pulse, 110 beats per min; respirations, 18 per min; temperature, 98.9°F. He appeared pale and slightly diaphoretic. His lungs were clear to auscultation, neck veins flat, and abdomen soft and non-tender with no peripheral edema. The remainder of his physical examination was unremarkable.

Management Course

On arrival, 2 large-bore IVs were established in the upper extremities while the primary examination was simultaneously performed. As part of his secondary survey, a rapid cardiac view by the subcostal window revealed a hyperdynamic heart. Repositioning of the transducer immediately revealed an enlarged abdominal aorta with an AP diameter of 7.1 cm (Figure 6–23). There was no free intraperitoneal fluid or fluid in either hemithorax. Surgical consultation was initiated.

Reassessment revealed a decline in blood pressure to 80/50 mm Hg. No other diagnostic maneuvers were

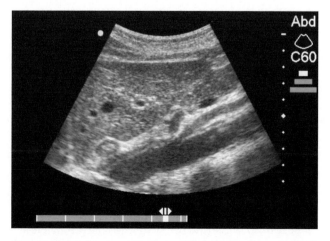

Figure 6–21. Long axis view of the aorta. A magnified view of the upper abdominal aorta shows the characteristic thick echogenic walls and anterior branching vessels. *(Courtesy of James Mateer, MD.)*

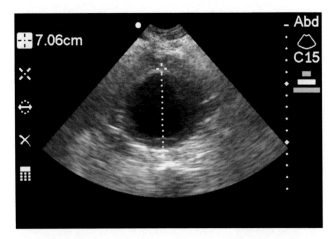

Figure 6–23. Transverse view of an AAA. The recorded measurement of 7.06 cm is less than the actual size because the caliper does not include the anterior wall of the aneurism. For accurate measurement of an AAA, the calipers should be placed on the anterior and posterior outer walls. *(Courtesy of James Mateer, MD.)*

employed and the patient was transported directly to the operating room for exploratory laparotomy. Operative findings included a 7.5 cm AAA that was successfully grafted.

Commentary

Case 1 was an example of a patient presenting to the emergency department with hemodynamic alteration from a rupturing AAA. This type of pre-hospital syncope followed by near-normalization of vital signs with subsequent decline in perfusion parameters is one of the most common presentations for ruptured AAA. This patient exemplifies an unstable hemodynamic profile that requires limited diagnostic evaluation and rapid surgical intervention. It is important to note that the same ultrasound was used to demonstrate marked global hyperkinesis of the heart, essentially excluding left ventricular failure as a cause of gradual hemodynamic decline. This was prior to performing either an electrocardiogram or chest radiograph.

Case 2

Patient Presentation

An obese 61-year-old man presented to the emergency department with acute onset of chest pain and shortness of breath. Pre-hospital management included detecting ST segment abnormalities on cardiac monitoring. The patient was given nitroglycerin 0.4 mg PO and aspirin 325 mg PO.

On physical examination, his blood pressure was 150/60 mm Hg, pulse was 110 beats per min; respirations were 18 per min. He was awake, alert, and complaining of increasing epigastric pain. The lungs were clear, neck veins were flat, and there was no peripheral edema. The cardiac sounds were normal with no murmur and peripheral pulses were symmetric.

Management Course

Electrocardiogram revealed 3 mm ST elevation in leads II, III, and AVF. An IV line was established and morphine sulfate 4 mg IV relived much of the patient's distress. Chest radiograph was non-specific. The patient had return of pain and IV thrombolytic therapy was initiated for an acute myocardial infarction. Approximately 12 min after thrombolytic therapy was initiated, the patient became pale and diaphoretic. Blood pressure was 90/40 mm Hg. A subxiphoid window revealed a hyperkinetic heart with no evidence of left ventricular failure or pericardial effusion. Immediate abdominal sonography revealed an enlarged abdominal aorta measuring 8.1 cm in AP diameter with no evidence of free intraperitoneal fluid. Thrombolytic therapy was discontinued and immediate surgical consultation was obtained. Medical records revealed evidence of abdominal aortic enlargement documented 4 years earlier and lost to follow-up. The patient was transported to the operating room where an 8-cm ruptured AAA was repaired. Serial electrocardiograms and cardiac markers revealed a concomitant acute myocardial infarction. The patient displayed no evidence of left ventricular failure on long-term follow-up.

Commentary

Case 2 in an example of a ruptured AAA presenting in a patient with significant comorbidity and appearing clinically as an isolated myocardial infarction. A significant number of patients suffering ruptured AAA have associated myocardial ischemia.[14] Patients with ruptured AAA may present with any combination of associated and often distracting clinical manifestations. The low threshold to apply aortic imaging in the emergency department led to the discovery of the AAA, thus allowing for timely intervention.

REFERENCES

1. Law MR, Morris J, Wald NJ. Screening for abdominal aortic aneurysms. J Med Screening 1994;1:110–116.
2. Rothrock S, Green S. Abdominal aortic aneurysms: current clinical strategies for avoiding disaster. Emerg Med Rep 1994;15:1–8.
3. Collin J, Araujo L, Walton J, et al. Oxford screening program for abdominal aortic aneurysm in men aged 65 to 74 years. Lancet 1988;2:613–615.
4. Bengtsson H, Bergqvist D, Sternby NH. Increasing prevalence of abdominal aortic aneurysms. A necropsy study. Eur J Surg 1992;158:19–23.
5. Sinzobahamvya N, Afriyie K, Shah S, et al. Ruptured abdominal aortic aneurysm in a 24-year-old African woman.

Unusual presentation—unknown etiology. Acta Chir Belg 1986;86:245–247.

6. Miller J. Small ruptured abdominal aneurysm diagnosed by emergency physician ultrasound. Am J Emerg Med 1999;17:174–175.

7. Burger T. Ruptured infrarenal aortic aneurysm—a critical evaluation. Vasa 1999;28:30–33.

8. Witkiewicz W, Czarnecki K. Primary aorto-intestinal fistula as a diagnostically difficult complication of ruptured abdominal aortic aneurysm. Wiad-Lek 1992; 45:852–856.

9. Craig SR, Wilson RG, Walker AJ, et al. Abdominal aortic aneurysm: still missing the message. Br J Surg 1993; 80: 450–452.

10. Harris LM, Faggioli GL, Fiedler R, et al. Ruptured abdominal aortic aneurysms: factors affecting mortality rates. J Vasc Surg 1991;14:812–815.

11. Darling RC, Messina CR, Brewster DC, et al. Autopsy study of unoperated abdominal aortic aneurysms: the case for early resection. Circulation 1977;56:161–164.

12. Marston WA, Ahlquist R, Johnson G, et al. Misdiagnosis of ruptured abdominal aortic aneurysms. J Vasc Surg 1992;16:17–20.

13. Lederle FA, Parenti CM, Chute EP. Ruptured abdominal aortic aneurysm: the internist as diagnostician. Am J Med 1994;96:163–165.

14. Johnson GA. Aortic dissection and aneurysm. In: Tintinalli JE, ed. Emergency medicine: a comprehensive study guide, 5th ed. New York: McGraw-Hill, 2000; 412–416.

15. Kiell CS, Ernst CB. Advances in the management of abdominal aortic aneurysm. Adv Surg 1993;26:73–76.

16. LaRoy LL, Cormier PJ, Matalon TA, et al. Imaging of abdominal aortic aneurysms. AJR 1989;152:785–790.

17. Kuhn M, Bonnin RL, Davey MJ, et al. Emergency department ultrasound scanning for abdominal aortic aneurysm: accessible, accurate, and advantageous. Ann Emerg Med 2000;36:219–223.

18. Pleumeekers HJ, Hoes AW, Mulder PG, et al. Differences in observer variability of ultrasound measurements of the proximal and distal abdominal aorta. J Med Screen 1998;5:104–108.

19. Shuman WP, Hastrup WJR, Kohler TR, et al. Suspected leaking abdominal aortic aneurysm: use of sonography in the emergency room. Radiology 1988;168:117–119.

20. Swedenborg J. Optimal method for imaging of abdominal aortic aneurysms. Ann Chir Gynaecol 1992; 81:158–160.

21. LaRoy LL, Cormier PJ, Matalo TA, et al. Imaging of abdominal aortic aneurysms. Am J Roentgenol 1989;152;785–792.

22. Muluk SC, Gertler JP, Brewster DC, et al. Presentation and patterns of aortic aneurysms in young patients. J Vasc Surg 1994;20:880–884.

23. VanMaele RG, DeBock L, Van Schil PE, et al. Limited acute dissections of the abdominal aorta: report of 5 cases. J Cardiovasc Surg 1992;33:298–304.

24. Lanne T, Bergqvist D. Aortocaval fistulas associated with ruptured abdominal aortic aneurysms. Eur J Surg 1992;158:457–465.

CHAPTER 7

Hepatobiliary

Simon Roy

Over the past 15 years, specific uses for ultrasonography in the emergency setting have evolved. These uses include detection of hemoperitoneum and hemopericardium in trauma, confirmation of intrauterine pregnancy, evaluation of aortic aneurysm, and others.[1–3] While limited bedside ultrasonography of the hepatobiliary system is an evolving entity, it clearly has direct utility in a growing number of specific clinical situations.

► CLINICAL CONSIDERATIONS

The diagnostic tools aiding clinicians in the evaluation of acute hepatobiliary disease include ultrasonography, computed tomography (CT) scan, endoscopic retrograde cholangiopancreatography (ERCP), oral cholecystography, and radionuclide studies (HIDA scan).[4–6] The major advantage of ultrasonography over all of these other modalities lies in the ability of the clinician to rapidly obtain diagnostic information without the time delays inherent in performing the other diagnostic studies mentioned. An ERCP requires involvement of a consultant and, often, conscious sedation and its associated risks. Radionuclide methods expose patients to radiation, an obvious concern in pregnant patients. Oral cholecystography requires oral intake without emesis and a subsequent time delay. CT scanning is frequently less sensitive and less informative than ultrasonography for a variety of hepatobiliary diseases, especially those involving cholelithiasis.

► CLINICAL INDICATIONS

The clinical indications for performing an emergency bedside hepatobiliary ultrasound examination by clinicians include:

- Evaluation of possible biliary colic
- Evaluation of possible cholecystitis
- Evaluation of acute jaundice
- Evaluation of possible hepatomegaly
- Detection and evaluation of ascites

Evaluation of Possible Biliary Colic

Gallstones are prevalent in most Western countries. In the United States, at least 20% of women and 8% of men over 40 years of age have been found to have gallstones at autopsy. It is estimated that 20 million persons in the United States have gallstones.[7]

Gallstones usually produce symptoms by causing obstruction or inflammation following their migration into the cystic duct or common bile duct. The most characteristic symptom of gallstone disease is described as biliary colic. This visceral pain is typically a severe and steady ache in the right upper quadrant or epigastric area of the abdomen. For patients with gallstones, the cumulative risk for the development of symptoms or complications requiring surgery is relatively low—10% at 5 yr, 15% at 10 yr, and 18% at 15 yr. Patients remaining asymptomatic for 15 yr have been found unlikely to develop symptoms during further follow-up.[7]

Biliary colic remains a clinical diagnosis and not a sonographic diagnosis. In an emergency or acute care setting, patients who present with right upper quadrant abdominal pain commonly require an ultrasound examination as part of their diagnostic evaluation. In cases where acute symptoms resolve with symptomatic treatment and the clinical presentation is not consistent with cholecystitis (i.e., no fever or leukocytosis), an emergency hepatobiliary ultrasound examination may not be required but may be beneficial for expediting diagnosis, disposition, or follow-up for the patient if gallstones are clearly demonstrated. However, the absence of gallstones on ultrasound does not exclude the diagnosis of biliary colic. Symptomatic patients with an unremarkable right upper quadrant ultrasound examination should be strongly encouraged to follow up with their primary physician for a repeat ultrasound examination. An algorithm that demonstrates how a limited ultrasound can be utilized for decision making in patients with possible biliary colic is outlined (Figure 7–1).

Schlager and co-workers reported a sensitivity, specificity, and positive and negative predictive value of 86%, 97%, 97%, and 85%, respectively, for emergency physicians in detecting cholelithiasis by ultrasound.[2] Lanoix and colleagues confirmed these findings in a study that noted a sensitivity, specificity, and positive and negative predictive value of 91%, 89%, 88%, and 92%, respectively, for the detection of cholelithiasis by emergency physicians.[1] The two studies dealt primarily with the ability of emergency physicians to detect gallstones in the gallbladder, and less so with the recognition of sonographic evidence of cholecystitis (e.g., gallbladder wall thickening, pericholecystic fluid, and the sonographic Murphy's sign). These reports are comparable to those obtained through a large meta-analysis of the ultrasound litera-

ture. The investigators found an estimated sensitivity and specificity of ultrasonography for cholelithiasis of 91% and 97%, respectively.[8]

Evaluation of Possible Cholecystitis

In patients with cholelithiasis, their clinical presentation, vital signs, time course of illness, white blood cell count, and liver function tests should assist the clinician in deciding whether the patient has biliary colic or acute cholecystitis. In a study of the ability of emergency physicians to detect sonographic evidence of cholecystitis, which was confirmed by cholecystectomy, Rosen and co-workers reported a sensitivity, specificity, and positive and negative predictive value of 91%, 66%, 70%, and 90%, respectively. Of note, the specificity was lower than the other statistical parameters since the sole criterion used in the diagnosis of acute inflammation was the presence of a sonographic Murphy's sign (pain elicited by pressing over the fundus of the gallbladder with an ultrasound probe). The investigators noted that other indicators of cholecystitis (wall thickening, pericholecystic fluid, etc.) were not used in the evaluation.[9]

In a meta-analysis, Shea and colleagues found an estimated sensitivity and specificity for ultrasound diagnosis of cholecystitis to be 91% and 79%, respectively.[8] The

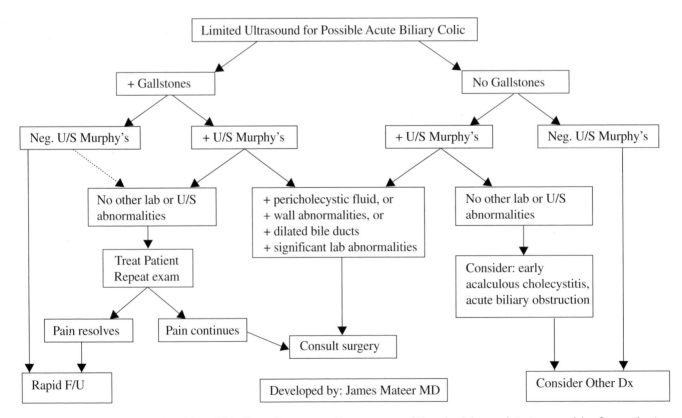

Figure 7–1. Biliary colic algorithm. This flow diagram outlines some of the decision points to consider for patient disposition based on clinical parameters and ultrasound findings. *(Courtesy of James Mateer, MD.)*

literature has established the accuracy of ultrasound-measured gallbladder wall thickness (in greater than 90% of cases, it correlates to within 1 mm of findings on postoperative specimens)[10] and that pericholecystic fluid can be detected by ultrasonography in 26% of cases of acute cholecystitis.[11] A 1985 article demonstrated that for diagnosing acute cholecystitis, a combination of gallstones and a sonographic Murphy's sign had a positive predictive value of 92.2%, whereas a combination of gallstones and gallbladder wall thickening had a positive predictive value of 95.2%.[12]

Evaluation of Acute Jaundice

In the evaluation of a patient with jaundice, when a predominantly direct hyperbilirubinemia (i.e., obstructive non-hemolytic jaundice) is detected, the next step centers on whether the clinical picture is consistent with an extra- or intrahepatic obstructive process. The role of ultrasonography in this situation is to detect dilated extrahepatic and/or intrahepatic ducts, which may indicate the level of obstruction. Once an extrahepatic process is detected, the next concern is whether the patient is presenting with clinical signs of cholangitis (fever, leucocytosis), which may precipitate the need for urgent ductal decompression (surgery, ERCP, transhepatic stenting). While ultrasonography may easily detect dilated extra- or intrahepatic ducts,[13] it is not the ideal diagnostic modality for determining the actual cause of an extrahepatic obstruction, and other modalities such as CT and ERCP are usually utilized.

Evaluation of Hepatomegaly

The differential diagnosis of hepatomegaly is broad and includes edematous states (acute hepatitis, right heart failure, systemic volume overload conditions), infiltrative processes, and intrinsic/metastatic tumors. The confirmation of hepatomegaly can be helpful for the overall assessment of a patient in the emergent setting. Although it may be helpful for the clinician to have an understanding of the sonographic appearance of various causes of hepatomegaly, the specific differentiation of these conditions lies outside the routine scope of practice for the clinician in the emergent setting.

Detection and Evaluation of Ascites

Detection of ascitic fluid is a useful diagnostic procedure when evaluating the patient with abdominal distention without signs of intestinal obstruction. On physical examination, the sensitivity of an abdominal fluid wave is low at best. In the emergency and acute care setting, determining whether a patient has ascites may influence the initial management and disposition. For example, in a patient with abdominal pain or fever, the presence of ascites would require the clinician to consider the possibility of bacterial peritonitis.

▶ ANATOMIC CONSIDERATIONS

A variety of solid and hollow organs are located in the right upper quadrant of the abdomen. The predominant organ is the liver, bordered superiorly by the diaphragm and coronary/triangular ligament confluence (Figure 7–2A), inferomedially by the duodenum and head of pancreas, and inferiorly by the gallbladder, hepatic flexure of the ascending colon, and superior pole of right kidney. The gastric fundus is located posterolateral to the left hepatic lobe. The liver is divided (Figure 7–2A) into right and left lobes by the major lobar fissure, which contains the middle hepatic vein and extends from the gallbladder fossa anteriorly to the inferior vena cava posteriorly. The right lobe is divided into anteromedial and posterolateral segments by the right hepatic vein, and the left lobe is divided into anterior and posterior segments by the left hepatic vein. After draining the liver of venous blood, all hepatic veins converge on the inferior vena cava posteriorly, just inferior to the atriocaval junction. The main portal vein courses from the intestinal venous drainage arcades, through the lesser omentum to the hepatic hilum, where it bifurcates into right and left branches and enters the liver (Figure 7–2B). The hepatic artery courses toward the hepatic hilum in the lesser omentum, occupying a position anterior to the main portal vein (Figure 7–2B). At the hilum, it divides into right and left branches and enters the liver parenchyma.

The biliary system begins with the intrahepatic right and left hepatic ducts, which course toward the hilum, uniting to form the extrahepatic common hepatic duct. After exiting the hilum, the common hepatic duct is joined by the cystic duct (from the gallbladder) to form the common bile duct, which courses anterior to the main portal vein, and usually to the right of the hepatic artery (Figure 7–2B) in the lesser omentum before entering the duodenum. It is important to remember the anatomic relationships of the hepatic artery, common bile duct, and main portal vein as they traverse the lesser omentum in the region of the hepatic hilum to form the main portal triad since this will aid in identification and differentiation during sonographic evaluation. Within the liver, branches of the main portal vein, proper hepatic artery, and biliary tree follow parallel pathways of distribution to the liver tissue in bundles known as lesser portal triads. Hepatic venous tributaries do not follow this system.

The gallbladder is divided into a fundus, body, and neck. The fundus may project below the inferior hepatic margin, illustrating the anatomic basis for a "sonographic Murphy's sign" (pain elicited by pressing over the fundus with the ultrasound probe). The body is contiguous with the inferior surface of the liver and narrows at the neck, which often contains spiral valves; these are occasionally misdiagnosed as impacted stones. The neck is continuous

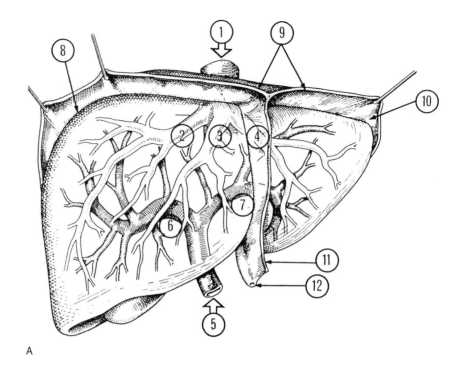

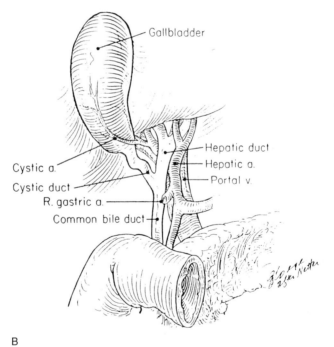

Figure 7–2. (A) Surgical anatomy of the liver: (1) inferior vena cava; (2) right hepatic vein; (3) middle hepatic vein; (4) left hepatic vein; (5) portal vein; (6) right branch portal vein; (7) left branch portal vein; (8) right triangular ligament; (9) coronary ligament; (10) left triangular ligament; (11) falciform ligament; (12) ligamentum teres. *(Reproduced from Feliciano et al. Trauma, 3rd ed. Norwalk, CT: Appleton & Lange, 1996;489.)* (B) Normal anatomy. The diagram depicts the relationships in the porta hepatis. The triangle of Calot is bordered by the edge of the liver, the cystic duct, and the hepatic duct. *(Reproduced from Schwartz et al. Principles of surgery, 6th ed. New York: McGraw-Hill, 1994;1368.)*

with the cystic duct, which empties into the common hepatic duct to create the common bile duct.

▶ TECHNIQUE AND NORMAL ULTRASOUND FINDINGS

Hepatobiliary ultrasound begins with proper patient preparation. A "nothing by mouth (NPO)" status is helpful for two main reasons. First, oral intake can generate upper abdominal gas and intestinal contents, creating a poor medium for ultrasound-wave transmission. Second, oral intake may stimulate gallbladder contraction by generating cholecystokinin, which decreases chances of adequate gallbladder visualization. Probe frequency selection is variable, but ranges from 2.5 to 5.0 MHz, with the higher frequency being used in the pediatric age group or for patients with thin abdominal walls where less depth of penetration is required and higher resolution images can be sought. Initially, the patient is typically positioned in the supine position, with the left lateral decubitus position or upright sitting position being used in technically difficult cases, or to document mobility of detected gallstones.

Evaluation of Biliary Colic and Acute Cholecystitis

If the focus of the examination is evaluating for possible biliary colic or cholecystitis, then the probe is placed under the right costal margin in the mid-clavicular line, with the probe tip directed toward the right shoulder and the probe axis marker oriented longitudinally. In this position, the operator can sweep the probe until an image of the gallbladder is obtained. This will usually be a transverse or oblique cut through the fundus.

The next step is to obtain a longitudinal profile of the presumptive gallbladder by gently rotating the ultrasound beam profile, keeping other three-dimensional aspects of the beam orientation constant. This is the technique of converting transverse or oblique sections of images into longitudinal cuts. If the gallbladder is not initially visualized from the subcostal view, the patient should be asked to take a deep breath and hold it in order to bring the gallbladder down from beneath the ribs and closer to the probe. Once this has been performed and a longitudinal image has been obtained, the final step is gentle image manipulation in order to demonstrate communication of the presumptive gallbladder with the main portal triad. The gallbladder neck should be traceable, along the echogenic major lobar fissure (visible in about 70% of patients) to the main portal triad (Figure 7–3). In the absence of gallstones, this is the only way to definitively prove the image obtained is the gall-

bladder and not a loop of bowel or an oblique section through the vena cava.

The main portal triad, made up of the main portal vein, common bile duct, and hepatic artery, is most easily identified by starting with a longitudinal view of the portal vein. The probe is positioned in the right epigastric area with the indicator generally pointing toward the right axilla. The portal vein can usually be visualized coursing toward the porta hepatis with portions of the common bile duct and/or hepatic artery above (Figure 7–4). By rotating the probe 90° counterclockwise from this view, a transverse image of the portal vein, with the associated common bile duct (anterior/lateral) and hepatic artery (anterior/medial) may be visualized (Figure 7–5A). This is the classic "Mickey Mouse sign." Dilatation of the common bile duct may occasionally be noted in this view as a sign of possible choledocholithiasis with obstruction. The site of common bile duct obstruction from stones is often near its termination close to the pancreatic head. This area may be visualized in a thin patient with little interfering gas (Figure 7–5B).

The gallbladder is then carefully scanned in multiple longitudinal and transverse planes, noting the presence or absence of gallstones, wall thickness, and the presence or absence of pericholecystic fluid. An accurate measurement of wall thickness is made on an anterior wall that is perpendicular to the imaging plane (usually less than 2 mm, with greater than 4 mm being abnormal) (Figure 7–6). If gallstones are detected, the patient is rolled or elevated into various body positions in an attempt to document movement versus impaction in the gallbladder neck and to evaluate the possibility of a calcified polyp

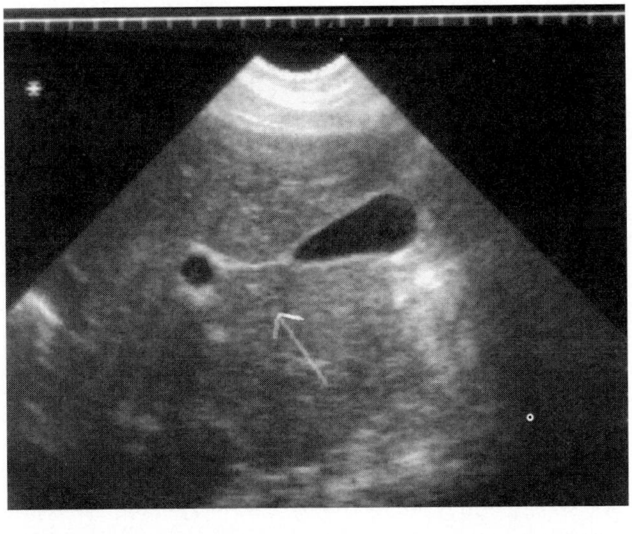

Figure 7–3. Long axis view of normal gallbladder. The main lobar fissure is seen between the gallbladder neck and right portal vein (arrow). *(Courtesy of Lori Sens and Lori Green, Gulfcoast Ultrasound.)*

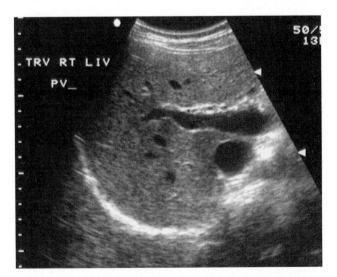

Figure 7–4. Long axis view of portal vein. The portal vein can be seen coursing towards the porta hepatis with portions of the non-distended common bile duct and/or hepatic artery above. The inferior vena cava is the large round vessel immediately below the portal vein. *(Courtesy of Lori Sens, Gulfcoast Ultrasound.)*

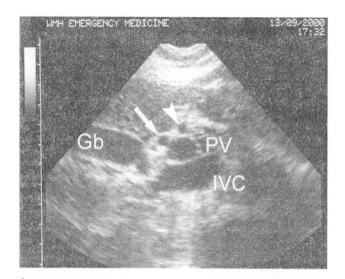

A

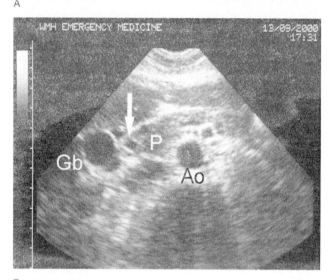

B

Figure 7–5. (A) Short axis view of the portal vein (PV), with the associated common bile duct (anterior/lateral) [arrow] and hepatic artery (anterior/medial) [arrowhead]. The relative positions of the gallbladder (Gb) and inferior vena cava (IVC) are noted. (B) Transverse view of the upper abdomen. The position of the common bile duct (arrow) near its termination by the pancreatic head (P) is noted along with the relative positions of the gallbladder (Gb) and aorta (Ao). *(Courtesy of James Mateer, MD.)*

or sessile mass. Finally, the probe tip is used to compress the gallbladder fundus in an attempt to elicit a "sonographic Murphy's sign."

For patients with significant intestinal gas or a gallbladder that is too superior to visualize using the subcostal technique, the intercostal oblique approach should be utilized. The probe is positioned in the seventh or eighth intercostal space near the anterior axillary line with the probe indicator pointing toward the axilla. The probe

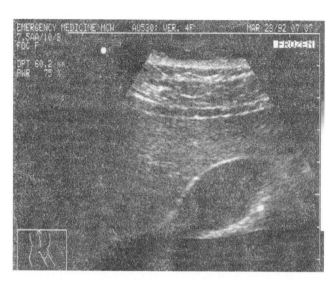

Figure 7–6. Longitudinal high-resolution image of the normal, thin anterior wall of the gallbladder. The posterior wall appears thickened due to posterior acoustic enhancement from the fluid-filled gallbladder. *(Courtesy of James Mateer, MD.)*

is then angled toward the gallbladder fossa. The liver is utilized as an acoustical window to avoid interfering bowel gas and both longitudinal and oblique views of the gallbladder can usually be obtained from this position.

Evaluation of Acute Jaundice

The initial step of this examination technique is to locate the main portal triad, which can be accomplished in two ways. The first method uses the portal vein as a landmark and is described above. The second method involves tracing more peripheral branches of the portal venous system as they course centrally toward the hilum. Their echogenic walls and their normal enlargement can identify portal venous branches as they course centrally toward the hilum to join the main portal vein in the main portal triad. They are clearly distinguished from the hepatic venous system, with its thin, hypoechoic walls and enlargement as it converges on the inferior vena cava posteriorly (Figure 7–7A, B). Hepatic arterial branches are rarely large enough to be visualized distal to the hilum. Intrahepatic bile ducts, although exhibiting echogenic walls and enlarging as they course centrally toward the hilum, can be distinguished from the portal venous system by tracing them to the common bile duct in the main portal triad at the hilum. In non-disease states, they are rarely visible within the hepatic parenchyma. Color Doppler techniques can also be used to differentiate between the portal and biliary trees by demonstrating flow within the former. Once the main portal triad has been identified, examination and measurement of the common duct is performed. The duct is usually normal if the transverse diameter, in millimeters, is less than one tenth of the pa-

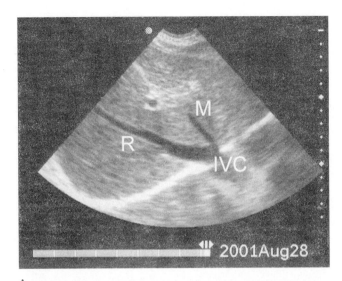

A

B

Figure 7–7. (A) Transverse view of the upper portion of the liver. The hepatic venous system, with its thin, hypoechoic walls and enlargement as it converges on the inferior vena cava (IVC) posteriorly is noted. The right hepatic vein (R) and a portion of the middle hepatic vein (M) are seen in this view. (B) Transverse/oblique view of the upper liver demonstrating the junction of the inferior vena cava (IVC) with the middle hepatic vein (M) and left hepatic vein (L). *(Courtesy of James Mateer, MD.)*

tient's age. After cholecystectomy, common ducts may normally range up to 1 cm.

The most convenient method for intrahepatic duct evaluation involves transverse imaging of the left lobe of the liver. Intrahepatic ducts run in the transverse plane in this location, allowing longitudinal images of the ducts to be obtained by orienting the beam axis transversely. Longitudinal imaging of the ducts allows easier detection and evaluation of abnormalities in the intrahepatic sys-

tem. Most examiners would agree that any visualization of intrahepatic ducts is probably pathologic. If duct dilatation is present, a brief search for the etiology is warranted with close attention to the porta hepatis and the head of the pancreas for possible masses.

Evaluation of Hepatomegaly

Sonographic evaluation of clinically suspected hepatomegaly begins with accurate documentation of enlargement, followed by parenchymal scanning to elucidate etiologies. The most convenient, although more qualitative, method of confirming hepatomegaly entails obtaining a right upper quadrant view of Morison's pouch (see Chapter 4). By demonstrating that the liver parenchyma of the right lobe extends to or beyond the inferior pole of the right kidney, hepatic enlargement is probable, and less is considered within normal range (Figure 7–8). An exception for this method occurs if the patient has a Reidel's lobe (an extension of the right lobe towards the iliac crest). Alternatively, a longitudinal scan is obtained at the mid-hepatic line, and the liver is measured from the dome (diaphragm) to the inferior margin. Enlargement is considered to be a measurement greater than 12.8 cm.[14] Since enlargement of the left lobe of the liver and splenomegaly can be confused on physical examination, the ultrasound evaluation for possible hepatomegaly should be completed with long axis views of the spleen. A measured length greater than 12 to 14 cm is considered abnormal.

Next, longitudinal and transverse images of the entire liver are obtained, and the general echo texture of the liver should be noted. The liver normally appears homogenous and moderately echogenic in nature (see Figure 7–8). This is compared to the degree of echogenicity of

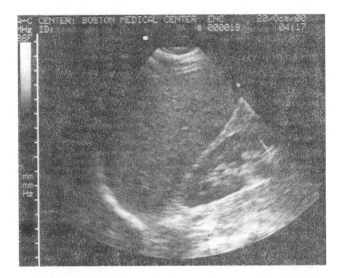

Figure 7–8. Right upper quadrant, longitudinal view of Morison's pouch area demonstrating normal relative echogenicity and size of the liver and kidney.

the spleen (isoechoic to liver), renal cortex (hypoechoic to liver), and pancreas (hyperechoic to liver in the elderly, isoechoic in the young). Focal abnormalities are then sought, and a general assessment as to whether the liver is diffusely or focally enlarged is made. If any lesions are detected attempts at localization to a specific lobe or segment can be performed by noting the lesion location with respect to the hepatic veins. This can be performed by obtaining a transverse image of the atriocaval junction where the hepatic veins empty into the inferior vena cava, and then noting the position of the lesion with respect to the lobes or segments defined by these vessels. Since the hepatic veins are not all located in the same plane, multiple views may be needed to follow each branch to the vena cava (see Figure 7–7).

Detection and Evaluation of Ascites

Ascites detection by ultrasound is useful in the patient presenting with abdominal distention where the differential diagnosis includes free intraperitoneal fluid versus dilated bowel. The ultrasound technique for detecting ascites is similar to that used in the FAST (focused abdominal sonography for trauma) examination (see Chapter 4). The clinician should carefully note the echo characteristics of any intraperitoneal fluid detected, as the possibilities include transudate, exudate, malignant, and infectious processes and blood.

▶ COMMON AND EMERGENT ABNORMALITIES

Gallbladder Disease

A commonly noted abnormality of the hepatobiliary system is cholelithiasis. Gallstones typically appear as echogenic foci with acoustic shadowing beneath the gallstone. They can range in size from that of a golf ball to the size of sand particles (Figures 7–9, 7–10, and 7–11A, B). The shadow is produced by ultrasound waves that are strongly reflected off of the gallstone. Shadowing may not be present if the gallstone diameter is less than 4 mm.[15] Unless extremely high in cholesterol content, gallstones will layer in the most dependent region of the gallbladder, and unless impacted in the neck or cystic duct, will move with patient positional changes. This is important, as non-shadowing stones may otherwise be difficult to distinguish from echogenic non-shadowing cholesterol polyps (fixed to the wall) (Figure 7–12). In patients with cholelithiasis and the appropriate clinical presentation, additional sonographic findings consistent with cholecystitis may include one or more of the following: wall thickness greater than 4 mm (Figure 7–13A, B), transverse gallbladder diameter greater than 5 cm, decreased wall echogenicity (as wall edema increases), pericholecystic fluid, and the presence

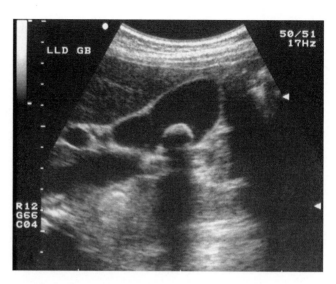

Figure 7–9. Longitudinal view of the gallbladder demonstrating a large solitary stone with prominent posterior acoustic shadowing. *(Courtesy of Lori Sens, Gulfcoast Ultrasound.)*

of a sonographic Murphy's sign.[16] When organisms that produce gas are involved, emphysematous changes in the gallbladder wall may be seen (Figure 7–14). Of note, thickening of the gallbladder wall is a nonspecific finding, and not always associated with cholecystitis. Other causes of gallbladder wall thickening include various systemic volume overload states, local liver disease, ascites, and myeloma. The WES (wall echo shadow) sign is commonly seen in gallstone-filled gallbladders. It consists of an anterior echogenic line arising from the near wall of the gall-

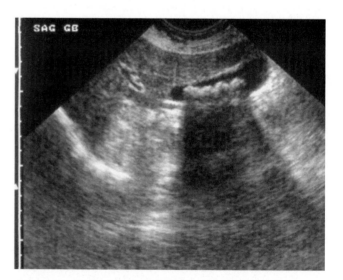

Figure 7–10. Longitudinal view of the gallbladder demonstrating multiple moderate-sized stones resembling "peas in a pod" also with prominent posterior acoustic shadowing. *(Courtesy of Lori Sens and Lori Green, Gulfcoast Ultrasound.)*

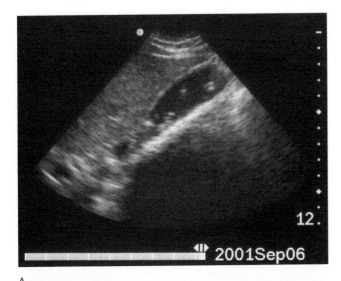

A

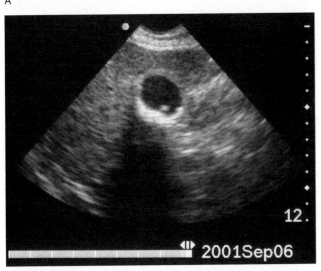

B

Figure 7–11. (A) Longitudinal view of the gallbladder shows multiple polyps suspended inside the wall. The dense posterior shadowing is from multiple tiny stones (sand-like) layering along the posterior wall of the gallbladder. This is best appreciated in the transverse view. (B) Transverse view. The posterior layering of the sand-like stones and the source of the shadowing is best appreciated in this view. *(Courtesy of James Mateer, MD.)*

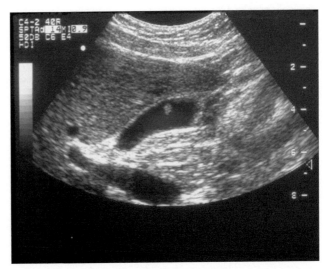

Figure 7–12. Longitudinal view of the gallbladder with solitary small polyp attached to the anterior wall. There was no shadowing and no movement with patient positioning. *(Courtesy of Lori Sens and Lori Green, Gulfcoast Ultrasound.)*

bladder, an intervening anechoic stripe generated from bile when present, and a posterior brightly echogenic line representing stone material followed by a prominent posterior acoustic shadow (Figure 7–15).

Jaundice and Biliary Obstruction

Biliary obstruction, regardless of underlying etiology, is often initially detected by demonstrating dilated biliary ducts on ultrasonography. Dilated extrahepatic ducts will

appear as an enlarged, anechoic tubular structure (with echogenic walls) in the main portal triad, anterior to and following the course of the main portal vein. This is referred to as the parallel channel sign (Figure 7–16). Dilatation of the extrahepatic ducts implies obstruction of the common bile duct. Common causes of extrahepatic obstructions include choledocholithiasis, pancreatic masses, and strictures (Figure 7–17A, B). Left untreated, an extrahepatic obstruction will eventually also lead to dilatation of the intrahepatic ducts. Dilated intrahepatic ducts appear as anechoic tubules with echogenic walls coursing through the hepatic parenchyma. Morphologically, they are described as "antler signs" (Figure 7–18). Dilatation of the intrahepatic ducts alone, suggests an obstructive process within the common hepatic duct or more proximal. Causes of primary intrahepatic obstruction include inflammatory conditions, intrahepatic masses, or biliary duct cancer (Figure 7–19A, B). As previously mentioned, although ultrasonography is sensitive in detecting ductal dilation, it may be less accurate for detecting the underlying cause of the obstruction. For example, ultrasonography has a sensitivity of 15 to 55% for detecting common duct stones.[17] The precise etiology is often determined by other modalities such as CT or ERCP.

Common causes of non-obstructive jaundice are hepatitis and cirrhosis. Sonographically, hepatitis usually appears as a relatively decreased parenchymal echogenicity secondary to the increased fluid content of the tissue.[18] The diaphragm and portal vessel walls are not involved in the edema, and remain brightly echogenic. Their relative "accentuated brightness" is the classic finding associated with acute hepatitis but this ultrasound finding is often not

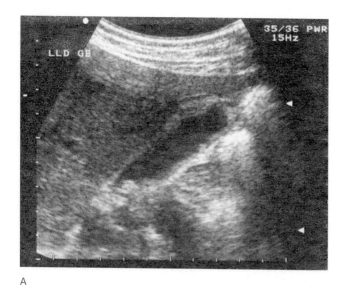

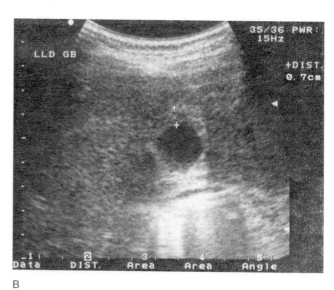

A

B

Figure 7–13. (A) Longitudinal view of a gallbladder with abnormal thickening of the wall. The bright echoes and shadowing below the gallbladder are from gas within the colon. (B) Transverse view. Wall thickness measures 7 mm. This patient was diagnosed with chronic cholecystitis. *(Courtesy of Lori Sens, Gulfcoast Ultrasound.)*

obvious. As inflammation becomes more chronic, and cirrhosis develops, the liver size decreases, parenchymal echogenicity and surface irregularity increase, and intrahepatic anatomy becomes distorted (Figure 7–20).

Hepatomegaly and Splenomegaly

By demonstrating that the liver parenchyma of the right lobe extends to or beyond the inferior pole of the right

kidney, hepatic enlargement is probable (Figure 7–21). If hepatomegaly is related to edema (acute hepatitis, right heart failure, systemic volume overload states), the liver will appear enlarged and relatively hypoechoic. If hepatomegaly is related to infiltrative processes (fatty liver, amyloid, hemochromatosis, etc.), the parenchyma appears dense and of relatively increased echogenicity.[20]

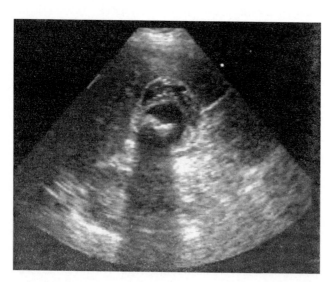

Figure 7–14. Transverse view of the gallbladder shows marked thickening of the anterior wall and associated edema separating the layers of the wall. Cholelithiasis with shadowing is obvious. This patient was diagnosed with acute cholecystitis.

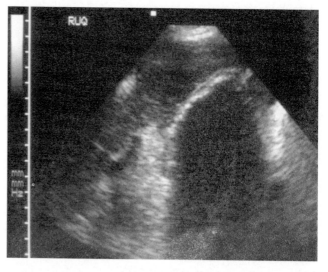

Figure 7–15. The WES sign (wall echo shadow). Note the superficial echogenic line arising from the near wall of the gallbladder, an intervening anechoic stripe generated from bile when present, and a posterior brightly echogenic line representing stone material, followed by a prominent posterior acoustic shadow. *(Courtesy of James Mateer, MD.)*

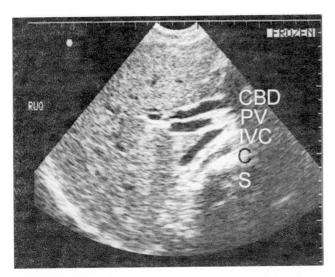

Figure 7–16. Parallel channel sign. Oblique view of the right upper quadrant. The dilated common bile duct (CBD) is located anterior to and following parallel to the course of the main portal vein (PV). Posterior to these structures is the inferior vena cava (IVC), crus of the diaphragm (C), and spine (S). *(Courtesy of James Mateer, MD.)*

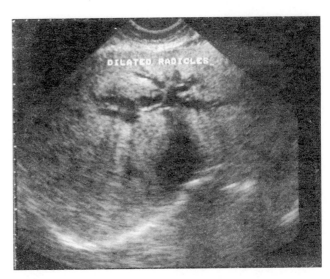

Figure 7–18. Antler signs. Transverse view of the liver. Dilated intrahepatic ducts appear as irregular anechoic tubules coursing through the hepatic parenchyma. *(Courtesy of Lori Sens and Lori Green, Gulfcoast Ultrasound.)*

Splenomegaly is confirmed when the length measured in long axis exceeds 12 to 14 cm (Figure 7–22).

Ascites

Transudative processes (hydrostatic and oncotic pressure related) create ascitic fluid with minimal, if any, in-

ternal echoes (see Figure 7–20). As fluid becomes more complex, variable echogenicity can develop. This is commonly noted in exudative processes (inflammation and malignancy related), especially those with high concentrations of white blood cells or malignant cells (Figure 7–23).[24] Fluid may be diffuse or loculated in proximity to a specific localized area of pathology. The conclusion should not be drawn, however, that fluid is a transudate

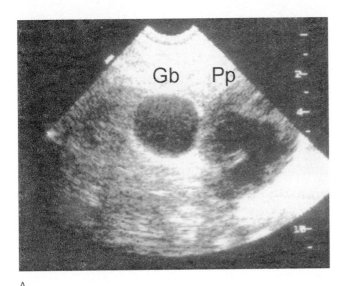

A

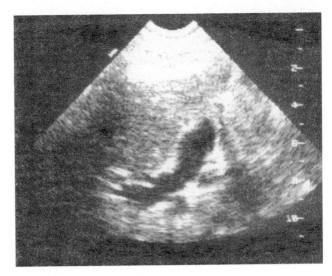

B

Figure 7–17. (A) Transverse view of the mid upper abdomen reveals a large pancreatic pseudocyst (Pp) just medial to the gallbladder (Gb). As both structures are of fluid density, there is significant posterior acoustic enhancement. (B) Long axis view of the common bile duct in this patient shows obvious evidence of obstruction. *(Courtesy of James Mateer, MD.)*

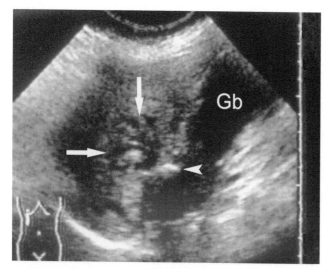

A

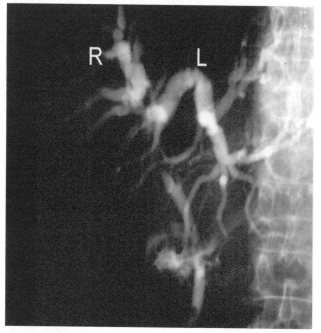

B

Figure 7–19. (A) Mirizzi syndrome. Longitudinal view of the gallbladder (Gb) reveals massive enlargement (hydrops) and evidence of dilated intrahepatic ducts (arrows). At laparotomy, a large stone was found in the gallbladder neck area (arrowhead) with surrounding inflammation resulting in common hepatic duct obstruction. This is an unusual cause of intrahepatic obstruction. (B) ERCP radiograph of the same patient demonstrates dilatation of the right (R) and left (L) hepatic ducts. (*Courtesy of James Mateer, MD.*)

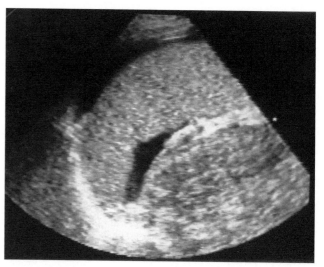

Figure 7–20. Cirrhosis of the liver. This oblique view of the right lobe demonstrates the findings of contracted size, increased echogenicity, and irregular texture of the liver. There is surrounding echo-free ascites.

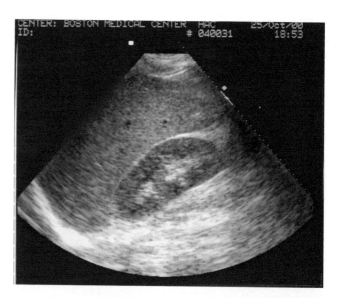

Figure 7–21. Longitudinal view of the liver and kidney shows possible hepatomegaly. The liver parenchyma of the right lobe extends to or beyond the inferior pole of the right kidney.

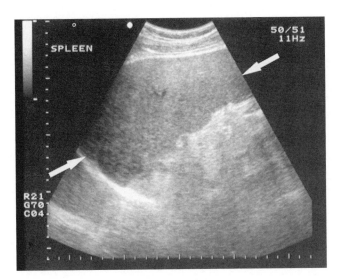

Figure 7–22. Long axis view of the spleen measures more than 17 cm. Calipers should be placed on the longest length from the diaphragm to the spleen tip (arrows). *(Courtesy of Lori Sens, Gulfcoast Ultrasound.)*

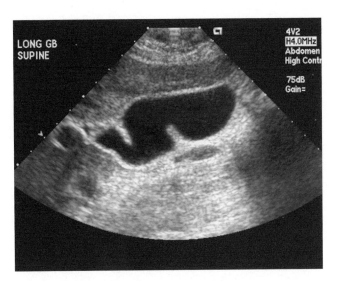

Figure 7–24. Longitudinal view of the gallbladder demonstrates non-shadowing mucosal folds on the mid posterior wall and the anterior neck areas *(Courtesy of James Mateer, MD, Waukesha Memorial Hospital.)*

if internal echoes are absent. Up to 25% of exudative fluid displays echo features consistent with simple transudative fluid.

▶ COMMON VARIANTS AND SELECTED ABNORMALITIES

A number of variants may be noted with respect to the gallbladder. Mucosal indentations may produce septations of the lumen (Figure 7–24), which can be mistaken

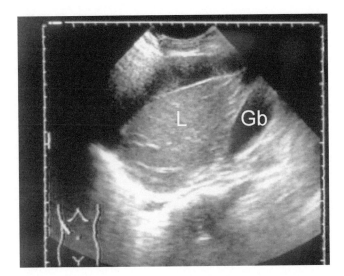

Figure 7–23. Coronal view of the right lobe of the liver (L) and gallbladder (Gb) shows echogenic ascites fluid with strand-like projections on the liver surface. The patient was diagnosed with bacterial peritonitis. *(Courtesy of James Mateer, MD.)*

for gallstones, although shadowing does not usually occur. Folds of the fundus may produce a phrygian cap (Figure 7–25A, B). Agenesis of the gallbladder has an incidence of less than 0.05%. Intrahepatic gallbladder, secondary to abnormal developmental migration of the gallbladder bud, should always be considered if not found in its typical location. Duplicated gallbladder occurs with an incidence of 0.02%. Biliary sludge may be detected as a dependent layer of variable non-shadowing echogenicity in the gallbladder (Figure 7–26). Although the sequelae of sludge are largely unknown, it is frequently detected in states associated with biliary stasis, such as limited oral intake.[25] Tumefactive sludge is non-layering, thickened, polypoid sludge that can be mistaken for a gallbladder wall tumor (Figure 7–27). A contracted gallbladder, commonly occurring in the postprandial patient, may be difficult to detect, and may demonstrate a non-pathologically thickened wall (Figure 7–28).

Riedel's lobe of the liver is a thin projection of otherwise normal hepatic tissue extending from the right lobe inferiorly toward the iliac crest (Figure 7–29). If not recognized, this could be mistaken for hepatomegaly. Simple hepatic cysts are often an incidental finding. Their features include sharp margins, no internal echoes, and increased "through transmission" (Figure 7–30).[22] Hepatic abscesses, although an uncommon finding, are worthy of mention. Sonographic features include thickened, poorly defined walls surrounding fluid of variable echogenicity, which is dependent on the nature of the internal pus (Figure 7–31).[23]

Intrinsic and metastatic tumors of the liver produce variable echo patterns, depending on histology and secondary tumor necrosis and hemorrhage.[21] Tumors can

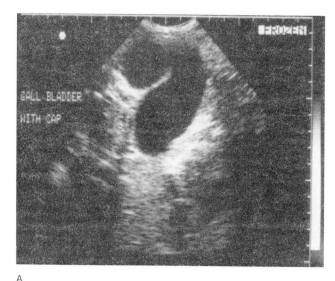

A

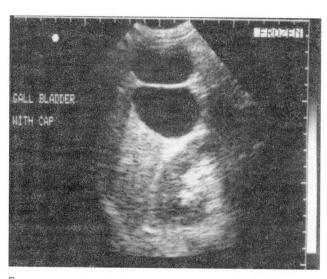

B

Figure 7–25. (A) Phrygian cap. Longitudinal view demonstrates a folded gallbladder at the fundus. (B) Transverse views of the same patient create the illusion of a double gallbladder in this plane. *(Courtesy of James Mateer, MD.)*

exhibit smooth, well-defined or irregular borders and can be of increased or decreased echogenicity relative to the general hepatic tissue. Necrosis produces areas of decreased echogenicity, whereas hemorrhage can create foci of increased or decreased echogenicity depending on the age and degeneration of blood. Common benign tumors include hemangiomas, with well-defined margins and a hyperechoic appearance (Figure 7–32), and hepatic adenomas, with well-defined margins and variable echogenicity (Figure 7–33). Common sources of metastatic lesions include colon, breast, and pancreas (Figure 7–34).

► PITFALLS

1. *Misidentifying the gallbladder.* Oblique sections through the vena cava and loops of small bowel can be mistaken for the gallbladder. The best way to avoid this mistake is by ensuring that the structure being identified as the gallbladder clearly communicates with the main portal triad via the major lobar fissure.
2. *Inadequate visualization of the gallbladder and biliary system.* Intestinal gas can interfere with

Figure 7–26. Biliary sludge is demonstrated as a dependent layer of non-shadowing mid-level echoes in this long axis view of the gallbladder. *(Courtesy of Lori Sens and Lori Green, Gulfcoast Ultrasound.)*

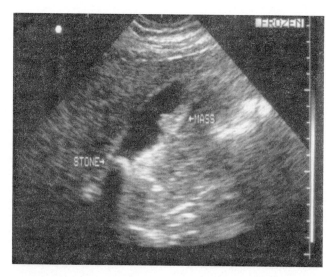

Figure 7–27. Tumefactive sludge. Dense polypoid sludge can be mistaken for a gallbladder wall tumor (<MASS). The patient also has a stone impacted in the gallbladder neck (STONE>). *(Courtesy of James Mateer, MD.)*

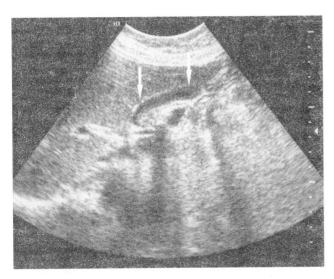

Figure 7–28. Contracted gallbladder. Can be difficult to detect (arrows), and may demonstrate a non-pathologically thickened wall. *(Courtesy of Lori Sens, Gulfcoast Ultrasound.)*

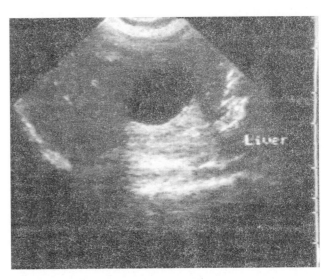

Figure 7–30. Liver cyst. Sharp margins, no internal echoes, and increased "through transmission" are demonstrated in this simple cyst of the right lobe of the liver. *(Courtesy of Lori Sens and Lori Green, Gulfcoast Ultrasound.)*

complete imaging of the gallbladder and biliary system. The fundus of the gallbladder is often obscured and may contain stones or localized wall thickening. Patient positioning or repeat scanning after patient instructions are given for proper bowel preparation may be necessary.

3. *Confusion with shadowing.* A common error after detecting shadowing is making the diagnosis of a small gallstone impacted in the gallbladder neck without actually visualizing a gallstone. Causes

of shadowing in the region of the gallbladder neck include the spiral valves of Heister (Figure 7–35), fat in the porta, duodenal gas, and edge artifacts from the gallbladder wall and fluid interface. A gallstone must be directly visualized before making this diagnosis. When a solitary gallstone is lodged in the neck of the gallbladder, however, it can be easily missed (Figure 7–36A, B). A persistent, clean shadow behind a rounded bright echo that is present from several viewing angles should be identified. A gallbladder packed with

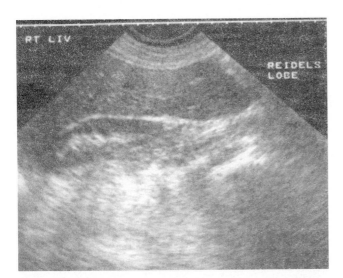

Figure 7–29. Reidel's lobe. Longitudinal view of the abdomen at the right anterior axillary line, centered over the kidney. A projection of normal hepatic tissue extends from the right lobe inferiorly toward the iliac crest. *(Courtesy of Lori Sens, Gulfcoast Ultrasound.)*

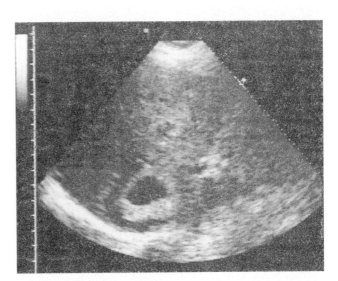

Figure 7–31. Liver abscess. An oblique view of the right lobe shows a fluid-filled cavity with thickened, poorly defined walls.

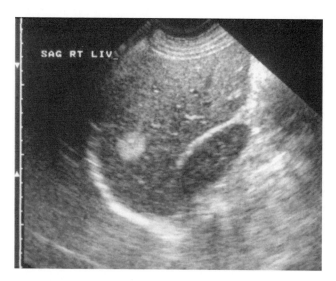

Figure 7–32. Hemangioma. Longitudinal view of the right lobe of the liver demonstrates the typical appearance. *(Courtesy of Lori Sens and Lori Green, Gulfcoast Ultrasound.)*

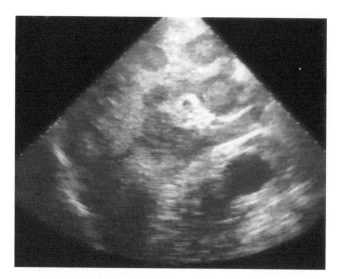

Figure 7–34. Metastatic tumors. Longitudinal view of the right lobe shows numerous target lesions. A cyst is also present within the lower pole of the kidney. *(Courtesy of Lori Sens and Lori Green, Gulfcoast Ultrasound.)*

stones and containing little or no liquid bile may be confusing due to dense shadowing in the area, which must be differentiated from shadowing caused by bowel gas (Figure 7–37A, B).

4. *Misdiagnosing cholelithiasis and cholecystitis.* Cholesterol polyps and mucosal folds can be mistaken for gallstones. Gallstones can be missed when they are small or when the entire gallbladder is not visualized due to intestinal gas or large mucosal folds. A thickened gallbladder wall

is a nonspecific finding, and may be consistent with cholecystitis, hepatitis, ascites, hypoalbuminemia, and systemic volume overload states (Figure 7–38A, B). The entire clinical picture should always be considered. In 5% of cases, cholecystitis may be diagnosed with the absence of gallstones (acalculous cholecystitis), which typically occur in patients who are chronically debilitated, diabetic, immunocompromised, on hyper-

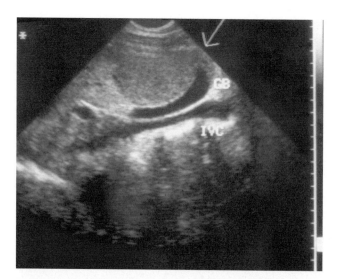

Figure 7–33. Hepatic adenoma. A hypoechoic liver mass (arrow) is seen compressing the gallbladder (GB) in this long axis view. *(Courtesy of Lori Sens and Lori Green, Gulfcoast Ultrasound.)*

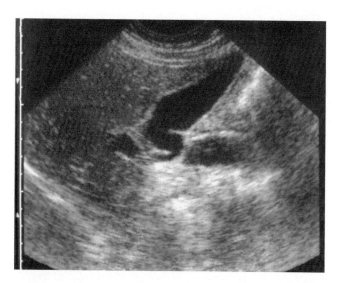

Figure 7–35. Hartman's pouch. Long axis view of the gallbladder neck (Hartman's pouch) demonstrates the spiral valves of Heister. *(Courtesy of Lori Sens and Lori Green, Gulfcoast Ultrasound.)*

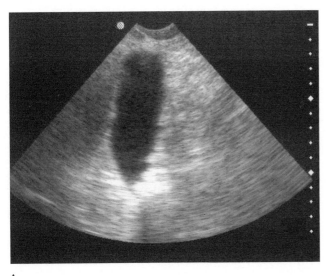 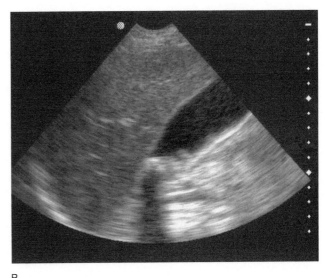

A   B

Figure 7–36. (A) Longitudinal view with the probe positioned at the tip of the gallbladder. Cholelithiasis is not obvious. (B) Intercostal oblique view of the same patient. Impacted stone in the gallbladder neck and prominent shadowing are more obvious in this view. *(Courtesy of James Mateer, MD.)*

alimentation, or recovering from a recent traumatic injury.

5. *Misdiagnosing dilated intrahepatic ducts.* Intrahepatic branches of the portal vein can be mistaken for dilated intrahepatic ducts as both have echogenic walls and become larger as they confluence toward the hepatic hilum. Care must be taken to trace the structures in question down to their parent structures at the main portal triad to

ensure the differentiation. Alternatively, color Doppler techniques may be employed, with flow being detected only in the vascular structures.

6. *Misdiagnosing ascites.* On ultrasound, ascites can be confused with hemoperitoneum, and vice versa. This can occur between simple transudative ascites and fresh blood (both typically echo free) and between complex exudative fluid and partially clotted blood (both with varying degrees

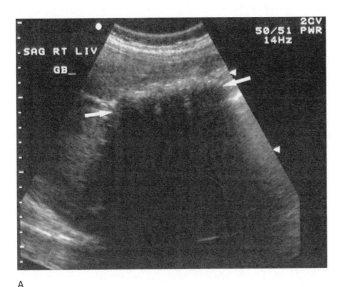 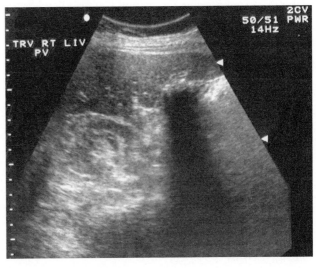

A   B

Figure 7–37. (A) Packed gallbladder. Longitudinal view of the gallbladder (arrows) shows dense shadowing from a collapsed gallbladder filled with stones. (B) Transverse views of the same patient clarify that the shadowing emanates from the gallbladder fossa. *(Courtesy of Lori Sens, Gulfcoast Ultrasound.)*

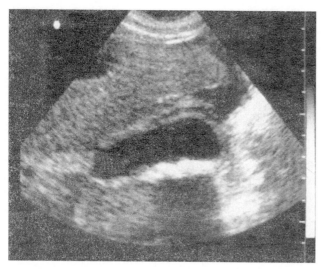

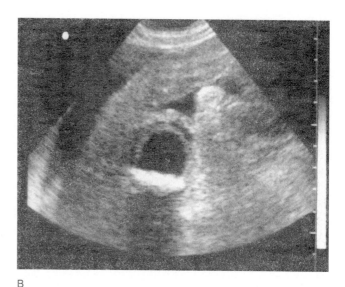

A

B

Figure 7–38. (A) Long axis view of the gallbladder shows typical ultrasound signs of cholecystitis: stones, a thickened wall, and pericholecystic fluid (B) Transverse views of the same patient demonstrate ascites as the cause for wall thickening. The patient did not have cholecystitis on further clinical evaluation. *(Courtesy of James Mateer, MD.)*

of echogenicity). Clinical correlation, along with fluid sampling, may be employed to make the correct diagnosis.

► CASE STUDIES

Case 1

Patient Presentation

A 56-year-old patient with a history of insulin-dependent diabetes, coronary artery disease, and chronic hepatitis B, presented to the emergency department with a 24-h history of epigastric and right upper quadrant abdominal pain. She noted a low-grade fever but no chills. She denied chest pain, shortness of breath, jaundice, bleeding, urinary symptoms, or abuse of gastric irritants. The patient felt this pain was similar to her hepatitis pain in the past.

Vital signs revealed temperature, 100.3°F; blood pressure, 90/60 mm Hg; pulse, 110 beats per min; and respirations, 32 per min. She appeared nontoxic but in moderate distress secondary to pain. There was no scleral icterus and the chest examination was normal. Abdominal examination revealed non-peritoneal tenderness in the right upper quadrant and epigastrium. Stool was guaiac negative. Pulses and aortic examination were normal.

Management Course

An ECG, chest radiograph, and urinalysis were normal. The white blood cell count was 16,000. Amylase, chemistry profile, and liver enzymes were remarkable only for mildly elevated transaminases, which were baseline for the

patient. The patient underwent right upper quadrant ultrasonography in the emergency department, which revealed gallstones and a thickened emphysematous gallbladder wall (see Figure 7–14). The biliary ducts were normal. The patient was administered intravenous antibiotics and taken to the operating room for cholecystectomy.

Commentary

The threshold for obtaining right upper quadrant sonography should be extremely low in patients at risk for complicated gallstone-related pathology. All urgent surgical pathology should be excluded in patients prior to making a nonoperative diagnosis such as hepatitis. Ultrasonography remains an excellent diagnostic tool for addressing these concerns in the emergency setting.

Case 2

Patient Presentation

A 45-year-old patient with a past medical history of alcoholic cirrhosis presented to the internal medicine clinic complaining of jaundice for the past 5 d. He also complained of pruritus, but denied abdominal pain, vomiting, or bleeding. Fever and chills were reported. He denied acute alcohol or acetaminophen use. He also reported a 30-lb weight loss over the past 3 months. The patient did report episodes of jaundice in the past after acute drinking episodes. He denied any history of gallstone-related disease.

Vital signs revealed temperature, 102.2°F; blood pressure, 85/60 mm Hg; pulse 120 beats per min; respirations, 24 per min. Physical examination revealed obvious scleral icterus and fullness in the upper abdomen, but no tenderness or fluid wave. Stool was guaiac negative.

Management Course

Plain radiographs of the chest and abdomen were normal. The complete blood cell count was normal but liver enzymes were remarkable for a total bilirubin of 14.3 with a direct bilirubin of 9.4. Alkaline phosphatase was 350 and GGT was 558. ALT was 110 and AST was 100. Medical staff members were planning on admitting the patient to the medical intensive care unit with a diagnosis of acute alcoholic hepatitis when a right upper quadrant ultrasound examination by an intensivist demonstrated a dilated common bile duct and intrahepatic ducts (see Figures 7–16 and 7–18 for intrahepatic ducts and "parallel channel sign"). A diagnosis of cholangitis was made, and the patient was admitted to the surgical intensive care unit where he was treated with intravenous antibiotics and fluids. An abdominal CT scan and ERCP demonstrated a mass on the head of the pancreas, which later was determined to be malignant.

Commentary

Direct hyperbilirubinemia should be assumed to be secondary to an extrahepatic obstructive process until proven otherwise, especially in the setting of fever and possible clinical cholangitis. Expeditious disposition between surgical and medical management is made by determining the presence or absence of dilated intra- and extrahepatic ducts consistent with an extrahepatic obstruction; hence, the expeditious utility of an ultrasound examination is warranted in these cases. In the case of an extrahepatic process and failure to respond to antibiotics, urgent ductal decompression via ERCP, transhepatic methods, or surgical means may be required.

Case 3

Patient Presentation

A 43-year-old male presented to an urgent care clinic with a chief complaint of progressive abdominal pain and distention over the past 2 weeks. He reported low-grade fever and nausea and vomiting. He denied change in bowel habits, urinary symptoms, or history of trauma. His past medical history was remarkable for progressive liver failure secondary to hepatitis B and C. He had undergone multiple laparotomies in the past for small bowel obstructions. There was no history of peptic ulcer disease, gallstones, pancreatitis, or any other intraabdominal pathology.

On examination, vital signs were remarkable only for a temperature of 99.9°F. He appeared in minimal distress. He had mild scleral icterus. Abdominal palpation revealed generalized distention with normoactive bowel sounds and mild diffuse tenderness with early peritonitis. No organomegaly, masses, or fluid waves were detected. Stool was guaiac negative.

Management Course

Laboratory studies were entirely normal. A plain kidney/ureters/bladder (KUB) radiograph revealed a single dilated small bowel loop in the mid-abdomen without cutoffs or free air. The patient was about to be transferred to a general surgeon's care with a diagnosis of partial small bowel obstruction when an ultrasound examination (see Figure 7–20) was performed. This examination demonstrated free intraperitoneal fluid and liver cirrhosis. Subsequent paracentesis revealed the ascites fluid to have a white blood count of 500 with gram-positive cocci organisms on Gram's stain, consistent with spontaneous bacterial peritonitis. The patient was then admitted to an internist's service. The patient's clinical symptoms resolved with intravenous antibiotics.

Commentary

Intraabdominal fluid is difficult to detect on a KUB radiograph, but simple to detect with ultrasonography. In non-traumatic patients presenting with vague abdominal complaints in conjunction with abdominal distention, ascites with spontaneous bacterial peritonitis should always be considered. This is especially true in patients with a history of liver failure. If plain abdominal radiographs reveal few findings consistent with bowel obstruction, ultrasonography in the emergency setting is the most appropriate next step. If peritoneal fluid is detected, paracentesis will be helpful with obtaining the diagnosis.

REFERENCES

1. Lanoix R, Leak LV, Gaeta T, et al. A preliminary evaluation of emergency ultrasound in the setting of an emergency medicine training program. Am J Emerg Med 2000;18:41–45.
2. Schlager D, Lazzareschi G, Whitten D, et al. A prospective study of ultrasonography in the ED by emergency physicians. Am J Emerg Med 1994;12:185–189.
3. Jehle D, Davis E, Evans T, et al. Emergency department sonography by emergency physicians. Am J Emerg Med 7:605–611.
4. Matolo N, Stadainik R, McGahan J. Comparison of ultrasonography, computerized tomography, and radionuclide imaging in the diagnosis of acute and chronic cholecystitis. Am J Surg 1982;144:676–681.
5. Shuman W, Mack L, Rudd T, et al. Evaluation of acute right upper quadrant pain. Am J Roentgenol 1982;139:61–64.
6. Burell MI, Zeman RK, Simeone JF, et al. The biliary tract: imaging for the 1990s. Am J Roentgenol 1991;157:223–233.
7. Johnston DE, Kaplan MM. Medical progress: pathogenesis and treatment of gallstones. N Engl J Med 1993;328:412–415.
8. Shea JA, Berlin JA, Escarce JJ, et al. Revised estimates of diagnostic test sensitivity and specificity in suspected biliary tract disease. Arch Int Med 1994;154:2573–2581.

9. Rosen CL, Brown DF, Chang Y, et al. Ultrasonography by emergency physicians in patients with suspected cholecystitis. Am J Emerg Med 2001;19:32–36.

10. Yeh HC. Update on the gallbladder. In: Sanders RL, ed. Ultrasound Annual 1982. New York: Raven Press, 1982.

11. Elyaderani MK, Gabriele OF. Cholecystosonography in detection of acute cholecystitis: the halo sign-a significant sonographic finding. South Med J 1983;76:174.

12. Ralls PW, Colletti PM, Lapin SA, et al. Real-time sonography in suspected acute cholecystitis. Prospective evaluation of primary and secondary signs. Radiology 1985;155:767–771.

13. Haubek A, Pedersen JH, Burcharth F, et al. Dynamic sonography in the evaluation of jaundice. Am J Radiol 1981;136:1071–1074.

14. Niederau C, Sonnenberg A. Liver size evaluated by ultrasound: ROC curves for hepatitis and alcoholism. Radiology 1984;153:503–505.

15. Good LI, Edell SL, Soloway RD, et al. Ultrasonic properties of gallstones. Gastroenterology 1979;77:258–263.

16. Ralls PW, Colletti PM, Lapin SA, et al. Real time sonography in suspected acute cholecystitis. Radiology 1985;155:767–771.

17. Laing FC, Jeffrey RB. Choledocholithiasis and cystic duct obstruction: difficult ultrasonographic diagnosis. Radiology 1983;146:475–479.

18. Kurtz AB, Rubin CS, Cooper HS, et al. Ultrasound findings in hepatitis. Radiology 1980;136:717–723.

19. Taylor KJ, Gorelick FS, Rosenfield AT, et al. Ultrasonography of alcoholic liver disease with histological correlation. Radiology 1981;141:157–161.

20. Behan M, Kazam E. The echographic characteristics of fatty tissues and tumors. Radiology 1978;129:143–151.

21. Green B, Bree RL, Goldstein HM, et al. Gray scale ultrasound evaluation of hepatic neoplasms: patterns and correlations. Radiology 1977;124:203–208.

22. Weaver RM, Goldstein HM, Green B, et al. Gray scale ultrasonographic evaluation of hepatic cystic disease. Am J Roentgenol 1978;130:849–852.

23. Kuligowska E, Connors SK, Shapiro JH. Liver abscess: sonography in diagnosis and treatment. Am J Roentgenol 1982;138:253–257.

24. Edell SL, Gefter WB. Ultrasonic differentiation of types of ascitic fluid. Am J Roentgenol 1979;133:111–114.

25. Angelico M, De Santis A, Capocaccia L. Biliary sludge: a critical update. J Clin Gastroenterol 1990;12:656–662.

CHAPTER 8

General Surgery Applications

Masaaki Ogata

Over the past two decades, abdominal sonography has become popular for surveying intraabdominal abnormalities such as hepatobiliary, vascular, urologic, and gynecologic disorders. With progress in the resolution of scanning devices, abdominal sonography has also been used for the evaluation of various acute gastrointestinal abnormalities. The operator-dependent nature of ultrasonography, however, may limit the application of the examination in the emergency setting. In the United States, ultrasonography has been a domain of radiology and, subsequently, the application of the examination for the acute abdomen in the emergency department has been somewhat limited. In most hospitals, the difficulty in providing 24-h service by expert sonographers has been a major factor in preventing ultrasonography from becoming a primary imaging modality in the emergency setting. It is quite important, however, to utilize the advantages of ultrasonography to improve patient evaluation in the emergency setting. Hence, bedside abdominal sonography performed by non-radiologist clinicians, such as emergency physicians or surgeons, will be increasingly necessary for the rapid investigation of the acute abdomen.

► CLINICAL CONSIDERATIONS

The evaluation of acute abdominal disorders begins with a careful history and physical examination. When required, the clinical findings may be supplemented by laboratory tests or conventional plain radiographs. Plain radiography may show some significant findings, such as pneumoperitoneum, bowel dilatation, calcified stones or bony disorders, but unsatisfactorily, it shows nonspecific findings in a significant number of patients. The development

of high resolution computed tomography (CT) and ultrasonography has greatly facilitated the identification of pathologies in many patients with an acute abdomen.

CT scanning is an excellent imaging modality to evaluate not only intraperitoneal disorders but also retroperitoneal abnormalities. CT scanning has a greater specificity than plain radiography but it has not been used as a routine screening tool for the acute abdomen because it is expensive and not immediately available in many hospitals. Both plain radiography and CT are non-invasive but are generally contraindicated in pregnant patients.

In contrast, sonography does not expose patients to ionizing radiation and is non-invasive, readily available, and repeatable at the bedside, and less expensive than CT scan. It has been accepted as a useful imaging modality for hepatobiliary, cardiovascular, urologic, or gynecologic disorders. In addition, recent studies have shown that sonography is applicable and may be accurate for acute gastrointestinal disorders such as acute appendicitis, acute colonic diverticulitis, intussusception, and bowel obstruction. It is also beneficial for patients who are hemodynamically unstable, who have unreliable physical findings due to drug intoxication or central nervous system disorders, or who have unexplained shock symptoms and an equivocal physical examination. Abdominal sonography, however, has some disadvantages, such as difficulty in visualizing intraperitoneal or retroperitoneal abnormalities in patients who are obese or who have excessive bowel gas.

The operator-dependent nature of ultrasonography has been identified as a factor influencing the reliability of emergency ultrasound performed by non-radiologist sonographers. Indeed, the clinical applications and results of emergency ultrasound are influenced by the clinical experience, skill, and interest of the sonographer. In several European countries and Japan, however, bedside ultrasound performed by non-radiologist clinicians has been accepted as a rapid and useful screening tool for the acute abdomen as well as for abdominal trauma. Physicians who are well trained to perform emergency ultrasound will significantly improve patient evaluation, initial treatment, selection of further diagnostic modalities, and timely consultation of surgeons or gastrointestinal specialists.

▶ CLINICAL INDICATIONS

In a general surgical setting, the clinical indications for applying an emergency ultrasound examination are:

- Acute abdominal pain
- Peritonitis
- Abdominal distention or mass
- Unexplained shock or sepsis

All patients who have been diagnosed with an acute abdomen on the basis of clinical findings are candidates for the examination. The common etiologies of acute abdomen are:

1. Hemorrhage
2. Gastrointestinal perforation
3. Bowel obstruction
4. Inflammatory disorder
5. Circulatory impairment

HEMORRHAGE

Active intraperitoneal and gastrointestinal hemorrhage are life-threatening etiologies for which rapid diagnosis and treatment are required. If patients are hemodynamically unstable, adequate resuscitation is the first priority. Rapid assessment for the approximate site of hemorrhage (intraperitoneal or gastrointestinal) should be made on the basis of clinical findings. The use of sonography for patients with massive hematemesis is limited in the emergency setting because they should be referred for emergency endoscopy. Patients who are hemodynamically unstable without gastrointestinal bleeding should be urgently examined for intraperitoneal hemorrhage. In this setting, abdominal sonography is very useful and reliable for the evaluation of intraperitoneal hemorrhage. It can be utilized during the resuscitation of the unstable patient in the emergency setting, whereas other imaging modalities, such as CT and angiography, require hemodynamic stability of patients.

Intraperitoneal Hemorrhage

Since intraperitoneal hemorrhage may be severe enough to produce hypovolemic shock, the rapid detection of

free intraperitoneal fluid is essential for patients who are suspected of having intraperitoneal hemorrhage on the basis of their clinical findings. For this purpose, the focused assessment with sonography for free peritoneal fluid is beneficial as in cases of abdominal trauma. As described in the Chapter 4, sonography has been recognized as a rapid, sensitive, and specific diagnostic modality for detecting free intraperitoneal fluid in many clinical studies.[1,2] Appropriately trained, non-radiologist clinicians, such as emergency physicians or surgeons, can accurately perform and interpret abdominal sonography for free intraperitoneal fluid in cases of acute abdomen as well as abdominal trauma. On the other hand, plain radiographs are insensitive and inappropriate for the early recognition of intraperitoneal hemorrhage since radiographic signs for the accumulation of peritoneal fluid, such as widening of the paracolic gutter or a "dog's ear" appearance, require a large amount of peritoneal fluid. CT scanning is unavailable for immediate use in some emergency departments and somewhat inappropriate for hemodynamically unstable patients; however, CT is very useful in detecting intraperitoneal hemorrhage and retroperitoneal hematoma.

In making a decision for surgical exploration, it is important to detect the presence and the amount of intraperitoneal hemorrhage even if primary lesions are not identified. As abdominal sonography can be used to estimate not only the amount but also the rate of intraperitoneal hemorrhage through serial examinations, it will supplement clinical findings in evaluating whether the hemorrhage is active or not.

Common sites where free peritoneal fluid accumulates are Morison's pouch, the rectovesical pouch, the pouch of Douglas, and bilateral subphrenic spaces. A small amount of free fluid may be seen between bowel loops. A large amount of free fluid can be seen above the bowels, located adjacent to the anterior peritoneum. On sonographic images, hemoperitoneum appears anechoic with coarse internal echoes as the blood is clotted. Bloody or purulent ascites or peritoneal fluid containing intestinal contents also may be shown as having similar images.[1,2] Although differentiating hemoperitoneum from ascites is not very difficult on the basis of a careful history and physical examination, paracentesis (guided by ultrasound if needed) can be applied for the definite diagnosis of hemoperitoneum.

The pathology causing intraperitoneal hemorrhage can be evaluated with abdominal sonography. While CT remains the gold standard for detecting specific intra-abdominal pathology, it is beneficial to utilize bedside sonography for this purpose, especially with unstable patients. Common causes of intraperitoneal hemorrhage are rupture of a hepatoma, aortic aneurysm, or ectopic pregnancy, or ovarian bleeding. Abdominal sonography can be performed as a rapid screening tool for detecting such specific lesions as hepatoma and abdominal aortic aneurysm. Early recognition of these etiologies is beneficial for selecting further examinations and making a strategy for treatment, which is either immediate surgery or interventional radiology. In young female patients who present with hypotensive shock and associated lower abdominal pain, gynecologic disorders, such as rupture of an ectopic pregnancy or ovarian bleeding unrelated to pregnancy, should be always taken into consideration. Although transabdominal sonography may demonstrate non-specific findings, massive hemorrhage warrants immediate surgical treatment.

Gastrointestinal Hemorrhage

Patients with an upper gastrointestinal hemorrhage generally present with various degrees of hematemesis or melena. However, some may present with only complaints of epigastric pain or with unexplained shock. Primary causes of upper gastrointestinal hemorrhage are duodenal ulcer, gastric ulcer, hemorrhagic gastritis, esophageal or gastric varices, and Mallory–Weiss syndrome. Patients who are suspected of having massive gastrointestinal hemorrhage should be referred for emergency endoscopy, which makes it possible to identify the bleeding source in up to 90% of cases of upper gastrointestinal hemorrhage. In contrast, other diagnostic modalities, such as plain radiography, sonography, CT, and gastrointestinal contrast studies, do not contribute to the diagnosis of acute gastrointestinal hemorrhage. When appropriate, emergency ultrasound may be applied for detecting adjunct findings such as liver cirrhosis and splenomegaly. Abnormalities of the gastroduodenal wall such as gastric cancer, peptic ulcer, and acute gastric mucosal lesion occasionally may be shown with sonography.[3,4]

In cases of massive lower gastrointestinal hemorrhage, direct endoscopic evaluation may be disturbed by a large amount of blood and stool in the colon. Furthermore, at times the causes of lower gastrointestinal hemorrhage originate in the small bowel. For these reasons, emergency angiography or scintigraphy is reserved for patients in whom colonoscopy is unsuccessful in locating the bleeding source. Abdominal sonography can be used as a screening tool to evaluate intraabdominal abnormalities suggesting a bleeding source (e.g., colon cancer, ischemic colitis) and its adjunct findings (e.g., liver cirrhosis, bowel obstruction, or abscess formation).

GASTROINTESTINAL PERFORATION

Gastrointestinal perforations are serious disorders requiring rapid diagnosis and treatment. Since they may be severe enough to produce septic or hypovolemic shock, rapid decision-making for urgent laparotomy is crucially important. The initial diagnosis is generally made on the basis of clinical symptoms and signs of peritonitis and then supplemented by plain radiography demonstrating pneumoperitoneum. Plain radiographs, however, may not always show pneumoperitoneum in cases of gastrointestinal perforation, and are useless in detecting underlying etiologies. The incidence of pneumoperitoneum appreciated on conventional radiographs was reported as 80 to 90% in cases of gastroduodenal perforation but only 20 to 30% and 30 to 50%, respectively, in cases of small bowel and large bowel perforation.[5,6] Moreover, in the elderly, signs of peritonitis on physical examination may be obscured and laboratory tests may show a normal white blood cell count. These clinical and radiographic features may cloud the diagnosis of gastrointestinal perforation in elderly patients. Consequently, any delay in making a decision for urgent laparotomy may lead to further deterioration in the clinical status of the patient, especially in cases of large bowel perforation. To avoid such delay in the diagnosis and treatment, therefore, conventional plain radiography should be supplemented with other diagnostic modalities, which include CT, sonography, contrast studies, and endoscopy. CT is more sensitive for demonstrating not only pneumoperitoneum but also ectopic gas in the retroperitoneal space. CT has been reported to demonstrate a very small pneumoperitoneum that was not appreciated on conventional plain radiographs.[7]

Abdominal sonography is not as sensitive as plain radiography for demonstrating pneumoperitoneum. It may be valuable, however, in complementing plain radiographs by rapidly identifying pneumoperitoneum in the supine patient.[8–12] Subphrenic free air can be identified as an echogenic line with posterior reverberation artifacts on the ventral surface of the liver. It should be discriminated, however, from gas in the gastrointestinal lumen or the lung to avoid a false diagnosis. Hyperventilation may interfere with the examination for clearly visualization of free air. Hepatodiaphragmatic interposition of the colon also may cause subphrenic gas echoes.

As for the underlying pathology, bedside ultrasound can be applied for the evaluation of specific lesions. It may detect a primary lesion, such as colon cancer, acute colonic diverticulitis, or an acute duodenal ulcer, and secondary abnormalities, such as free peritoneal fluid, a localized abscess, or paralytic ileus. Upper gastrointestinal perforation is not very difficult to diagnose on the basis of clinical and radiographic findings. If required, emergency endoscopy can be adopted for identifying gastroduodenal lesions. Therefore, it is not essential to detect images of a peptic ulcer or gastric cancer by sonography or CT. As a screening tool available at bedside, however, abdominal sonography may occasionally demonstrate a duodenal ulcer or gastric cancer as hypoechoic wall thickening.[3,4]

The strategies for treatment of a peptic ulcer, which is the leading cause of upper gastrointestinal perforation, have changed in recent years. Nonoperative treatments using anti-ulcerative agents have been successful in selected patients with a perforated duodenal ulcer. This new option for treating perforated peptic ulcers may influence the use of diagnostic modalities. A patient with a perforated duodenal ulcer can be a candidate for non-operative treatments when signs of peritonitis are localized in the right upper quadrant. In this setting, consequently, pneumoperitoneum itself is not considered to be an absolute indication for immediate surgery. Serial examinations with sonography can be used as follow-up studies to evaluate the accumulation of peritoneal fluid or occurrence of any other abnormalities when non-operative treatments are adopted for a perforated duodenal ulcer.

On sonographic images of gastrointestinal perforation, free peritoneal fluid often contains gray level echoes inside an anechoic space in the pelvis or Morison's pouch, or adjacent to intestinal loops. The image is regarded as showing turbulent, purulent, or feculent peritoneal fluid. Gas echoes may be occasionally identified as echogenic spots inside an anechoic space. Although the nature of peritoneal fluid cannot be ascertained strictly on ultrasound, such sonographic images can be helpful in making a decision for surgical intervention when pneumoperitoneum is not identified.

BOWEL OBSTRUCTION

Bowel obstruction is a common etiology of acute abdomen. The clinical picture of a patient with bowel obstruction varies depending on location, form, etiology, and degree of the obstruction. Thus, strategies for treatment should be carefully determined on the basis of clinical findings, laboratory tests, and imaging methods. Generally, plain radiography is conventionally used as an initial imaging method when bowel obstruction is considered. It serves to confirm the distribution of gaseous dilated bowel and the approximate site of obstruction. However, it is widely known that plain radiography cannot reliably differentiate strangulation from simple obstruction and is useless to demonstrate causative lesions for bowel obstruction.[13,14]

For years, the application of sonography for bowel obstruction had been regarded as inappropriate and unreliable because of the significant artifact arising from gastrointestinal gas. This misconception has prevented not only radiologists but also surgeons and emergency physicians from utilizing sonography for the evaluation of bowel obstruction. With progress in the resolution of scanning devices, however, abdominal sonography has become more popular for the evaluation of gastrointestinal diseases.[15,16] Sonography's role in recognizing fluid-filled distended bowel was reported in the literature during the latter half of 1970s.[17,18] Fleischer and co-workers first introduced sonographic patterns of distended, fluid-filled bowel both in vivo and in vitro in 1979.[17] Since

the latter half of 1980s, abdominal sonography has gained increasing popularity for the evaluation of bowel obstruction in Japan and Germany. Some studies have shown the usefulness of abdominal sonography for demonstrating a radiograph-negative small bowel obstruction, and for differentiating between a small bowel obstruction and a paralytic ileus.[19–22] In the 1990s, the use of sonography for the differentiation between strangulation and simple small bowel obstruction was reported.[23-25] Ogata and colleagues introduced the usefulness of sonography in identifying radiograph-negative large bowel obstruction, and Ogata and Mateer prospectively demonstrated that initial bedside ultrasound was as sensitive and more specific than plain radiographs for the diagnosis of bowel obstruction in an emergency department setting.[26,27]

The pathophysiologic appearances of bowel obstruction are characterized primarily by the accumulation of fluid and electrolytes in the gastrointestinal tract proximal to the obstruction.[28] With further progression, the bowel loops become distended with accumulated fluid in the lumen. In addition, the bowel wall may be thickened with interstitial edema, and free fluid may accumulate in the peritoneal cavity. Taking these features into consideration, abdominal sonography as well as CT may be appropriate and applicable to the diagnosis of bowel obstruction because it is superior to plain radiographs in visualizing accumulated fluid. Furthermore, real-time sonography can provide a dynamic view of intestinal peristalsis, which can not be recognized by CT. These advantages of real-time sonography have made a revolutionary progress in the diagnosis of bowel obstruction, especially in the early recognition of strangulated small bowel obstruction.

Strangulated small bowel obstruction involves compromise of blood supply to the strangulated loop of bowel and requires early surgical intervention. A number of clinical studies have shown that it is difficult to recognize the early stages of strangulation because of the lack of reliable criteria.[13] Difficulty in making the early diagnosis of strangulation has resulted in a recommendation for early surgical intervention. While this strategy seems logical in reducing delays in surgical repair, it increases the number of surgical cases for nonstrangulated obstruction that could have been relieved without operative therapy. On the other hand, in order to safely elect non-operative treatment, the exclusion of strangulation is essential. Ogata and associates reported that abdominal sonography was useful in revealing the presence of strangulation that was not suspected by clinical judgment. Abdominal sonography was also useful for excluding the presence of strangulation in patients with simple obstruction who were clinically suspected of having strangulation.[23] According to their report, the sensitivity and specificity of sonography for strangulation were 90% and 92%, respectively, in the study of 231 patients with small bowel obstruction by adhesions. The use of sonography to differentiate strangulation from simple obstruction may permit earlier operative intervention for strangulation while also allowing wider use of nonoperative management for cases that are simple small bowel obstruction.

When abdominal sonography is applied for the evaluation of bowel obstruction, it is clinically important to analyze the following factors in each case.

1. To identify the evidence of mechanical bowel obstruction
2. To locate the level of obstruction
3. To differentiate strangulation from simple obstruction
4. To evaluate the etiology of bowel obstruction
5. To estimate the severity of bowel obstruction
6. To survey the whole abdomen for other abnormalities

Mechanical Bowel Obstruction versus Ileus

The clinical manifestations of a mechanical bowel obstruction depend on the level of the obstruction (proximal or distal small bowel or large bowel) and the blood supply to the affected loop of bowel (simple or strangulated obstruction). The evidence of a mechanical bowel obstruction is confirmed by demonstrating a distinct point of transition between dilated proximal bowel and collapsed distal bowel with an imaging modality such as plain radiography, sonography, or CT. In contrast, the diagnosis of ileus is based on the absence of such a distinct point of transition along with a clinical presentation consistent with ileus. Abdominal sonography, as well as plain radiography and CT, can be used for the differentiation of a mechanical bowel obstruction versus an ileus.[19,27,29] In the early stage of ileus, slightly dilated small bowel loops (less than 25 mm wide in diameter) are often recognized on ultrasound. Gas echoes, which are more dominant than fluid collection inside the bowel, are featured in the sonographic images of ileus. Also, other abnormalities suggesting the primary etiology of ileus may be shown on ultrasound. In the advanced stage of ileus, real-time sonography may occasionally show fluid-filled, dilated bowel loops without peristaltic activity.

Small Bowel Obstruction versus Large Bowel Obstruction

Initially, abdominal sonography was used in suggesting the diagnosis of small bowel obstruction in patients with atypical plain radiographs, such as a "pseudotumor" appearance or a totally "gasless" abdomen, and also in demonstrating an intussusception in patients with an abdominal mass suspected of the entity. Recent studies have suggested, however, that real-time bedside ultrasound may be used as an initial imaging method for the evaluation of small bowel obstruction.[20,22,24] According to

the report by Ogata and colleagues, sonography was not diagnostic due to interference by gastrointestinal gas in only 3 of 231 patients with a small bowel obstruction by adhesions.[23]

As for patients clinically suspected of having a large bowel obstruction, plain radiographs are routinely used as the initial imaging procedure as it serves to confirm the diagnosis and locate the obstruction in the majority of the cases. However, plain radiographs may show an isolated small bowel dilatation but no gaseous colonic dilatation in approximately 15% of patients with a large bowel obstruction.[14,26] In such cases, it is difficult to differentiate a large bowel obstruction from a small bowel obstruction on plain radiographs alone. The use of sonography for the diagnosis of large bowel obstruction has not yet been fully evaluated due to the belief that accumulated gas in the colon interferes with the examination. Indeed, it is difficult to evaluate the gaseous distended colon with sonography. In cases of large bowel obstruction, however, abdominal sonography often reveals dilated colon as filled with dense spot echoes, which seem to represent feculent, liquid contents including small bubbles of gas. According to the study by Ogata and associates, abdominal sonography provided a diagnosis of large bowel obstruction in 33 of 39 patients with this condition, and proved useful in detecting radiograph-negative colonic dilatation that was occasionally seen in patients with large bowel obstruction proximal to the splenic flexure.[26]

Strangulation versus Simple Obstruction

Strangulation small bowel obstruction is most commonly caused by adhesive bands. The strangulated, closed loop may be occasionally shown as a "pseudotumor" appearance on plain radiographs. Numerous studies have shown the value and effectiveness of sonography in demonstrating the closed loop filled with fluid. Real-time sonography also can provide a dynamic view of peristalsis in the obstructed loops.

The sonographic criteria for simple small bowel obstruction include the presence of dilated small bowel proximal to collapsed small bowel or ascending colon and the presence of peristaltic activity in the entire dilated proximal small bowel. The peristaltic activity is appreciated as peristalsis of the bowel wall or to-and-fro movements of spot echoes inside the fluid-filled dilated small bowel. The criteria for early strangulation include: (1) the presence of an akinetic dilated loop, (2) the presence of peristaltic activity in dilated small bowel proximal to the akinetic loop, and (3) rapid accumulation of peritoneal fluid after the onset of obstruction. An established strangulation is recognized by asymmetric wall thickening (more than 3 mm) with increased echogenicity in the akinetic loop, or a large amount of peritoneal fluid containing scattered spot echoes indicating bloody ascites. Although the presence of peritoneal fluid is not specific for strangulation, the quantitative evaluation of peritoneal fluid will be helpful in differentiating strangulation from simple obstruction.

Specific Etiologies of Obstruction

Abdominal sonography offers the advantage of providing additional information about specific etiologies of obstruction that is not obtained with plain radiographs. Although adhesions obstructing the small bowel cannot be visualized, sonography can image the specific etiologies of small bowel obstruction, which include cecal carcinoma, intussusception, external hernias, inflammatory bowel diseases (tuberculosis, Crohn's disease, or radiation enteritis), small bowel tumors, afferent loop obstruction following Billroth II gastrectomy, and gallstone ileus. Except intussusception and incarceration of an external hernia, the specific etiologies are relatively rare but should be considered.

Intussusception is a common etiology of bowel obstruction in children but relatively rare in adults, accounting for only about 5% of all intussusception cases and 1 to 3% of adult patients with bowel obstruction. Unlike in children, the causative lesion can be identified in more than 80% of adult patients. The most common cause of intussusception is a polypoid tumor of the small bowel. Ileocolic intussusception is the most common form (more than 70%), followed by enteroenteric and colocolic intussusception. Plain radiographs rarely define the intussusception as a mass of soft tissue density, and show no evidence of bowel obstruction in the acute stage. In contrast, abdominal sonography can present the characteristic appearances of intussusception. The cross-sectional image is well known as the "multiple concentric ring sign" or "target sign."[30,31] The multi-laminar structure also can be demonstrated in the long axis planes. It is very rare, however, to demonstrate the causative lesion itself (i.e., tumor or diverticulum) with sonography. The sonographic appearance of bowel obstruction may not yet be established when the diagnosis of intussusception is obtained.

Incarceration, which is a common complication of external hernias, produces a bowel obstruction and impairs the blood supply to the entrapped bowel segment. It occurs more frequently in cases of femoral hernia than with inguinal hernia. The clinical symptoms and physical examination findings depend on the degree of the obstruction and the blood supply to the herniated bowel segment. The diagnosis is not difficult to make on the basis of a careful physical examination in most cases. If physical examination findings are equivocal, abdominal sonography can be used to demonstrate an incarcerated hernia, showing an entrapped bowel segment without peristaltic activity.

As for the etiologies of large bowel obstruction, obstructing colon carcinoma, which is by far the most common cause of large bowel obstruction, may be detected as an irregular-shaped hypoechoic mass with echogenic core inside or a localized circular wall thickening. Intraluminal tumor obstructing the lumen may be occasionally demonstrated with sonography. Ogata and co-workers reported that sonography demonstrated the obstructing lesion in 14 of 35 patients with primary or metastatic colorectal carcinoma.[26] Even when the obstructing lesion is not visualized, detecting the associated lesions such as metastatic liver tumors would be useful in making the diagnosis. In volvulus of the sigmoid colon, however, sonography shows only vast gas echoes that spread beneath the abdominal wall because the twisted and obstructed colon loop is markedly distended with excessive gas. Plain radiography is diagnostic of this entity by presenting the classic "coffee bean" sign. In volvulus of the entire small bowel, a rare entity in the Western countries, sonography may show fluid-filled, dilated loops with mural thickening and peritoneal fluid. Peristaltic activity dwindles as the intestinal infarction progresses.

INFLAMMATORY DISORDERS

Various kinds of inflammatory disorders are included in the etiologies of acute abdomen. Abdominal sonography can be used for evaluating the site, extent, or severity of the inflammatory disorder by visualizing interstitial edema or hemorrhage, and peritoneal fluid. Segmental wall thickening of the bowel may be demonstrated in inflammatory gastrointestinal disorders such as appendicitis, diverticulitis, infectious enterocolitis, ischemic colitis, or Crohn's disease. Also, wall thickening of the gallbladder can show the severity of acute cholecystitis, and the echogenicity of the pancreas can vary according to the degree of interstitial edema or hemorrhage in acute pancreatitis.

Acute Appendicitis

Acute appendicitis is the most common cause of the acute abdomen in Western countries. The diagnosis is straightforward in most patients who present with typical clinical symptoms and signs. It is not uncommon, however, to face difficulties in making a diagnosis of appendicitis in patients who have an equivocal presentation. Abdominal sonography has been increasingly used for differentiating acute appendicitis from other abdominal disorders.

Conventional radiographs present non-specific findings, such as regional bowel dilatation, in most cases of acute appendicitis. The most specific finding on plain radiographs is the presence of a calcified appendicolith, which is noted in about 10% of adults with appendicitis. On the other hand, abdominal sonography for acute appendicitis is considered to be useful for (1) direct visualization of the inflamed appendix, (2) assessment of the degree of inflammatory changes, (3) identification of abscess formation or free peritoneal fluid, (4) differentiation from other acute abdominal disorders, and (5) application to pregnant patients.

Since Puylaert reported that high-resolution ultrasound with a graded compression technique was successful in visualizing the abnormal appendix in a high percentage of cases, many physicians have adopted the technique and confirmed high diagnostic accuracy of the technique for acute appendicitis.[32-36] The sensitivity and specificity of graded compression sonography in experienced hands was reported to be 76 to 90% and 90 to 98%, respectively, in prospective studies. In the United States, abdominal CT scan is commonly utilized for evaluating patients with possible appendicitis; its accuracy for confirming or ruling out appendicitis has been reported to be 93 to 98%.

The accuracy of sonography is examiner dependent. Practically, inexperienced sonographers will face difficulties obtaining such a high accuracy in the diagnosis of acute appendicitis.[37,38] The most important reason for a false-negative study is overlooking the inflamed appendix. Dilated bowel loops due to an associated ileus may obscure the appendix. Optimal images may not be obtained because of the inability to achieve adequate compression of the right lower quadrant. This is caused by severe pain or marked obesity. False negative studies may also occur in patients with retrocecal or perforated appendicitis. A false positive diagnosis can be made if a normal appendix is mistaken for an inflamed one or if a terminal ileum is confused with an enlarged inflamed appendix. With adequate training and enough experience, however, non-radiologist sonographers can obtain an acceptable accuracy rate comparable to experienced radiologists.[39-42]

Sonography is more sensitive for the detection of an appendicolith than plain radiographs, and has been reported as detecting intraluminal fecalith in up to 30% of cases. In general, a normal appendix (about 6 mm or smaller) can rarely be visualized by graded compression sonography although some investigators have reported that in the majority of patients a normal appendix can be identified with modern equipment in experienced hands.[43,44]

Acute appendicitis may present in various stages at the time of diagnosis: catarrhal, phlegmonous, gangrenous, or perforated accompanying pericecal abscess or purulent peritonitis. Abdominal sonography can be used to evaluate the pathologic severity of acute appendicitis by delineating the layer structure of thickened appendiceal wall. In cases of catarrhal or phlegmonous appendicitis, a swollen appendix maintains the mural lamination. In contrast, focal loss of the layer structure is often observed in patients with gangrenous appendicitis. A pericecal ab-

scess can be demonstrated as a fluid collection with a thick, non-compressible wall. With a pericecal abscess secondary to perforated appendicitis, it may be quite difficult to identify the gangrenous appendix itself. Even if an inflamed appendix is not detected, identifying an abscess or free peritoneal fluid in the pelvis or the pericecal region can be valuable for surgeons to make a decision for urgent exploration. On the other hand, it is still controversial whether surgical intervention or conservative treatment with antibiotics should be adopted in the early stage of appendicitis. In general, sonographic findings should be correlated with both clinical and laboratory findings in order to determine an indication for surgery.

Acute appendicitis in pregnant women can be rather difficult to diagnose because of the deviated location of the appendix and equivocal presentation. Abdominal sonography can be applied for the evaluation of appendicitis in pregnant patients. In this setting, it is important to take the deviated location of appendix into consideration.

Sonography is also useful for establishing an alternative diagnosis in patients examined with suspicion of appendicitis. The spectrum of differential diagnoses includes mesenteric lymphadenitis (particularly in children), right-sided adnexal pathology in young women, enterocolitis, diverticulitis, Crohn's disease, cholecystitis, and colon cancer.

Acute Colonic Diverticulitis

The prevalence of colonic diverticulosis increases with age. Although approximately 80 to 90% of all diverticula remain asymptomatic for life, acute colonic diverticulitis is a relatively common etiology of an acute abdomen in elderly patients. The rectosigmoid colon is the most frequently involved segment in acute diverticulitis. Diverticulitis in the ascending colon and cecum is less frequently involved, and is rather difficult to diagnose clinically since it has the same features as appendicitis.

Plain radiographs are of little value in obtaining direct findings of acute diverticulitis; however, it may demonstrate pneumoperitoneum, mechanical bowel obstruction, or ileus in complicated cases. The use of contrast barium enema for demonstrating the extent of the disease is limited to the cases of clinically mild diverticulitis because it is hazardous in cases of possible colonic perforation. Water-soluble contrast enema is safe and available in complicated cases, although the quality of images is inferior to barium contrast enema.

Abdominal sonography can be applied for the initial evaluation of possible diverticulitis. The sensitivity and specificity of sonography for this etiology was reported as more than 80% when the examination was performed by experienced sonographers.[45,46] Abdominal ultrasound may reveal additional findings such as pericolonic abscess or free peritoneal fluid in complicated cases. CT is more optimal, however, in demonstrating not only colonic diverticula but also extracolonic complications including pericolonic or pelvic abscess, free perforation, or colovesical fistula.

Acute Pancreatitis

Acute pancreatitis is defined as an inflammation of the pancreas associated with typical abdominal complaints and elevated serum and urinary pancreatic enzymes, and may be classified according to the clinical picture, etiologic factors, or pathologic changes. The clinical course ranges from a mild, benign process to a severe, fulminant process that may lead to fatal outcomes. The two most common etiologic factors are alcoholism and biliary stone disease, although up to 10 to 30% of patients with acute pancreatitis may present without a history of either.

The pathologic forms are classified generally as edematous and necrotizing pancreatitis. Edematous pancreatitis is characterized by interstitial edema and mild pancreatic and peripancreatic inflammation, and accounts for 80 to 85% of cases. The mortality rate is less than 2%. Necrotizing pancreatitis is characterized by interstitial hemorrhage, fat necrosis, extensive extrapancreatic infiltration, and suppuration. Bacterial infection occurs in up to 40% of patients with necrotizing pancreatitis and is gradually manifested within several weeks after the onset of pancreatitis. On the whole, necrotizing pancreatitis is a far more severe form of acute pancreatitis that often requires hemodynamic support and mechanical ventilation, and leads to severe complications and mortality rates of 10 to 40%.[47,48] Although it is clinically important to distinguish patients with either edematous or necrotizing pancreatitis in terms of therapy and prognosis, it is rather difficult at the early stage of their clinical course. Quantitative assays of serum pancreatic enzymes may be useful in diagnosing acute pancreatitis but the degree of the enzyme abnormality does not correlate with the severity of acute pancreatitis. Plain radiographs may show non-specific findings such as the "sentinel loop sign," "colon cut-off sign," or a generalized ileus but are of little use in evaluating acute pancreatitis.

Direct imaging of the pancreas with CT or sonography may provide morphologic information to establish the diagnosis of pancreatitis and its complications.[48–50] In general, CT is clearly superior to sonography in demonstrating complex extrapancreatic involvement as well as contour irregularities or focal changes in the pancreas. Ultrasound examinations are frequently disturbed by excessive gastrointestinal gas caused by an accompanying ileus, especially in cases of severe pancreatitis. Therefore, the main role of emergency ultrasound is to evaluate the biliary tree for gallstone disease as a remediable cause. Sonographic diagnosis of choledocholithiasis or significant dilatation of the common bile duct may obviate the need for invasive diagnostic procedures.

Abdominal sonography can also be used for the initial survey of acute pancreatitis. The echogenicity of the pancreas generally decreases in acute pancreatitis as a result of interstitial edema. In some patients, the echogenicity is normal or increased. Cotton and co-workers noted that the echogenicity of the pancreas compared to the liver was increased in 16% of patients and normal in 32% of patients with acute pancreatitis.[49] The variability may be caused by pancreatic hemorrhage, necrosis, or fat saponification. Enlargement of the pancreas in acute pancreatitis is also variable; significant individual variations are recognized in pancreatic dimensions. Therefore, enlargement is of limited value for the diagnosis of acute pancreatitis. Clinically important findings obtained with sonography are peripancreatic fluid collections or echogenic pancreatic masses, which suggest the progress of necrotizing pancreatitis. Such sonographic findings should be confirmed with both contrast and non-contrast CT for the definitive diagnosis.

Extrapancreatic fluid collections are most commonly detected in the superior recess of the lesser sac and the anterior pararenal space. Fluid collections are generally visualized as hypoechoic images on ultrasound. CT is more advantageous in locating fluid collections to specific anatomic compartments. It is difficult, however, to distinguish pancreatic abscess from uninfected necrosis or fluid collections, although pancreatic abscess are often associated with extensive, ill-defined multi-compartmental changes. CT-guided fine-needle aspiration is used to make an early diagnosis of pancreatic abscess.

On the other hand, acute peripancreatic fluid collections resolve with conservative therapy in 70 to 90% of the cases. The remaining fluid collections persist long enough (at least 6 weeks) to develop a fibrous wall, and then are called pancreatic pseudocysts. Pseudocysts may develop in association with chronic pancreatitis, or after pancreatic surgery or trauma. Uncomplicated small pseudocysts (smaller than 6 cm) may allow persistent observation, but larger pseudocysts should be drained by surgical, endoscopic or percutaneous means to reduce the risk of complications, which include secondary infection, rupture, and hemorrhage.[47,48] Serial examinations with CT or sonography can document the gradual development of pseudocysts. The advantage of sonography is the lower cost of follow up studies. On sonographic images, pancreatic pseudocysts are generally visualized as cystic masses of various sizes, which are well defined by adjacent organs and a visible capsule. However, small well-defined cystic masses should be examined with color Doppler scanning to exclude a pancreatic pseudoaneurysm, which may occasionally develop 2 to 3 weeks after the onset of severe pancreatitis.

Acute Cholecystitis

Since acute cholecystitis may lead to serious complications such as sepsis, pericholecystic abscess, or bilious peritonitis secondary to gallbladder perforation, immediate surgery often is required. It is critically important to make the rapid and definite diagnosis of acute cholecystitis and to determine the indication for surgical intervention. Abdominal sonography is a rapid and reliable technique for establishing or excluding the diagnosis of acute cholecystitis, even though sonographic findings should always be correlated with clinical and laboratory findings (see also Chapter 7).

There are three important indirect signs to establish the diagnosis of acute cholecystitis.[51,52] Gallstones are the prime etiologic factor since approximately 90% of cases with acute cholecystitis develop as a complication of cholelithiasis. The identification of impacted gallstones in the gallbladder neck or cystic duct is highly specific for acute calculus cholecystitis, although sonography may be unable to detect a small impacted gallstone in a few cases of calculous cholecystitis. Biliary sludge along with the absence of gallstones in the expanded gallbladder can be identified in cases of acalculous cholecystitis. The most specific sign of acute cholecystitis is the "sonographic Murphy's sign," which corresponds to the spot of maximum tenderness directly over the gallbladder (Murphy's sign is elicited with focal tenderness over the gallbladder with inspiratory arrest). According to the report by Ralls and associates, 99% of patients with acute cholecystitis had calculi and a positive sonographic Murphy's sign.[52]

In cases of acalculous cholecystitis, however, focal tenderness over the gallbladder may be difficult to obtain. Thickening of the gallbladder wall to more than 3 mm is another sign for acute cholecystitis, although it is not specific as long as the wall maintains a distinct trilaminar structure with a hypoechoic band surrounded by two hyperechoic lines. Irregular sonolucent layers in the gallbladder wall may be indicative of more advanced cholecystitis. The presence of asymmetric thickening of the gallbladder wall or intraluminal membranes parallel to the gallbladder wall may be identified in patients with acute gangrenous cholecystitis. Localized pericholecystic fluid collection may be caused by gallbladder perforation and abscess formation. The site of the perforation may occasionally be visualized as a defect in the gallbladder wall. These sonographic findings can be indicative of the need for immediate surgery.

CIRCULATORY IMPAIRMENT

Another relatively common and clinically important entity is ischemic bowel disease, which can be lethal if not promptly diagnosed and surgically treated. Embolism of the superior mesenteric artery and ischemic colitis are the most commonly encountered events in the emergency setting.

Embolism of the Superior Mesenteric Artery

Acute mesenteric ischemia is notoriously difficult to diagnose early in its clinical course, and subsequently often results in delayed surgical intervention in a number of cases. Patients with this entity present with sudden onset of abdominal pain, diarrhea, and vomiting; the symptoms, however, are nonspecific and there may be a striking disparity between the severity of symptoms and the lack of direct physical findings. Progressive signs of shock may be apparent in the initial stage. Therefore, it is clinically important to suspect an embolism of the superior mesenteric artery (SMA) when elderly patients with mitral valve disorders or atrial fibrillation present with non-specific abdominal symptoms.

Routine abdominal sonography can provide no specific findings in cases of a SMA embolism. In the initial stage, fluid-filled dilatation of the small bowel is minimal. Peritoneal fluid and mural thickening in the small bowel without peristaltic activity are non-specific, but suggest the possibility of acute mesenteric ischemia. Color Doppler can be used to demonstrate an occlusion of the main trunk of the SMA.[53] CT may directly demonstrate an occluding thrombus within the SMA, pneumatosis of the bowel wall, or gas in the portal vein in conjunction with peritoneal fluid, bowel wall thickening, or dilatation of fluid-filled loops of the small bowel. When the disease is suspected, immediate angiography should be applied for the definite diagnosis of SMA embolism.

Ischemic Colitis

Ischemic colitis is characterized by the abrupt onset of crampy abdominal pain and diarrhea, which often contains blood. Since the clinical features are non-specific and few symptoms may be present initially, it is especially important to consider the diagnosis of ischemic colitis in elderly patients. Unlike small bowel ischemia, most cases of colonic ischemia are not associated with a visible arterial occlusion. The pathophysiology is believed to relate to decreased perfusion of the colon wall due to peripheral vasoconstriction (e.g., in cardiac failure), sepsis, or hypovolemia. Age-related atherosclerotic disease is a predisposing factor. The effects range from reversible mucosal ischemia to transmural infarction. Strictures and stenoses can follow the resolution of conservatively managed cases.

Abdominal sonography may suggest the diagnosis by demonstrating segmental wall thickening of the affected colon. Colonoscopy and contrast studies remain the primary methods to evaluate patients with clinically suspected ischemic colitis. The most common site of involvement is the distal colon within the vascular territory of the inferior mesenteric artery. The proximal colon to the splenic flexure area (the so-called "watershed zone") may be involved. As sonography cannot reliably differentiate inflammatory changes from ischemic changes, color Doppler should be applied for the differentiation between colonic diverticulitis and ischemic colitis.[54] Mural blood flow is diminished in the affected segment of ischemic colitis. Both routine sonography and color Doppler scanning can be used for a follow-up study of ischemic colitis. In cases of reversible mucosal ischemia, wall thickening is gradually reduced in approximately 1 week. In cases of transmural infarction, sonography may show rapid accumulation of peritoneal fluid. CT can be used for the same purpose and is more sensitive for complications such as perforation or abscess formation.

▶ ANATOMIC CONSIDERATIONS

Free Peritoneal Fluid

The site of accumulation of peritoneal fluid, which is discussed in the Chapter 4, is dependent on the position of the patient and the etiology that causes free fluid to accumulate. In the supine patient, peritoneal fluid in the pelvis or Morison's pouch is most easily detected by sonography.

Stomach

The gastric antrum is generally located posterocaudally to the left lobe of the liver. The proximal stomach is usually difficult to delineate due to the significant artifact arising from gas in the stomach. When filled with liquid contents, the proximal stomach can be identified medially to the splenic hilum with left intercostal or coronal scanning.

Duodenum

The duodenal bulb is located medially to the gallbladder, posterior to the liver, and anterior to the pancreatic head. The inferior vena cava is another landmark located posterior to the duodenal C-loop.

Small Bowel

Normal small bowel loops are generally recognized as a tubular structure with peristalsis. However, the sonographic images of the small bowel vary depending on the nature and volume of the intestinal contents.

Large Bowel

The ascending colon is easily demonstrated anterior to the right kidney in the right flank. The transverse colon can be identified caudally to the gastric antrum in a sagittal plane. The descending colon can be demonstrated anterior to the lower pole of the left kidney in the left flank. The sigmoid colon may be difficult to examine. The rectum can be demonstrated posterior to the uterus or prostate. The normal colonic wall thickness is up to 3 mm.

Appendix Vermiformis

The position of the appendix is highly variable. The most common position is caudal to the cecum and terminal ileum (31 to 70%), followed by a retrocecal position (25 to 60%). Other less common positions are deep within the pelvis (4%), lateral to the cecum (2%), and mesocecal (1%). The psoas muscle and the external iliac artery and vein are important anatomic landmarks when examining the appendix.

Pancreas

The pancreas is easily located by its vascular landmarks. In transverse planes, the pancreas lies posterocaudal to the left lobe of the liver and crosses over the aorta and the inferior vena cava. The splenic vein is a useful landmark for identifying the pancreas as it runs along the posterior surface of the pancreas. In sagittal planes, the pancreatic body is located posterior to the gastric antrum and the left lobe of the liver, and anterior to the splenic vein and the superior mesenteric artery. The pancreatic head lies anterior to the inferior vena cava and caudal to the portal vein. The pancreatic duct runs along the length of the gland, and is best imaged in the pancreatic body. With modern ultrasound equipment, the duct can be frequently visualized as a tubular structure with reflective walls with maximum diameter up to 2 mm. The anteroposterior diameters of the head and body are in general less than 3 and 2 cm, respectively. Wide normal variations are noted in pancreatic dimensions, and tend to decrease with age. The normal pancreas is homogeneous with the echogenicity greater than or equal to the adjacent liver.

▶ TECHNIQUE AND NORMAL ULTRASOUND FINDINGS

In the emergency and acute care setting, a rapid, focused inspection and systematic survey of the entire abdomen are required for obtaining useful information. Among a number of factors that influence the accuracy of emergency ultrasound, the most critical is the sonographer's experience, which includes not only the technique of scanning but also the knowledge of the clinical and pathologic findings in acute abdominal disorders.

Positioning of the patient during the emergency ultrasound examination is important for obtaining optimal images. A patient is generally placed in the supine position. To avoid interference by gas echoes, they may be placed in the semi-lateral, lateral, or semi-erect positions. Oblique or coronal planes are more frequently used than sagittal or transverse planes, especially in patients who have a bowel obstruction or ileus. The standard examination is performed using a sweeping motion with a 3.5 MHz probe. A higher frequency (greater than 7 MHz) probe should be used for delineating the laminar structure of the appendix, intestinal wall, or specific lesions of the abdominal wall.

Acute Abdomen

For cases of an **acute** abdomen, a rapid inspection for free peritoneal fluid should be performed in a manner similar to the FAST examination (see also Chapter 4). The right intercostal and coronal views should be used to examine for free peritoneal fluid in Morison's pouch and the right subphrenic space. From these views, the right kidney and the right lobe of the liver can be inspected briefly. The left intercostal and left coronal views should be used to examine for free fluid in the subphrenic space and the splenorenal recess. From these views, the spleen and the left kidney can be inspected briefly. Then, the pelvic (sagittal and transverse) views should be used to examine for free fluid in the pelvis. From these views, the bladder and the prostate or uterus can be inspected briefly. Next, a focused inspection for acute abdominal disorders should be performed in a systematic fashion. The areas to be examined first should be determined ac-cording to the clinical findings, but the entire abdomen should be surveyed to exclude less suspicious disorders in the differential diagnosis. Subphrenic free air is best visualized on the ventral surface of the liver with right intercostal scanning. The patient may be placed in the semi-lateral position elevating the right flank.

Epigastric Region

In scanning the epigastric region, the gastric antrum can be demonstrated anterior to the pancreatic body and caudal to the left lobe of the liver (Figure 8–1). The five-layer structure of the gastric wall can be demonstrated using a high-frequency probe. The duodenal bulb may be visualized between the gallbladder and the gastric antrum. It is difficult to clearly visualize the duodenal C-loop except when it is dilated with accumulated fluid (Figure 8–2). It may be visualized anterior to the inferior vena cava in a coronal or oblique plane from the right anterior flank.

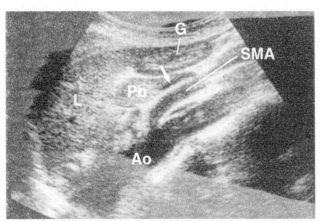

A

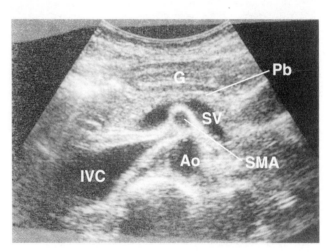

B

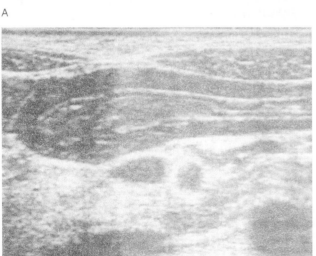

C

Figure 8-1. A normal gastric antrum. (A) In an epigastric sagittal plane, the cross-section of antrum (G) is visualized anterior to the pancreatic body (Pb) and caudal to the left lobe of the liver (L). The pancreatic body is located anterior to the splenic vein (arrow) and the superior mesenteric artery (SMA). (B) In a transverse plane, the gastric antrum is demonstrated anterior to the pancreatic body. (C) Five-layer structure of the gastric wall is demonstrated in a transverse plane using a high-frequency probe. Ao = aorta, IVC = inferior vena cava, SV = splenic vein.

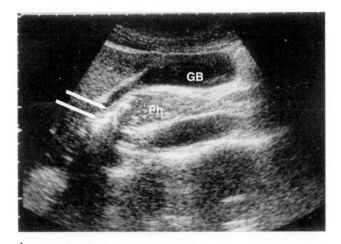

A

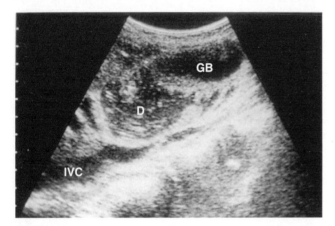

B

Figure 8–2. A duodenum. (A) A normal proximal duodenum (arrows) is visualized between the gallbladder (GB) and the pancreatic head (Ph). The posterior wall of the duodenum is usually impossible to demonstrate because of the gas in the lumen. (B) A slightly dilated duodenal C-loop (D) is visualized anterolateral to the inferior vena cava (IVC) and posterior to the gallbladder.

Bowel Obstruction

For cases of possible bowel obstruction, the examination begins with scanning the ascending colon and the hepatic flexure in the right flank. The hepatic flexure is viewed at the ventral side of the right kidney, and then the longitudinal views of the ascending colon are obtained by positioning the probe caudally in the mid- to posterior axillary line. A sequence of gas echoes separated with the haustra folds can be seen inside the hypoechoic wall (Figure 8–3). When a distended ascending colon is identified, the scanning proceeds to the left flank to inspect the descending colon. The approximate site of obstruction can be evaluated on the basis of whether or not the descending colon is distended. When an ascending colon is not

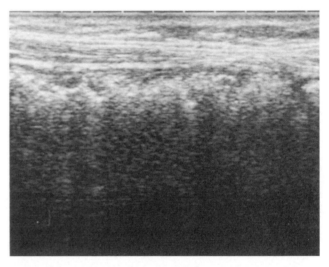

Figure 8–3. A normal ascending colon. A sequence of gas echoes separated with the Haustra folds is seen inside the hypoechoic wall.

distended, the ileocecal region should be carefully examined to guard against overlooking collapsed ileal loops or specific lesions. The scanning then proceeds to survey the degree of dilatation, peristaltic activities, wall thickening, or specific lesions in the small bowel loops, and peritoneal fluid between the loops. When appropriate, a high-frequency probe may be used to demonstrate the layer structure of the bowel wall (Figure 8–4). Real-time sonography may demonstrate peristaltic activity as peristalsis of the bowel wall or to-and-fro movements of intestinal contents. Akinesis of the loop can be established with observation for a several minutes or serial observations in order to avoid overlooking intermittent peristaltic activity.

Appendicitis

For cases of possible appendicitis, the standard examination with a 3.5 or 3.75 MHz probe is initially performed to survey the anatomic orientation in the right lower quadrant. The psoas muscle and the external iliac artery and vein are important landmarks when searching for the appendix (Figure 8–5). A graded-compression technique with a high-frequency probe is usually applied when searching for an inflamed appendix. Gentle, progressive application and withdrawal of pressure is important in order not to elicit peritoneal irritation for the patient. Graded compression can express all overlying fluid or gas from normal bowel to visualize the inflamed non-compressible appendix. The terminal ileum can be recognized as crossing over the psoas muscle to the cecum. Just caudal to this area is the cecal tip. To locate a tip of the appendix, a careful inspection with a graded-compression technique should be done to the point of maximal abdominal tenderness.

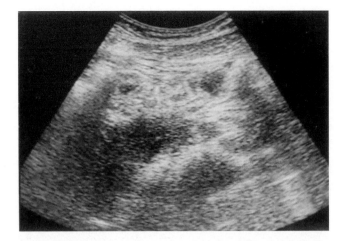

A

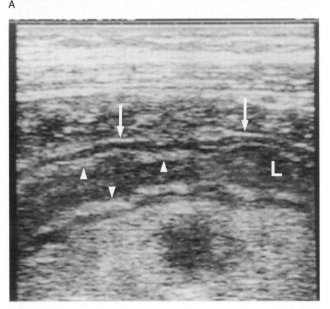

B

Figure 8–4. Normal small bowel loop. (A) No unified images of the small bowel are obtained with routine sonography using a 3.5 MHz probe. (B) Wall structure of the small bowel is demonstrated with a high-frequency probe. The lumen (L) is bounded by the broad hyperechoic layer (arrowheads), and then surrounded by the hypoechoic muscular layer, which is bounded externally by the fine, hyperechoic reflection from the serosa (arrows).

Pancreatitis

For cases of possible pancreatitis, it may be difficult to obtain optimal sonographic images of the pancreas in the emergency setting because of the significant artifacts arising from gastrointestinal gas. To avoid such interference, the semierect position can be adopted to visualize the pancreatic head and body. In this position, gas in the stomach rises to the fundus and the left lobe of the liver

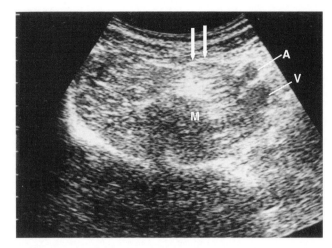

Figure 8–5. Ultrasonogram with a transverse plane in the right lower quadrant. The psoas muscle (M) and external iliac artery (A) and vein (V) are important anatomic landmarks to search for the appendix. The terminal ileum (arrow) crosses over the psoas muscle to the cecum.

often provides an acoustic window for imaging the pancreas and the lesser sac. The standard planes are sagittal and transverse along the vascular landmarks (Figure 8–1A and 8–6). The tail of the pancreas can be best visualized with a coronal view in a right posterior oblique position. The spleen is used as an acoustic window in this position. The anterior pararenal space is best imaged through a coronal flank approach.

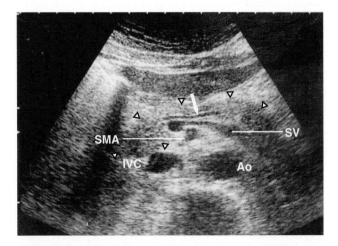

Figure 8–6. A normal pancreas. In a transverse plane the pancreas (arrowheads) lies caudal to the left lobe of the liver and crosses over the aorta (Ao) and the inferior vena cava (IVC). The splenic vein (SV) runs along the posterior surface of the pancreas. The pancreatic duct (arrow) is visualized as a tubular structure with reflective walls. SMA = superior mesenteric artery.

▶ COMMON AND EMERGENT ABNORMALITIES

Free Peritoneal Fluid

Free intraperitoneal fluid is delineated as an anechoic stripe with sharp edges (Figure 8–7). Intraperitoneal hemorrhage, bloody or purulent ascites, or peritoneal fluid containing intestinal contents may be shown as having gray level echoes inside.

Pneumoperitoneum

Subphrenic free air can be identified as an echogenic line with posterior reverberation artifacts on the ventral surface of the liver, separate from gas echoes in the gastro-

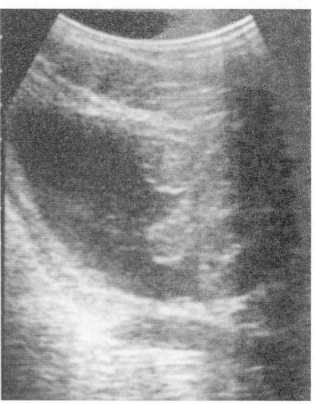

A

Figure 8–7. Free peritoneal fluid. (A) Free peritoneal fluid with internal echoes is demonstrated in the pelvic space in a patient with intraperitoneal hemorrhage secondary to ovarian bleeding. (B) Bloody ascites secondary to strangulation small bowel obstruction is demonstrated as an anechoic space with fine internal echoes in the pouch of Douglas. (C) A large amount of ascites is shown in a case of peritoneal carcinomatosis.

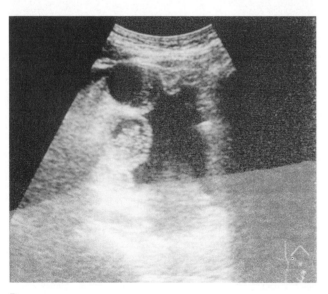

B

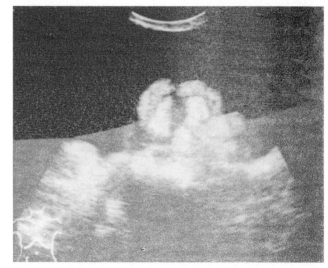

C

intestinal lumen at the caudal side and those in the lung at the cephalic side (Figure 8–8).

Gas in the abscess or free intraperitoneal fluid may be occasionally recognized as echogenic spots inside the anechoic or hypoechoic fluid (Figure 8–9).

Small Bowel Obstruction

In cases of small bowel obstruction, dilated small bowel proximal to collapsed small bowel or ascending colon can be identified (Figure 8–10). Dilated small bowel is usually visualized as fluid-filled dilated loops with the maximal diameter greater than 25 mm (usually greater than 30 mm) at the time of diagnosis of small bowel ob-

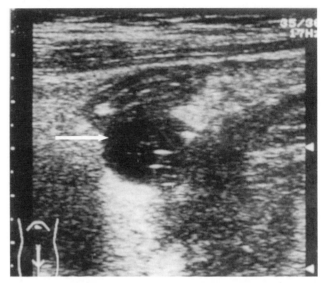

Figure 8–9. Gas in an abscess. Gas in a paracolonic abscess is demonstrated as echogenic spots inside the hypoechoic fluid (arrow) in a case of perforated colonic diverticulitis.

struction. In the early stage of distal small bowel obstruction, no dilated loops may be observed in the proximal jejunum. The sonographic images of dilated loops vary depending on the degree of distention and the nature of intestinal contents (Figure 8–11). The well-known "keyboard sign" is not essential for the diagnosis of small bowel obstruction. The sonographic appearance of

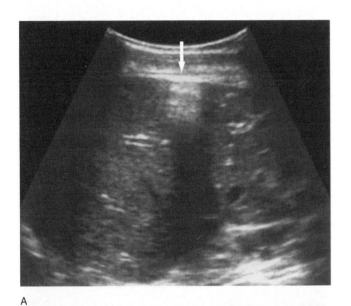

A

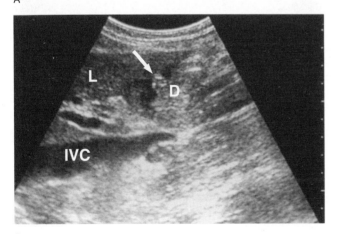

B

Figure 8–8. Pneumoperitoneum. (A) Subphrenic free air (arrow) is recognized at the ventral side of the liver in a case of perforated duodenal ulcer. (B) A perforated duodenal ulcer (arrow) is delineated as deformity of the duodenal bulb (D) with echogenic lumen. L = liver, IVC = inferior vena cava.

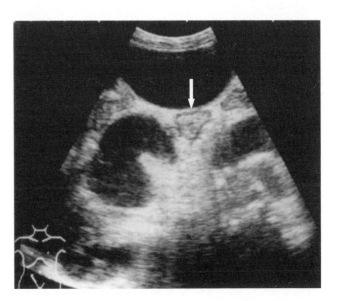

Figure 8–10. Mechanical small bowel obstruction. Both dilated small bowel and a collapsed one (arrow) are demonstrated in the right lower abdomen.

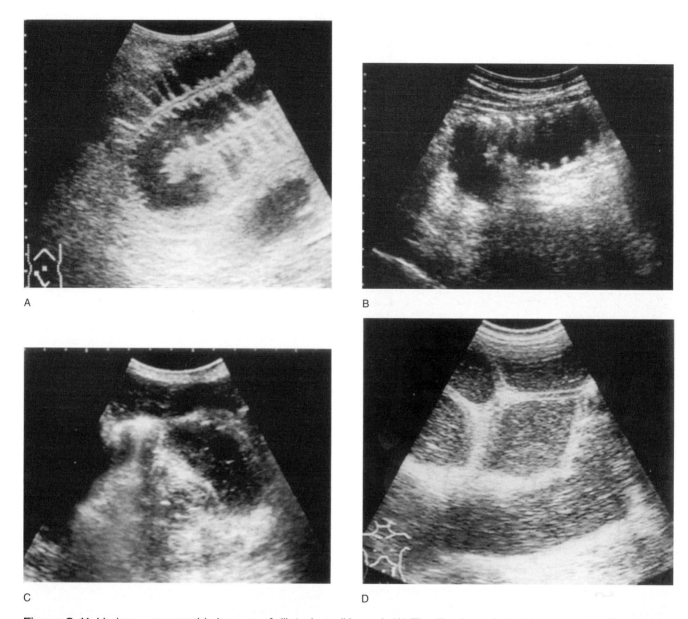

Figure 8–11. Various sonographic images of dilated small bowel. (A) The "keyboard sign" is characteristic of fluid-filled, dilated jejunum. (B) The sonographic image of small bubbles of gas entrapped between the Kerckring's folds inside dilated small bowel loops is similar to the "string of beads sign" on plain radiographs. (C) In mild or early stages of small bowel obstruction, gas echoes may be more dominant than anechoic fluid in the dilated loops. (D) Dilated small bowel may be filled with spot echoes when intestinal contents become more feculent.

Kerckring's folds varies depending on scanning planes and intestinal contents, and in the distal small bowel they are rarely visualized.[17] The criterion for simple obstruction is the presence of peristaltic activity in the entire dilated proximal small bowel (Figure 8–12).

Strangulation Obstruction

A strangulated loop is demonstrated as an akinetic dilated small bowel loop with real-time sonography (Figure 8–13A and B). In contrast, peristaltic activity can be recognized in the dilated small bowel proximal to the akinetic loop. Peritoneal fluid can be demonstrated in most cases and rapidly accumulates after the onset of

obstruction. In cases of an established strangulation, real-time sonography may demonstrate wall thickening with increased echogenicity and flattened folds within the akinetic loop, and/or a large amount of peritoneal fluid (Figure 8–13C).

Large Bowel Obstruction

In cases of large bowel obstruction, the dilated colon proximal to the obstruction is usually delineated as filled with dense spot echoes around the periphery of the abdomen (Figure 8–14A); whereas, the dilated small bowel loops are located more centrally. Haustral indentations may be visualized as widely spaced in the dilated as-

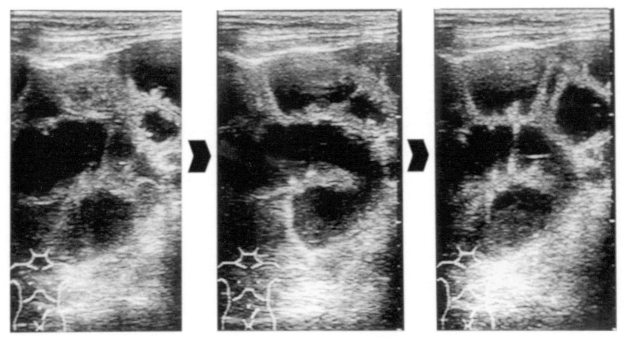

Figure 8–12. Simple small bowel obstruction. Real-time sonography reveals intermittently increased peristaltic activity of the entire dilated small bowel proximal to the obstruction.

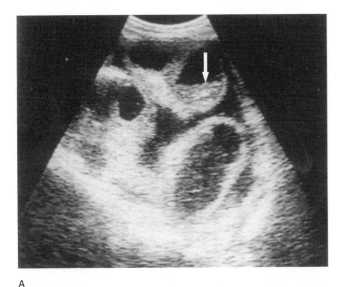

A

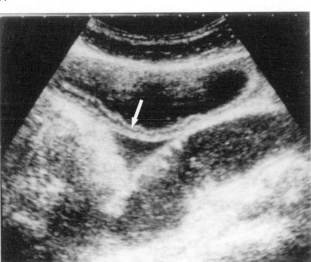

B

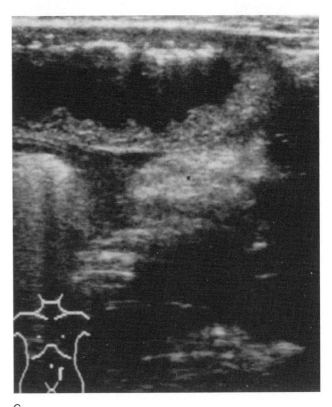

C

Figure 8–13. Strangulation small bowel obstruction. (A) Real-time sonography reveals an akinetic dilated loop accompanied by a large amount of peritoneal fluid in the cul-de-sac. Inside the akinetic loop, spot echoes are demonstrated as deposited like sludge (arrow). (B) Submucosal edema caused by mild strangulation is demonstrated as a hypoechoic layer (arrow) of the wall. (C) In a case of established strangulation with hemorrhagic necrosis, wall thickening with increased echogenicity and flattened folds is visualized within the akinetic loop (7.5 MHz).

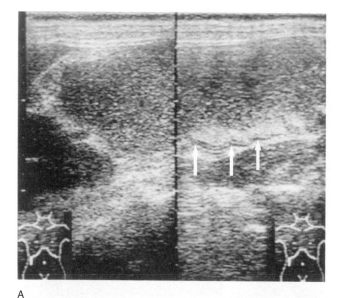

A

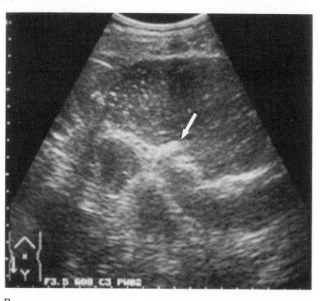

B

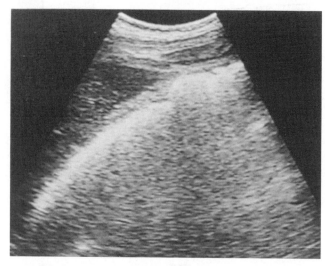

C

Figure 8–14. Dilated ascending colon. (A) A dilated ascending colon filled with feculent, liquid contents is delineated as filled with dense spot echoes. Haustral indentations (arrows) may be visualized in the dilated ascending colon. (B) To-and-fro movements of the internal spot echoes through the ileocecal valve (arrow) are occasionally identified with real-time sonography. (C) A dilated ascending colon with excessive gas inside is recognized as wide gas echoes around the periphery of the abdomen.

cending colon. Real-time sonography can occasionally reveal to-and-fro movements of the intestinal contents through the ileocecal valve when the valve is incompetent (Figure 8–14B). In cases of large bowel obstruction distal to the splenic flexure, however, sonography may show a dilated colon simply as wide gas echoes around the periphery of the abdomen (Figure 8–14C).

The criterion for large bowel obstruction is the presence of dilated colon proximal to normal or collapsed large bowel. Ascending colon and descending colon are the initial checkpoints for the sonographic evaluation of large bowel obstruction. The site of obstruction can be estimated on the basis of distribution of the dilated colon (greater than 50 mm for the ascending colon). Clinically, it is unnecessary to strictly define the accurate site or cause of obstruction with sonography because water-soluble

contrast enema demonstrates the degree and level of obstruction and helps to clarify its cause.

Specific Etiologies of Bowel Obstruction

Intussusception

The cross-sectional image of intussusception is known as the "multiple concentric ring sign" or "target sign" (Figure 8–15A). Multi-laminar structures may be demonstrated with scanning along the long axis of the intussusception (Figure 8–15B).

Incarcerated Hernia

An incarcerated small bowel segment can be demonstrated as entrapped within the hernia sac (Figure 8–16).

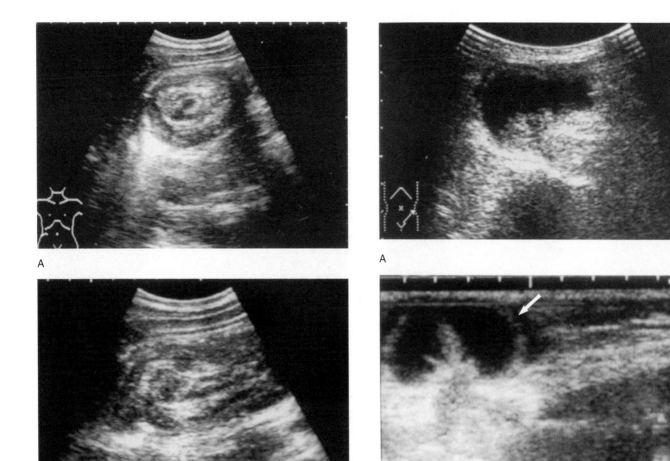

A

B

Figure 8–15. Ileocolic intussusception in an adult patient. (A) A cross-sectional image of intussusception is demonstrated as a "multiple concentric ring sign". (B) Multiple layer structure of intussusception in the long axis plane is demonstrated.

A

B

Figure 8–16. Incarcerated hernia. (A) An incarcerated femoral hernia is demonstrated as a herniated small bowel segment with fluid accumulation within the hernia sac in the inguinal region. (B) In an incarcerated incisional hernia, a herniated small bowel segment (arrow) is demonstrated in the mid-abdomen, accompanied by dilated loops proximal to the incarceration.

Afferent Loop Obstruction

Afferent loop obstruction after a Billroth II gastro-jejunostomy may result from adhesions or recurrent carcinoma. Abdominal sonography can show a dilated duodenum and jejunum proximal to the anastomosis (Figure 8–17). The diagnosis of afferent loop obstruction can be made on the basis of the sonographic features and the clinical findings consistent with acute pancreatitis in patients with a prior history of a Billroth gastrectomy.

Gallstone Ileus

Gallstone ileus is a rare complication of acute cholecystitis. The sonographic features diagnostic of gall-stone ileus include pneumobilia, small bowel obstruction, and a large calculus (average diameter greater than 3 cm) obstructing the small bowel (Figure 8–18). The most common site of impaction is the ileocecal valve. Biliary-enteric fistula may be suggested by gas echoes inside the intra- or extrahepatic biliary tree.

Small Bowel Tumor

It is rare for a small bowel tumor to cause a bowel obstruction. Malignant small bowel tumor, such as metastatic carcinoma, malignant lymphoma, or leiomyo-

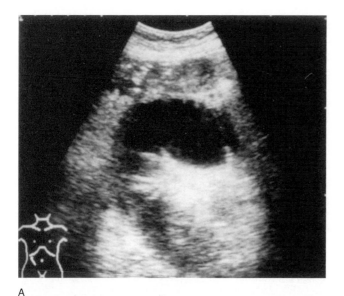

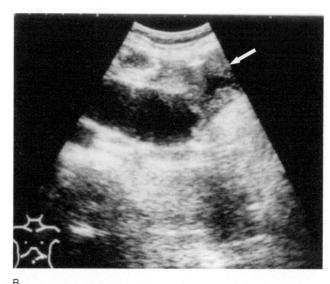

A

B

Figure 8–17. Afferent loop obstruction. (A) Dilated duodenal C-loop and (B) dilated jejunum proximal to the anastomosis are demonstrated in a case of recurrent carcinoma (arrow) at the site of anastomosis.

sarcoma, may occasionally be identified by sonography (Figure 8–19).

Inflammatory Bowel Disease

Segmental wall thickening of the small bowel may be identified in cases of inflammatory bowel disease such as intestinal tuberculosis, Crohn's disease, or radiation enteritis (Figure 8–20).

Colon Cancer

Colorectal cancer is by far the most common cause of large bowel obstruction, and may be detected as an ir-

regular-shaped hypoechoic mass with echogenic core inside (Figure 8–21A) or a localized circular wall thickening (Figure 8–21B and C). Intraluminal tumor obstructing the lumen may occasionally be demonstrated (Figure 8–21D).

Ileus

In the early stages of an ileus, slightly dilated small bowel loops (less than 25 mm wide in diameter) may be recognized on ultrasound. Gas echoes are more dominant than fluid collection inside the bowel (Figure 8–22).

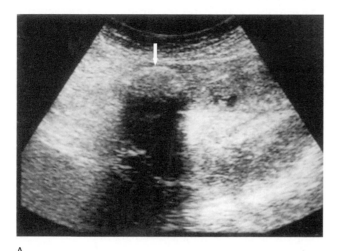

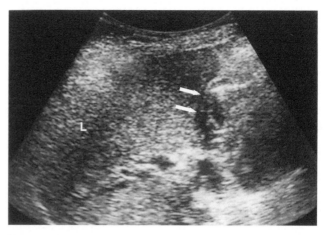

A

B

Figure 8–18. Gallstone ileus. (A) The impacted gallstone (arrow) obstructing the small bowel is directly visualized with a prominent acoustic shadow inside the dilated small bowel. (B) Gas echoes in the atrophic gallbladder (arrows) are recognized as showing the presence of a biliary-enteric fistula between the gallbladder and the duodenum (or less commonly the stomach, jejunum). L = liver.

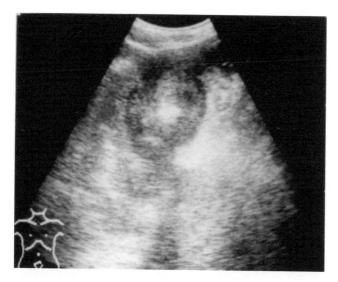

Figure 8–19. Small bowel tumor. A leiomyosarcoma causing a small bowel obstruction is recognized as an oval-shaped mass with a mosaic image.

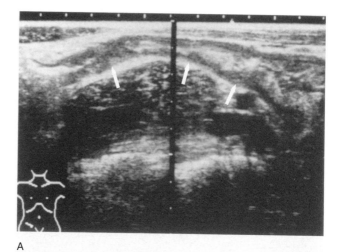

A

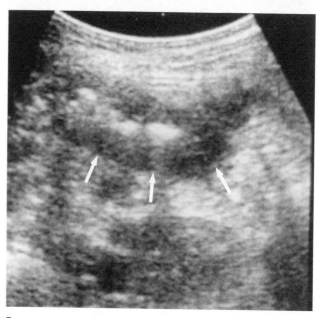

B

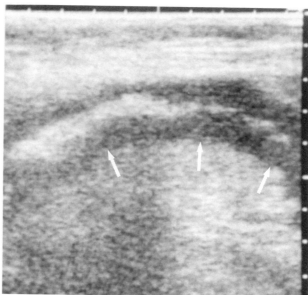

C

Acute Appendicitis

Demonstration of a swollen, non-compressible appendix greater than 6 mm in diameter is the prime sonographic criterion for the diagnosis of acute appendicitis (Figure 8–23). The typical appearance of an inflamed appendix is a tubular structure with one blind end. Maximal outer diameter ranges from 7 to 16 mm. Sonography may also demonstrate an appendicolith with acoustic shadowing. The presence of appendicolith is always indicative of acute appendicitis in patients with acute right lower quadrant abdominal pain.

In cases of catarrhal or phlegmonous appendicitis, a swollen appendix maintains the layer structure of the wall. In cases of gangrenous appendicitis, a progressive loss of mural lamination and organ contours can be demonstrated as a result of gangrene. With progression of the inflammation, the inflamed appendix or pericecal abscess may often be observed as surrounded by reflective fatty tissue that represents the mesentery or omentum. Atony of the terminal ileum may be seen as well as swelling of the cecal wall. A pericecal abscess can be demonstrated as fluid collection with a thick, non-compressible wall (Figure 8–24). Free peritoneal fluid in the pelvis is another common finding.

Acute Colonic Diverticulitis

On ultrasound, acute diverticulitis is shown as hypoechoic mural thickening (5 to 18 mm in thickness) of the affected

(text continues on page 186)

Figure 8–20 (at right). Inflammatory bowel diseases. A segmental wall thickening (arrows indicate posterior wall) of the small bowel is demonstrated in cases of (A) intestinal tuberculosis (7.5 MHz), (B) Crohn's disease (3.5 MHz), or (C) radiation enteritis (3.5 MHz).

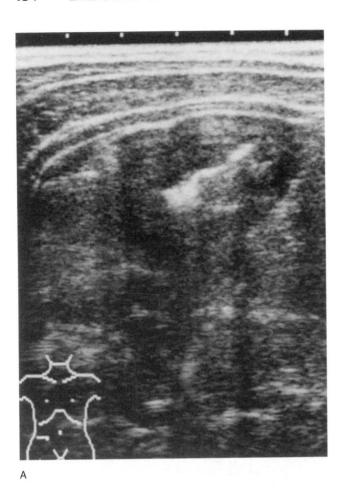

A

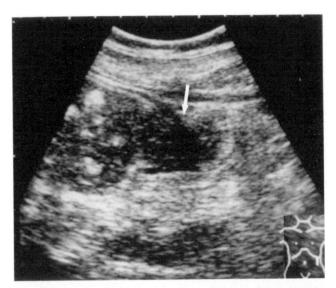

B

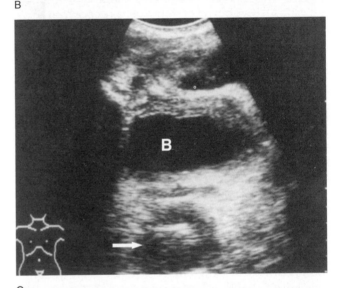

C

Figure 8–21. Colon carcinoma. (A) A colon cancer is often demonstrated as an irregular-shaped hypoechoic mass with an echogenic core inside, which is called the "pseudokidney sign" (7.5 MHz). (B) An obstructing colon cancer (arrow) is demonstrated as circular wall thickening at the site of obstruction, where dilated colon filled with dense spot echoes is tapering (3.5 MHz). (C) Circular wall thickening of the rectum (arrow) is demonstrated in a case of recurrent gastric carcinoma (3.5 MHz). (D) Occasionally, a prominent tumor (arrow) obstructing the lumen may be demonstrated (3.5 MHz). B = urinary bladder.

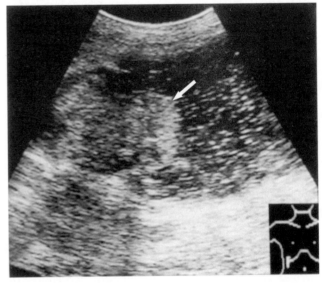

D

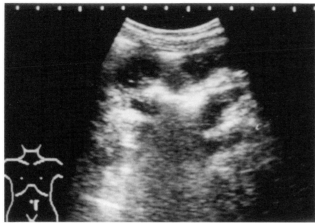

Figure 8–22 (at left). Ileus. Slightly dilated small bowel is demonstrated in a case of peritonitis secondary to perforated appendicitis.

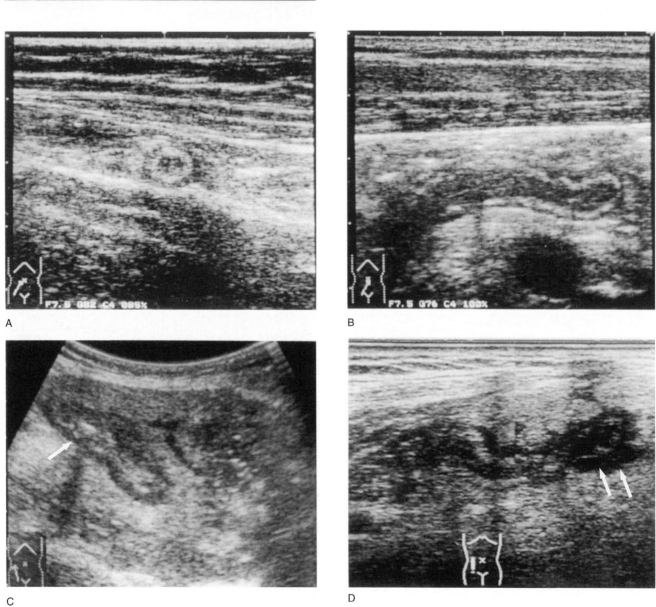

A

B

C

D

Figure 8–23. Acute appendicitis. A non-compressible, inflamed appendix is shown in (A): a cross-sectional view (7.5 MHz), and (B): a longitudinal section (7.5 MHz). Mural lamination of the swollen appendix is maintained in the early stages of acute appendicitis. (C) An appendicolith (arrow) with acoustic shadowing is demonstrated (5 MHz). (D) A focal loss of mural lamination in the appendiceal tip (white arrows) is demonstrated as a result of gangrene (9 MHz).

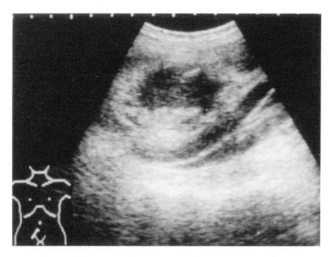

Figure 8-24. Pericecal abscess. A pericecal abscess secondary to perforated appendicitis is demonstrated as a hypoechoic fluid collection with a thick, non-compressible wall.

segment (Figure 8-25A). Graded compression over the site of tenderness is a simple method of localizing any inflammatory mass. Diverticulum may be demonstrated as a focal, hypoechoic prominence with a hyperechoic fecalith or gas echoes inside, although it is not always identified in all cases of acute colonic diverticulitis (Figure 8-25B). Pericolonic abscess or purulent peritoneal

fluid may be recognized in cases of complicated diverticulitis (see Figure 8-9).

Acute Pancreatitis/Pancreatic Pseudocyst

Diffuse swelling of the pancreas is often recognized in cases of acute edematous pancreatitis. Decreased echogenicity of the pancreas represents interstitial edema (Figure 8-26A). In cases of severe pancreatitis, peripancreatic fluid collections or echogenic pancreatic masses may be demonstrated (Figure 8-26B and C). Pancreatic pseudocysts are generally visualized as well-defined cystic masses in which sludge-like echoes may be identified (Figure 8-27).

Acute Cholecystitis

Irregular sonolucent layers in the gallbladder wall are indicative of serious cholecystitis (Figure 8-28A). The presence of asymmetric thickening of the gallbladder wall or intraluminal membranes parallel to the gallbladder wall can be identified in patients with acute gangrenous cholecystitis. Pericholecystic fluid collection can be caused by gallbladder perforation or abscess formation (Figure 8-28B).

Acute Mesenteric Ischemia

Wall thickening of the small bowel associated with a significant amount of peritoneal fluid is non-specific but suggestive of acute mesenteric ischemia as well as peritonitis and peritoneal carcinomatosis (Figure 8-29).

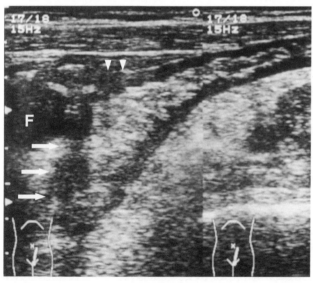

A

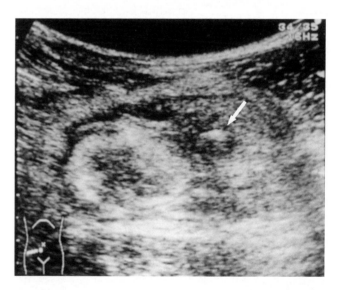

B

Figure 8-25. Acute colonic diverticulitis. (A) Longitudinal view shows segmental, hypoechoic wall thickening (arrowheads) of the sigmoid colon. Posterior shadowing from gas within a diverticulum is indicated (arrows) (7.5 MHz). F = paracolonic fluid. (B) On transverse views a solitary diverticulum (arrow) is shown as a focal, hypoechoic prominence with gas echoes inside at the maximum point of tenderness (7.5 MHz).

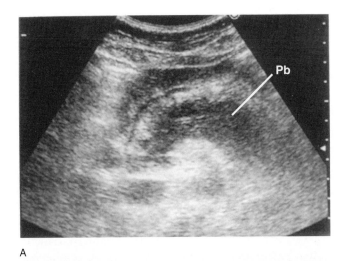

A

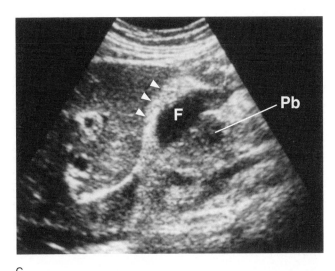

C

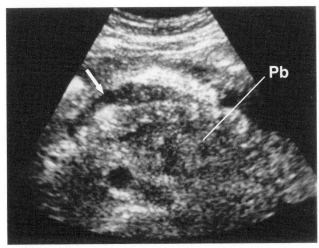

B

Figure 8–26. Acute pancreatitis. (A) Diffuse, homogeneous swelling of the pancreatic body (Pb) with decreased echogenicity is demonstrated in a case of acute edematous pancreatitis. (B) In a case of acute necrotizing pancreatitis the pancreatic body is visualized as a heterogenous mass with unclear border. Hypoechoic inflammatory exudate (arrow) is demonstrated anterior to the pancreatic body. (C) Peripancreatic fluid collection (F) is demonstrated between the hypoechoic pancreatic body and reflective fatty tissue (arrowheads).

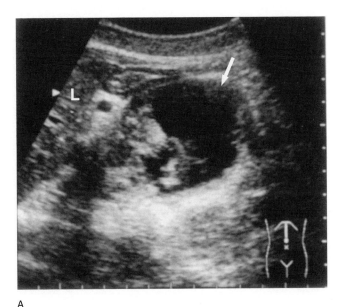

A

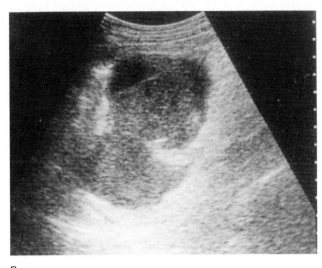

B

Figure 8–27. Pancreatic pseudocyst. (A) A well-defined cystic mass (arrow) is demonstrated posterior to the gastric antrum. (B) An irregular-shaped cystic mass filled with spot echoes is demonstrated medial to the splenic hilum in a case of infected pseudocyst. L = liver.

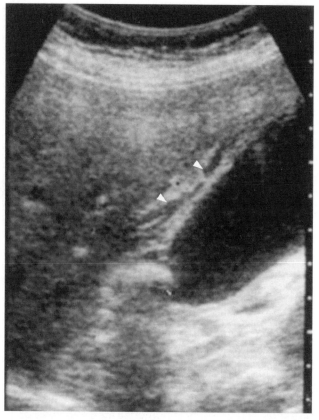

A

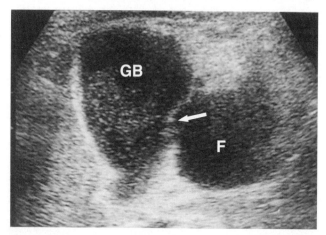

B

Figure 8–28. Acute cholecystitis. (A) Irregular sonolucent layers (arrowheads) in the swollen gallbladder wall are accompanied by an impacted stone in the gallbladder neck. (B) Pericholecystic fluid collection (F) with a defect (arrow) in the gallbladder wall, which represents a gallbladder perforation, is directly visualized with sonography. GB = gallbladder.

Ischemic Colitis

In cases of ischemic colitis, hypoechoic wall thickening is often demonstrated in the affected segment especially from the splenic flexure to the rectosigmoid junction (Figure 8–30).

► COMMON VARIANTS AND SELECTED ABNORMALITIES

Common normal variants that may be erroneously identified as free peritoneal fluid are discussed in Chapter 4. Fluid in the stomach when examining the perisplenic views and fluid in a collapsed bladder or an ovarian cyst when examining the pelvic views may be erroneously identified as free intraperitoneal fluid. Also, premenopausal women can occasionally have a small amount of free fluid in the pouch of Douglas.

Collapsed small bowel can be visualized similarly to a swollen appendix vermiformis, leading to a false-positive diagnosis of acute appendicitis (Figure 8–31). Peristaltic activity is not observed in the appendix while it should be recognized in the small bowel.

Gastric Outlet Obstruction

Gastric outlet obstruction can be demonstrated with emergency ultrasound (Figure 8–32). It can be caused by a variety of lesions including gastric cancer, peptic ulcer, and pancreatic cancer. To confirm the diagnosis, endoscopy and contrast studies are usually applied after decompression of the distended stomach.

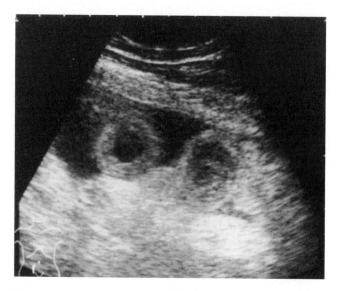

Figure 8–29. Acute mesenteric ischemia. Slightly dilated small bowel with wall thickening and peritoneal fluid are non-specific but suggestive of acute mesenteric ischemia.

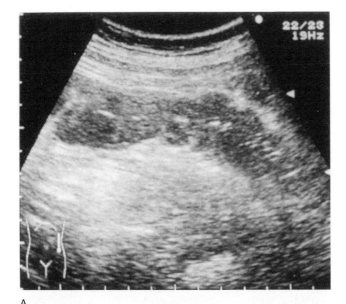

A

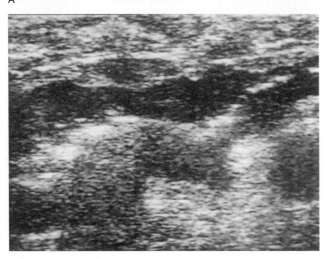

B

Figure 8–30. Ischemic colitis. (A) Hypoechoic wall thickening is delineated in the descending colon (3.5 MHz). (B) An irregular contour of the wall of the affected segment with decreased echogenicity is visualized in the advanced stage of ischemic colitis (7.5 MHz).

Torsion of the Pedicle of Ovarian Tumor

Ovarian torsion rarely occurs in patients without ovarian tumors or enlarged cysts. The clinical symptoms and physical findings may be confused with appendicitis, salpingitis, or gastroenteritis. The sonographic findings may be nonspecific and demonstrate a complex or cystic-appearing mass accompanied by free fluid in the pouch of Douglas (Figure 8–33). With a hemorrhagic infarction, the ovarian tumor can be hyperechoic.

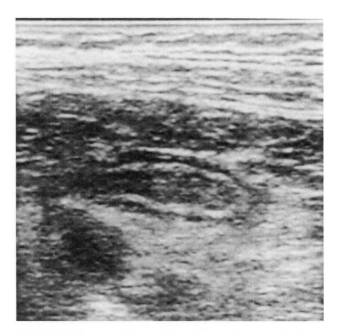

Figure 8–31. Normal collapsed ileum. A normal ileum may be misdiagnosed as a swollen appendix vermiformis (7.5 MHz). Peristaltic activity is recognized in the normal small bowel, while it is not observed in the appendix.

Rectus Sheath Hematoma

Acute or subacute hematoma in the rectus sheath, generally confined to the upper or lower quadrant, can occasionally be experienced without trauma in a patient who has a bleeding diathesis or after strenuous physical exertion. It is not always easy to differentiate rectus sheath hematoma from intraabdominal pathology because most

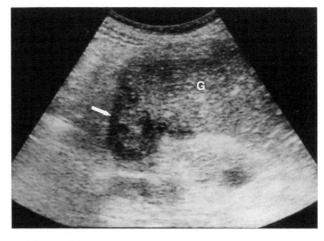

Figure 8–32. Gastric outlet obstruction. Distended stomach (G) filled with spot echoes is demonstrated proximal to the circular, hypoechoic wall thickening (arrow) in the pylorus, which represents a gastric cancer.

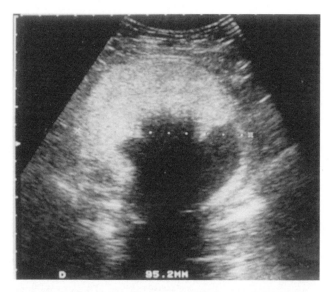

Figure 8–33. Torsion of the pedicle of an ovarian tumor. A solid and cystic tumor is demonstrated in the pouch of Douglas. The dense central shadowing suggests calcified components. The mixed components may represent a Dermoid tumor. Significant tenderness on the tumor suggests possible torsion of the pedicle. Color Doppler may be helpful if available.

patients with the hematoma present with significant abdominal swelling and tenderness. Without suspicion of this pathologic entity, a non-therapeutic laparotomy might be performed for an acute abdomen when conservative treatment or percutaneous drainage is indicated. Abdominal sonography is useful in this clinical situation by demonstrating the hematoma within the abdominal wall (Figure 8–34).

Acute Enterocolitis

Imaging modalities have seldom been used in cases of acute enterocolitis. Recently, sonography has been increasingly applied for infectious enterocolitis. Only slightly dilated bowel loops with normal wall thickness and increased peristalsis can be obtained with sonography in cases of mild enterocolitis. Mural thickening of the terminal ileum and colon accompanied with enlarged mesenteric lymph nodes may be identified in more severe cases (Figure 8–35).

▶ PITFALLS

1. *Contraindication.* For cases of acute abdomen, there is no absolute contraindication to performing the emergency ultrasound examination. A rapid ultrasound examination can be applied even while the resuscitation efforts are performed on patients in shock. An unnecessary, time-consuming examination for obtaining unfocused findings should be avoided so as not to delay patient treatment.

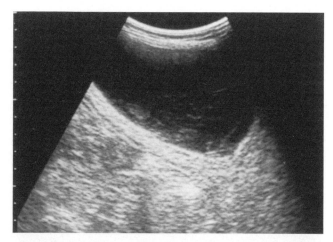

A

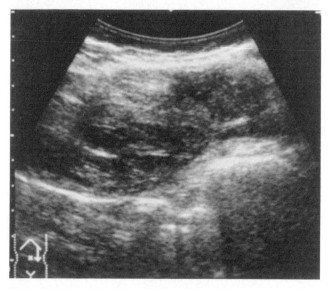

B

Figure 8–34. Rectus sheath hematoma. (A) Sonography shows a large hematoma as a circumscribed fluid collection within the abdominal wall. (B) In the early stage rectus sheath hematoma may be shown as a heterogeneous image.

2. *Over-reliance on the emergency ultrasound examination.* A pitfall is the over-reliance of an initial negative ultrasound examination in caring for patients with acute abdomen. Each examination is a single data point in the overall clinical picture. As the clinical symptoms and findings change, serial ultrasound examinations should be applied to evaluate any changes of sonographic findings. If the ultrasound examination presents equivocal, non-specific findings, abdominal CT, other radiographic procedures using contrast media, or endoscopy should be utilized.

3. *Limitations of the emergency ultrasound examination.* Limitations include difficulty in imaging patients who are morbidly obese or have an immense amount of gastrointestinal gas. Various ar-

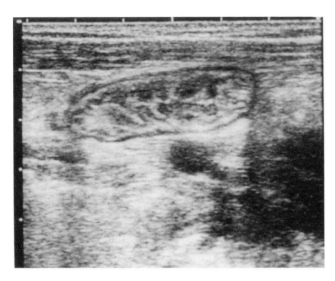

Figure 8–35. Infectious enterocolitis. Mural thickening of the ileum is regarded as reflective of inflammatory changes in the intestinal wall (7.5 MHz).

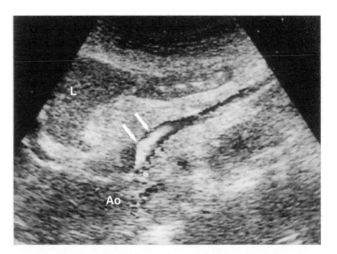

Figure 8–36. Application of color Doppler ultrasound technique. A color Doppler ultrasound shows the blood flow through the SMA on longitudinal view (arrow). The aorta is not well visualized in this plane but the approximate location is indicated (Ao).

tifacts may interfere with the examination in obtaining optimal images. Also, it may be difficult to determine the nature of free intraperitoneal fluid. If clinically required, an ultrasound-guided paracentesis of the fluid can be applied to clarify the issue. Another limitation is that ultrasound is an operator-dependent examination for both obtaining and interpreting the images.

4. *Limitations associated with pregnancy.* In pregnant patients, the distortion of usual landmarks caused by the presence of a gravid uterus can complicate the identification of an inflamed appendix. Interpreting sonographic images of extrauterine vasculature may be difficult for inexperienced sonographers. Non-obstructive dilatation of the renal collecting system may occur after 6-week in a normal pregnancy.

5. *Technical difficulties with the emergency ultrasound examination.* Many clinicians will not have enough experience initially to confidently apply sonography for the diagnosis of gastrointestinal disorders such as bowel obstruction, acute appendicitis, or acute diverticulitis. Significant tenderness, peritoneal irritability, or hyperventilation may interfere with the examination.

6. *Etiologies undetected by sonography.* Certain etiologies that can cause an acute abdomen may not be detected initially by the emergency ultrasound examination. These include perforation of a vesical bladder or gastrointestinal tract, embolism of the SMA, colonic volvulus, and gastrointestinal hemorrhage. Color Doppler can potentially be used to evaluate blood flow through the SMA in a patient suspected to have a SMA embolism (Figure 8–36).

► CASE STUDIES

Case 1

Patient Presentation

A 68-year-old man presented to the emergency department with complaints of intermittent epigastric pain, nausea, and vomiting. He felt the sudden onset of pain prior to dinner. The pain increased intermittently and was accompanied by emesis of bilious fluid. He denied hematemesis, abdominal distention, and constipation. He had a bowel movement earlier in the day. He had a medical history of gastrectomy for gastric cancer and cholecystectomy for gallstone disease.

On physical examination, his blood pressure was 160/90 mm Hg; pulse, 82 beats per min; respirations, 16 per min; temperature 37.1°C. His head, neck, pulmonary, and cardiovascular examinations were unremarkable. His abdomen was soft and flat but had moderate tenderness to palpation and rebound tenderness in the epigastric region. No muscle guarding was appreciated. On rectal examination, his stool was guaiac negative.

Management Course

While his plain radiographs showed no apparent subphrenic free air, they revealed dilated small bowel with multiple air-fluid levels. His urinalysis was normal. Laboratory tests revealed an elevated serum glucose level (171 mg/dL) and leukocytosis (WBC 10,300/μl). His serum CPK, amylase, and liver enzymes were within normal range. An emergency ultrasound examination revealed dilated loops of small bowel with peristaltic activity in the entire abdomen and collapsed loops localized in the right lower quadrant (Figure 8–37A). The maximal diameter of visualized dilated loops was 34 mm. A small amount of

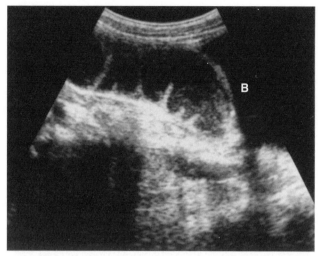

A

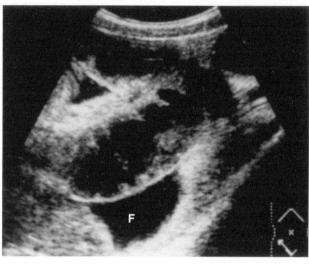

B

Figure 8–37. Sonograms of case 1. (A) An initial ultrasound examination revealed dilated loops of small bowel with peristaltic activity. (B) Reexamination with sonography revealed an aperistaltic, dilated loop with slight mural thickening and increased amount of peritoneal fluid (F) in the pelvis.

peritoneal fluid was also identified between the dilated loops. No evidence of hepatobiliary disorders, splenomegaly, or pancreatitis was found.

The patient was admitted with the diagnosis of small bowel obstruction by adhesions and treated conservatively with nasogastric tube decompression and intravenous fluids. Although his symptoms were relieved after the nasogastric tube decompression, sonographic appearances of small bowel obstruction were slightly progressive. Three days after admission, a long intestinal tube was inserted for decompression of dilated small bowel and for a contrast study to confirm the site and degree of the obstruction. A small amount of water-soluble contrast

medium was passed through the obstruction to the ascending colon, and thus the patient was suspected of having a partial obstruction on radiograph findings. At the time, laboratory tests showed only slight elevation of serum C-reactive protein (CRP) level (2.0 mg/dL). The WBC count was 7100/μl. However, more than 1,000 mL of intestinal fluid was drained via the long intestinal tube in 24 h. Re-examination with sonography revealed an aperistaltic, dilated loop with slight mural thickening in the right lower abdomen, and increased amount of peritoneal fluid (Figure 8–37B). Slowly progressing strangulation obstruction was suspected on sonographic images contrary to his minimal clinical and radiograph findings. He was taken to the operating room for surgical intervention, which revealed a large amount of serobloody ascites and a congestive, hemorrhagic loop of bowel that was twisted and strangulated by an adhesive band. The strangulated loop was still viable and relieved by adhesiolysis.

Commentary

Case 1 was an example of a patient who had a slowly progressing strangulation obstruction. The clinical picture of a strangulation obstruction varies by the severity of circulatory impairment, the length of strangulated loop, and the period after the onset. Diagnosis of strangulation small bowel obstruction is difficult preoperatively unless the patient presents with severe pain or peritoneal signs. In general, laboratory tests and plain radiographs are not diagnostic in the early stages of strangulation. Real-time sonography, however, can evaluate not only the morphologic changes but also the physiologic changes observed in bowel obstruction. An aperistaltic, dilated loop distal to dilated loops with peristaltic activity is essential in the sonographic diagnosis of strangulation small bowel obstruction. The increase in the amount of peritoneal fluid, which is also diagnostic for strangulation, can be assessed by serial ultrasound examinations. In this particular case, the information provided by serial examinations was crucial in the decision process to proceed with an urgent laparotomy, and this prevented an enterectomy for hemorrhagic necrosis of the strangulated loop.

Case 2

Patient Presentation

A 55-year-old man presented to the emergency department with a 5-d history of lower abdominal pain and watery diarrhea. He denied nausea and vomiting. He had a medical history of chronic hepatitis and cerebral infarction, and was a heavy smoker and heavy drinker.

On physical examination, his blood pressure was 145/84 mm Hg; pulse, 110 beats per min; and temperature, 38.4°C. His head, neck, pulmonary, and cardiovascular examinations were unremarkable. The abdominal examination was soft, diffusely tender, and without peritoneal signs.

Management Course

The patient remained hemodynamically stable in the emergency department. An upright chest radiograph and abdominal radiographs showed no evidence of bowel obstruction or gastrointestinal perforation. His urinalysis was normal. His laboratory tests showed an elevated serum CRP level (4.5mg/dL) and leucocytosis (WBC 11,000/μl). An emergency ultrasound examination revealed no free intraperitoneal fluid but slightly thickened wall of the sigmoid colon (Figure 8–38A). Blood flow through the SMA was recognized on color Doppler. An abdominal CT scan was negative for intraperitoneal and retroperitoneal pathology. The patient was admitted for observation and treated conservatively with antibiotics and intravenous fluid therapy. Two days after the admission, he complained of having severe abdominal pain; a repeat bedside ultrasound examination revealed mural thickening of the sigmoid colon and turbulent peritoneal fluid, including gas echoes in the anterior pelvis (Figure 8–38B, C). He was taken to the operating room for an urgent laparotomy, which revealed feculent peritonitis due to perforative diverticulitis of the sigmoid colon.

Commentary

The patient in case 2 had an initial negative ultrasound examination and CT scan. Re-examination with bedside ultrasound revealed turbulent free peritoneal fluid and wall thickening of the sigmoid colon. These findings were suggestive of a sigmoid colon perforation due to acute diverticulitis, and thus, negated the need for a repeat CT scan while making a decision for surgical intervention. As abdominal sonography is available at the bedside, it should be repeated for a patient with an acute abdomen whose etiology is not yet defined.

Case 3

Patient Presentation

A 26-year-old pregnant woman presented to the emergency department with complaints of right lower quadrant

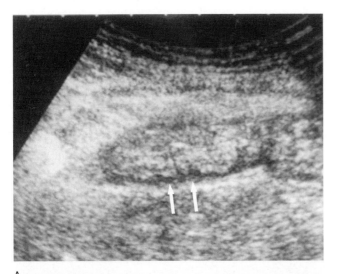

A

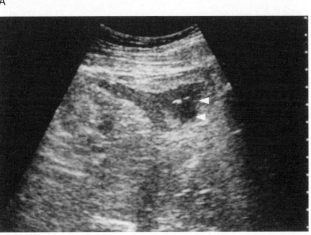

C

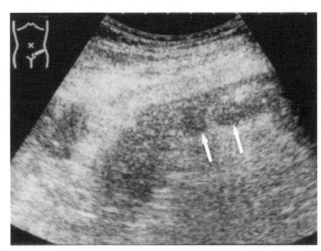

B

Figure 8–38. Sonograms of case 2. (A) No free peritoneal fluid but slightly thickened wall of the sigmoid colon (arrows) was revealed with an initial ultrasound examination. (B) Mural thickening of the sigmoid colon (arrows) was identified with re-examination. (C) Turbulent peritoneal fluid (arrowheads) including gas echoes was recognized in the anterior pelvis.

abdominal pain radiating to the right flank. She initially experienced epigastric pain accompanied by nausea and vomiting, which was followed by right lower quadrant pain. She denied urinary retention, dysuria, hematuria, diarrhea, and constipation. She was 18 wk pregnant and had no vaginal bleeding. She denied any significant past medical history.

On physical examination, her blood pressure was 128/78 mm Hg; pulse, 94 beats per min; respirations, 18 per min; and temperature, 37°C. She was anicteric. Her pulmonary and cardiovascular examinations were normal. The abdominal examination was soft but had significant peritoneal signs localized in the right lower quadrant laterally and superiorly deviated from McBurney's point. She also felt a severe pain on percussion in the costovertebral angle and right lumbar region. A gravid uterus, 3 cm below the umbilicus, was noted. The rectal examination revealed guaiac negative stool.

Management Course

The patient remained hemodynamically stable in the emergency department. No radiographs were taken because she was pregnant. Her urinalysis showed no red blood cells or bacteria. Her laboratory tests demonstrated leukocytosis (WBC 12,000/μl) and elevated CRP level (10 mg/dL). An emergency ultrasound examination using a standard probe revealed a target figure of the appendix that was draped over by omental tissues (Figure 8–39A), dilated pyelocaliceal system in the right kidney (Figure 8–39B), and the fetus moving actively within the gravid uterus. There was no evidence of peritoneal fluid. The obstetrics and urology consultants agreed with the attending surgeon's clinical and sonographic findings. The patient was suspected of having an acute appendicitis accompanied with acute hydronephrosis on the basis of clinical and sonographic findings. Further diagnostic modalities to define the etiology of urinary system disorders were limited because she was pregnant. For the purpose of differential diagnosis and treatment, the urologist performed a retrograde ureteral catheterization under cystoscopic procedures. No evidence of pyuria or apparent obstructive lesions was confirmed, and subsequently, the patient was suspected of having a non-obstructive dilatation of the renal collecting system, which is occasionally recognized in pregnant women. The patient was taken to the operating room for an urgent laparotomy, which revealed an acute gangrenous appendix without abscess or apparent retroperitoneal infiltration. An appendectomy was performed and her postoperative course was uneventful. The right hydronephrosis was slightly reduced but lasted throughout pregnancy.

Commentary

Case 3 was an example of a pregnant patient who presented with an acute abdomen. She had acute appendicitis with puzzling symptoms and signs. The sonographic findings were compatible with her complicated clinical findings. The diagnosis of acute appendicitis in pregnant patients can be challenging even when they present with a typical clinical picture for the disease. Abdominal sonography should be utilized for pregnant women with abdominal pain and can assist physicians with their management strategy.

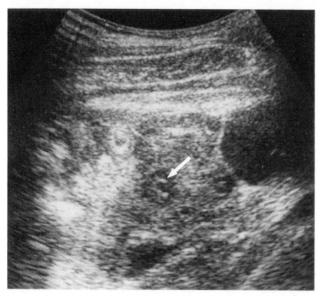

A

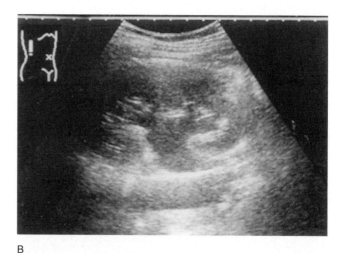

B

Figure 8–39. Sonograms of case 3. (A) An emergency ultrasound examination using a standard probe revealed a target figure of the appendix (arrow), which was draped over by omental tissues, in the right lower flank. (B) A coronal view in the right upper flank showed moderately dilated pyelocaliceal system in the right kidney.

Non-obstructive dilatation of the collecting system occurs in normal pregnancy after 6 to 10 wk, with both hormonal factors and pressure of the gravid uterus on the ureters considered to be likely causes. The dilatation is more marked on the right than on the left, and increases in severity throughout pregnancy. In this case, the retroperitoneal involvement of the inflammation from the appendicitis may have caused paresis of the ureter and, consequently, aggravated urinary retention.

► ACKNOWLEDGMENT

The author wishes to thank the staff of the section of ultrasound in the Kobe Nishi City Hospital and the Kobe City General Hospital for their assistance in obtaining the images used in this chapter.

REFERENCES

1. Gore RM, Gore MD. Ascites and peritoneal fluid collections. In: Gore RM, Levine MS, eds. Textbook of gastrointestinal radiology, 2nd ed. Philadelphia: WB Saunders, 2000:1969.
2. Jeffrey RB, McGahan JP. Gastrointestinal tract and peritoneal cavity. In: McGahan JP, Goldberg BB, eds. Diagnostic ultrasound—a logical approach. Philadelphia: Lippincott-Raven, 1998:511.
3. Lim JH, Lee DH, Ko YT. Sonographic detection of duodenal ulcer. J Ultrasound Med 1992;11:91.
4. Garcia SJM. Direct sonographic signs of acute duodenal ulcer. Abdom Imaging 1999;24:226.
5. Winek TG, Mosely HS, Grout G, et al. Pneumoperitoneum and its association with ruptured abdominal viscus. Arch Surg 1988;123:709.
6. Williams N, Everson NW. Radiological confirmation of intraperitoneal free gas. Ann R Coll Surg Engl 1997;79:8
7. Jeffrey RB, Federle MP, Wall S. Value of computed tomography in detecting occult gastrointestinal perforation. J Comput Assist Tomogr 1983;7:825.
8. Meiser G, Meissner K. Clinical relevance of sonography in acute diagnosis of perforated gastroduodenal ulcers. Langenbecks Arch Chir 1986;368:197.
9. Chanda D, Kedar RP, Malde HM. Sonographic detection of pneumoperitoneum: an experimental and clinical study. Australas Radiol 1993;37:182.
10. Kainberger P, Zukriegel M, Sattlegger P, et al. Ultrasound detection of pneumoperitoneum based on typical ultrasound morphology. Ultraschall Med 1994;15:122.
11. Braccini G, Lamacchia M, Boraschi P, et al. Ultrasound versus plain film in the detection of pneumoperitoneum. Abdom Imaging 1996;21:404.
12. Grechenig W, Peicha G, Clement HG, et al. Detection of pneumoperitoneum by ultrasound examination: an experimental and clinical study. Injury 1999;30:173.
13. Corn I. Intestinal obstruction. In: Berk JE, ed. Bockus gastroenterology, 4th ed, vol. 3. Tokyo: WB Saunders, 1985:2056.
14. Ziter FMH Jr, Markowitz SK. Radiologic Diagnosis. In: Welch JP, ed. Bowel obstruction: differential diagnosis and clinical management. Philadelphia: WB Saunders, 1990:96.
15. Stephanie R, Wilson MD. Ultrasonography of the hollow viscera. In: Gore RM, Levine MS, eds. Textbook of gastrointestinal radiology, 2nd ed. Philadelphia: WB Saunders, 2000:67.
16. Peck R. The small bowel. In: Meire H, Cosgrove D, Dewbury K, et al., eds. Clinical ultrasound (Vol. 2, abdominal and general ultrasound), 2nd ed. New York: Churchill Livingstone, 1999:823.
17. Fleischer AC, Dowling AD, Weinstein ML, et al. Sonographic patterns of distended, fluid-filled bowel. Radiology 1979;133:681.
18. Scheible W, Goldberger LE. Diagnosis of small bowel obstruction: The contribution of diagnostic ultrasound. AJR 1979;133:685.
19. Meiser G, Meissner K. Ileus and intestinal obstruction: ultrasonic findings as a guideline to therapy. Hepatogastroenterology 1987;34:194.
20. Cho KC, Hoffman-Tretin JC, Alterman DD. Closed-loop obstruction of the small bowel: CT and sonographic appearance. J Comput Assist Tomogr 1989;13:256.
21. Truong S, Arlt G, Pfingsten F, et al. Importance of sonography in diagnosis of ileus. A retrospective study of 459 patients. Chirurg 1992;63:634.
22. Schmutz GR, Benko A, Fournier L, et al. Small bowel obstruction: role and contribution of sonography. Eur Radiol 1997;7:1054.
23. Ogata M, Imai S, Hosotani R, et al. Abdominal ultrasonography for the diagnosis of strangulation in small bowel obstruction. Br J Surg 1994;81:421.
24. Ogata M. Ultrasonographic findings in the intestinal wall with hemorrhagic necrosis caused by strangulation ileus. Jpn J Med Ultrasonics 1990;17:19.
25. Czechowski J. Conventional radiography and ultrasonography in the diagnosis of small bowel obstruction and strangulation. Acta Radiol 1996;37:186.
26. Ogata M, Imai S, Hosotani R, et al. Abdominal sonography for the diagnosis of large bowel obstruction. Jpn J Surg 1994;24:791.
27. Ogata M, Mateer JR, Condon RE. Prospective evaluation of abdominal sonography for the diagnosis of bowel obstruction. Ann Surg 1996;223:237.
28. Russell JC, Welch JP. Pathophysiology of bowel obstruction. In: Welch JP, ed. Bowel obstruction: differential diagnosis and clinical management. Philadelphia: WB Saunders, 1990:28.
29. Suri S, Gupta S, Sudhakar PJ, et al. Comparative evaluation of plain films, ultrasound and CT in the diagnosis of intestinal obstruction. Acta Radiol 1999;40:422.
30. Weissberg DL, Scheible W, Leopold GR. Ultrasonographic appearance of adult intussusception. Radiology 1977;124:791.
31. Holt S, Samuel E. Multiple concentric ring sign in the ultrasonographic diagnosis of intussusception. Gastrointest Radiol 1978;3:307.

32. Puylaert, JBCM. Acute appendicitis: US evaluation using graded compression. Radiology 1986;158:335.

33. Jeffrey RB, Laing FC, Lewis FR. Acute appendicitis: high-resolution real-time US findings. Radiology 1987;163:11.

34. Jeffrey RB, Laing FC, Townsend RR. Acute appendicitis: Sonographic criteria based on 250 cases. Radiology 1988;167:327.

35. Schwerk WB, Wichtrup B, Rothmund M, et al. Ultrasonography in the diagnosis of acute appendicitis: a prospective study. Gastroenterology 1989;97:630.

36. Douglas DD, Macpherson NE, Davidson PM, et al. Randomised controlled trial of ultrasonography in diagnosis of acute appendicitis, incorporating the Alvarado score. BMJ 2000;321:919.

37. Skaane P, Schistad O, Amland PF, et al. Routine ultrasonography in the diagnosis of acute appendicitis: a valuable tool in daily practice? Am Surg 1997;63:937.

38. Pohl D, Golub R, Schwartz GE, et al. Appendiceal ultrasonography performed by nonradiologists: does it help in the diagnostic process? J Ultrasound Med 1998;17:217.

39. Amgwerd M, Rothlin M, Candinas D, et al. Ultrasound diagnosis of appendicitis by surgeons—a matter of experience? A prospective study. Lagenbecks Arch Chir 1994;379:335.

40. Williams RJ, Windsor AC, Rosin RD, et al. Ultrasound scanning of the acute abdomen by surgeons in training. Ann R Coll Surg Engl 1994;76:228.

41. Zielke A, Hasse C, Sitter H, et al. Influence of ultrasound on clinical decision making in acute appendicitis: a prospective study. Eur J Surg 1998;164:201.

42. Chen SC, Wan HP, Huang PM, et al. Accuracy of ED sonography in the diagnosis of acute appendicitis. Am J Emrg Med 2000;18:449.

43. Puylaert JBCM, Rioux M, Oostayen JA. The appendix and small bowel. In: Meire H, Cosgrove D, Dewbury K, et al., eds. Abdominal and general ultrasound, 2nd ed. New York: Churchill Livingstone, 1999:841.

44. Simonovsky V. Sonographic detection of normal and abnormal appendix. Clin Radiol 1999;54:533.

45. Schwerk WB, Schwarz S, Rothmund M. Sonography in acute colonic diverticulitis. A prospective study. Dis Colon Rectum 1992;35:1077.

46. Zielke A, Hasse C, Kisker O, et al. Prospective evaluation of ultrasonography in acute colonic diverticulitis. Br J Surg 1997;84:385.

47. Glazer G, Mann D. Acute pancreatitis. In: Monson J, Duthie G, O'Malley K, eds. Surgical emergencies. Oxford, Blackwell Science, 1999:134.

48. Balthazar EJ. Pancreatitis. In: Gore RM, Levine MS, eds. Textbook of gastrointestinal radiology, 2nd ed. Philadelphia: WB Saunders, 2000:1767.

49. Jeffrey RB. The pancreas. In: Jeffrey RB, ed. CT and sonography of the acute abdomen. New York: Raven Press, 1989:111.

50. Cosgrove DO. The pancreas. In: Meire H, Cosgrove D, Dewbury K, et al., eds. Clinical ultrasound (Vol. 1, abdominal and general ultrasound), 2nd ed. New York: Churchill Livingstone, 1999:349.

51. Laing F. Ultrasonography of the acute abdomen. Radiol Clin North Am 1992;30:389.

52. Ralls PW, Colletti PM, Lapin SA, et al. Real-time sonography in suspected acute cholecystitis. Radiology 1985;155:767.

53. Danse EM, Laterre PF, Van Beers BE, et al. Early diagnosis of acute intestinal ischaemia: contribution of colour Doppler sonography. Acta Chir Belg 1997;97:173.

54. Teefey SA, Roarke MC, Brink JA, et al. Bowel wall thickening: differentiation of inflammation from ischemia with color Doppler and duplex US. Radiology 1996;198:547.

CHAPTER 9

Renal

Stuart Swadron and Diku Mandavia

The kidney and bladder are two of the most sonographically accessible organs. Both are easily recognizable to those that are new to ultrasound and thus the urinary tract can be a simple starting point for learning focused sonography in the acute care setting.

The primary focus of renal ultrasonography in the emergency setting has been to determine the presence or absence of hydronephrosis.[1,2] As with other areas of emergency ultrasound, physicians using the modality for this specific goal have begun to explore new indications for imaging the urinary tract. The determination of bladder volume is one such indication.[3–10] Another important consideration that has arisen with the focused use of renal ultrasound is the management of unexpected or incidental findings, such as masses and cysts.[11–13]

▶ CLINICAL CONSIDERATIONS

For years, the standard diagnostic test in cases of suspected renal colic has been the intravenous pyelogram (IVP). Although IVP is more specific than ultrasound for the detection and characterization of a renal stone, it has several disadvantages in the emergency and acute care settings.[14–18] Intravenous contrast dye, even in low ionic formulation, carries a small but real risk of allergy and nephrotoxicity.[19–22] For this reason, in patients with a known allergy to contrast, diabetes mellitus, renal insufficiency, or pregnancy, renal ultrasound becomes the preferred modality. Because of the inherent risk involved with intravenous contrast, clinicians may be required to give the injection themselves, which takes valuable time and presence away from other patients. Although routine determination of renal function tests in patients presenting with flank pain and hematuria is controversial, many radiology departments require these measurements before an IVP can be performed. This also adds time and expense to the modality.

Ultrasound can be performed safely and quickly at the bedside with essentially no risks. Although it does not provide information about renal function, the presence of unilateral hydronephrosis or hydroureter in the setting of hematuria and flank pain is very sensitive for the presence of a renal stone. Recent studies that combine the use of emergency renal ultrasound with a single plain abdominal film have found a sensitivity of 64 to 97% using IVP as a comparative standard.[14,15,17,18,23,24] Moreover, the degree of hydronephrosis, in combination with the patient's history, is helpful in determining the need for urgent consultation with the urologist. In this respect, bedside ultrasound often provides sufficient information to efficiently guide the treatment and disposition of the patient. Whereas a patient with mild to moderate hydronephrosis can, with few exceptions, be managed on an outpatient basis, the presence of severe hydronephrosis should prompt urgent consultation and further definition of the obstruction by computed tomography (CT) or IVP.

Furthermore, ultrasound has the added value of providing anatomic information and detecting abnormalities that may be missed on IVP. In the course of utilizing ultrasound of the urinary tract to detect obstruction, practitioners can identify other such abnormalities with increasing frequency. Some of these represent life- or kidney-threatening processes and can prompt timely definitive treatment. Ultrasonography is especially sensitive for the presence of cysts and for distinguishing between solid and cystic masses.[25]

Because the differential diagnosis in patients with flank or abdominal pain involves other organs visualized well by bedside ultrasound, invaluable additional information may be available that cannot be obtained with IVP. Specifically, if no hydronephrosis is seen on ultrasound examination, the physician may proceed to examine the gallbladder, common bile duct, and abdominal aorta.

Spiral CT has emerged as an important modality in the emergency and acute care settings for the evaluation of suspected renal colic.[26,27] Not only does CT provide excellent visualization of the urinary tract and of renal stones, it provides similar detail for other abdominal structures. Many physicians are now using CT in the place of both ultrasound and IVP, especially in older patients where the risk of abdominal aortic aneurysm (AAA) is greater. CT can reliably exclude this life-threatening entity from the differential diagnosis. The sensitivity of CT scan in the detection of renal stone disease varies from 86 to 100%.[28–36] However, CT scanning remains less accessible, involves a considerable exposure to radiation, and probably is not necessary in younger patients with a straightforward clinical presentation of renal colic.

► CLINICAL INDICATIONS

Possible indications for ultrasound examination of the urinary tract in the emergency and acute care setting are:

- Suspected renal colic
- Acute urinary retention
- Acute renal failure
- Acute pyelonephritis and/or abscess
- Possible renal mass
- Trauma

Suspected Renal Colic

A focused emergency ultrasound examination of the kidneys is presently indicated for evaluation of the patient with suspected renal colic. Because of the prevalence of renal stone disease, this diagnosis is in the differential diagnosis of any patient presenting with abdominal or flank pain. While ultrasonography is primarily utilized in patients presenting with flank pain and hematuria, its use also may be considered in the broader group of patients with undifferentiated abdominal pain and the absence of hematuria since renal stone disease may present in this fashion as well. While ultrasonography most frequently does not detect an actual renal stone, its ability to detect hydronephrosis, an important consequence of obstructive uropathy, makes it an invaluable tool in the emergency setting.[37]

In the largest study comparing IVP with renal ultrasound, 288 patients admitted to a hospital for intractable flank pain were studied.[23] Using IVP as the gold standard, the sensitivity of ultrasound alone for detecting renal stone

disease was 93%, its specificity 83%, positive predictive value 93%, and negative predictive value 83%. When a kidney/ureter/bladder (KUB) radiograph was added to ultrasound, its specificity improved to 100%. In a study of 180 patients in the emergency department setting, Dalla Palma and co-workers found a sensitivity of 95% for the detection of renal stone disease using the combination of ultrasound and a KUB radiograph. The high negative predictive value of a KUB radiograph and ultrasound in this study (95%) led these researchers to conclude that IVP need not be performed when these are both negative.[15]

If microscopic hematuria is present and no hydronephrosis is seen, the consideration of other diagnoses should be made even though the diagnosis of renal stone is still possible. Those diagnoses that are immediately life-threatening, such as a ruptured AAA, must be considered. Once the clinician is satisfied that more serious disease entities are not present, the patient may be discharged home for further evaluation as necessary on an outpatient basis, which may include an IVP, CT scan, or renal stone analysis, if collected. The presence of a solitary kidney, renal failure, or urinary tract infection can be indications for admission or further investigation, even without significant hydronephrosis, when the diagnosis of renal stones is still under consideration. An algorithm for the evaluation of renal colic that incorporates the use of focused ultrasonography is outlined in Figure 9–1.

Patients who are dehydrated may fail to show the signs of hydronephrosis on ultrasound[38,39]; thus, oral or intravenous hydration is recommended before obstructive hydronephrosis can be excluded. Conversely, a patient with a full bladder may have the appearance of bilateral hydronephrosis; if such a situation is encountered, the ultrasound examination should be repeated after the patient voids.[40,41] Because of these variations with state of hydration and bladder volume, it is extremely important to obtain images of both kidneys for comparison and to correlate the images with the clinical picture.

In a patient with no hematuria, a negative KUB radiograph, and a negative bedside ultrasound examination for hydronephrosis, the diagnosis of renal colic becomes extremely unlikely; the negative predictive value of this combination is high, ranging from 75 to 95%.[14,16,23]

The persistence of bilateral hydronephrosis may indicate bladder outlet obstruction and further study is indicated. With long-standing hydronephrosis, a thinning of the medulla and cortex begin to occur.[25] The presence of right-sided hydronephrosis is a common finding in pregnancy and should not be confused for pathology.[41] Occasionally, the finding of calyceal rupture will be noted by the presence of perinephric fluid with mild to moderate hydronephrosis. The finding of urinary extravasation is significant and should prompt urgent urological consultation.

An evolving technique in the evaluation of renal outflow obstruction involves the imaging of ureteral jets.[42,43]

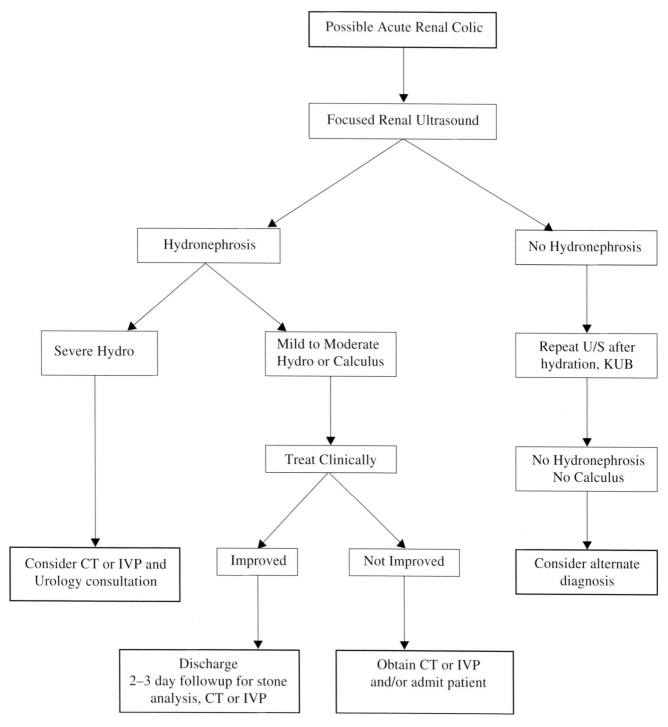

Figure 9–1. Algorithm for the evaluation of renal colic.

In the normal bladder, the intermittent ejection of urine into the bladder from the ureters can be visualized during real-time examination. In the presence of unilateral obstruction, ureteral jet flow to the ipsilateral side is impaired or not present. This can provide information on renal tract function and may be particularly useful when contrast dye administration is contraindicated.

Acute Urinary Retention

Bedside ultrasound can assist in the evaluation of patients with symptoms of acute urinary retention. At times, it can be difficult to ascertain, from the history alone, whether or not the patient has developed acute urinary retention. Although the physical examination of the abdomen can demonstrate a distended bladder, this may not be reliable, especially in obese patients. Therefore, the placement of a urinary catheter for residual urine, both as a diagnostic and therapeutic procedure, has been the traditional approach when the diagnosis of acute urinary retention is being considered. Although this approach does quantify the amount of urine retained, it is uncomfortable for patients and incurs a risk of infection. Most clinicians would prefer to avoid this diagnostic procedure unless it is clear that urinary retention exists.

Ultrasound can immediately confirm and quantify the degree of obstruction and retention by imaging the urinary bladder and estimating its size. Many of the studies examining bladder volume have been performed by urologists in conjunction with urodynamic measurements.[3,5–10,44–47] In this setting, even small degrees of error may be unacceptable. By contrast, a qualitative estimate of bladder size may be very helpful in the emergency setting. Bedside ultrasound can easily classify the bladder volume as small, medium, or large, thus aiding the clinician in determining the need for emergent urinary catheterization. The presence of a large, distended bladder mandates emergency urinary catheterization; whereas, an empty or small bladder on ultrasound suggests another cause for the patient's symptoms. Whenever the bladder is imaged in this fashion, the kidneys should be examined for bilateral hydronephrosis, which is a concerning complication of long-standing bladder outlet obstruction.

Acute Renal Failure

Renal ultrasound can be a useful adjunct in the evaluation of acute renal failure. The clinical evaluation of acute renal failure begins with a determination of whether the cause is proximal to the kidneys (prerenal failure), distal to the kidneys (post-renal failure), or intrinsic to the kidneys ("renal" failure). Since post-renal causes, such as obstruction of either ureteric or urethral outflow, are readily reversible if identified in a timely fashion, these are most often considered first in the evaluation. Ultrasound is clearly an effective tool in the identification of post-renal obstruction, easily detecting bilateral hydronephrosis and bladder distention. If only a solitary kidney is visualized and hydronephrosis is present, the need for acute decompression becomes particularly urgent. Moreover, prostatic enlargement, one of the most common causes of lower tract obstruction, can be identified on ultrasound.

After a post-renal cause has been excluded, renal ultrasound may provide further diagnostic information. Whereas prerenal causes of renal failure will not generally cause ultrasonographic abnormalities, several causes of acute and acute-on-chronic intrinsic renal failure will manifest themselves on ultrasound examination. Small, atrophic and hyperechoic kidneys suggest chronic pathologic processes such as hypertensive nephropathy and chronic glomerulonephritis. The finding of enlarged kidneys with multiple cysts distorting the renal architecture suggests polycystic kidney disease as the cause of renal failure. Unfortunately, many causes of acute renal failure that are intrinsic, such as acute glomerulonephritis and acute tubular necrosis, may have non-specific or minimal sonographic findings. Furthermore, different clinical entities may have different sonographic manifestations at different stages in their presentation. For this reason, other clinical methods, such as volume status determination, response to fluid therapy, microscopic urinalysis, and measurement of the fractional excretion of sodium, must be utilized to distinguish between prerenal and intrinsic causes of renal failure to guide therapy. Renal biopsy, which is often necessary to establish a definitive diagnosis, may be facilitated by ultrasound guidance.

Acute Pyelonephritis and Renal Abscess

Acute pyelonephritis, an extremely common emergency diagnosis, does not necessarily require imaging. In fact, the sonographic appearance of the kidney in acute pyelonephritis is most commonly normal.[37] However, in complex cases or those not responding to medical management, ultrasound may be helpful in excluding complications of pyelonephritis that do require surgical management. For example, the formation of a renal abscess may complicate pyelonephritis. Renal abscesses are typically solitary, round hypoechoic masses, often with internal septations or mobile debris and a degree of posterior acoustic enhancement.[37,41] Suspicious lesions identified in the course of the emergency ultrasound may prompt consultation with a urologist, a formal ultrasonographic study, or, in some cases, CT scanning to further characterize the lesion and formulate a treatment plan.[48] Perinephric abscesses, which extend beyond the kidney, can be visualized on ultrasound, but are better evaluated with CT scanning. This modality should be sought for further evaluation of renal lesions or suspected perirenal abscesses.[37]

One rare but life-threatening infection, emphysematous pyelonephritis, deserves special mention. Gas formation in the kidney by bacteria will cause echogenic areas that obscure the deeper structures. These echogenic areas could potentially be confused with renal stone disease; however, in the setting of pyelonephritis, this finding should prompt emergent surgical consultation. Patients with this infection are most frequently diabetic or immunocompromised for other reasons. Because patients with emphysematous pyelonephritis may have toxic and nonspecific presentations, suggestive findings on emergency ultrasound may prompt surgical intervention (either percutaneous drainage or open nephrectomy) that would have otherwise been overlooked or unduly delayed.[49,50]

Renal Masses

Renal masses are being seen with increasing frequency as a result of both emergency sonography and the incorporation of screening abdominal ultrasound into periodic health evaluations.[11,51–54] There is no question that the mortality and morbidity of malignancies detected in this incidental fashion are greatly reduced.[55–57] Although there is concern regarding the cost effectiveness of routine use of ultrasound in the absence of specific symptomatology, a mechanism for the follow-up of abnormalities found in the emergency and acute care setting must be available. It cannot be overemphasized that the focused use of ultrasound to evaluate a patient for hydronephrosis is not a substitute for formal sonography or other follow up studies. Moreover, renal masses discovered on ultrasound almost always require further characterization with another modality, usually CT.[37] The majority of malignancies seen in the kidney are renal cell carcinoma (RCC).[12,54,58] These tumors are extremely heterogeneous in their sonographic appearance and may be isoechoic, hyperechoic, or hypoechoic to the adjacent parenchyma. It is also important to note that many of these tumors have a cystic presentation and may be mistaken for a simple benign cyst.[37]

Another common tumor seen in the kidney is the angiomyolipoma (AML).[37,58] These tumors are mostly benign and may be treated conservatively.[59] Whereas they are usually well demarcated and brightly echogenic on ultrasound, there is a significant overlap in their sonographic appearance with that of echogenic renal cell carcinoma.[60] This serves to underscore the caution that is required in the interpretation of any mass found incidentally during ultrasound. Any such finding requires follow up with a formal ultrasound examination, CT scan, or urologic consultation if appropriate.

Other tumors that are commonly seen on ultrasound are lymphomas and metastatic malignancies, which commonly appear as irregular nodules, either single or multiple. These may also be diffuse, grossly disturbing the renal architecture or infiltrative, extending into the perirenal and surrounding structures.[37] Transitional cell carcinoma (TCC), which is more commonly found in the bladder and ureter than in the renal pelvis, is frequently not visible on renal ultrasound. This is because it is frequently symptomatic (with gross hematuria) before sufficient tumor mass can be seen in the renal pelvis. Its sonographic appearance is one of a hypoechoic mass within the highly echogenic renal sinus.[37]

Renal cysts are an extremely common finding on ultrasound. Although simple cysts are benign, malignancies may present with a cystic appearance.[61] For this reason, caution needs to be exercised before dismissing a lesion seen on sonography as a simple cyst.

Polycystic kidney disease (PCKD) can be recognized as an abundance of cysts of varying sizes that both enlarge and distort the regular renal architecture.[37,41,61] Ultrasound is the modality of choice to evaluate this heritable disorder, which may present with hematuria, flank pain, hypertension, and renal failure. Cysts are frequently present in multiple organs in the body and there is an association with cerebral aneurysms.[61] Urology or nephrology referral is indicated upon discovery of this disorder. Patients with chronic renal failure undergoing long-term dialysis also tend to develop multiple renal cysts. This disorder, known as acquired renal cystic disease (ARCD), is characterized by a huge increase in the incidence of renal malignancies and, for this reason, regular surveillance of this condition is indicated.[37,61]

Renal Trauma

On grayscale sonography, the primary indicator of major renal trauma is a subcapsular hematoma or perinephric hematoma. These findings may be recognized on the initial trauma ultrasound screening examination or on subsequent examinations. Multiple trauma patients in whom injury of the renal pedicle injury is suspected are best evaluated with contrast CT scan, which provides information about renal function and is considered the modality of choice.[62] If CT is not available, newer ultrasound techniques, such as power color Doppler, may provide immediate bedside information about renal tissue perfusion. These techniques have not been thoroughly evaluated in the trauma setting, but are promising and deserve further study.[63]

Ultrasound may also have a role in the follow-up and management of patients with identified parenchymal injury, such as hematomas and lacerations. These lesions are often well visualized by ultrasonography and can be evaluated periodically to monitor their resolution.

Ultrasound may have a role in screening patients with minor trauma. In minor trauma patients with microscopic hematuria, the clinician must decide whether to follow the patient clinically or to do a CT scan (which is usually negative for any process requiring intervention). Some clinicians may utilize limited ultrasound as a less costly alternative to CT scan in these patients. Patients without signs of renal trauma are followed for normalization of the hematuria. Those with an abnormal ultrasound examination, persistent hematuria, or a mechanism that suggests risk of renal pedicle injury require CT scanning.

▶ ANATOMIC CONSIDERATIONS

Compartments of the Retroperitoneum

Before describing the gross anatomy of the kidney, ureter, and bladder, it is important to review where these structures lie within the abdominal cavity and their relation to their surroundings.

The retroperitoneal cavity is divided into three distinct compartments, with the kidneys occupying the middle or *perirenal* compartment. The anterior compartment contains the duodenum, pancreas, descending colon, celiac trunk, and superior mesenteric vessels, as well as associated fat. The posterior compartment, which lies anterior to the quadratus lumborum and psoas muscles, simply contains fat. The anterior and posterior compartments are also referred to as the *pararenal* compartments.

The perirenal compartment is bounded by *Gerota's fascia* both anteriorly and posteriorly, although many authors refer to the posterior component of the renal fascia as *Zuckerkandl's fascia*. This fascia, which invests the kidneys, adrenal glands, renal hila, proximal collecting system, and perinephric fat, merges laterally to form the lateroconal fascia that extends to the parietal peritoneum of the lateral paracolic gutter. This completes the separation of the anterior and posterior retroperitoneal compartments. Thus, the kidneys are surrounded by two distinct layers of fat: the *perinephric fat,* which lies immediately outside the true fibrous capsule of the kidney, bounded by Gerota's fascia, and the *paranephric fat,* which lies in the pararenal compartments outside of Gerota's fascia.

This compartmentalization of the retroperitoneum is important clinically as it serves to localize various pathologic processes. It also creates a barrier to the progression of various pathologic processes such as hemorrhage and infection. Collections of fluid in the anterior pararenal compartment, for example, are commonly related to pancreatitis or trauma, whereas collections of fluid in the posterior pararenal compartment are uncommon, usually representing spontaneous hemorrhage in patients with coagulopathy or related to trauma. Figure 9–2 illustrates the compartments of the retroperitoneum.

Anatomic Relationships of the Urinary System

There is significant asymmetry in the position of the two kidneys within the abdominal cavity. The right kidney is bounded anteriorly by the liver, which serves as an excellent acoustic window for sonography. The right kidney is usually slightly larger and slightly inferior to the left kidney. The left kidney is bounded anteriorly by several structures, including the pancreas, stomach, spleen, and large and small bowel, making it somewhat more difficult to image, as only the spleen serves as an acoustic window of equal quality to the liver. Superiorly and posteriorly, both kidneys have symmetrical relationships, with the diaphragms superiorly and the musculature of the retroperitoneum (psoas and quadratus) posteriorly.

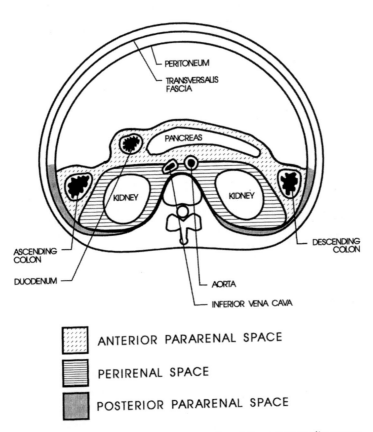

Figure 9-2. Anatomic compartments of the retroperitoneum. *(Reprinted, with permission, from Williamson M. Essentials of ultrasound. Philadelphia: WB Saunders, 1996.)*

In the supine position, the superior pole of the left kidney is at the level of the 12th thoracic vertebrae and the inferior pole is at the level of the third lumbar vertebrae. However, it is important to realize that the kidneys are mobile structures within the retroperitoneum, moving with changes in position and with the phases of respiration. Figure 9–3 illustrates the anatomic relationships of the two kidneys.

The renal *hilum* is the specific area of the sinus where the renal artery enters and the renal vein and ureter exit the kidney on its medial concave surface. The ureters, which arise from the hila of each kidney, travel inferiorly toward the bladder in close relation to the psoas muscle, just anterior to the transverse process of the lumbar spine. As they enter the pelvis, they course medially to cross the iliac vessels and then laterally once again to parallel the margins of the bony pelvis before inserting posteriorly into the bladder.

The bladder, when empty, abuts the posterior aspect of the pubis. As it fills, it expands to fill more of the pelvis, displacing bowel loops into the abdomen. A distended bladder moves into the lower abdomen and gains relationships to the anterior abdominal wall.

Renal Anatomy

The kidneys are paired structures that lie obliquely with respect to every anatomic plane. They are situated so that their inferior poles are anterior and lateral to their superior poles. In addition, each hilum is directed obliquely as well, in an anteromedially rather than simple medial orientation. The sonographic significance of this orientation is that the technique for imaging the kidneys must involve adjusting the probe obliquely in each plane to match the anatomy.[39,40]

Each kidney is between 9 and 13 cm in its maximum longitudinal measurement, and they decrease in size with advanced age and chronic renal failure. The approximate width and depth of the kidneys is 5 cm and 3 cm, respectively. Each kidney is surrounded by a true fibrous capsule and can be divided into two parts, the renal *parenchyma* and the renal *sinus*. The renal parenchyma, which surrounds the sinus on all sides except at the hilum, is composed of the outer *cortex,* consisting of the filtration components of the nephrons and the inner *medulla,* consisting of the reabsorptive components (loop of Henle). The cone-shaped medullary pyramids are oriented with their apices, or *papillae,* protruding inward toward the renal sinus. Thus, the functional unit of the kidney, or renal lobe, consists of a medullary pyramid and its surrounding cortex. Urine is filtered by the cortex and then excreted through the papillae into the collecting system. There are between 8 and 18 such lobes in each kidney, bounded by interlobar arteries and veins. The arcuate arteries, which branch from these interlobar arteries, are

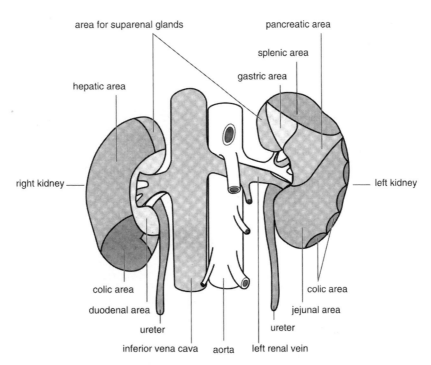

Figure 9–3. Anatomic relationship of the kidneys. *(Reprinted, with permission from Curry AC, Tempkin BB. Ultrasonography: an introduction to normal structure and functional anatomy. Philadelphia: WB Saunders, 1995.)*

found at the base of the medullary pyramids and can serve as important landmarks in the interpretation of sonographic images.

The renal sinus, the central portion of the kidney, begins where the renal papillae empty their urine into the smallest subunit of the collecting system, the minor calyces. There are, therefore, between 8 to 18 minor calyces in each kidney corresponding to the pyramids. These minor calyces in turn coalesce into two to three major calyces. The major calyces merge with the renal *pelvis,* which is the dilated proximal end of the ureter as it joins the kidney. In addition to the collecting system, the renal sinus also contains the renal artery and vein, as well as fatty tissue, which is an extension of the perinephric fat bounded by Gerota's fascia. Figure 9–4 illustrates the gross anatomy of the kidney.

▶ TECHNIQUE AND NORMAL ULTRASOUND FINDINGS

The kidneys are usually imaged using a 3.5 MHz transducer, although the 5.0 MHz transducer may be used to yield greater anatomic detail in thin patients or in those patients with a transplanted kidney located in the pelvis. Images of both the affected and unaffected kidney in both the longitudinal and transverse planes should be obtained. As with other structures, it is necessary to carefully scan through the kidneys in both of these planes to ensure that all of the parenchyma is imaged.[40] It is important to image both kidneys for comparison to normal, and to exclude congenital or surgical absence. A limited ultrasound examination of the urinary tract should also include views of the bladder to access total filling and identify possible abnormalities.

Right Kidney

The right kidney can usually be imaged with the patient supine using the anterior subcostal approach. It may be necessary to have the patient turn toward the left side or prone. From a position inferior and lateral to the edge of the right costal margin, the transducer is moved incrementally medially and inferiorly until the right kidney comes into view. Because of the kidney's oblique lie, it will be necessary to rotate the transducer to obtain the image of the kidney in its maximal length. This is the longitudinal axis, and once obtained, the transducer is moved medially and laterally to scan all of the parenchyma and sinus in this axis. In many patients, it will not be possible to view the entire kidney longitudinally in one window, and separate images are often required of the superior and inferior poles. It also may be necessary to obtain some of the images using intercostal windows or by having the patient briefly

Figure 9–4. Gross anatomy of the kidney. *(Reprinted, with permission from Curry AC, Tempkin BB. Ultrasonography: an introduction to normal structure and functional anatomy. Philadelphia: WB Saunders, 1995.)*

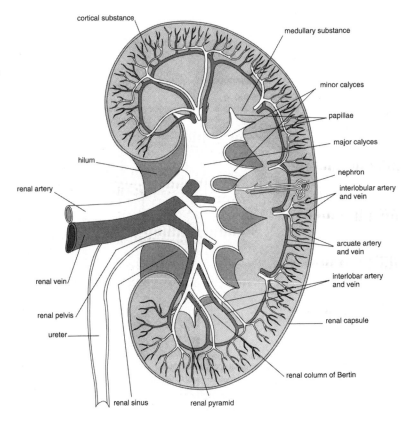

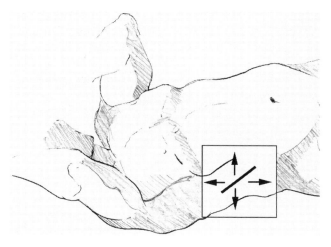

Figure 9–5. Sonographic technique for the right kidney.

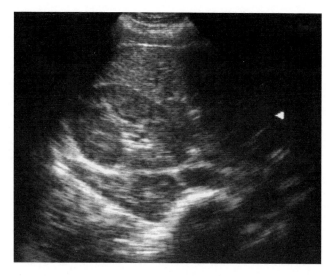

Figure 9–7. Transverse ultrasound view of the normal right kidney.

hold their breath, moving the kidneys inferiorly to a subcostal window.

To obtain the transverse plane images, the transducer merely needs to be rotated 90° from the longitudinal plane. Once in the transverse plane, the transducer can be moved, either superiorly and medially, or inferiorly and laterally, to locate the renal hilum, with images superior representing the superior pole and images inferior representing the inferior pole. Figure 9–5 demonstrates the technique for sonography of the right kidney with corresponding longitudinal (Figure 9–6) and transverse images (Figure 9–7).

If intestinal gas is interfering with anterior views, coronal views of the right kidney should be used. This technique is described in detail in Chapter 4.

Left Kidney and Bladder

To obtain images of the left kidney, the sonographer may have to contend with the interference of air in the stomach and intestine. This may be circumvented by finding a more posterior window (usually through the spleen), with the patient turning toward the examiner in the right lateral decubitus position, if possible.[39,40] To obtain the longitudinal images of the left kidney, the transducer first should be placed in the midcoronal plane, moving between the costal margin superiorly and the iliac crest inferiorly to find the kidney. As with the right kidney, it will be necessary to find the longest axis first before scanning the kidney throughout in this plane. With respect to imaging the entire left kidney, the same guidelines apply as for the right kidney. A combination of intercostal and subcostal views and, subsequently obtaining transverse images by rotating the transducer, may be needed. The coronal view is particularly helpful for imaging the inferior pole of the left kidney, which is often obscured by overlying gas within the descending colon. This technique is described in detail in Chapter 4. Figure 9–8 illustrates the technique for sonography of the left kidney with corresponding longitudinal and transverse images (Figure 9–9).

The bladder, which is ideally moderately filled at the time of the examination, should be imaged with the transducer placed suprapubically. Like the kidney, the bladder should be scanned thoroughly in both sagittal and transverse planes.

Sonographic Appearance of the Kidney, Ureter, and Bladder

Each kidney is well demarcated by a brightly echogenic fibrous capsule surrounded by a variable amount of

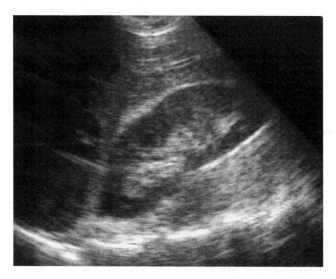

Figure 9–6. Longitudinal ultrasound view of the normal right kidney.

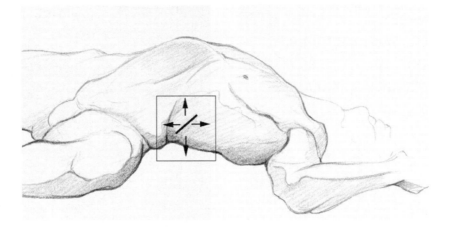

Figure 9–8. Sonographic technique for the left kidney.

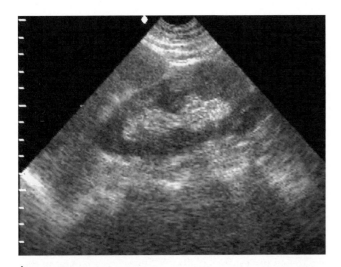

A

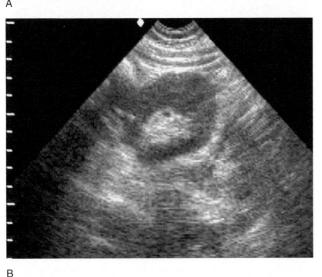

B

Figure 9–9. Normal left kidney. Longitudinal (A) and transverse (B) ultrasound views.

perinephric fat. The parenchyma typically has an echogenicity somewhat less than that of the liver. Within the parenchyma, the cortex can often be distinguished from the medullary pyramids, which because of their urine filled tubules cut a less echogenic, saw-toothed ribbon deep to the margin of the cortex. The sinus, which lies deep to the parenchyma, is highly echogenic due to its high fat content. In well-hydrated patients, anechoic pockets of urine may be seen within the brightly reflective sinus. When scanned in real-time, the continuity of these pockets within the renal pelvis can be demonstrated. Figures 9–6 and 9–7 show normal longitudinal and transverse images, respectively, of the right kidney. Although the normal ureter is not seen on ultrasound, a proximally distended ureter can often be visualized. The shape and relationships of the bladder on ultrasound examination depend on its degree of filling (Figure 9–10).

With urine in the bladder, its wall appears as a thin echogenic line surrounding an anechoic cavity. The normal prostate gland may be recognized as an ovular mass at the bladder neck (Figure 9–11). This is often best seen on transverse views angled caudad, with a normal prostate size of up to 5 cm in width.

In patients with normal hydration and no ureteral obstruction, ureteral flow jets can be observed near the trigone area as urine flows into a filled bladder. These can be visualized with grayscale sonography but are more obvious using color Doppler techniques (Figure 9–12).

▶ COMMON AND EMERGENT ABNORMALITIES

Obstructive Uropathy

In hydronephrosis, large, echo-free areas representing urine can be seen within the echogenic renal sinus. The

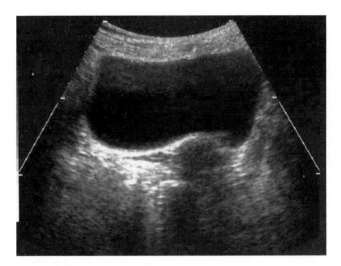

Figure 9–10. Transverse view of filled female bladder with uterus and echoes from bowel gas in the far field.

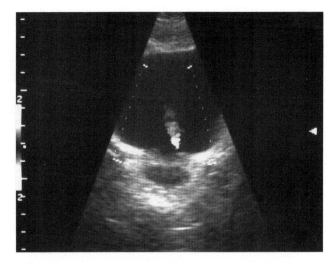

Figure 9–12. Transverse view of the male bladder reveals a normal ureteral flow jet on color Doppler (gray-scale image) arising from the trigone area. A transverse view of the hypoechoic prostate gland is seen immediately below the bladder.

degree of hydronephrosis seen is a continuum, although arbitrary designations of mild, moderate, and severe hydronephrosis are commonly used (Figures 9–13, 9–14, and 9–15). Occasionally, hydronephrosis with perinephric fluid, signifying a ruptured calyx, will be noted (Figures 9–16 and 9–17).

Although stones in the ureter are rarely visualized, they may be seen within the kidney (Figure 9–18) at the ureteropelvic junction (Figures 9–19) or ureterovesicular junctions, two common locations of obstruction. As with gallstones, they have a strongly echogenic appearance and cause acoustic shadowing. Figures 9–20 and 9–21

show ureteral stones, which are not commonly identified on ultrasound.

Bladder Volume Measurement

This technique involves measuring the bladder in its maximal width, depth, and length, and then inserting the product of these measurements into a complex mathematical formula. It has been used for more than 25 years and was first performed using B-mode imaging.[3,8] With real-time ultrasound, most current machines contain automated calculators for volume measurement (Figure 9–22). As an alternate, the simple formula (length X width X height X 0.75) can be used to estimate bladder volume.[9] Because of the inherent variability of bladder shape and the variation in this shape with differing degrees of filling, bladder volume measurements obtained in this fashion may have an error of between 15 and 35%.[3,7–10]

Renal Abscess

Renal abscesses are typically solitary, round hypoechoic masses, often with internal septations or mobile debris and a degree of posterior acoustic enhancement. When these rupture or extend into the perinephric space, complex fluid may be appreciated surrounding a portion of the kidney.

Renal Masses

Renal cell carcinoma (RCC) tumors (Figure 9–23) are extremely heterogeneous in their sonographic appearance *(text continues on page 211)*

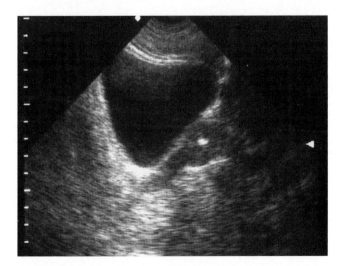

Figure 9–11. Longitudinal view of the male bladder reveals the prostate posteriorly which contains a small central calcification.

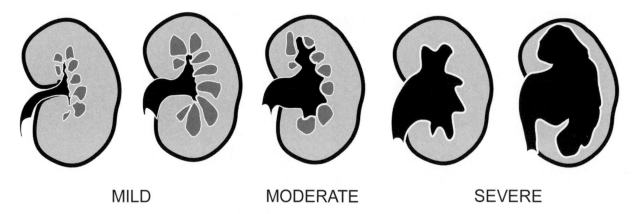

MILD   MODERATE   SEVERE

Figure 9–13. Grades of hydronephrosis.

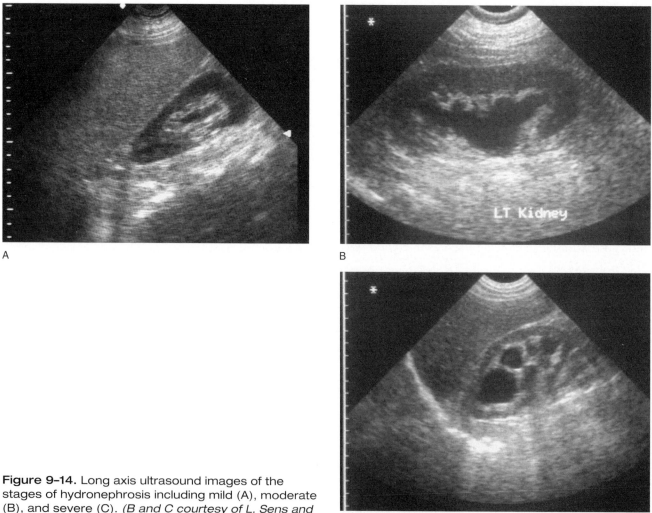

A

B

C

Figure 9–14. Long axis ultrasound images of the stages of hydronephrosis including mild (A), moderate (B), and severe (C). *(B and C courtesy of L. Sens and L. Green, Gulfcoast Ultrasound.)*

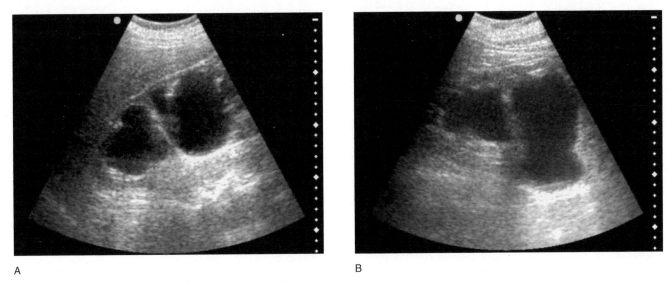

A   B

Figure 9–15. Chronic severe hydronephrosis. Coronal views of the kidney show severe hydronephrosis and cortical atrophy (A). Another view of the same kidney demonstrating severe urinary distention of the renal pelvis (B). *(Courtesy of James Mateer, MD.)*

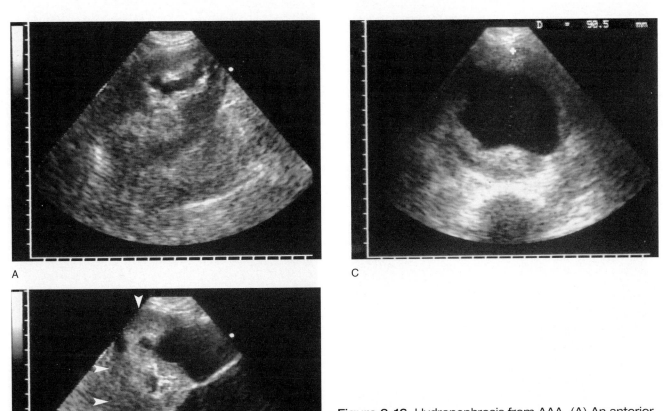

A

C

B

Figure 9–16. Hydronephrosis from AAA. (A) An anterior coronal view of the inferior pole of the left kidney reveals mild hydronephrosis. (B) A posterior coronal view of the lower flank (angled superiorly) in the same patient shows a septated fluid collection that communicates with the collecting system of the kidney. The renal borders are outlined (arrowheads). The contained fluid collection is a perinephric urinoma secondary to ureteral compression with calyceal rupture from a large (9.5 cm) AAA. *(Courtesy of James Mateer, MD.)*

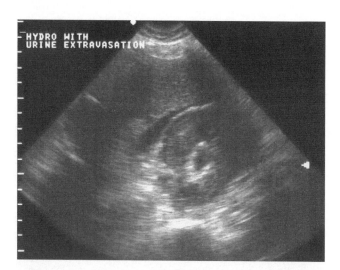

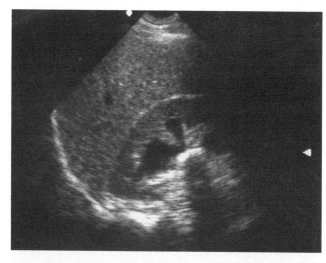

Figure 9–17. Hydronephrosis with acute calyceal rupture. Transverse view of right kidney (outlined by rib shadows) with hydronephrosis and urinary extravasation into the perirenal space.

Figure 9–19. Longitudinal view of right kidney shows moderate hydronephrosis and a large stone within the renal pelvis.

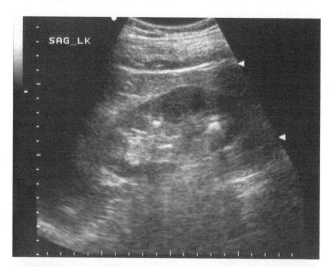

A

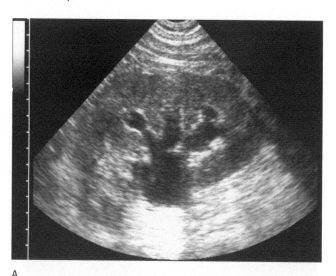

A

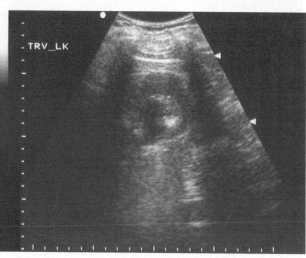

B

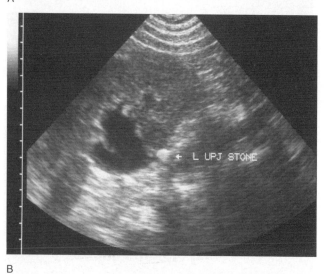

B

Figure 9–18. Longitudinal (A) and transverse (B) views of the left kidney show intrarenal stones (with posterior shadowing below the larger of the two stones). *(Courtesy of L. Sens, Gulfcoast Ultrasound).*

Figure 9–20. Ureteropelvic junction stone. Coronal view of the kidney (A) shows moderate hydronephrosis. A slightly different angle of the same kidney demonstrates a ureteropelvic junction stone (with posterior shadowing) as the cause of the urinary obstruction. *(Courtesy of James Mateer, MD.)*

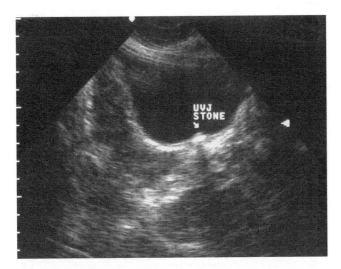

Figure 9–21. Ureterovesicular junction stone. Ureteral stone seen at the ureterovesical junction through a transverse view of the bladder.

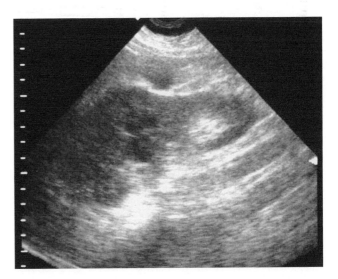

Figure 9–23. Renal cell carcinoma. Long axis view through the right kidney showing renal cell carcinoma with enlargement of the upper pole including both solid and cystic elements.

and may be isoechoic, hyperechoic, or hypoechoic to the adjacent parenchyma. It is also important to note that these tumors may have a cystic presentation and be mistaken for a simple benign cyst.[37]

Another common tumor seen in the kidney is the *angiomyolipoma* (AML). Whereas this tumor is usually well demarcated and brightly echogenic on ultrasound, there may be a significant overlap in its sonographic appearance and that of echogenic renal cell carcinoma.[60]

Renal Cysts

Renal cysts (Figure 9–24) are a common finding on ultrasound. A benign cyst must meet all of the following criteria:[37,39,41]

1. Smooth, round, or oval shaped
2. No internal echoes or solid elements
3. Well-defined interface between the cyst and the adjacent renal parenchyma in all planes and orientations
4. Posterior echo enhancement beyond the cyst

Renal Trauma

At present, sonography is not the definitive modality in the evaluation of renal trauma. The indicators of major renal trauma, subcapsular and perinephric hematomas (Figure 9–25), must be differentiated from fluid in the hepatorenal

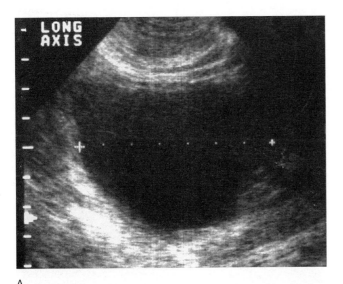

A

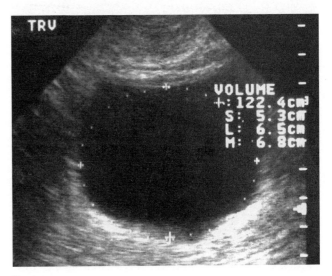

B

Figure 9–22. Longitudinal (A) and transverse (B) views of the bladder show the use of a software calculation program to determine bladder volume.

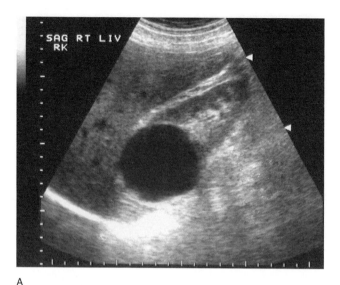

A

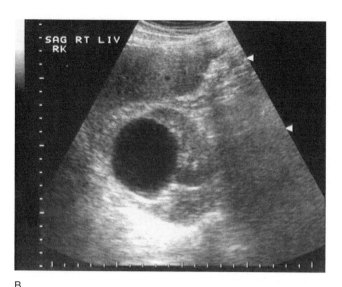

B

Figure 9–24. Renal cyst. Longitudinal (A) and transverse (B) views of the right kidney demonstrate the usual features of a simple cyst. *(Courtesy of L. Sens, Gulfcoast Ultrasound.)*

space or in the posterior pararenal compartment of the retroperitoneum, which are not specific for renal trauma (Figure 9–26). Fluid in the anterior pararenal space is often difficult to visualize with ultrasound due to overlying bowel gas and lack of a distinct interface with solid organs.

► COMMON VARIANTS AND SELECTED ABNORMALITIES

Sonolucent Pyramids

In some patients, the medullary pyramids appear so sonolucent that they may be mistaken for the anechoic

collections of urine seen with hydronephrosis.[39] They can be differentiated from distended calyces by the presence of cortex between them, by their triangular shape, and sometimes by the appearance of arcuate arteries, which appear as bright echogenic dots at the base of the pyramids (Figure 9–27).

Renal Pseudotumors

The term "pseudotumor" is used to refer to several anatomic variants that can simulate a renal mass, the most frequent of which are hypertrophied column of Bertin and the dromedary or splenic hump. Although the identification of renal masses is not a goal of focused emer-

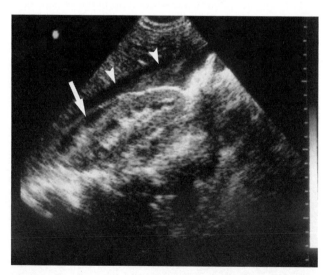

Figure 9–25. Renal trauma. Longitudinal view of the right upper quadrant shows fluid and clots in Morison's pouch (arrowheads) from hepatic injury and capsular elevation and a subcapsular hematoma of the kidney (arrow) related to blunt renal trauma. *(Courtesy of James Mateer, MD.)*

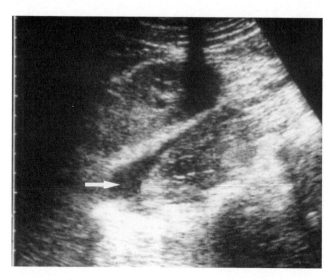

Figure 9–26. Coronal view of the kidney and psoas muscle demonstrates fluid in the posterior pararenal space (arrow). *(Courtesy of James Mateer, MD.)*

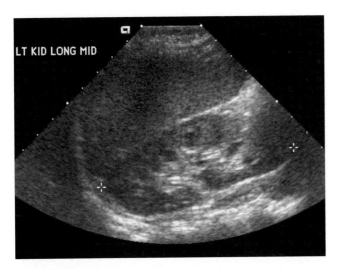

Figure 9–27. Right kidney in long axis with sonolucent renal pyramids. This corresponds to the medullary portions of the kidney. *(Courtesy of James Mateer, MD; Waukesha Memorial Hospital.)*

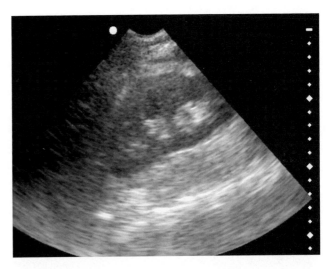

Figure 9–29. Long axis view of the left kidney demonstrating the typical morphology of a dromedary hump. *(Courtesy of James Mateer, MD.)*

gency ultrasound of the kidney, these anomalies deserve special mention because of their potential to be mistaken for a renal mass.

A "hypertrophied column of Bertin" refers to an invagination of renal cortical tissue into the renal sinus (Figure 9–28). This invagination can mimic a mass because it can cause an indentation and splaying of the sinus structures. It does, however, have the same echogenicity as the renal cortex and can be seen to be continuous with the cortex in real time. In addition, these columns should not alter the outer contour of the kidney, as commonly occurs with RCC.[37,39,41,61]

The dromedary (splenic) hump occurs on the left kidney as a symmetrical, rounded enlargement of the

center portion of the cortex with homogenous echotexture. Since the contour of the kidney is altered, it is more difficult to confidently exclude RCC and a follow up study is recommended (Figure 9–29).

Duplication of the Collecting System

A duplex collecting system is one of the most common congenital renal anomalies and the degree of duplication can vary. A partial duplex collecting system can be detected sonographically as two central echogenic sinuses with normal bridging renal parenchyma between them (Figure 9–30). Hydronephrosis of the upper pole sinus

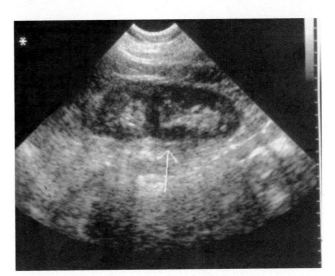

Figure 9–30. Partial duplex collecting system. Long axis view of the kidney shows a distinct separation between the upper and lower portions of the collecting system within the kidney. *(Courtesy of L. Sens and L. Green, Gulfcoast Ultrasound.)*

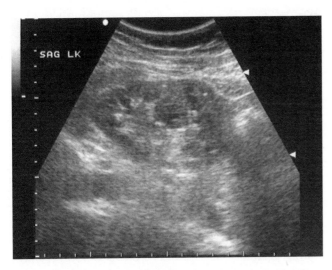

Figure 9–28. Long axis of the left kidney demonstrating a column of Bertin displacing the sinus structures. *(Courtesy of L. Sens, Gulfcoast Ultrasound.)*

with visualization of two distinct collecting systems and ureters is diagnostic of a complete duplication.

Ectopic Kidney

If the kidney is not located on examination of the flank, then congenital abnormalities such as horseshoe kidney (Figure 9–31), pelvic kidney (Figure 9–32), or congenital absence of a kidney must be entertained. In any of these circumstances, consideration of formal imaging and specialty consultation is indicated. All of these abnormalities place the patient with obstructive uropa-

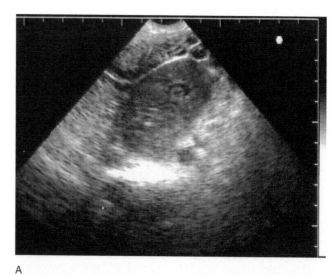

A

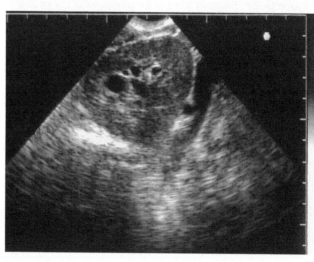

B

Figure 9–32. Pelvic kidney. Endovaginal image with a 7.5-MHz probe. Left adnexal mass is noted to be kidney shaped (A). Detail views demonstrated normal renal architecture and a position adjacent to the iliac vein (B). *(Courtesy of James Mateer, MD.)*

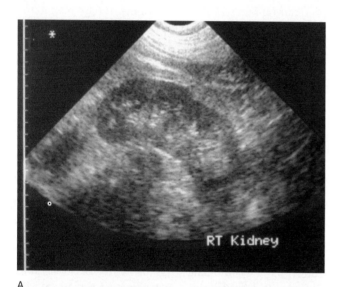

A

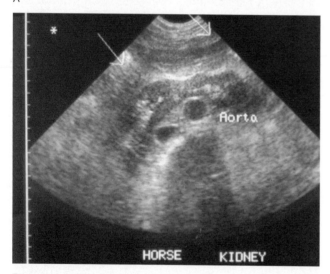

B

Figure 9–31. Horseshoe kidney. Longitudinal view of the right kidney shows a slightly unusual shape and an indistinct lower pole (A). The horseshoe kidney could have been missed if transverse views had not been done. Transverse views (B) clearly demonstrated a connection of the lower poles of both kidneys in the midline over the aorta (labeled). *(Courtesy of L. Sens and L. Green, Gulfcoast Ultrasound.)*

thy (and other renal pathologies) at increased risk for complications.

Prostate Enlargement

An enlarged prostate gland may be seen while imaging the bladder on transabdominal ultrasonography. It can be recognized as a hyperechoic ovular mass at the bladder neck with a transverse diameter greater than 5 cm (Figure 9–33).

Polycystic Kidneys

Polycystic kidney disease can be recognized as an abundance of cysts of varying sizes that both enlarge and distort the regular renal architecture (Figure 9–34).

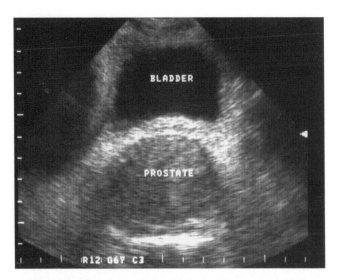

Figure 9–33. Transverse view of the bladder showing an enlarged prostate posteriorly.

Chronic Renal Disease

The most common sonographic finding in chronic renal failure is that of bilaterally small and hyperechoic kidneys. A variety of pathologic processes, ranging from glomerular disease (e.g., glomerulonephritis), infection, and renal vascular disease, may result in this sonographic finding. It is not specific to any particular etiology (Figure 9–35).

Adrenal Mass

Although the normal adrenal glands may not be visualized during focused ultrasound of the urinary tract in the acute care setting, moderate and large adrenal masses can be seen anteromedially to the upper pole of the kidney. Because of the excellent acoustic window provided by the liver, right-sided masses are often better visualized. The appearance of adrenal masses is varied, as is

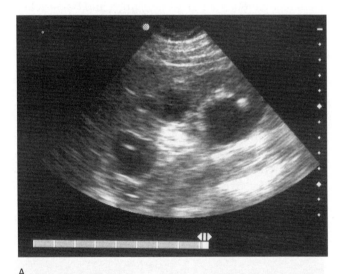

A

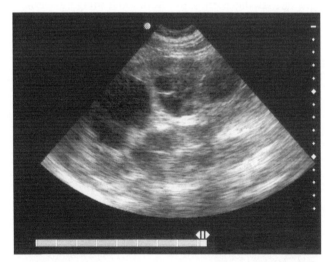

B

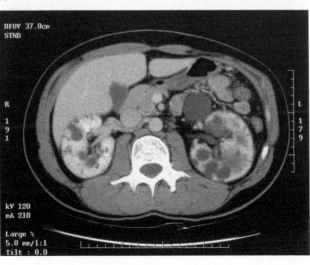

C

Figure 9–34. Polycystic kidneys. Coronal views of the right (A) and left (B) kidneys demonstrate adult polycystic kidney disease. CT scan of the same patient (C) for comparison. *(Courtesy of James Mateer, MD.)*

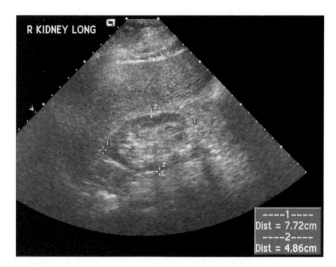

Figure 9–35. Chronic renal disease. This kidney demonstrates thinning of the cortex and a contracted size from chronic renal disease. *(Courtesy of James Mateer, MD; Waukesha Memorial Hospital.)*

the underlying pathology. Additional imaging with CT and biopsy may both be required to make a definitive pathologic diagnosis (Figure 9–36).

Bladder Mass

Bladder masses, both benign and malignant, may present as focal bladder wall thickening (Figure 9–37) or as an irregular echogenic mass projecting into the lumen (Figure 9–38). If such a mass is visualized, the possibility of upper tract obstruction should be addressed by visualizing the kidneys as well examining for hydronephrosis. Further imaging and biopsy are required to make a definitive diagnosis. A bladder hematoma may

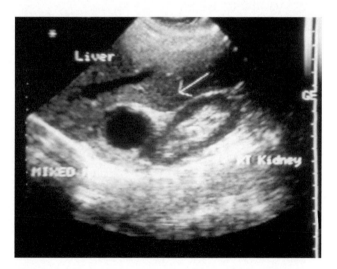

Figure 9–36. Adrenal mass. The right adrenal mass (arrow) has a thickened ring of tissue surrounding a cystic central portion. *(Courtesy of L. Sens and L. Green, Gulfcoast Ultrasound.)*

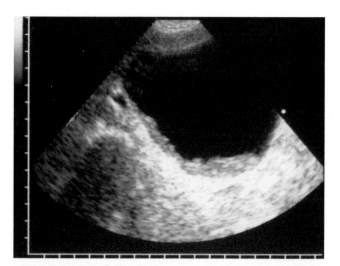

Figure 9–37. Bladder wall tumor. Transverse view of the bladder reveals a localized irregular thickening of the posterolateral bladder wall. *(Courtesy of James Mateer, MD.)*

form in a patient with gross hematuria and be mistaken for a solid mass (Figure 9–39).

▶ PITFALLS

1. *Bedside ultrasound is limited in scope.* Any additional abnormalities that are recognized require close follow-up for further evaluation.
2. *Hydronephrosis may be mimicked.* Several fairly common processes may mimic the presence of hydronephrosis, which include prominent medullary pyramids, renal cortical cysts, an overdistended bladder, and pregnancy. Techniques to distinguish these conditions from hydronephrosis are outlined in this chapter. Renal parapelvic cysts

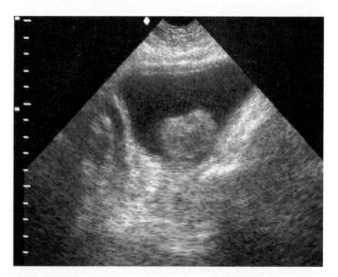

Figure 9–38. Large polypoid bladder mass noted in posterior bladder on an oblique view.

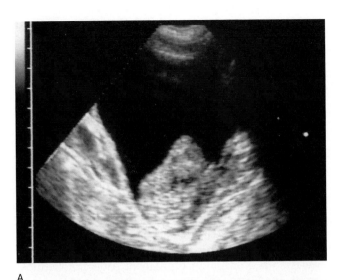

A

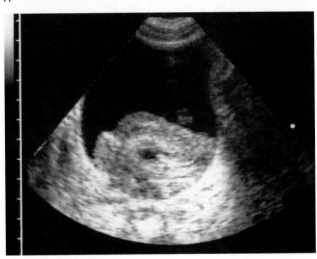

B

Figure 9–39. Bladder hematoma. Longitudinal view of an enlarged bladder showing a posterior mass (A). Transverse views suggesting a laminar structure of the mass (B). This mass resolved following bladder irrigation. *(Courtesy of James Mateer, MD.)*

are less common but are easily confused with hydronephrosis due to their central location within the renal sinus. They can be differentiated from hydronephrosis due to their round shapes and their lack of communication with the fluid-filled renal pelvis. Extrarenal pelvis is a congenital variant in which the renal pelvis lies outside of the kidney. It can be confused with hydronephrosis. The visible anechoic area will be anatomically related to the sinus but will lie outside of the body of the kidney.[38] Both kidneys should always be scanned for comparison and the bladder should be evaluated for degree of filling.

3. *Presence of hydronephrosis may be masked by dehydration.* If ureterolithiasis is suspected, im-

ages should be obtained after the patient receives either an intravenous or oral fluid bolus.

4. *Patients with an acute AAA often present with flank pain.* A rupturing AAA can present with a clinical picture similar to that of acute renal colic. A large AAA can potentially compress the ureter and cause hydronephrosis. In patients older than 50 years of age suspected of having renal colic, clinicians should image the aorta in addition to the urinary tract.

▶ CASE STUDIES

Case 1

Patient Presentation

A 38-year-old man presented to the emergency department at 3 AM after 2 h of excruciating left flank pain and vomiting. He had similar pain the day prior but it was not as intense and subsided after a short period of time. He denied hematuria or dysuria. He had no previous history of renal colic.

On physical examination, he was noted to be in significant pain with difficulty getting comfortable. His blood pressure was 140/80 mm Hg, heart rate 110 beats per min, respirations 16 per min, and his temperature was 37.5°C. Head, neck, chest, and cardiovascular examinations were within normal limits. Examination of the abdomen revealed no significant anterior abdominal tenderness but he was noted to have tenderness at the left costovertebral angle. External genitourinary examination was normal.

Management Course

The patient was administered an intravenous narcotic for acute pain control and an antiemetic. Intravenous saline was initiated and basic laboratory tests were sent, including urinalysis. While awaiting laboratory tests, a bedside focused ultrasound of the kidneys was performed by the treating physician. Ultrasound revealed moderate hydronephrosis of the left kidney confirming the clinical impression of acute renal colic (Figure 9–40). Two hours later, he was pain-free and urinalysis revealed 10 to 20 RBCs/hpf with no pyuria. He was given urology follow-up for the following day and oral analgesics on discharge.

Commentary

Case 1 is a classic presentation of acute renal colic in a young adult. Many investigators would recommend no testing except urinalysis in this scenario while others would argue for an imaging study for all cases. Even in classic presentations, a confirmatory test is desirable. Of the available modalities, ultrasound is the least expensive, fastest, and requires no ionizing radiation. This patient presented at 3 AM, which further complicates the case because of the limited imaging resources usually available at this hour. This patient may need further de-

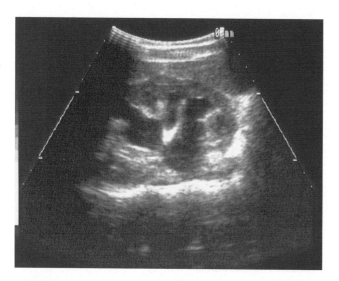

Figure 9–40. Case 1. Moderate hydronephrosis of the left kidney.

finitive imaging, but bedside ultrasound provides enough information for acute diagnosis and disposition for emergency purposes.

Case 2

Patient Presentation

A 26-year-old woman, gravida 2 para 1 at 11-weeks gestation, presented to the emergency department with acute left flank and left lower quadrant pain. She had mild nausea but no vomiting. She denied any vaginal bleeding or any acute urinary symptoms and was previously healthy with no previous operations.

Physical examination revealed a young woman in moderate pain with a blood pressure of 100/60-mm Hg, heart rate 100 beats per min, respirations 14 per min, and temperature 37°C. Head, neck, chest, and cardiovascular examinations were normal. Abdominal examination revealed left costovertebral angle tenderness and mild left lower quadrant tenderness without peritoneal signs. Pelvic examination revealed a nontender enlarged uterus with no cervical or adnexal tenderness.

Management Course

Intravenous saline was started and the patient received a small dose of intravenous narcotic for analgesia. Basic laboratory testing, including urinalysis, was obtained followed by a bedside ultrasound performed by the treating physician. The pelvis was quickly scanned through a transabdominal approach, revealing a live intrauterine pregnancy with no evidence of free pelvic fluid or abnormal mass. The left kidney revealed large hydronephrosis while mild hydronephrosis was seen in the right kidney (see Figure 9–14). Urinalysis revealed 20 to 50 RBCs/hpf and 1 to 2 WBC/hpf with no bacteriuria.

Blood work was normal but she had persistent pain and admission to the antepartum ward was arranged along with urologic consultation. Within 24 h, she was feeling much better and repeat sonography at that time revealed resolving hydronephrosis. She was discharged home and had an uncomplicated delivery 6 months later.

Commentary

This case illustrates the complex nature of evaluating abdominal pain in pregnancy. The physician has to consider an expanded differential diagnosis to include pregnancy-related conditions, while simultaneously being limited to fewer diagnostic adjuncts. In this case, the radiation and dye load associated with intravenous pyelography or CT is a relative contraindication to their use. Ultrasound provides ideal imaging for pregnant patients. The most important initial priority, the exclusion of an ectopic pregnancy, was done within minutes of arrival using a transabdominal scan. Hydronephrosis of the left kidney that was greater than the physiological hydronephrosis on the right side was significant in this case. Repeat sonography was also used to follow resolution of this patient's hydronephrosis.

Case 3

Patient Presentation

A 78-year-old man presented to the emergency department with left flank pain of 2-h duration. He denied nausea, vomiting, or any urinary symptoms. Past history was significant for chronic hypertension and nephrolithiasis requiring basket extraction 10 years prior.

Physical examination revealed an elderly man in moderate distress. Vital signs revealed a blood pressure of 160/90-mm Hg, heart rate 110 beats per min, respirations 12 per min, and temperature 37.7°C. Head, neck, chest, and cardiovascular examinations were within normal limits. Abdominal examination revealed an obese abdomen with diffuse tenderness without any definite discrete masses. External genitourinary examination was normal, as was the rest of the physical examination.

Management Course

Intravenous access and blood work was immediately ordered. Cardiac monitor revealed sinus tachycardia and 12-lead electrocardiogram showed nonspecific ST changes. The emergency physician performed a focused abdominal ultrasound examining both the aorta and kidneys. The aorta was dilated with a maximum diameter of 8.9 cm and both kidneys appeared within normal limits (Figure 9–41). The diagnosis of AAA was made and he was taken emergently to surgery within 40 min of arrival. At laparotomy, the aneurysm was noted to have extensive retroperitoneal rupture but the patient had a successful repair and was discharged from the hospital 7 d later.

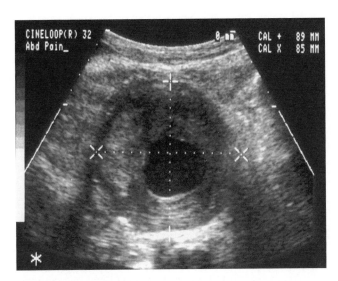

Figure 9-41. Case 3. Short axis view of abdominal aortic aneurysm measuring 8.9 cm.

Commentary

Though uncomplicated renal colic itself does not present as an acute life-threatening emergency, the major differential in the elderly is asymptomatic AAA. In the illustrated case, the patient had a history of previous renal colic complicating the clinical picture but bedside ultrasound was used to quickly evaluate both the kidneys and the aorta, and thus clarified the emergent diagnosis of AAA.

REFERENCES

1. American College of Emergency Physicians. Policy statement: use of ultrasound imaging by emergency physicians. Ann Emerg Med 1997;30:364–365.
2. Brown DF, Rosen CL, Wolfe RE. Renal ultrasonography. Emerg Med Clin North Am 1997;15:877–893.
3. Kiely EA, Hartnell GG, Gibson RN, Williams G. Measurement of bladder volume by real-time ultrasound. Br J Urol 1987;60:33–35.
4. Krupnick AS, Teitelbaum DH, Geiger JD, et al. Use of abdominal ultrasonography to assess pediatric splenic trauma. Potential pitfalls in the diagnosis. Ann Surg 1997;225:408–414.
5. Mainprize TC, Drutz HP. Accuracy of total bladder volume and residual urine measurements: comparison between real-time ultrasonography and catheterization. Am J Obstet Gynecol 1989;160:1013–1016.
6. Topper AK, Holliday PJ, Fernie GR. Bladder volume estimation in the elderly using a portable ultrasound-based measurement device. J Med Eng Technol 1993; 17:99–103.
7. Poston GJ, Joseph AE, Riddle PR. The accuracy of ultrasound in the measurement of changes in bladder volume. Br J Urol 1983;55:361–363.
8. Hartnell GG, Kiely EA, Williams G, Gibson RN. Real-time ultrasound measurement of bladder volume: a comparative study of three methods. Br J Radiol 1987;60:1063–1065.
9. Chan H. Noninvasive bladder volume measurement. J Neurosci Nurs 1993;25:309–312.
10. Ireton RC, Krieger JN, Cardenas DD, et al. Bladder volume determination using a dedicated, portable ultrasound scanner. J Urol 1990;143:909–911.
11. Spouge AR, Wilson SR, Wooley B. Abdominal sonography in asymptomatic executives: prevalence of pathologic findings, potential benefits, and problems. J Ultrasound Med 1996;15:763–767.
12. Ozen H, Colowick A, Freiha FS. Incidentally discovered solid renal masses: what are they? Br J Urol 1993;72: 274–276.
13. Zagoria RJ, Dyer RB. The small renal mass: detection, characterization, and management. Abdom Imaging 1998;23:256–265.
14. Henderson SO, Hoffner RJ, Aragona JL, et al. Bedside emergency department ultrasonography plus radiography of the kidneys, ureters, and bladder vs intravenous pyelography in the evaluation of suspected ureteral colic. Acad Emerg Med 1998;5:666–671.
15. Dalla Palma L, Stacul F, Bazzocchi M, et al. Ultrasonography and plain film versus intravenous urography in ureteric colic. Clin Radiol 1993;47:333–336.
16. Rosen CL, Brown DF, Sagarin MJ, et al. Ultrasonography by emergency physicians in patients with suspected ureteral colic. J Emerg Med 1998;16:865–870.
17. Haddad MC, Sharif HS, Shahed MS, et al. Renal colic: diagnosis and outcome. Radiology 1992;184:83–88.
18. Ghali AM, Elmalik EM, Ibrahim AI, et al. Cost-effective emergency diagnosis plan for urinary stone patients presenting with ureteric colic. Eur Urol 1998;33:529–537.
19. Gerlach AT, Pickworth KK. Contrast medium-induced nephrotoxicity: pathophysiology and prevention. Pharmacotherapy 2000;20:540–548.
20. Morcos SK. Contrast media-induced nephrotoxicity—questions and answers. Br J Radiol 1998;71:357–365.
21. Waybill MM, Waybill PN. Contrast media-induced nephrotoxicity: identification of patients at risk and algorithms for prevention. J Vasc Interv Radiol 2001;12:3–9.
22. Berg KJ. Nephrotoxicity related to contrast media. Scand J Urol Nephrol 2000;34:317–322.
23. Gorelik U, Ulish Y, Yagil Y. The use of standard imaging techniques and their diagnostic value in the workup of renal colic in the setting of intractable flank pain. Urology 1996;47:637–642.
24. Sinclair D, Wilson S, Toi A, Greenspan L. The evaluation of suspected renal colic: ultrasound scan versus excretory urography. Ann Emerg Med 1989;18:556–559.
25. Zagoria R TG. Genitourinary radiology: the requisites. In: Radiology yearbook. St Louis: Mosby, 1997:415–417.
26. Fielding JR, Silverman SG, Rubin GD. Helical CT of the urinary tract. AJR Am J Roentgenol 1999;172:1199–1206.
27. Spencer BA, Wood BJ, Dretler SP. Helical CT and ureteral colic. Urol Clin North Am 2000;27:231–241.
28. Boulay I, Holtz P, Foley WD, et al. Ureteral calculi: diagnostic efficacy of helical CT and implications for treatment of patients. AJR Am J Roentgenol 1999;172:1485–1490.
29. Chen MY, Zagoria RJ. Can noncontrast helical computed tomography replace intravenous urography for evaluation

of patients with acute urinary tract colic? J Emerg Med 1999;17:299–303.

30. Chen MY, Zagoria RJ, Saunders HS, Dyer RB. Trends in the use of unenhanced helical CT for acute urinary colic. AJR Am J Roentgenol 1999;173:1447–1450.

31. Dalrymple NC, Verga M, Anderson KR, et al. The value of unenhanced helical computerized tomography in the management of acute flank pain. J Urol 1998;159:735–740.

32. Fielding JR, Steele G, Fox LA, et al. Spiral computerized tomography in the evaluation of acute flank pain: a replacement for excretory urography. J Urol 1997;157:2071–2073.

33. Sheley RC, Semonsen KG, Quinn SF. Helical CT in the evaluation of renal colic. Am J Emerg Med 1999;17:279–282.

34. Sheafor DH, Hertzberg BS, Freed KS, et al. Nonenhanced helical CT and US in the emergency evaluation of patients with renal colic: prospective comparison. Radiology 2000;217:792–797.

35. Smith RC, Verga M, McCarthy S, Rosenfield AT. Diagnosis of acute flank pain: value of unenhanced helical CT. AJR Am J Roentgenol 1996;166:97–101.

36. Vieweg J, Teh C, Freed K, et al. Unenhanced helical computerized tomography for the evaluation of patients with acute flank pain. J Urol 1998;160:679–684.

37. Thurston W, Wilson S. The urinary tract. In: Rumack C, Wilson S, Charboneau J, eds. Diagnostic ultrasound. St. Louis: Mosby, 1997:378–389.

38. Hagen-Ansert S. Urinary system. In: Hagen-Ansert S, ed. Textbook of diagnostic ultrasound. St. Louis: Mosby, 1995:893–919.

39. Anderhub B. General sonography: A clinical guide. In: Radiology yearbook. St. Louis: Mosby, 1995:123–140.

40. Tempkin B. Ultrasound scanning: principles and protocols. In: Williamson M, ed. Essentials of ultrasound. Philadelphia: WB Saunders, 1996:45–59.

41. Williamson M. Renal ultrasound. In: Williamson M, ed. Essentials of ultrasound. Philadelphia: WB Saunders, 1996:562–579.

42. Burge HJ, Middleton WD, McClennan BL, Hildebolt CF. Ureteral jets in healthy subjects and in patients with unilateral ureteral calculi: comparison with color Doppler US. Radiology 1991;180:437–442.

43. Strehlau J, Winkler P, de la Roche J. The uretero-vesical jet as a functional diagnostic tool in childhood hydronephrosis. Pediatr Nephrol 1997;11:460–467.

44. Alnaif B, Drutz HP. The accuracy of portable abdominal ultrasound equipment in measuring postvoid residual volume. Int Urogynecol J Pelvic Floor Dysfunct 1999;10:215–218.

45. Riccabona M, Nelson TR, Pretorius DH, Davidson TE. In vivo three-dimensional sonographic measurement of organ volume: validation in the urinary bladder. J Ultrasound Med 1996;15:627–632.

46. Marks LS, Dorey FJ, Macairan ML, et al. Three-dimensional ultrasound device for rapid determination of bladder volume. Urology 1997;50:341–348.

47. Ozawa H, Chancellor MB, Ding YY, et al. Noninvasive urodynamic evaluation of bladder outlet obstruction using Doppler ultrasonography. Urology 2000;56:408–412.

48. Yen DH, Hu SC, Tsai J, et al. Renal abscess: early diagnosis and treatment. Am J Emerg Med 1999;17:192–197.

49. Huang JJ, Tseng CC. Emphysematous pyelonephritis: clinicoradiological classification, management, prognosis, and pathogenesis. Arch Intern Med 2000;160:797–805.

50. Wan YL, Lo SK, Bullard MJ, et al. Predictors of outcome in emphysematous pyelonephritis. J Urol 1998;159:369–373.

51. Mandavia DP, Pregerson B, Henderson SO. Ultrasonography of flank pain in the emergency department: renal cell carcinoma as a diagnostic concern. J Emerg Med 2000;18:83–86.

52. Siepel T, Clifford DS, James PA, Cowan TM. The ultrasound-assisted physical examination in the periodic health evaluation of the elderly. J Fam Pract 2000;49:628–632.

53. Ueda T, Mihara Y. Incidental detection of renal carcinoma during radiological imaging. Br J Urol 1987;59:513–515.

54. Tosaka A, Ohya K, Yamada K, et al. Incidence and properties of renal masses and asymptomatic renal cell carcinoma detected by abdominal ultrasonography. J Urol 1990;144:1097–1099.

55. Lanctin HP, Futter NG. Renal cell carcinoma: incidental detection. Can J Surg 1990;33:488–490.

56. Sweeney JP, Thornhill JA, Graiger R, et al. Incidentally detected renal cell carcinoma: pathological features, survival trends and implications for treatment. Br J Urol 1996;78:351–353.

57. Smith SJ, Bosniak MA, Megibow AJ, et al. Renal cell carcinoma: earlier discovery and increased detection. Radiology 1989;170:699–703.

58. Charboneau JW, Hattery RR, Ernst EC, et al. Spectrum of sonographic findings in 125 renal masses other than benign simple cyst. Am J Roentgenol 1983;140:87–94.

59. Belldegrun A, deKernion J. Renal tumors. In: Campbell M, Walsh P, eds. Campbell's Urology. Philadelphia: WB Saunders, 1998:349–366.

60. Forman HP, Middleton WD, Melson GL, McClennan BL. Hyperechoic renal cell carcinomas: increase in detection at US. Radiology 1993;188:431–434.

61. Drago J, Cunningham J. Ultrasonography of renal masses. In: Resnick M, Rifkin M, eds. Ultrasonography of the urinary tract. Baltimore: Williams & Wilkins, 1991:239–245.

62. McGahan JP, Richards JR, Jones CD, Gerscovich EO. Use of ultrasonography in the patient with acute renal trauma. J Ultrasound Med 1999;18:207–213.

63. Fang YC, Tiu CM, Chou YH, Chang T. A case of acute renal artery thrombosis caused by blunt trauma: computed tomographic and Doppler ultrasonic findings. J Formos Med Assoc 1993;92:356–358.

CHAPTER 10

Testicular

Michael Blaivas

Acute testicular pain represents approximately 0.5% of the complaints presenting to an average emergency department each year.[1] Patients complaining of acute testicular pain can elicit some anxiety on the part of the emergency physician. Causes of acute testicular pain include trauma, epididymitis, orchitis, torsion of the testicular appendage, and hemorrhage; however, testicular torsion is the diagnosis of greatest concern in the emergency setting.

Previously, most young men who presented to an emergency or urgent care setting with a complaint of acute onset testicular pain were suspected of having testicular torsion.[2] Over the last decade, this misconception has been dispelled and it is now know that the most common etiology of acute testicular pain is epididymitis.[2] However, the evaluation of acute testicular pain still presents a considerable challenge for emergency physicians since fully 50% of young men presenting to an emergency department with testicular torsion have already waited over 6 h and are well on their way toward losing the torsed testicle.[3]

The issue of acute testicular pain is further complicated by the high potential for litigation associated with the loss of a testicle or infertility associated with torsion or disruption of the testicle from severe trauma. When the diagnosis of testicular torsion is missed, the majority of patients have been incorrectly classified as epididymitis.[4] Despite the fact that the two disease processes would seem to be easily differentiated on the basis of history and physical examination, research and practice have demonstrated this not to be the case.[4]

► CLINICAL CONSIDERATIONS

The most important concern with testicular torsion is the potential for loss of the testicle or infertility. Other disease processes that may present with scrotal pain include torsion of the testicular appendage, epididymitis, orchitis, testicular trauma, hemorrhage into a testicular mass, and herniation of abdominal contents into the scrotum. High-resolution color Doppler ultrasonography has become widely accepted as the test of choice for evaluating acute scrotal pain, replacing scintigraphy in most institutions.[5] While scintigraphy requires less technical skill on the part of the radiologist consulted to evaluate the patient, there are major drawbacks to the technique. Scintigraphy is a time-consuming process that can add an hour or more to the evaluation of a patient who may already be several hours into experiencing testicular torsion.[5] Further, the resultant hyperemia of the scrotal skin during testicular torsion can mask a lack of blood flow to the testicle itself and lead to a misdiagnosis in less experienced hands.[6] This nuclear medicine study also provides no information regarding testicular anatomy.

A careful history and physical examination are important and have been thought to enable an emergency physician to virtually exclude the diagnosis of testicular torsion without further testing in the majority of cases.[3] In practice, historical features of several disease processes can overlap. For example, duration of pain in testicular torsion, epididymitis, orchitis, and torsion of a testicular appendage frequently overlap.[7] In up to 20% of cases, testicular torsion is associated with trauma or physical exertion, such as heavy lifting.[8] Adding to the difficulty of making a diagnosis by history alone is the resistance of many young men to provide accurate histories regarding trauma. The author can recall several cases where the young teenager in question was too embarrassed to recall a swift kick to the groin from his sister or "friend" until just after the diagnosis was made on ultrasound examination.

Typical textbook clinical features of epididymitis, such as dysuria and urethral discharge, cannot be uniformly relied upon. Up to 50% of patients with acute epididymitis may present with no dysuria or urethral discharge.[4] Furthermore, many patients with epididymitis seem to complain of the acute onset of pain. This is probably due to poor recall or the need for a threshold of discomfort to be crossed prior to the patient's recognition of pain. Also, some patients simply tell the emergency physician what they think he or she wants to hear. Many experienced emergency physicians can recall a patient with epididymitis who insisted that they noticed the onset of pain suddenly just prior to presentation. Patients with testicular torsion who were initially misdiagnosed as epididymitis are most commonly misdiagnosed due to the presence of dysuria, pyuria, urethral discharge, or a history of prior vague testicular pain giving the impression of a less acute process.[1]

Ultrasonography of the acute scrotum is a relatively new application for bedside use in the emergency and acute care setting. Due to the time-sensitive nature of testicular torsion, ultrasonography is a tool to consider for the bedside diagnosis of possible torsion. Time is of the essence in diagnosing testicular torsion. Since inadequate funding and personnel limits have hurt the off-hours diagnostic imaging services provided by many hospitals, bedside ultrasonography for this indication should become a tool used by emergency physicians, urologists, and other interested clinicians. This chapter presents some aspects of bedside ultrasonography as applied to the evaluation of acute scrotal pain in the emergency and acute care setting.

▶ CLINICAL INDICATIONS

The clinical indications for emergency bedside ultrasound evaluation of the testicle include:

- Testicular pain
- Scrotal mass
- Trauma

Testicular Pain

An ultrasound examination of the testicle is indicated whenever testicular torsion is in the differential diagnosis after the history and physical examination. The etiology of testicular torsion is related to laxity found in a redundant spermatic cord that allows the testicle to twist about its own axis. The redundant cord can be highly mobile and twist about its axis. Further increasing the likelihood of testicular torsion is a history of an undescended testicle.[9] Once blood flow is interrupted to the testicle, infarction and loss of the testicle can occur quickly. The urologic literature demonstrates that salvage rates are approximately 100% at 3 h, 83 to 90% at 5 h, 75% at 8 h, and 50 to 70% at 10 h. When a testicle has been torsed for

more than 10 h, the rates of salvage decrease to 10 to 20%. After 24 h, salvage of a testicle is rarely seen unless there has been intermittent detorsion.[10]

In general, urologists are reluctant to take patients to the operating room and explore a painful testicle based only on the clinical examination. The urology literature has made arguments that such patients should not be routinely explored and that accurate diagnosis should be provided with color and spectral Doppler testing of the involved testicle.[11] A practical issue is that of getting a urologic specialist, who may have spent the last 16 h in an operating room, to come into the emergency department during off hours for a case that may not be testicular torsion.

For the detection of testicular torsion, the sensitivity and specificity of ultrasonography approaches 100% for experienced sonologists. However, the literature regarding testicular ultrasound use by emergency physicians at the bedside is relatively limited.[12–15] This is due, in part, to the fact that the technology needed to accurately diagnose or exclude testicular torsion includes both color and spectral Doppler. The price for this technology, although now found on basic machines for less than $30,000, was often out of reach for many emergency departments and clinics.

The sonographic evaluation of acute testicular pain by emergency physicians has been studied.[12] The investigators evaluated a total of 36 patients with acute testicular pain and found a sensitivity and specificity of 95% and 94%, respectively, for testicular torsion when using surgical follow-up and radiology imaging as the criterion standard. All three patients with testicular torsion were correctly identified. Other diagnoses found included epididymitis, orchitis, hemorrhage, and herniation. The investigators demonstrated that emergency physicians could evaluate and diagnose a broad range of testicular pathology using ultrasonography. Prospective studies are currently in progress and should provide for larger sample sizes.

A major limitation for any individual attempting to get enough experience with testicular ultrasonography may be the frequency of acute scrotal pain presentation at his or her facility. A recently presented abstract did show that testicular torsion could easily be simulated for training purposes by digital compression of the spermatic cord unilaterally, and this holds promise as an educational tool.[15]

The clinician benefiting most from scrotal ultrasonography would be the one without radiologic or urologic backup during a portion of the day. Determination that a testicle is intact or that normal testicular blood flow is present could allow avoiding, or at least delaying, costly or difficult transport to another facility.

Scrotal Mass

Painless scrotal masses are unlikely to represent an acute disease process. By history, patients often admit that the involved testicle had been slowly enlarging for some time and they had simply ignored it or grown accustomed to the difference until some factor finally made them seek medical assistance. The vast majority of soft, nontender scrotal masses are hydroceles that may develop due to a number of disease processes or idiopathically. Many are congenital and result from a direct communication with the abdominal cavity. Hydroceles can result from trauma, infection, neoplasm, radiation therapy, and undiagnosed torsion.[16]

Firm, nontender testicular masses commonly represent neoplasms that should be directed for expeditious follow-up with the urologist. When the patient presents complaining of pain from the testicular mass, it may be from hemorrhage into the neoplasm itself. If a large intratumor hemorrhage is detected, then immediate urologic consultation may be needed. Patients who present with large painless testicular masses that may have been developing for years require careful consideration regarding discharge, as most testicular tumors are malignant.

Trauma

Blunt trauma to the scrotum can lead to damage of the testicle or associated structures. Assault, sports injury, bicycle crashes, and motor vehicle crashes are the most common causes of blunt testicular trauma. Injuries can be in the form of laceration, hemorrhage, or contusion of the testicle. Clinical features of testicular injury are a tender swollen testicle, often accompanied by ecchymosis. Accurate diagnosis by physical examination alone is often difficult secondary to marked swelling and pain in the traumatized scrotum, thus making ultrasound imaging a requisite. The goals of emergency ultrasound in patients presenting with acute trauma to the scrotum is to evaluate whether the testicle is damaged and the need for consultation and possible operative intervention. Although a contusion localized to the scrotum requires simple follow up, findings that suggest a possible capsular rupture of the testicle may require surgical intervention. Furthermore, since trauma can lead to testicular torsion, blood flow should be evaluated as well. High-resolution ultrasound is sensitive for detecting evidence of major trauma to the testicles and, therefore, can be useful for screening patients. While the diagnostic accuracy of ultrasound for specific traumatic findings (such as capsular rupture) is heavily operator dependent, determining the presence or absence of significant injury (such as hematocele or intratesticular hematoma) is relatively straightforward.[17,18]

▶ ANATOMIC CONSIDERATIONS

The normal adult testes are located in the scrotum and are oval in shape. Average measurements obtained are 4 cm X 3 cm X 2.5 cm on ultrasound. Each testicle weighs

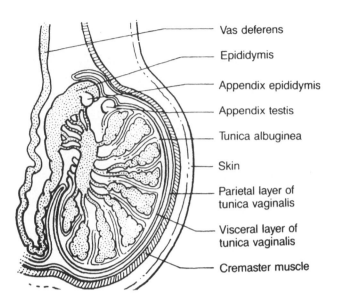

Figure 10–1. Normal testicular and scrotal anatomy. *(Reprinted with permission from Cohen HL. Hematocele. In: Cohen HL, Civit CJ, eds. Fetal and pediatric ultrasound: a casebook approach. New York: McGraw-Hill, 2001:541.)*

between 10 to 19 g. The testes are surrounded by the tunica vaginalis (Figure 10–1). Multiple septations arise from the tunica albuginea and run through the testicle. These septations result in the separation of the testicle into multiple lobules. The epididymis, an extratesticular structure, is made up of the head, body, and tail. The tail of the epididymis turns into the vas deferens as it travels superiorly out of the scrotum. In turn, the vas deferens travels in the spermatic cord. The spermatic cord contains a number of important structures, including the testicular artery, cremasteric artery, deferential artery, lymphatic structures, and the genitofemoral nerve.

Sonographically, a testicle appears quite homogeneous in echotexture (Figure 10–2). The echogenicity of

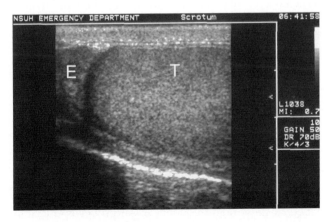

Figure 10–2. Longitudinal view of the normal testes. E = head of the epididymis; T = testicle.

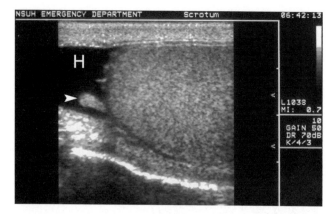

Figure 10–3. A small hydrocele outlines the appendix testis in this patient presenting for chronic testicular pain. Appendix testes (arrowhead); H = hydrocele.

the testes is sometimes compared with that of the liver. Many structures, such as the tunica albuginea, are not seen under normal circumstances. The epididymis can be readily identified from the rest of the testicle in normal as well as pathologic instances. It has similar echogenicity to the testicle but can appear slightly brighter. While the head of the epididymis is readily seen, the body and tail may be harder to differentiate when no inflammation is present. The appendix testis is a small oval structure and is normally hidden by the epididymal head, thus making it nearly impossible to differentiate in normal examinations. If a hydrocele is present, the appendix testis often becomes outlined by the fluid and is seen as a defined structure (Figure 10–3). However, when torsed, it may cause not only local inflammation but also an epididymitis-like appearance due to diffuse inflammation.

Most of the arterial blood supply received by a testicle comes from the abdominal aorta by way of the testicular artery. A small portion of the arterial supply comes from the deferential and cremasteric arteries, which anastomose with the testicular artery. The deferential and cremasteric arteries supply the extratesticular structures of the scrotum, including the epididymis. Color and power Doppler can easily detect blood flow in these vascular structures in both normal and most pathologic states.

▶ TECHNIQUE AND NORMAL ULTRASOUND FINDINGS

When evaluating the testes, a 7.5 to 10 MHz probe is required in most situations, with a 5.0 MHz probe being utilized for large masses or very edematous testes (Figure 10–4). The increased resolution and magnification provided by these high-frequency linear probes is crucial in not only examining the parenchyma of the testicle but also the blood flow within it. The use of high-resolution

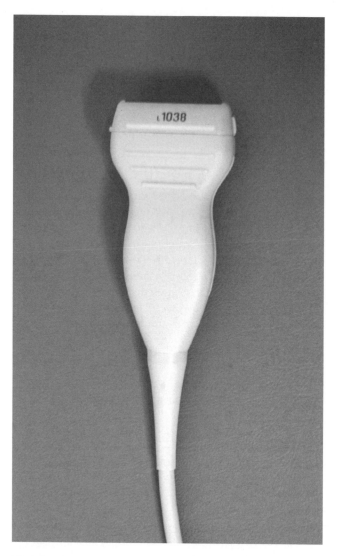

Figure 10–4. An example of a high-resolution linear array that can be used for testicular sonography.

linear array transducers has been described with increasing frequency in the emergency medicine literature. Common applications include detection of foreign bodies, central line placement, and for the evaluation of lower extremity deep venous thrombosis.[19–21]

In addition to a high-resolution probe, color and spectral Doppler are required when evaluating a patient for torsion. On more basic ultrasound machines, adding color Doppler often leads to the greatest cost increase for an ultrasound unit. Power Doppler, a nondirectional version of color Doppler, is thought to be more sensitive for detecting blood flow but omits the directional information.[5] It can, however, improve the sensitivity of the test, especially in the testicle, where blood flow tends to occur through relatively small diameter vessels and at lower speed. Spectral Doppler is also an important component of the evaluation, especially when incomplete torsion is present. It allows for documentation of both venous and arterial blood flow within the testicle. It is the venous component that is initially lost early in testicular torsion. The cost of color and spectral Doppler technology is now more afford-able than ever and is in reach of most emergency departments. Training in scrotal ultrasound applications is also an issue that has been largely solved. Training courses are available at commercially offered conferences as well as at ultrasonography meetings throughout the country.

Prior to performing a testicular ultrasound examination, the patient may need reassurance and analgesia. Ideally, warmed ultrasound gel should be available. Cold gel may make the patient more uncomfortable by eliciting a cremasteric reflex. The patient should be draped to preserve modesty and the scrotum placed in a sling designed from a towel to provide support and improve exposure (Figure 10–5). A frog-leg position for the patient is preferred by most sonologists. It is best to examine the unaffected testicle initially. This provides a comparison of anatomy and blood flow as well as helping to reassure the patient.

Both testes should be imaged in long and short axis in their entirety (Figure 10–6A and B). The epididymis should be visualized as well (see Figure 10–2). For the long axis view, the image is usually adjusted so that the epididymal head is on the left side of the screen. The need for standardized imaging will be apparent to most emergency sonologists when they show their images to colleagues familiar with testicular ultrasound. To adequately evaluate blood flow, the Doppler parameters should be adjusted to their most sensitive settings (Figure 10–6C). The wall filter should be set at the lowest selection possible and the PRF (pulse repetition frequency) should be minimized as well. The novice sonographer should guard against raising the color gain too much or

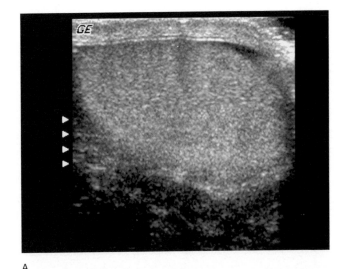

A

B

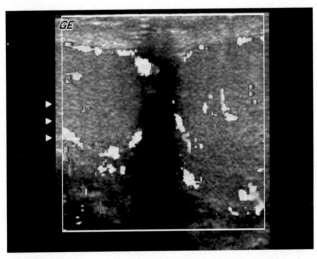

C

Figure 10–6. Normal long axis (A) and short axis (B) views of the testicle. (C) An example of blood flow picked up on power Doppler in normal testicles. The amount of blood flow seen will vary from testicle to testicle and a comparison with the contralateral side must be made. *(Courtesy of James Mateer, MD, Waukesha Memorial Hospital.)*

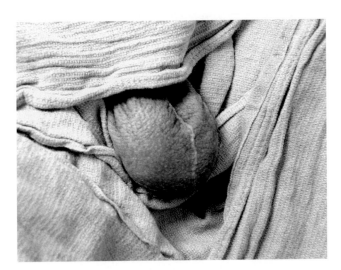

Figure 10–5. A properly exposed and draped patient with the scrotum supported in a sling of towels for improved patient comfort and visualization.

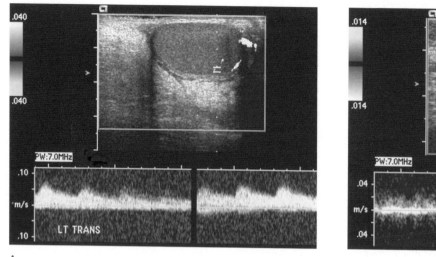

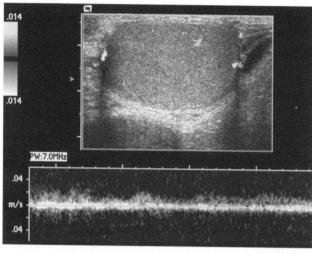

Figure 10–7. Spectral Doppler of the testicles. A typical arterial waveform is demonstrated (A). A common waveform pattern for venous flow is shown (B). *(Courtesy of James Mateer, MD, Waukesha Memorial Hospital.)*

the appearance of blood flow may be created in an avascular mass or torsed testicle. Spectral Doppler waveforms should be obtained in several areas of blood flow detected by color Doppler to document both arterial and venous flow patterns (Figure 10–7).

▶ COMMON AND EMERGENT ABNORMALITIES

Epididymitis

Infection of the epididymis or testicle usually results from retrograde spread of bacteria from the bladder or prostate

via the vas deferens. Epididymitis is the most common type of scrotal inflammatory process and is thought to be a disease of adults.[3] Epididymitis is being diagnosed more commonly in adolescents as this age group continues to engage in sexual activity at an earlier age. Other inflammatory processes that can present with signs and symptoms of epididymitis include torsion of the testicular appendage.

Sonographically, the affected epididymis appears enlarged, which is usually confirmed by measuring both the affected and unaffected side (Figure 10–8). It will often have decreased echogenicity on standard B-mode examination. Occasionally, focal inflammation of a region of the epididymis is seen leading to an area of well-defined swell-

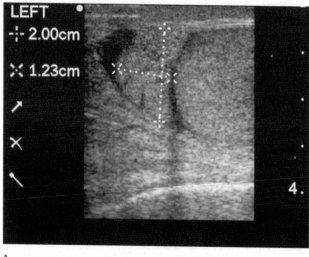

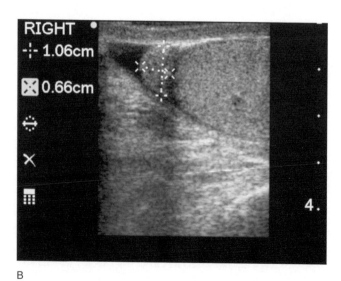

Figure 10–8. Epididymitis. The left epididymal head is enlarged (A). Measurements for normal comparison on the right are included (B). *(Courtesy of James Mateer, MD.)*

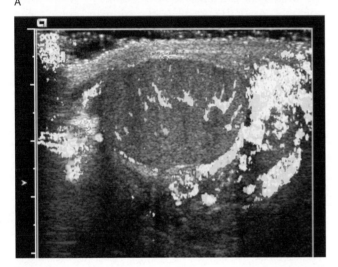

A

B

Figure 10-9. Epididymitis. Longitudinal view of the affected testicle shows enlargement of the tail of the epididymis (A). With color Doppler, marked flow is seen in the tail of the epididymis of the same patient (B). *(Courtesy of James Mateer, MD, Waukesha Memorial Hospital.)*

Orchitis

Orchitis is an acute infection of the testicle; most cases follow an initial episode of epididymitis.[3] The typical presentation includes a markedly tender and inflamed testicle. Standard B-mode ultrasound is not a reliable method to differentiate between orchitis and torsion unless the torsion is advanced and prominent changes are noted. For both orchitis and torsion, inflammation and edema can lead to enlargement and decreased echogenicity of the testis. Performing color or power Doppler, however, will quickly assist in differentiating between the two diagnoses since testicular blood flow will increase as a result of inflammation (Figure 10–10).

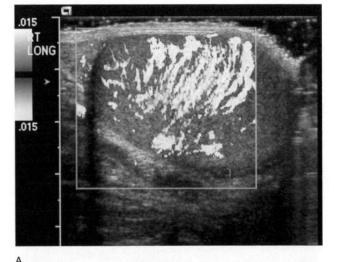

A

B

Figure 10-10. Orchitis. Marked increase in blood flow is seen throughout the testicle. Comparison view of the same patient demonstrating normal flow. *(Courtesy of James Mateer, MD, Waukesha Memorial Hospital.)*

ing or enlargement. This is usually either the head or body of the epididymis. Epididymitis can cause accumulation of a reactive hydrocele similar to testicular torsion or torsion of the appendix. Thus, the presence of a small or moderate amount of fluid in the hemiscrotum is not a reliable sign for differentiating between the disease processes.

Epididymal inflammation, either idiopathic or infectious, usually leads to increased blood flow that is easily noted on color Doppler when compared to the unaffected side (Figure 10–9). What clearly separates epididymitis from testicular torsion is this presence of normal blood flow in the testicle when compared to the contralateral side. Increased blood flow may be seen if the inflammation is spreading to the testicle (see "Orchitis").

Testicular Torsion

A normal testicle has a diffusely homogenous sonographic appearance. B-mode ultrasound allows for a good evaluation of the testicular parenchyma. This method, however, will detect torsion only when signs of edema or necrosis are already present. Color or power Doppler will reveal blood flow within the normal testicle. When blood flow is absent or severely compromised in the affected testicle, the diagnosis of testicular torsion is clear (Figure 10–11A, B, and C). When the degree of flow is similar between the affected and comparison testicle, spectral Doppler tracings should be obtained to confirm both arterial and venous flow (see Figure 10–7). Color Doppler alone will not assure the sonologist that both venous and arterial flow are present. The absence of a venous pattern by spectral Doppler on the affected side suggests early torsion. This is better understood by reviewing the mechanism of torsion and loss of blood supply to the testicle.

During torsion, the testicle begins to twist around the axis of the spermatic cord. As the twisting progresses, venous flow is lost, initially due to easily collapsible vessel walls and a lower pressure system. Venous obstruction is followed by a drop in arterial inflow that eventually progresses to complete obstruction of blood flow. Thrombosis occurs in the arteries and veins and results in necrosis of testicular tissue. Experimental studies have shown that complete arterial occlusion occurs at about 450 to 540° of torsion.[22] Once the spermatic cord is fully torsed and no blood flow is present, the testicle will begin to take on a diffusely edematous appearance on ultrasound (see Figure 10–11C). With the completion of testicular torsion, no color Doppler signal will be seen in the testicle (see Figure 10–11A and C).

If the diagnosis is in doubt due to continued pain or if torsion-detorsion is suspected, performing serial examinations at the bedside is helpful. Closely following the blood flow can allow the practitioner to detect worsening torsion or the presence of torsion and detorsion in a patient that may otherwise have been sent home. Repeated color/power Doppler imaging along with spectral Doppler examination in 45 min to an hour could

A

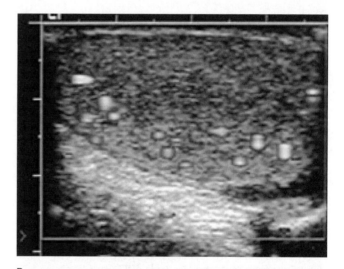

B

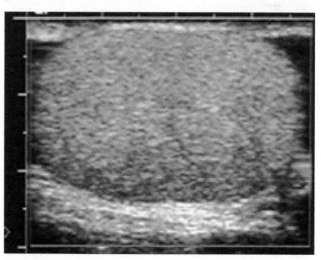

C

Figure 10–11. Testicular torsion, Doppler and gray-scale findings. Scrotal ultrasound. (A) Transverse plane through both testes. The Doppler image of the scrotum demonstrates right testicular perfusion. The swollen left testis is not perfused. There is therefore left testicular torsion. (B) Normal right testicle. Sagittal plane. This image confirms the finding of flow in the normal right testicle. (C) Torsive left testicle. Sagittal plane. Despite the presence of a flow box around the entire left testicle and the use of the same technique that enabled flow to be seen on the right, no flow is noted in the left testicle. It is not perfused. *(Reprinted, with permission from Paltiel HJ. Acute left testicular torsion in an adolescent. In: Cohen HL, Civit CJ, eds. Fetal and pediatric ultrasound: a casebook approach. New York: McGraw-Hill; 2001;535.)*

catch subtle progression of torsion in a patient with continued suggestive pain but a normal initial examination. Finally, the emergency physician will have to make a clinical decision on whether to discharge the patient with close follow-up or obtain a urology consultation should the suggestive testicular pain continue. A critical (and occasionally overlooked) point regarding evaluating for testicular torsion is providing patients with discharge instructions that specify immediate return to the emergency department for worsening pain.

Scrotal Trauma

Scrotal trauma may result in damage to both the testes and/or the extratesticular structures. Visualization of a normal testicle on ultrasound examination virtually excludes any significant injury. However, since surgical intervention is generally required for capsular rupture of the testicle, any significant abnormalities identified with bedside ultrasound should be considered evidence of possible testicular rupture. In these cases, further diagnostic intervention and/or urology consultation is mandated.

Ultrasound findings that directly suggest testicular rupture are inhomogeneity of testicular echotexture with irregularity of the testicular outline[17] (Figure 10–12). When a fracture line can be seen crossing the capsule, surgical

intervention is required. A significant hematocele is an indirect finding for possible rupture (Figure 10–13) and an indication by itself for exploration according to some investigators.[18] A hematocele may be differentiated from a simple, new onset hydrocele because the high frequency transducers used for scrotal ultrasound will demonstrate low level echoes or clots within a hematocele. A chronic hydrocele, however, may develop internal echoes from cholesterol crystal formation. If a complete ultrasound ex-

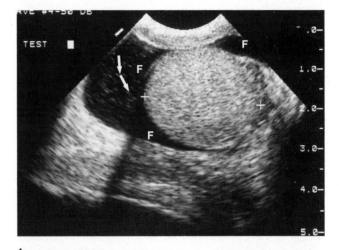

A

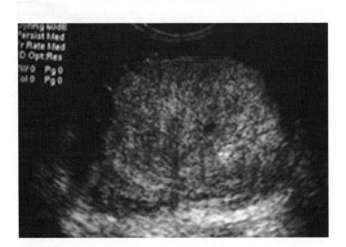

Figure 10–12. Testicular fracture—contour irregularity. Left testicle. Longitudinal plane. There is a contour irregularity (arrow) in the superior portion of the testicle, suggesting rupture of the tunica albuginea and a need for surgery to repair and salvage the testicle. Some 90% of ruptured testes can be salvaged if surgery is performed within 72 h. This 18-year-old's injury was due to a gunshot wound that went through the scrotum. Asymmetrical vascular flow within the testicle also suggested significant injury, which was confirmed at surgery. *(Reprinted, with permission from Cohen, HL. Hematocele. In: Cohen HL, Civit CJ, eds. Fetal and pediatric ultrasound: a casebook approach. New York: McGraw-Hill, 2001;541.)*

B

Figure 10–13. Hematocele. (A) Right hemiscrotum. Longitudinal plane. Bright echoes (arrows) are seen in fluid (F) surrounding, but predominantly superior to, a normal right testicle (marked off by crosses). This was due to hematocele from trauma that occurred the day prior to examination. (B) Transverse plane superior to testicle. Many echoes are seen in the large amount of fluid within the superior scrotum. Excellent through transmission (arrows) confirms the fluid nature of the hematocele. *(Reprinted with permission from Cohen, HL. Hematocele. In: Cohen HL, Civit CJ, eds. Fetal and pediatric ultrasound: a casebook approach. New York: McGraw-Hill, 2001;540.)*

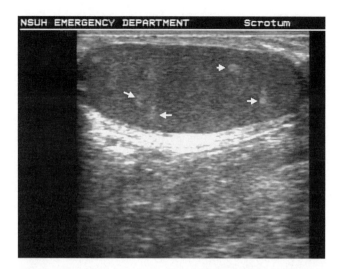

Figure 10–14. Arrows point to small focal hemorrhages after a blow to the groin. The patient was found to have no other testicular injury and recovered uneventfully.

amination of the testicle shows that the capsule of the testicle is intact, then conservative treatment may be recommended. The sensitivity and specificity for ultrasound detection of testicular fracture varies in multiple studies and some disagreement still persists regarding the utility of ultrasound.

Hemorrhage within the testicle can have an inconsistent appearance depending on the age of the hemorrhage. Acute hemorrhage will appear inhomogeneously echogenic (Figure 10–14), but will later develop large anechoic regions within it (Figure 10–15). Although grayscale sonography can occasionally confuse hematomas and tumors, the use of color Doppler usually differentiates the

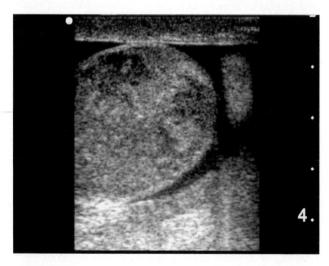

Figure 10–15. Intratesticular hemorrhage. A longitudinal view of the testicle demonstrates focal hypoechoic areas due to evolving intratesticular hematoma of 4-d duration. *(Courtesy of James Mateer, MD.)*

two processes (Figure 10–16). Tumors are usually vascular structures, whereas hematomas will not reveal blood flow signals. A mixture of findings can occur when a patient hemorrhages into a testicular mass.

► COMMON VARIANTS AND SELECTED ABNORMALITIES

Mediastinum Testis

This is a normal finding and is well visualized in some patients. The mediastinum testis is very echogenic and is formed from an inward extension of the testicular capsule (Figure 10–17).

Hydrocele

There is a potential space between the visceral and parietal layers of the tunica vaginalis that can collect fluid, resulting in a hydrocele (see Figure 10–1). Hydroceles are usually visualized in the anterolateral aspect of the scrotum and may be bilateral or unilateral. Their location is due to the attachment of the tunica to the testicle and scrotum posteriorly. Many hydroceles are congenital and result from a direct communication with the abdominal cavity. Hydroceles can also result from trauma, infection, neoplasm, radiation therapy, and undiagnosed torsion.[16] A hydrocele can be seen as an isolated finding or in conjunction with acute or chronic pathology. They are occasionally seen as a lone finding in a patient who complains of acute scrotal pain.

On ultrasound examination, a hydrocele appears as an echo-poor or dark area surrounding the testicle (Figures 10–3 and 10–18). In a hydrocele of recent onset, low-level spot echoes within the fluid suggest the presence of blood or inflammatory cells (see Figure 10–13). A history of trauma or surgery would suggest a hematocele. A chronic hydrocele, however, may also develop internal echoes from cholesterol crystal formation. Subacute and chronic hydroceles may contain loculations, especially when an inflammatory process or hematocele is present (Figure 10–19). Chronic hydroceles that have developed slowly tend to be larger than those developing acutely from trauma or torsion.

Varicocele

Varicoceles occur in the presence of abnormal dilation and tortuosity of the veins in the pampiniform plexus located in the spermatic cord. Nearly 99% of all varicoceles are on the left side but they can present bilaterally.[20] The bilateral presentation is due to the drainage of the spermatic vein on the right directly into the inferior vena cava. The left spermatic vein first drains into the left renal vein at nearly a 90°angle. This sharp angle prevents the spermatic vein from forming a valve.

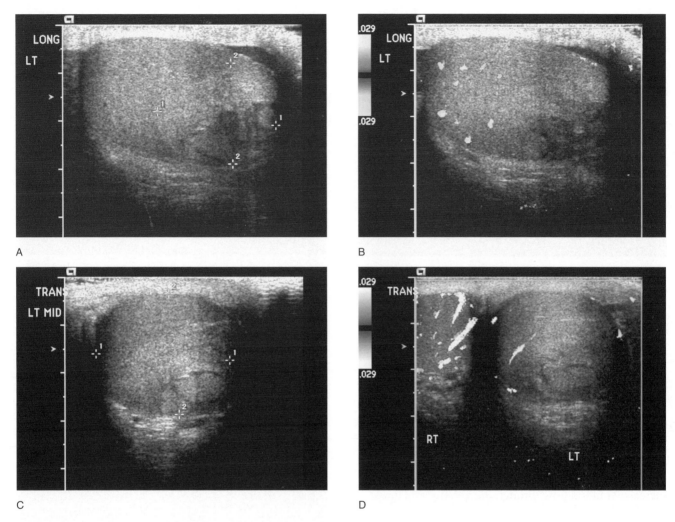

Figure 10–16. Testicular contusion. Longitudinal view of the testicle reveals inhomogeneous echogenicity in the lower pole (A) with decreased tissue color Doppler flow in the area of the contusion (B). A transverse grayscale view (C) and color Doppler view (D) of the same patient demonstrates normal comparative flow for the non-injured testicle. *(Courtesy of James Mateer, MD, Waukesha Memorial Hospital.)*

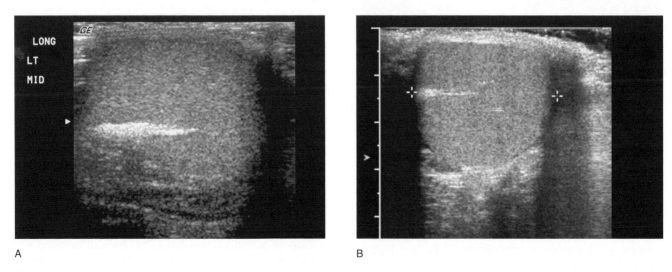

Figure 10–17. Mediastinum testis. Longitudinal oblique view of the testicle (A) reveals a brightly echogenic linear structure within the normal testicular tissue. A transverse view shows the usual appearance (B). *(Courtesy of James Mateer, MD, Waukesha Memorial Hospital.)*

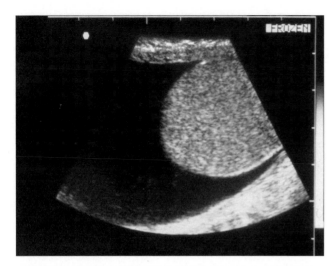

Figure 10–18. Hydrocele. A longitudinal view of the scrotum reveals a large hydrocele and the superior pole of a normal testicle. *(Courtesy of James Mateer, MD.)*

Varicoceles are associated with decreased sperm motility and low sperm count. Acute thrombosis is a concern in young men and may lead to surgical intervention. On ultrasound examination, varicoceles appear as an extratesticular bundle of tubular structures (Figure 10–20). Occasionally, varicoceles may be confused with inflammation of the epididymal tail or bowel content in the scrotum. Having the patient perform a Valsalva maneuver may cause distention of the varices, and an obvious increase in blood flow through the venous structures.

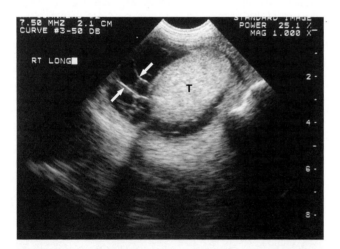

Figure 10–19. Hydrocele with septations. Longitudinal plane through right hemiscrotum. A normal right testicle is surrounded by fluid. Septations (arrows) are seen within the fluid superior to the testicle. This finding is consistent with the patient's history of old trauma and hematocele. *(Reprinted with permission from Cohen, HL. Hematocele. In: Cohen HL, Civit CJ, eds. Fetal and pediatric ultrasound: a casebook approach. New York: McGraw-Hill, 2001;542.)*

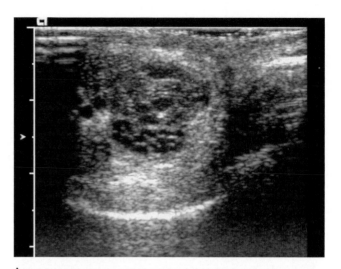

A

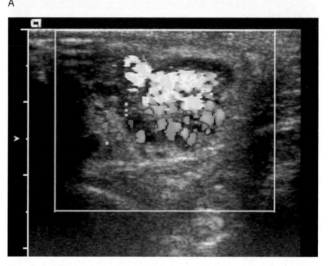

B

Figure 10–20. Varicocele. Transverse plane of the upper scrotum shows a cross-section view of multiple tubular structures near the epididymal head (A). Color Doppler of the same patient confirms the vascular nature of these structures (B). *(Courtesy of James Mateer, MD, Waukesha Memorial Hospital.)*

Herniation

Herniation of abdominal contents into the scrotum may lead to a patient presenting with acute testicular pain. In some cases, the patient's history will be negative for previous hernias. The scrotum may be swollen and painful, thus simulating testicular torsion, epididymitis, or orchitis. Ultrasound evaluation can help identify the testes and often allows the examiner to visualize abdominal content, such as bowel loops or omentum. Occasionally, a loop of bowel can be clearly seen on ultrasound examination. The emergency sonologist will need to be guided by artifacts from gas within the loop of bowel. Omental fat can also be herniated into the scrotum and can become strangulated just like bowel, leading to necrosis.

Testicular Masses

Testicular masses can present as either acute onset pain, especially if there is hemorrhage into a tumor, or chronic and painless testicular enlargement. Most testicular tumors are malignant germ cell neoplasms, with only 5% being benign tumors.[23] Testicular tumors without acute hemorrhage are often hypoechoic and disrupt the normal testicular architecture (Figure 10–21). Testicular tumors can also be isoechoic, echogenic, or polypoid in nature (Figure 10–22A). Testicular malignancies can metastasize to the paraspinous lymphatics, which may also be visible by ultrasound (Figure 10–22B).

Extratesticular masses can be encountered in emergency practice. Those masses most often seen are benign cysts of the albuginea, epididymal cysts, or spermatoceles. Cysts of the albuginea typically present as small palpable masses and are seen to be without echo on ultrasound. They are frequently located near the rete testis and epididymis. Epididymal cysts (Figure 10–23) can be seen in up to one-third of asymptomatic adults.[23] Spermatoceles are cystic collections of seminal fluid and are also fairly common. They are typically found within an efferent duct near the head of the epididymis and can result from trauma, inflammation, or vasectomy. Sonographic appearance is frequently that of multiple cystic fluid collections. Torsion of the appendix testis can present with similar symptoms to testicular torsion but is often noted in a younger age group. Torsion of the ap-

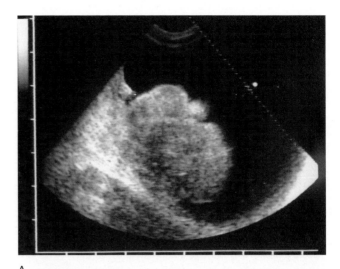

A

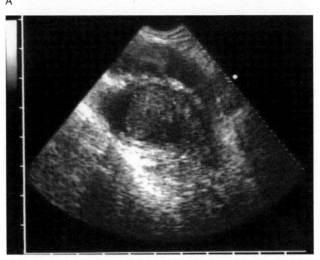

B

Figure 10–22. Testicular malignancy with metastasis. Oblique view of the upper portion of the testicle (A) reveals a slightly hyperechoic and polypoid mass that was malignant. A semicoronal view of the left lower quadrant (LLQ) of the abdomen (B) shows a 5-cm soft tissue density mass near the psoas muscle representing lymphatic extension of the tumor. This 35-year-old male presented with a complaint of back pain. The LLQ and scrotal masses were found incidentally on physical examination. *(Courtesy of James Mateer, MD.)*

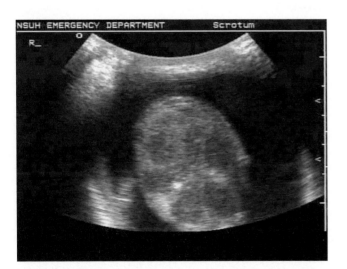

Figure 10–21. Testicular tumor. A long axis view of the testicle reveals a surrounding hydrocele and multiple hypoechoic areas, which replace the normal architecture. This tumor was discovered in a patient presenting complaining of acute testicular enlargement. On further questioning the patient admitted that his testicle was slowly enlarging for over 2-yr.

pendix testis often results in inflammation of the epididymis and apparent epididymitis (Figure 10–24).

▶ PITFALLS

1. *Contraindication.* There are no absolute contraindications to evaluating the testicle with ultrasound. Examinations may be limited by severe

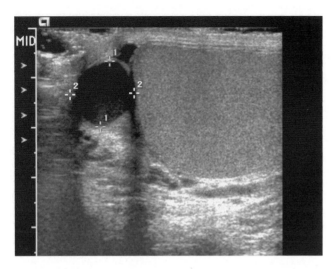

Figure 10–23. Longitudinal view of the upper pole of the testes demonstrates a typical singular epididymal cyst. *(Courtesy of James Mateer, MD, Waukesha Memorial Hospital.)*

pain, though, and analgesia will occasionally be required. Since minimal pressure is applied during the evaluation of the acute testicle, damage to a fractured testicle is not a concern.

2. *Prepubescent and infant boys.* Testicular blood flow in prepubescent boys and infants can be very difficult to detect. In cases of trauma, the testicular anatomy can still be accurately evaluated. However, it may require very sensitive equipment and considerable expertise to evaluate prepubescent testes. Some radiology departments even prefer to have nuclear medicine studies performed when experienced attending staff or sonographers are not available.

3. *Incomplete torsion.* Complete torsion occurs at approximately 450° of twisting of the spermatic cord. Venous flow initially disappears followed by arterial blood flow. Careful comparison between the two sides is important to exclude incomplete torsion. Diagnosing torsion early in the disease process when it is still incomplete can be challenging with color Doppler alone; this method relies on subtle differences between the two testicles. Use of spectral Doppler to document both venous and arterial waveforms is optimal.

4. *Torsion and detorsion.* Some patients may exhibit torsion and detorsion. This usually presents as a waxing and waning pain that results from intermittent ischemia. This entity can make for a challenging diagnosis if the ultrasound examination is performed during a period of detorsion. Shortly after detorsion, hyperemia may be detected as increased blood flow in the affected testicle. This will usually not last much longer than 15 min and may be missed. Bedside ultrasonography may be helpful to evaluate this possibility as it allows for serial examinations. With the clinical acumen to observe the patient and perform serial ultrasound examinations, the emergency physician should be able to avoid this pitfall.

► CASE STUDIES

Case 1

Patient Presentation

A 21-year-old man presents to the emergency department with a complaint of right testicular pain. He states the pain started suddenly 5 h prior to presentation. Since then, he has also noted some swelling on the right. The patient denies being sexually active but does note being struck in the genitals the day before during a basketball game. He has an unremarkable medical history and does not smoke. The patient denies any history of sexually transmitted diseases and states he is not having any urinary symptoms or urethral discharge.

Physical examination reveals a healthy young male in mild distress with normal vital signs. The abdominal examination is unremarkable, with no obvious hernias or costovertebral angle tenderness. Testicular examination reveals an erythematous right hemiscrotum with moderate swelling. The testicle is enlarged and painful to the touch. The epididymis is tender and slightly enlarged on examination. The testicle has a horizontal lie and the cremasteric reflex cannot be elicited. No cremasteric reflex is elicited on the contralateral side where the testicular and hemiscrotum examinations are normal.

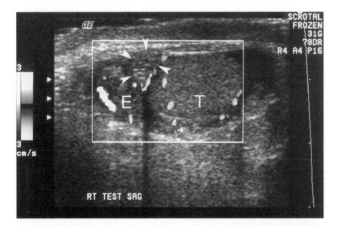

Figure 10–24. While increased flow was seen in the epididymis and testicle of this 8-year-old patient, no flow was noted within the suspected torsed appendix testis outlined by arrowheads. E = epididymis; T = testicle.

Management Course

The urine dip is negative. No urology service is available and the only radiology studies available at night are plain films, which are read by the emergency physician. A tertiary care hospital is approximately 90 min away by ambulance. Bedside emergency ultrasonography is available to the emergency physician. She performs an examination of the scrotum, noting enlargement and greatly increased blood flow to the right testicle and epididymis, with the epididymis being double the width compared to the contralateral side (see Figures 10–8A and B and 10–9A and B). A diagnosis of epididymitis with orchitis is made and the patient is discharged home with antibiotics, analgesics, and close follow-up and return instructions.

Commentary

Case 1 represents an example of the non-specific signs, symptoms, and history that may be associated with the presentation of acute testicular pain. The patient acutely became aware of testicular discomfort and swelling, although the disease process was probably slower in onset. The history of minor testicular trauma was a red herring but could not be ignored. The physical examination is often less helpful than described in many textbooks, especially when orchitis is present and the entire testicle is tender and swollen. Without the availability of bedside ultrasonography to evaluate the testicle, the emergency physician would have had to decide if transfer to an outside facility was mandated. If a lack of flow was seen in the testicle, arrangements could have been made for immediate transfer to a urology consultant and manual detorsion attempted. In this case, the diagnosis was made at the bedside with the aid of ultrasonography. An unnecessary transfer was avoided and the patient was discharged home with appropriate treatment and follow-up instructions.

Case 2

Patient Presentation

An 18-year-old man presents to the emergency department 3 d after being kicked in the groin during a soccer match. The patient was seen at an outside facility shortly after the injury, at which time an evaluation, including an ultrasound examination, revealed a small to moderate sized area of hemorrhage and no rupture through the testicular capsule. The patient was evaluated by the urologist and discharged home. He presents today because of increased swelling of the testicle. The scrotal skin is firm and erythematous, according to the mother, who is a pediatrician. The hydrocodone the patient was prescribed no longer relieves his pain. He denies any hematuria or other urinary symptoms.

Physical examination reveals an uncomfortable appearing man. The patient's vital signs are within normal limits. The cardiac, lung, and abdominal examinations are normal. Testicular examination reveals a swollen,

enlarged, and erythematous left hemiscrotum that is markedly tender to the touch. The testicle is clearly enlarged but difficult to differentiate within the scrotum. The contralateral testicle is nontender and appears to be of normal size. A urinalysis shows no white or red blood cells and is within normal limits. The mother insists something has changed since his injury; however, when she contacted the urologist, he asked that she see him in 2 d and recommended increasing the patient's analgesic dose.

Management Course

An ultrasound examination in the medical imaging department is not available after hours. The nuclear medicine technician is in-house performing a V/Q scan and could be ready for this patient in 60 to 90 min. The emergency physician performs a bedside ultrasound examination and this reveals a large heterogeneous testicle with areas of acute and old hemorrhage. Normal color Doppler flow is present in the portion of the testicle that appeared normal. A fracture line could be defined through the parenchyma of the testicle and appears to go through the capsule of the testicle (Figure 10–25). The urologist on call is contacted regarding the patient and comes in for evaluation. After a brief evaluation and review of the ultrasound examination on videotape, the patient is taken to the operating room for exploration. Surgical exploration reveals several areas of hemorrhage and a testicular rupture that is repaired. The patient is admitted overnight. Follow-up shows slow resolution of the injury with 80% function of the testicle at 30 days. No further surgical intervention is required.

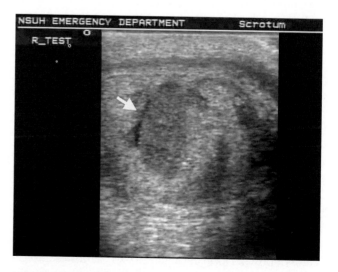

Figure 10–25. Significant testicular trauma was suffered by this teenager during a martial arts tournament. The testicle is fractured with a large amount of hemorrhage seen as an echo-poor area within the testicle, arrow.

Commentary

Case 2 illustrates the utility of ultrasound in defining testicular anatomy. The patient had already been scanned almost 3 d ago and no severe pathology was noted. However, he bled more into the testicle and a fracture line going through the capsule was defined on reexamination. The patient harbored a finding that led directly to operative intervention. However, it would have been tempting to simply discharge him home for follow up with his urologist once pain was better controlled. After all, the patient had already been imaged after the injury. The nuclear medicine scan may not have revealed any abnormalities as it is limited in defining anatomy.

Case 3

Patient Presentation

A 14-year-old male, accompanied by his parents, presents to the emergency department complaining of abdominal pain. The patient states his lower abdomen started hurting about 9 h ago. He did not want to tell his parents but the pain became increasingly intolerable. The patient denies fever or urinary symptoms but notes he is nauseated from the pain. He is crying intermittently and with his entire hand sweeps over a wide area below his umbilicus as to the source of his pain.

Physical examination reveals a patient in moderate distress with a respiratory rate of 24 and heart rate of 112 beats per min, and a normal temperature. Examination of the heart, lungs, and abdomen are unremarkable except for tachycardia and tachypnea. The genitourinary examination shows a slightly erythematous scrotum, more so on the left. There is moderate swelling of the left testicle and it is exquisitely tender. It has an oblique lie and the epididymis cannot be reliably palpated, in part, due to the patient's lack of cooperation. The cremasteric reflex is elicited with difficulty bilaterally. After the parents are asked to leave the examination room, the patient admits to sexual activity. He denies any recent trauma.

Management Course

A urinalysis shows 3 red blood cells per high-powered field and 25 white blood cells. No bacteria are seen. A urethral swab is taken for culture but no discharge is present. The evaluating emergency physician performs a bedside emergency ultrasound examination. The right testicle is found to have normal echotexture, size, and blood flow. The left testicle is moderately enlarged and appears less echogenic than the contralateral, unaffected side. No blood flow is seen within the testicle with either color or power Doppler (Figure 10–26). The urologist on call is notified and arrives to evaluate the patient, booking an operating room on her way into the hospital. The patient is taken for exploration and found to have a torsed left testicle. Detorsion leads to some improvement in the appearance of the testicle. At 1-wk follow-up, the

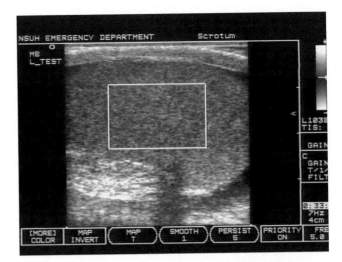

Figure 10–26. The left testicle was moderately enlarged and appeared less echogenic than the contralateral, unaffected side. No blood flow is seen within the testicle with either color or power Doppler.

urologist states that approximately 50% of the function has been preserved and orchiectomy was not necessary.

Commentary

The patient in this case is a good example of a teenager seen in the emergency department for acute testicular pain. The presentation is often late and the history is sketchy. Signs, symptoms, and the single laboratory test are nonspecific. The ability to detect the absence of blood flow in the testicle leads to rapid action by the attending emergency physician. The decreased echogenicity indicates edema and, in this case, progression of injury due to torsion. Even patients with delayed presentations can sometimes have partial recovery of testicular function. Urologic consultation must be expeditious. Taking such a patient directly to the operating suite without immediate ultrasound could easily have resulted in exploration of a patient with epididymitis or orchitis, and not testicular torsion.

REFERENCES

1. Lewis AG, Bukowski TP, Jarvis PD. Evaluation of acute scrotum in the emergency department. J Pediatric Surg 1995;30:277–280.
2. Fernandez MS, Dominguez C, Sanguesa C. The use of color Doppler sonography of the acute scrotum in children. Cir Pediatr 1997;10:25–27.
3. Zoller G. Genitourinary trauma. In: Rosen P, Barkin R, eds. Emergency medicine concepts and clinical practice, 4th ed. St Louis: Mosby, 1997;2243–2245.
4. Knight PJ, Vassy LE. The diagnosis and treatment of the acute scrotum in children and adolescents. Ann Surg 1984;200:664–666.

5. Albrecht T, Lotzof K, Hussain HK, et al. Bruyn: Power Doppler US of the normal prepubertal testis: does it live up to its promises? Radiology 1997;203:227–231.

6. Fenner MN, Roszhart DA, Texter JH. Testicular scanning: evaluating the acute scrotum in the clinical setting. Urology 1991;10:25.

7. Jefferson RH, Perez LM, Joseph DB. Critical analysis of the clinical presentation of acute scrotum: a 9-year experience at a single institution. J Urol 1997;158:1198, 1201.

8. Cos LR, Rabinowitz R. Trauma-induced testicular torsion in children. J Trauma 1982;22:223–225.

9. Prater JM, Overdorf BS. Testicular torsion: a surgical emergency. Am Fam Emerg Physician 1991;44:834–840.

10. Lee TF, Winter DB, Madsen FA, et al. Conventional color Doppler velocity sonography versus color Doppler energy sonography for the diagnosis of acute experimental torsion of the spermatic cord. AJR 1996;167:785–790.

11. Kass EJ, Stone KT, Cacciarelli AA, Mithcell B. Do all children with an acute scrotum require exploration? J Urol 1993;150:667–669.

12. Blaivas M, Sierzenski P, Lambert M. Emergency evaluation of patients presenting with acute scrotum using bedside ultrasonography. Acad Emerg Med 2001;8:90–93.

13. Blaivas M, Sierzenski P. Emergency ultrasonography in the evaluation of the acute scrotum. Acad Emerg Med 2001;8:85–89.

14. Blaivas M, Batts M, Lambert M. Ultrasonographic diagnosis of testicular torsion by emergency emergency physicians. Am J Emerg Med 2000;18:198–200.

15. Sierzenski P, Blaivas M. Belden M, et al. Manual compression of the spermatic cord to simulate testicular torsion on ultrasound. A teaching model for emergency physicians. Acad Emerg Med 2000;7:493.

16. Stewart R, Carroll B. The scrotum. In: Rumack CM, Wilson SR, Charboneau JW, eds. Diagnostic ultrasound. Vol 1. St. Louis: Mosby, 1991;565–589.

17. Micallef M, Ahmad I, Ramesh N, et al. Ultrasound features of blunt testicular injury. Injury 2001;32:23–26.

18. Corrales JG, Corbel L, Cipolla B, et al. Accuracy of ultrasound diagnosis after blunt testicular trauma. J Urol 1993;150:1834–1836.

19. Blaivas M, Lambert JM, Harwood RA, et al. Lower extremity Doppler for deep venous thrombosis—can emergency physicians be accurate and fast? Acad Emerg Med 2000;7:120–126.

20. Hilty WM, Hudson PA, Levitt MA, Hall JB. Real-time ultrasound-guided femoral vein catheterization during cardiopulmonary resuscitation. Ann Emerg Med 1997;29:331–337.

21. Hill R, Conron R, Greissinger P, Heller M. Ultrasound for the detection of foreign bodies in human tissue. Ann Emerg Med 1997;29:353–356.

22. Netter F. Scrotum: reproductive system. West Caldwell: CIBA, 1989;73.

23. Hill MC, Sanders RC. Sonography of benign disease of the scrotum. In: Sanders RC, Hill M, eds. Ultrasound annual. New York: Raven Press, 1986;197–237.

CHAPTER 11

First Trimester Pregnancy

Robert F. Reardon and Marc L. Martel

Ultrasonography is the primary imaging modality used in pregnancy.[1,2] In first trimester patients who present with vaginal bleeding or abdominal pain, ultrasound can be used to distinguish ectopic pregnancy from threatened abortion or embryonic demise. The primary goal of emergency sonography of the pelvis in the first trimester is to identify an intrauterine pregnancy, which essentially excludes the diagnosis of ectopic pregnancy.[3] Secondary objectives are to detect extrauterine signs of an ectopic pregnancy, estimate the viability of an intrauterine pregnancy, and characterize other causes of pelvic pain and vaginal bleeding. In addition, sonographic detection of free fluid outside of the pelvis can help emergency physicians expedite the care of a patient with a ruptured ectopic pregnancy.[4] Emergency bedside sonography is not intended to define the entire spectrum of pelvic pathology in early pregnancy. A "formal" pelvic ultrasound examination, by medical imaging or obstetric specialists, may be indicated after an initial emergency bedside screening examination.

► CLINICAL CONSIDERATIONS

Abdominal or pelvic pain and vaginal bleeding are common complaints during early pregnancy. Challenges to emergency or acute care physicians include making the diagnosis of pregnancy and then using available diagnostic tools to determine the etiology of the patient's complaint.

The development of sensitive pregnancy tests has made a missed diagnosis of early pregnancy unlikely. Modern qualitative urine tests for beta-human chorionic gonadotropin (β-hCG) have a threshold of about 20 IU/L and allow detection of pregnancy as early as 1 week postconception (3 weeks gestational age). False negative

urine tests may occur when the urine is very dilute (specific gravity less than 1.010), and obtaining a quantitative serum β-hCG should be considered in such cases.[5]

Once pregnancy is recognized in a symptomatic or high-risk patient, complications of early pregnancy, particularly ectopic pregnancy, must be considered. Those patients with pelvic or abdominal pain, vaginal bleeding, dizziness, syncope, or any risk factors for ectopic pregnancy need to have the status of their pregnancy evaluated. The location, viability, and gestational age of the pregnancy are important factors in establishing a diagnosis. Other findings, such as free intraperitoneal fluid in the pelvis or a pelvic mass, may also impact the patient's management.

Many diagnostic tests can be used to detect complications of early pregnancy. Serum β-hCG and progesterone levels, suction curettage, culdocentesis, and laparoscopy yield some information, but none can identify the entire spectrum of pathology like pelvic sonography. Furthermore, other imaging modalities, like CT and MRI, are not commonly used for detecting complications of early pregnancy.

The hormone β-hCG is produced by the trophoblasts during early pregnancy. Serum β-hCG levels rise exponentially in early pregnancy and can be used as a marker to date normal pregnancies. However, abnormal pregnancies have widely varying β-hCG levels, so a single level cannot differentiate a normal intrauterine pregnancy from an ectopic pregnancy or other abnormality.[6]

Progesterone is produced by the corpus luteum in early pregnancy and serum levels remain relatively high during a normal pregnancy. Serum levels are generally lower in abnormal pregnancies, including ectopic pregnancy, and fall with pregnancy failure. Clinicians who do not have bedside ultrasound immediately available have utilized progesterone levels to help differentiate between a normal pregnancy and a possible ectopic with some success.[7,8] These methods, however, have not proven to be as efficient or as accurate as protocols that incorporate initial transvaginal sonography. Preliminary reports suggest that progesterone may have a role in further categorizing patients who have an initial indeterminate transvaginal ultrasound. Patients with a progesterone level at or above 11 ng/mL are significantly more likely to have an early intrauterine pregnancy rather than an ectopic or an abortion (sensitivity 91%, specificity 84%).[9]

Suction curettage of the uterus can provide a definitive diagnosis of an intrauterine pregnancy if chorionic villi are identified. However, this test terminates an intrauterine pregnancy, making it useful only when termination is desired or the pregnancy has obviously failed. Because it is invasive and other tests can provide similar information, suction curettage is rarely useful in the initial emergency evaluation during early pregnancy.

Culdocentesis is needle aspiration of the pelvic cul-de-sac through the posterior fornix of the vagina. Aspiration of blood is considered indicative of an ectopic pregnancy. However, culdocentesis is not very sensitive, especially for detecting nonruptured ectopic pregnancies.[3,10–12] It now has a very limited role and is only recommended when ultrasound is not available.[13]

Laparoscopy is an excellent test for visualizing extrauterine pelvic pathology, especially ectopic pregnancy.[14] However, it does not give any information about intrauterine contents or fetal viability. Recently laparoscopy has been utilized less frequently because sonography is noninvasive and can provide more information.[11] Laparoscopy can be used as a therapeutic tool and a diagnostic adjunct when sonography is nondiagnostic.

There are many advantages to using sonography in the first trimester of pregnancy. It is an ideal diagnostic tool in this setting since it can visualize both intrauterine contents and the extrauterine pelvic pathology. When used judiciously, ultrasound has no known adverse effects on the embryo and can be repeated as needed. Unlike curettage or culdocentesis, ultrasound is noninvasive and well tolerated by most patients.[15] Unlike curettage or laparoscopy, ultrasound can directly visualize the intrauterine or extrauterine location of a pregnancy.[16] Unlike serum markers, ultrasound can immediately identify an abnormal pregnancy or evaluate fetal viability. Also, ultrasound can accurately measure the gestational age of a pregnancy; whereas, serum markers can only give a gross estimation. Finally, patients with an ectopic pregnancy can be risk-stratified using ultrasound by estimating the size of an extrauterine mass or the amount of free intraperitoneal blood.

A disadvantage of using ultrasound in early pregnancy is that a pregnancy may not be visible between 3 and 5 weeks gestational age. During this time, sensitive urine pregnancy tests are positive but the gestation is usually too small to identify, even with transvaginal ultrasound. Another disadvantage of using ultrasound is that it is equipment and operator dependent. Clinicians who make important patient management decisions based on ultrasound results must know the limitations of each study based on who is performing the examination and what type of equipment is being used.

▶ CLINICAL INDICATIONS

Any patient who is at risk for complications of early pregnancy is a candidate for pelvic sonography. Symptoms and physical examination findings include pelvic or abdominal pain or tenderness, vaginal bleeding, dizziness, syncope, a pelvic mass, or uterine size that does not correlate with the gestational age. Risk factors for ectopic pregnancy include pelvic inflammatory disease, tubal ligation, tubal surgery, increased maternal age, intrauterine contraceptive devices, prior ectopic pregnancy, and a history of infertility.[17] Most patients with an ectopic pregnancy present with abdominal or pelvic pain, vaginal bleeding, or dizziness, but some are relatively asymptomatic. Since no specific sign or symptom is absolute, physicians must have a high index of suspicion so that subtle presentations are not overlooked. Also, any woman of childbearing age who presents with shock of unknown etiology should have an immediate abdominal and pelvic ultrasound examination, even before a pregnancy test is completed.[4]

The main indication for emergency pelvic sonography in the first trimester is to differentiate an intrauterine pregnancy from an ectopic pregnancy. Sonography can immediately establish one of these diagnoses in most patients with first trimester complaints.[16]

- Intrauterine pregnancy
- Ectopic pregnancy

Emergency pelvic sonography is also useful for the diagnosis of the following conditions in the first trimester of pregnancy:

- Pregnancy loss
- Multiple pregnancy
- Pelvic mass
- Ovarian torsion
- Gestational trophoblastic disease

INTRAUTERINE PREGNANCY

A normal intrauterine pregnancy is the most common sonographic finding during the first trimester. Even novice sonographers can use pelvic ultrasound effectively because identifying an intrauterine pregnancy is simple and this finding virtually eliminates the possibility of an ectopic pregnancy.[18] About 70% of patients who present with abdominal pain or vaginal bleeding in the first trimester will have an intrauterine pregnancy visualized with bedside ultrasound and will not require further testing.[19] Care must be taken when using sonography between 3 and 5 weeks gestational age because it is easy to confuse sonographic signs of an early intrauterine pregnancy with those of an ectopic pregnancy.

Identifying an intrauterine pregnancy with cardiac activity can give patients some reassurance about the outcome of their pregnancy. Those patients with a finding of embryonic cardiac activity have a much lower incidence of pregnancy loss than other patients with similar symptoms.[20,21] However, physicians should be careful not to give patients false hope about their pregnancy. Even when a normal intrauterine pregnancy is discovered, it is prudent to inform patients that emergency bedside sonography is a screening examination only and will not detect fetal anomalies. Also, patients with abdominal pain or vaginal bleeding still have a significant chance of pregnancy loss.

Dating an intrauterine pregnancy is not as important as excluding an ectopic pregnancy. However, when the uterine size does not correlate with the gestational age or when the last menstrual period is unknown, sonography is indicated to date the pregnancy. This is very common because about half of all pregnant women cannot remember their last menstrual period. Pregnancy dating is simple and rapid with modern ultrasound equipment. Sonographic dating during the first trimester is more accurate than dating later in pregnancy. A few minutes spent measuring an embryo will be much appreciated by the patient's obstetrician, especially in patients who have unclear menstrual dates or are noncompliant with prenatal care. This early measurement becomes more important near term when the obstetrician is considering induction of labor in a patient whose uterine size does not correlate with gestational age.

ECTOPIC PREGNANCY

Ectopic pregnancy occurs in about 2% of all pregnancies in the United States.[11,12] However, symptomatic patients who present to an emergency setting have a much higher incidence, as high as 7.5 to 13% in some reports.[7,22] The incidence of ectopic pregnancy has quadrupled in the last 20 years.[12] During the same period of time, the case-fatality rate for ruptured ectopic pregnancies has decreased significantly. This decrease is due to earlier diagnosis and treatment secondary to increased awareness and improved diagnostic capabilities, such as transvaginal sonography.[11] Despite these improvements, a significant percentage of ectopic pregnancies are still missed.[23] Also,

ectopic pregnancy remains the leading cause of maternal death during the first trimester of pregnancy.[24]

Heterotopic pregnancy, which is a concomitant intrauterine and extrauterine pregnancy, has also become more common in the last few decades. In 1948, the incidence of heterotopic pregnancy was estimated to be one per 30,000 pregnancies, based on a theoretical calculation and assuming an ectopic pregnancy rate of 0.37%.[25] Now that the ectopic pregnancy rate is about 2%, it is reasonable to expect that the rate of heterotopic pregnancy is higher than previously estimated. Although precise data are lacking, the current incidence of heterotopic pregnancy in the general obstetric population is probably greater than one per 8,000 pregnancies.[25–30] The incidence is much higher in patients taking ovulation-inducing medications or undergoing *in vitro* fertilization (as high as 1 per 100 pregnancies).[31,32]

Emergency or acute care physicians have an important role in preventing morbidity and mortality from ectopic pregnancy.[33] Early diagnosis of ectopic pregnancy allows conservative treatment options, like methotrexate therapy.[11,34] Pelvic ultrasound is the main diagnostic modality that allows an early diagnosis to be made.

When emergency physicians perform bedside transvaginal sonography, pregnant patients have a shorter length of stay in the emergency department.[35–37] Also, bedside pelvic ultrasound screening by clinicians is more cost effective than ordering "formal" pelvic sonography on every patient with a possible ectopic pregnancy.[38] Most importantly, a protocol, which includes bedside transvaginal ultrasound by emergency physicians, has been shown to decrease the incidence of discharged patients returning with a subsequent ruptured ectopic pregnancy.[19,22,39]

Algorithm with Transvaginal Sonography and β-hCG Discriminatory Zone

Prior to the development of ectopic pregnancy algorithms and the widespread use of transvaginal sonography, the diagnosis of about half of all ectopic pregnancies were missed, and about half of those ruptured prior to their next presentation.[22,40,41] In the 1980s, ectopic pregnancy was one of the leading causes of emergency physician malpractice suits.[42,43] Algorithms that incorporate transvaginal sonography and a β-hCG discriminatory zone have improved diagnostic accuracy and reduced the incidence of patients who are discharged and subsequently present with a ruptured ectopic pregnancy.[16,22]

One algorithm utilizes emergency bedside transvaginal sonography as the initial diagnostic step for all patients at risk for ectopic pregnancy, before a quantitative serum β-hCG is obtained (Figure 11–1).[2,22,39,41,44–53] Transvaginal sonography can establish a diagnosis of intrauterine pregnancy or ectopic pregnancy in 75% of patients at the time of their initial presentation.[16] If emergency bedside sonography demonstrates an intrauterine

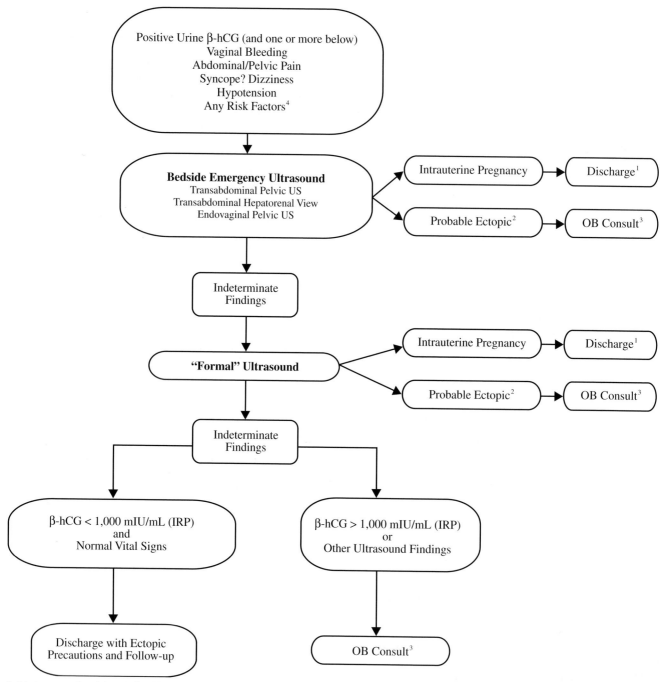

1. Unless patient is on fertility medications or undergoing IVF.
2. US criteria for probable ectopic pregnancy: extrauterine yolk sac or embryo, tubal ring, complex mass, or free fluid.
3. Surgery may be required if the patient has hypotension, a large ectopic sac (>4 cm), a large amount of pelvic free fluid, or hepatorenal free fluid.
4. Risk factors include: PID, tubal surgery or ligation, IUD's, prior ectopic, infertility, advanced age.

Figure 11–1. Ectopic pregnancy algorithm.

pregnancy or an ectopic pregnancy, then the work-up is complete. When no intrauterine pregnancy or ectopic pregnancy is identified, then the bedside ultrasound examination is indeterminate, and at this point a quantitative serum β-hCG level and a "formal" pelvic ultrasound examination should be ordered. Again, if the "formal"

study shows an intrauterine pregnancy or an ectopic pregnancy, then the work-up is complete. If either the bedside or "formal" ultrasound examination demonstrates nonspecific signs of an ectopic pregnancy, then the risk is very high. Therefore, this situation should be managed in the same manner as a clear ectopic pregnancy and an obstetrics consult should be obtained. If both sonograms show no intrauterine pregnancy and no signs of an ectopic pregnancy, then the management depends on the serum β-hCG level. Patients with an indeterminate ultrasound examination and a β-hCG level above the discriminatory zone (β-hCG higher than 1000 mIU/mL) have a presumed ectopic pregnancy or embryonic demise and require an immediate obstetrics consultation. Those with an indeterminate ultrasound examination and a β-hCG level below the discriminatory zone (β-hCG < 1,000 mIU/mL) may have either a small ectopic pregnancy, a very early intrauterine pregnancy, or embryonic demise. If stable, these patients can be discharged home without an obstetrics consult but they should be given clear ectopic pregnancy discharge instructions and scheduled for close follow-up in 2–3 days for a repeat ultrasound examination and serum β-hCG level.

Similar algorithms, incorporating emergency bedside transvaginal sonography, have been shown to improve the quality of patient care and to be more cost effective than other approaches.[16,22,38,39]

Quantitative Serum β-hCG and Discriminatory Zone

Serum β-hCG rises exponentially and predictably during the first 6 to 8 weeks of pregnancy and peaks at about 100,000 mIU/mL in a normal pregnancy. Serial β-hCG levels are useful for differentiating normal pregnancies from abnormal pregnancies. The serum level should increase by at least 66%, multiplying by 1.6, every 48 h. An abnormally slow rise in β-hCG indicates an abnormal pregnancy, either an ectopic pregnancy or embryonic demise.

Quantitative β-hCG measurements are currently standardized in relation to the International Reference Preparation (IRP). The reference standard for all β-hCG levels discussed in this chapter is the IRP. The standard method for reporting IRP β-hCG levels is in mIU/mL. Other reference standards are referred to in the literature and it is important to distinguish between them since they are not equivalent. The Second International Standard is roughly equal to one half of the IRP and the Third International Standard is roughly equal to the IRP. In this chapter, β-hCG concentrations are reported in relation to the IRP, in mIU/mL.

A single serum β-hCG level is not as useful as serial levels because it does not differentiate a normal early intrauterine pregnancy from an ectopic pregnancy. Rarely is a single level helpful.[54] A common misconception is that a very low β-hCG level rules out ectopic pregnancy. Recent studies show that about 40% of ectopic pregnancies present with a β-hCG level less than 1000 mIU/mL and about 20% present with a β-hCG level less than 500 mIU/mL.[16,55] In fact, patients who present with a β-hCG level less than 1000 mIU/mL have a higher risk of ectopic pregnancy than other patients.[16,56] Furthermore,

a low β-hCG level does not predict a benign course. Approximately 30 to 40% of ectopic pregnancies with a β-hCG level less than 1000 mIU/mL will be ruptured at the time of diagnosis.[16,55,56]

The "discriminatory zone" is a concept that was developed to allow the complimentary use of pelvic ultrasound and a single serum β-hCG level to help determine the likelihood of ectopic pregnancy. The discriminatory zone is the β-hCG level above which an intrauterine pregnancy can be consistently visualized by pelvic sonography. Patients with a β-hCG level above the discriminatory zone who do not have an intrauterine pregnancy on ultrasound examination are presumed to have an ectopic pregnancy until proven otherwise. This is the concept that led to the use of the discriminatory zone in previous ectopic pregnancy algorithms. Older algorithms used the β-hCG discriminatory zone to limit the use of pelvic sonography since it was thought that only patients with levels greater than 1000 mIU/mL would benefit from an ultrasound examination.[41,44] When older algorithms are applied, however, a significant percentage of ectopic pregnancies will be missed.[41]

Recent studies clearly show the benefit of performing pelvic sonography on all patients with a possible ectopic pregnancy, regardless of their β-hCG level.[16,22,48,55,56] Although a normal pregnancy will not be visualized when the β-hCG level is low, many ectopic pregnancies are easily identified when the β-hCG level is less than 1000 mIU/mL. In fact, transvaginal sonography can detect about half of ectopic pregnancies with β-hCG levels less than 1000 mIU/mL.[16,55,56]

In this chapter's algorithm, the discriminatory zone serum β-hCG level is used to help guide the management of patients with indeterminate pelvic ultrasound examinations. The discriminatory zone β-hCG level of 1000 mIU/mL was chosen because this is the level above which an intrauterine pregnancy can be consistently visualized by "formal" transvaginal sonography.[24,47,55,57] Individual hospitals and clinics should choose their own discriminatory zone in collaboration with their obstetrics consultants and those who will perform their "formal" ultrasound studies.

Indeterminate Ultrasound Examinations

An "indeterminate" ultrasound examination in early pregnancy demonstrates no signs of intrauterine pregnancy or an ectopic pregnancy. Dart and co-workers attempted to subclassify patients with an indeterminate ultrasound examination based on their intrauterine findings.[58] Patients with a completely empty uterus and normal thin midline stripe had a 27% chance of an ectopic pregnancy and a 10% chance of an intrauterine pregnancy. Those with a nonspecific endometrial fluid collection had a 13% chance of an ectopic pregnancy and a 25% chance of an intrauterine pregnancy. Patients with intrauterine echogenic material had a 5% chance of ectopic pregnancy and none had an intrauterine pregnancy.

Approximately 15% of patients who are evaluated for a possible ectopic pregnancy have a β-hCG level greater than 1000 mIU/mL and an indeterminate ultrasound examination.[16,58] Roughly 20% of these patients have an ectopic pregnancy.[52,53,58,59]

Management and Disposition

Patients diagnosed with an ectopic pregnancy have traditionally required surgery, which is usually a laparoscopic procedure. Recently, medical therapy has become more popular, with a single-dose intramuscular methotrexate therapy being the most common regimen. This regimen has a success rate of about 90%.[11] Clinical and sonographic criteria can help obstetricians decide which patients are candidates for medical therapy instead of surgery. Higher serum β-hCG levels are associated with failure of methotrexate therapy, especially levels above 10,000 mIU/mL.[34] Also, an adnexal mass greater than 4 cm in diameter, the presence of embryonic cardiac activity, a large amount of pelvic free fluid, and severe pain should be considered relative contraindications to medical management.[11,60] Clinical signs of shock along with free intraperitoneal fluid outside of the pelvis, such as in the hepatorenal space, are indications for surgery and contraindications to medical therapy.[4,11,24]

Patients with an unclear diagnosis of ectopic pregnancy need serial sonography and serial β-hCG levels. Obstetricians may be unwilling to initiate therapy in such patients for fear of interrupting an intrauterine pregnancy. Patients who have a β-hCG level greater than 1000 mIU/mL and unclear or questionable sonographic findings should ideally be observed in the hospital. Repeat sonography and β-hCG level at 12 to 24 h will make the diagnosis more clear. Those with no mass, free fluid, or other signs of ectopic pregnancy and a β-hCG level less than 1000 mIU/mL are safe to be discharged with early follow-up for repeat sonography and β-hCG level in 24 to 48 h.[11,41,46,48]

A small percentage of ectopic pregnancies will spontaneously resolve without any treatment.[61] Therefore, expectant management may be reasonable in selected cases. Candidates for expectant management must have minimal symptoms, a small ectopic mass, and a low β-hCG level. Excellent clinical, sonographic, and laboratory follow-up must be assured if expectant management is attempted. About 10% of ectopic pregnancies can be successfully managed in this manner.[62]

PREGNANCY LOSS

Diagnosing pregnancy loss is not as urgent as excluding an ectopic pregnancy. It is important, however, for emergency or acute care physicians to be aware of the sonographic features of pregnancy loss. It is helpful to know the risks of pregnancy loss related to specific ultrasound findings. This information will allow physicians to do a better job of counseling patients and making reasonable management plans for those with a threatened abortion.

Vaginal bleeding, or "threatened abortion," is a very common presentation and occurs in about 25% of all clinically apparent early pregnancies.[57,63,64] About 40 to 50% of these patients will eventually be diagnosed with pregnancy loss.[16,24,65–67] A threatened abortion is a significant source of anxiety for pregnant patients. Concern for the viability of the pregnancy is usually the primary reason for presentation. Pelvic sonography is very useful in patients with a threatened abortion because it provides an immediate diagnosis in about half of all patients with subsequent pregnancy loss.[67] Those without a definitive diagnosis require serial pelvic sonography and β-hCG levels.

Spontaneous abortion refers to expulsion of a nonviable pregnancy from the uterus before 20 weeks gestational age. Microscopic identification of chorionic villi or obvious products of conception are required to make a definitive diagnosis. A completed spontaneous abortion can be diagnosed when all products of conception have been expelled. This usually occurs shortly after embryonic demise but may be delayed for days to weeks. Sonographically, an empty uterus should be seen after a completed spontaneous abortion. This finding indicates that the patient can be managed expectantly without curettage.[68–70]

Incomplete abortion is a non-specific term used when a pregnancy has failed but all of the products of conception have not been expelled from the uterus. The terms embryonic demise, blighted ovum, and retained products of conception are all synonymous with incomplete abortion. Patients with an incomplete abortion may experience continued bleeding, infection, and anxiety, so it is important to make the diagnosis as soon as possible after embryonic demise has occurred. Patients with an incomplete abortion may require curettage to remove retained products of conception.[70,71] Sonography is the only diagnostic modality that can directly assess intrauterine contents before a curettage is performed.

The term inevitable abortion implies that expulsion of uterine contents is in progress. Patients with an inevitable abortion have an open cervical os on physical examination. Pelvic sonography may show a separated gestational sac lying low within the uterus.[57]

It is reasonable for physicians to use bedside pelvic sonography to help make initial management decisions in patients with a threatened abortion. However, it is prudent to confirm the diagnosis of embryonic demise with a "formal" pelvic ultrasound prior to evacuation of intrauterine products. Also, it is important not to give patients false reassurance. Even when a completely normal intrauterine pregnancy is seen, they should be aware that there is still a chance of subsequent pregnancy loss.

Sonographic signs of a normal intrauterine pregnancy are reassuring and decrease the likelihood that a pregnancy will be lost.[20,67,72–74] In asymptomatic patients, those without threatened abortion, the rate of first trimester pregnancy loss decreases as the gestational age increases and as more normal structures can be identified with sonography.[72] The rate of loss after only a gestational sac is identified is 11.5%. The rate decreases to 8.5% after a yolk sac is identified and to 7.2% after an embryo (2 to 5 mm) is identified. When a larger embryo is seen, the loss rate is even lower: 3.3% with a 6 to 10 mm embryo and 0.5% with an embryo greater than 10 mm.[72] Additionally, there is a 2% risk of pregnancy loss after the first trimester in pregnancies that previously appeared viable by ultrasound.[72]

As stated previously, patients presenting with a first trimester threatened abortion have a 40 to 50% chance of pregnancy loss.[16,24,65–67] If embryonic cardiac activity can be seen, however, the rate of subsequent pregnancy loss is lower at 15 to 20%.[20,67] Also, as the gestational age and the size of the embryo increase, cardiac activity is more reassuring. Very early in the first trimester, when the embryo is less than 5 mm long, patients with a threatened abortion and cardiac activity have a loss rate of about 24%.[74] Those with a threatened abortion and cardiac activity near the end of the first trimester have a very low rate of pregnancy loss.[21]

MULTIPLE PREGNANCY

Characterizing a multiple pregnancy (twins, triplets, etc.) seems to be outside the realm of emergency medicine. However, timely pelvic sonography is indicated when menstrual dates do not correlate with the size of the patient's uterus. In such cases, sonographic pregnancy dating and evaluation for multiple pregnancy or molar pregnancy should be performed. Also, multiple pregnancies are often an incidental finding when sonography is performed for other indications, like ruling out an ectopic pregnancy. Regardless of the indication for the sonogram, finding a multiple pregnancy is significant since the pregnancy will then be categorized as high risk and the patient will need close follow-up with an obstetrician.

Twin pregnancies are more likely to have fetal anomalies, premature delivery, and low birth weight. Early sonographic evaluation of a multiple pregnancy is important because differentiating dichorionic from monochorionic twins is much easier during the first trimester. Fraternal (dizygotic) twins are always dichorionic and diamnionic but identical (monozygotic) twins may be dichorionic, monochorionic, diamnionic, or monoamnionic depending on when the zygote splits. Determining chorionicity is important since monochorionic twins have a mortality rate two to three times higher than dichorionic twins. Monochorionic twins share a single placenta, so they are at risk of twin transfusion syndrome, twin embolization syndrome, and acardiac parabiotic twin syndrome.

In addition, determining amnionicity is important since monoamniotic twins are at risk for cord knots, wrapping of the cord around a co-twin, or locking of twins during delivery.

When imaging a multiple pregnancy, physicians should try to record quality images that clearly show the chorionicity and amnionicity. If chorionicity and amnionicity cannot be determined, then the patient should have a "formal" sonogram within several days. Also, it is important to inform patients that about 25% of twin pregnancies diagnosed during the first trimester will become singleton pregnancies by the second trimester.[75,76]

PELVIC MASSES

A pelvic mass may be noted in the first trimester of pregnancy during the physical examination or routine pelvic ultrasound examination. Physicians who perform bedside sonography need to have some basic knowledge of pelvic masses so they can make reasonable management plans. Most pelvic masses found in the first trimester are benign and require no treatment. They all, however, require close follow-up with serial sonography because some masses are at risk of hemorrhage, torsion, rupture, dystocia, and malignancy. Surgery will be required in about 1 per 1300 pregnancies to exclude malignancy or to deal with one of the above complications.[77] About 3% of all masses discovered during pregnancy have malignant potential.[77]

In general, patients with masses less than 5 cm in diameter in early pregnancy are treated conservatively and followed with serial sonography. Those presenting with peritoneal signs or severe pain may need immediate surgery because of rupture or torsion of a mass. Masses that are large, cause pain, or grow rapidly may require surgery. Those containing large solid areas, solid irregular areas, papillary excrescences, and irregular septae are at higher risk of malignancy. Also, the presence of ascites, in addition to a cystic pelvic mass, increases the chance of malignancy.[78] If surgery is required, then the optimal period is during the second trimester, when maternal and fetal risks are smallest.

The most common mass seen in early pregnancy is a corpus luteum cyst. The corpus luteum secretes progesterone to support the early pregnancy. A corpus luteum cyst is usually less than 5 cm in diameter and appears as a thin-walled unilocular structure surrounded by normal ovarian parenchyma. The appearance may vary substantially and the size may be greater than 10 cm. Hemorrhage into a corpus luteum cyst can cause the appearance of internal echogenic debris and septae.[24] Corpus luteum cysts usually regress spontaneously prior to 18 weeks of gestation.

A theca lutein cyst is an exaggerated corpus luteum and occurs in patients with very high β-hCG levels. Theca lutein cysts are commonly seen in patients with gestational trophoblastic disease and ovarian hyperstimulation from fertility medications. They appear as large multiseptated cystic masses. Theca lutein cysts usually resolve spontaneously once the abnormal stimulus is removed.

Uterine leiomyomas, or fibroids, are solid pelvic masses that are very common and may enlarge during pregnancy because of increased estrogen levels. They usually appear as relatively hypoechoic masses within the uterine wall and are sometimes confused with a simple muscular contraction of part of the uterine wall. Fibroids can have many different appearances depending on the amount of smooth muscle and hyaline they contain and whether they have undergone hemorrhagic degeneration. They may contain calcifications or cystic areas of degeneration. Small fibroids tend to enlarge during the first and second trimesters but larger fibroids tend to enlarge only during the first trimester.[79] All fibroids tend to decrease in size during late pregnancy. Patients with multiple fibroids have a higher risk of bleeding, premature contractions, malpresentation, and retained products.[78] Large fibroids located in the lower part of the uterus during late pregnancy can obstruct labor and necessitate a cesarean section.

The most common complex mass seen in early pregnancy is a teratoma, or dermoid cyst.[77,78] These tumors arise from germ cells within the ovary and contain heterologous tissue like fat, skin, hair, and teeth. Sebaceous material within a dermoid can appear as a fluid-fluid level and teeth are very echogenic with distal shadowing. Dermoids are prone to torsion and rupture. Leaking of dermoid fluid can cause granulomatous peritonitis and sudden rupture can cause an acute abdomen.[78]

Mucinous and serous cystadenomas are ovarian epithelial neoplasms; they are the most common cystic tumors that enlarge during pregnancy.[80] Both of these tumors can appear as multicystic masses. Mucinous cystadenomas usually contain multiple thick internal septations and serous cystadenomas usually appear as unilocular structures. Again, pelvic masses that have internal septations and papillary excrescences are more likely to have malignant potential.[78]

It is not the emergency or acute care physician's job to characterize pelvic masses using sonography. However, these physicians will inevitably discover pelvic masses as incidental findings. When this occurs, most patients will need a "formal" ultrasound examination and close follow-up with an obstetrician. Patients should be informed when a mass is found, and they should understand that bedside sonography is a screening tool and that further work-up is needed.

ADNEXAL TORSION

Adnexal torsion is uncommon but about 20% of all cases occur during pregnancy.[81,82] Also, most cases occur during the first trimester.[77,83] Pregnant patients may be predisposed to torsion because of increased ovarian arterial flow

and decreased ovarian venous flow, causing ovarian edema and enlargement. Torsion almost always occurs in the setting of an enlarged ovary or an ovarian mass; torsion rarely occurs in a normal size ovary. Recently, ovarian hyperstimulation from fertility medications has been recognized as a risk factor for adnexal torsion.

Pain is the most common symptom of adnexal torsion. The diagnosis of torsion may be easily missed during pregnancy because pain may be attributed to the gravid uterus, the round ligament, or an adnexal mass. Further delay may occur because of the poor accuracy of Doppler ultrasound, which may miss up to 60% of cases of adnexal torsion.[84] Also, when a cystic ovarian mass is present, blood flow to the ovary may be difficult to visualize using Doppler, even though torsion has not occurred.

Simple grayscale pelvic sonography may be of some help in diagnosing adnexal torsion.[85] Finding a unilaterally enlarged ovary with multifollicular enlargement or any adnexal mass makes torsion more likely. Most patients with torsion have free fluid in the pelvic cul-de-sac, probably as a result of obstruction of venous and lymphatic drainage.[85,86] Finding normal-size ovaries and no pelvic free fluid makes the diagnosis of adnexal torsion unlikely.

Most diagnoses of adnexal torsion are delayed due to atypical clinical presentations and poor sensitivity of diagnostic modalities.[87] This may be especially detrimental in pregnancy causing maternal morbidity and fetal mortality. Therefore, it is prudent to have a high index of suspicion when there is no clear etiology for abdominal, pelvic, flank, or groin pain. Also, when the diagnosis is strongly suspected, negative diagnostic studies should not deter consultation and further evaluation.[88] Laparoscopy has been used during pregnancy as both a diagnostic and therapeutic modality.

GESTATIONAL TROPHOBLASTIC DISEASE

Gestational trophoblastic disease (GTD) is a proliferative disease of the trophoblast. It occurs in about 1 per 1700 pregnancies in the United States but is much more common in some other parts of the world.[89] GTD may occur with an intrauterine pregnancy or an ectopic pregnancy, or after a spontaneous abortion or full term pregnancy. Most cases of GTD (80%) present as a benign hydatidiform mole. More malignant forms of GTD, invasive mole (12 to 15%) and choriocarcinoma (5 to 8%), may develop after a hydatidiform mole. Hydatidiform moles usually involve the entire placenta but a mole involving only part of the placenta can be associated with a live pregnancy.

Early in pregnancy, GTD may present with vaginal bleeding, uterine size that is too large for dates, persistent severe hyperemesis gravidarum, or early preeclampsia. Sometimes, the first clue to the diagnosis is a markedly elevated serum β-hCG level, usually greater than 100,000 mIU/mL. GTD is often discovered during routine pelvic sonography for pregnancy dating or other indications.

Ultrasound is the preferred modality for diagnosing GTD and both transabdominal and transvaginal sonography are usually diagnostic.[90] The classic finding, described as having a grape-like appearance, is an intrauterine echogenic mass containing diffuse small hypoechoic vesicles. In the first trimester, GTD may not be as obvious and can be confused with an incomplete abortion. In about half of cases of GTD, a theca lutein cyst is seen in the adnexa.

Early diagnosis and prompt treatment is the key to a favorable outcome. A hydatidiform mole usually resolves completely with evacuation of the uterus. Choriocarcinoma can metastasize to the lung, liver, and brain. It is very sensitive to chemotherapy but morbidity and mortality depend on the extent of metastases and early aggressive treatment.

▶ ANATOMIC CONSIDERATIONS

The uterus is located in the center of the true pelvis between the bladder anteriorly and the rectosigmoid colon posteriorly. The uterus is a thick-walled muscular structure that is about 6 to 7 cm long and about 3 to 4 cm in transverse and anterior to posterior (AP) diameters. It is shaped like an inverted pear and the uterine body is the widest portion. The cervix is the narrowest portion and is anchored to the posterior bladder by the parametrium. The cervix meets the vagina at the level of the bladder angle and protrudes into the anterior wall of the vagina. When the uterus is in the normal anteflexed position, the longitudinal axes of the uterus and vagina create an angle of about 90°. The fallopian tubes enter the body of the uterus laterally, in an area called the cornua. The fundus is the most superior portion of the uterine body above the cornua.

The uterine body and fundus lie inside the peritoneal cavity so intraperitoneal potential spaces exist both anterior and posterior to the uterus. The anterior cul-de-sac, between the bladder and uterus, is usually empty but can contain loops of bowel or free fluid. The posterior cul-de-sac, between the uterus and the rectosigmoid colon, is also known as the "pouch of Douglas" and it usually contains bowel loops. The posterior cul-de-sac is the most dependent intraperitoneal region when the patient is supine; therefore, it is the most common site for pooling of free pelvic fluid.

Lateral to the uterus, the peritoneal reflection forms the two layers of the broad ligament. The broad ligament extends from the uterus to the lateral pelvic sidewalls. The fallopian tubes extend laterally from the body of the uterus in the upper free margin of the broad ligament. The ovaries are attached to the posterior surface of the broad ligament. They are also attached to the body of the uterus by the ovarian ligaments and to the lateral pelvic sidewalls by the suspensory ligaments of the ovary. Normal ovaries are about 2 cm wide and 3 cm long. The ovaries are usually located in a depression on the lateral pelvic walls called the ovarian fossa. However, since the ligaments are not rigid structures, the ovaries may be seen in a number of other locations, especially in women who have previously been pregnant.

▶ TECHNIQUE AND NORMAL ULTRASOUND FINDINGS

Transabdominal and transvaginal sonography are complimentary imaging techniques and should be used together. In general, transvaginal imaging should not be performed without also performing a transabdominal scan. Transvaginal imaging allows the probe tip to be placed very close to the organ of interest so that high-frequency probes can be used to generate high-resolution images. However, transvaginal probes have a limited field of view and objects more than a few cm away from the probe tip may not be seen. Transabdominal sonography uses lower frequency probes so the field of view is much larger and a better overview of pelvic structures can be obtained. The main drawback of transabdominal scanning is that the resolution is lower, so details of small pelvic structures are not discernible, particularly ovaries and early pregnancies.

Normal Nonpregnant Pelvis

Transabdominal Scanning

Transabdominal scanning is usually accomplished using a 3.5 to 5 MHz ultrasound probe. The bladder is used as a window in transabdominal scanning, so the bladder should be full to obtain optimal images. In the emergency setting, transabdominal scanning is often done without a full bladder because it is not practical to have patients drink fluid and wait for an hour while their bladders fill. High-quality images are usually obtained without bladder filling in thin women and those with an anteflexed uterus. Gentle pressure on the probe can also be used to produce good quality transabdominal images without filling the bladder.

The best transabdominal view for evaluating the uterus and its contents is the standard midline sagittal view (Figure 11–2). To obtain this view, the probe is placed on the abdominal wall in the midline just above the pubic bone, with the marker-dot pointing cephalad (Figure 11–3). By convention, the marker-dot on the probe should correlate with the left side of the monitor so that in sagittal images cephalad structures are on the left side. This view provides a longitudinal image of the uterus and the entire midline stripe should be visible. The cervix is seen just posterior to the bladder angle with the body of the uterus to the left of the angle and the vaginal stripe to the right. The ovaries may be seen by sliding the probe laterally, with the marker-dot still pointing cephalad, and aiming the beam toward the contralateral adnexa, using the

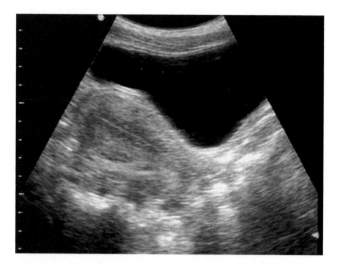

Figure 11–2. Transabdominal midline sagittal ultrasound view of the normal pelvis.

bladder as a window. Sometimes when the bladder is very full or a large pelvic mass is present, better images can be obtained by placing the probe directly over the adnexa.

It may be easier to visualize the ovaries and other adnexal structures with the standard transabdominal transverse view (Figure 11–4). This view is obtained by placing the probe in the midline of the abdominal wall just above the pubic bone, with the marker-dot pointing to the patient's right side (Figure 11–5). This view provides a transverse image of the uterus and allows the midline of the uterus and the adjacent adnexa to be seen in the same image. In transverse images, anatomic structures have the same orientation as on a CT scan: right-sided structures are on the left side of the monitor and left-sided structures are on the right. To examine the entire pelvis in transverse planes, the probe should be kept in the midline suprapubic region with the marker-dot pointed to the patients right and the beam should be aimed caudad and cephalad. This motion will allow the uterus to be viewed in transverse sections from the cervix to the fundus respectively.

The ovaries are most commonly found between the body of the uterus and the pelvic sidewall (see Figure 11–4B). In their normal location, the ovaries are bound posteriorly by the internal iliac artery and superiorly by the external iliac vein. These structures can be identified and used to help locate the ovaries. Normal ovaries appear as small discrete hypoechoic structures. Individual ovarian follicles are often not visible with transabdominal imaging. Normal ovaries are not always seen with transabdominal sonography because they are relatively small and may be camouflaged by bowel or other surrounding structures with similar echogenicity. However, adnexal masses are often larger and very easy to identify with transabdominal imaging (see Figure 11–4C).

Transvaginal Sonography

Transvaginal scanning is different from other ultrasound techniques because the ultrasound probe is placed inside the vagina and very close to the organs of interest. Transvaginal sonography is accomplished using a specialized probe with a 5 to 7.5 MHz transducer. The probe has a marker-dot, similar to other ultrasound probes, which should correlate to the left side of the monitor screen. The sound beams may emanate straight out from the tip of the probe (end-fire) or at an angle from the tip of the probe (offset). End-fire probes are more versatile and make imaging planes easier to understand. This dis-

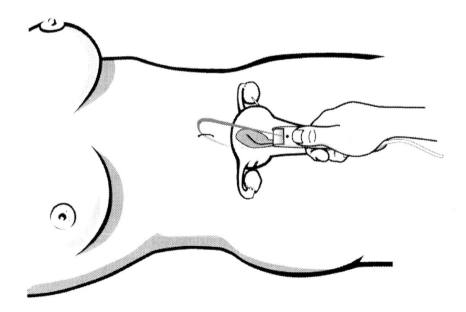

Figure 11–3. Probe position for the transabdominal midline sagittal view. The marker dot is pointed cephalad.

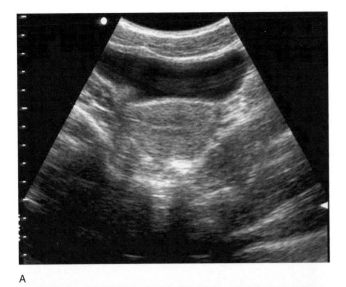

A

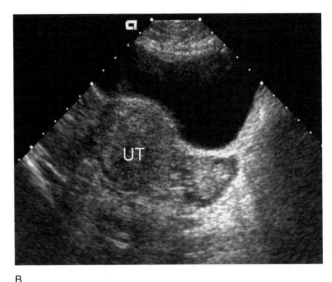

B

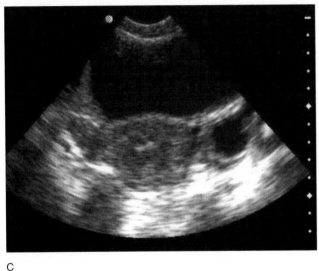

C

Figure 11–4. (A) Transabdominal transverse ultrasound view of the normal pelvis. (B) Transabdominal transverse ultrasound view of the left ovary. UT = uterus. Transabdominal transverse ultrasound view of the uterus and both ovaries. (C) The right ovary is small and of similar echogenicity as the uterus, the left ovary is more prominent due to a contained cyst. *(Courtesy of James Mateer, MD.)*

cussion of scanning planes will assume that an end-fire probe is being used.

Before the transvaginal probe is used, it must be thoroughly cleansed and covered by a rubber or vinyl sheath. Conducting gel should be placed inside the sheath before the probe is covered so that air bubbles in the tip of the sheath are eliminated. Many sonographers use specially made latex condoms as probe covers, but these are usually too big and allow air bubbles into the tip. Many sonographers prefer to use vinyl gloves as probe covers since they provide a better fit and allow less air into the tip.[91] Water-based lubricant, not conducting gel, should be used to lubricate the outside of the sheath before insertion into the vagina. Ultrasound conducting gel may be irritating to the vaginal mucosa.

Patients should empty their bladder before transvaginal scanning is performed. A full bladder will straighten the angle between the uterus and vagina and move the body of the uterus away from the probe. Patient posi-

tioning is important in obtaining good transvaginal scans. The operator must be able to aim the probe anterior enough to see the fundus of an anteverted uterus. Scanning is best accomplished while the patient is in lithotomy stirrups or by elevating her pelvis on a pillow while she is in a frog-leg position. Many clinicians prefer to use lithotomy stirrups and perform transvaginal sonography as part of their pelvic examination, after the speculum and bimanual examinations.

Before inserting the transvaginal probe, the procedure should be explained to the patient. It is usually best to explain that transvaginal sonography is similar to the bimanual pelvic examination but visual rather than tactile information is obtained. Transvaginal sonography should not be painful and is usually very well tolerated by patients. Anxious patients may be given the option of inserting the probe into the vagina themselves.

The probe is initially inserted with the marker-dot pointed toward the ceiling (Figures 11–6 and 11–7). The

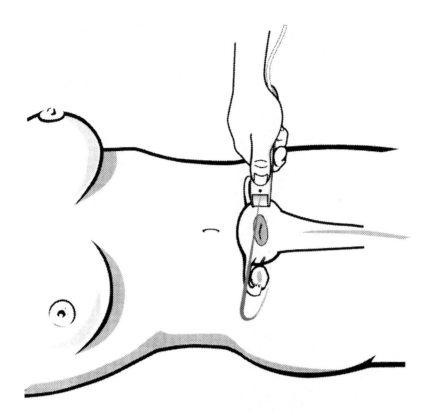

Figure 11–5. Probe position for the transabdominal transverse view. The marker dot is pointed toward the patient's right side.

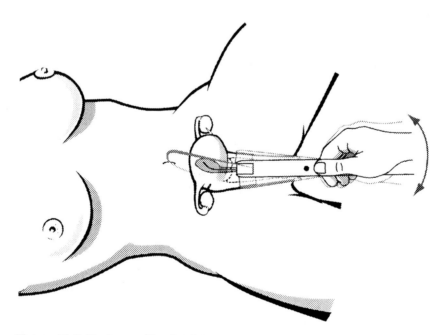

Figure 11–6. Probe position for the transvaginal saggital view. The marker dot is pointed toward the ceiling.

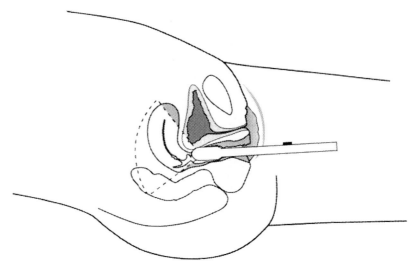

Figure 11–7. Probe position for the transvaginal saggital view. The marker dot is pointed toward the ceiling.

uterus is easily recognized upon insertion of the probe. This is the standard transvaginal sagittal view; it produces a longitudinal image of the uterus similar to the trans-abdominal sagittal view but rotated 90° counterclockwise (Figure 11–8). The entire uterine midline stripe should be seen in this view. If the uterus is not seen immediately, then it may be extremely anteverted and the probe should be aimed upward toward the anterior abdominal wall, keeping the marker-dot pointed toward the ceiling. Lateral movement of the probe can be used to scan from side to side through the entire pelvis (see Figure 11–6). The uterus appears as a relatively hypoechoic structure with thick walls and a well-defined border. The

endometrial midline stripe is thin during the initial proliferative (preovulatory) phase (see Figure 11–8) and progressively thickens and becomes more echogenic during the secretory (postovulatory) phase of the menstrual cycle (Figures 11–9 and 11–10). The cervix can be seen by pulling the probe back a few cm and aiming the probe tip downward toward the patient's back (Figure 11–11). In this view, the posterior cul-de-sac should be inspected for any evidence of free fluid.

After the uterus is identified, the ovaries can be found by their position relative to the uterus. They are usually found just lateral and posterior to the body of the uterus, between the uterus and the lateral pelvic wall.

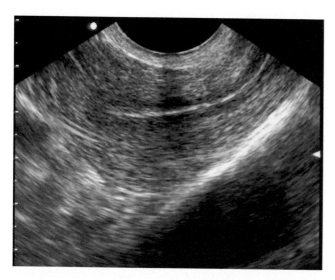

Figure 11–8. Transvaginal midline sagittal ultrasound view of the normal pelvis. The thin endometrial stripe represents the early proliferative phase.

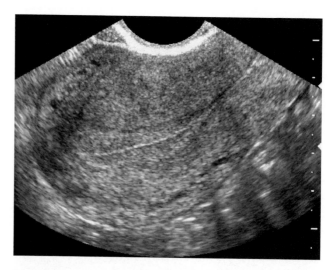

Figure 11–9. Transvaginal midline sagittal ultrasound of the uterus during the late proliferative menstrual phase. The endometrial stripe is slightly thickened, but not very echogenic.

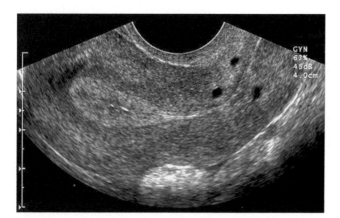

Figure 11–10. Transvaginal midline sagittal ultrasound of the uterus during the secretory menstrual phase. The endometrium is thickened and echogenic. Three nabothian cysts are seen in the cervix.

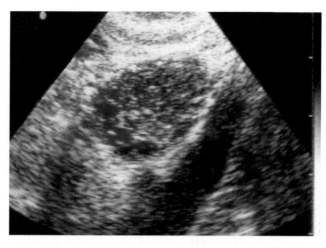

Figure 11–12. Transvaginal view of a normal left ovary. The ovary is recognized by the oval shape, peripheral follicles, and echogenicity similar to the myometrium of the uterus. This ovary is adjacent to the iliac vein. *(Courtesy of James Mateer, MD.)*

The sonographic appearance of the ovaries is distinct. They are relatively hypoechoic structures containing multiple anechoic follicles (Figures 11–12 and 11–13). To find the ovaries in sagittal oblique planes, the probe is aimed laterally, with the marker-dot still toward the ceiling (see Figure 11–6). The internal iliac artery and external iliac vein can often be identified and used as a guide because the normal position of the ovary is adjacent to these structures (Figures 11–14). Sometimes the ovaries cannot be identified with transvaginal sonography.[92]

The standard transvaginal coronal view may be better for surveying the entire pelvis. This view is obtained by turning the marker-dot toward the patient's right side (Figures 11–15 and 11–16). The coronal view gives a transverse image of the uterus and allows the uterus and ovaries to be seen in the same plane. The entire pelvis can be explored with oblique coronal planes by aiming the probe up toward the anterior abdominal wall and down toward the patient's back, keeping the marker-dot pointing toward the patient's right side (Figure 11–17).

Transvaginal sonography is a dynamic imaging technique. To visualize structures, they need to be very close to the tip of the probe. When structures are not readily visualized, operators should use their free hand to palpate the patient's anterior abdominal wall, similar to performing a bimanual pelvic examination.[24,57,91] Pressure on the anterior abdominal wall will often bring an ovary or mass into the field of view. Also, the abdominal hand and the transvaginal probe can be used together to ma-

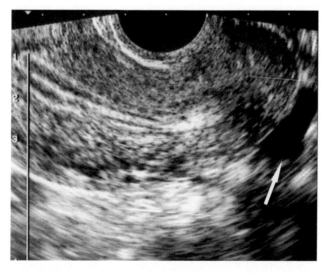

Figure 11–11. Transvaginal sagittal view of the uterine body and cervix. A small (physiologic) fluid collection is present in the posterior cul-de-sac (arrow).

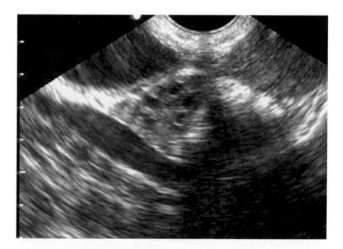

Figure 11–13. Transvaginal view of a normal ovary. This ovary (center of the image) is surrounded by the bladder (above left), iliac vein (below), intestine with gas and shadows (below-right) and the uterus (above-right).

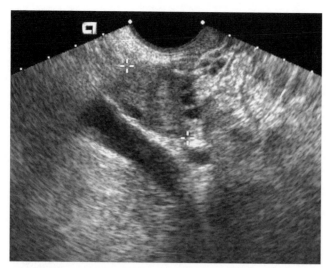

Figure 11–14. Transvaginal ultrasound of the normal right ovary in long axis. The external iliac vein is below and to the left of the ovary on the image while a cross section of the internal iliac artery (or vein) is directly below and to the right. *(Courtesy of James Mateer, MD; Waukesha Memorial Hospital.)*

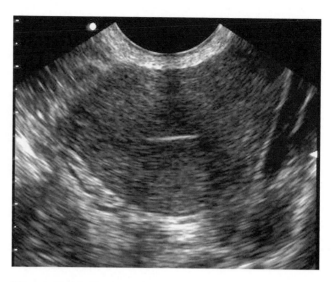

Figure 11–16. Transvaginal coronal ultrasound view of the normal pelvis.

nipulate pelvic contents and observe how the organs move in relation to one another. An ovary may be easier to identify if it is seen as a discrete structure moving independently from adjacent loops of bowel. Also, structures that appear as complex masses may be comprised of multiple smaller structures that move independent of each other. Holding the transvaginal probe very still and observing for bowel peristalsis is a good method for differentiating bowel from other pelvic structures. Finally,

the tip of the transvaginal probe can be used to try to localize pelvic pain. This may help the physician narrow the differential diagnosis when a mass or other abnormality is visualized.

Although several standard imaging planes have been described, the pelvis can often be scanned without being concerned about specific planes. Once an organ or mass is identified, the probe can be turned in any direction that helps the operator obtain better images. Also, as long as the entire pelvis is imaged in a systematic organized manner, the use of specific planes is probably not crucial.[93]

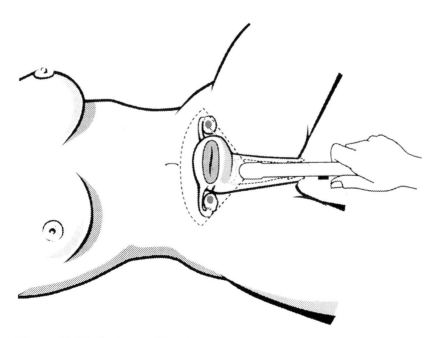

Figure 11–15. Probe position for the transvaginal coronal view. The marker dot is pointed toward the patient's right side.

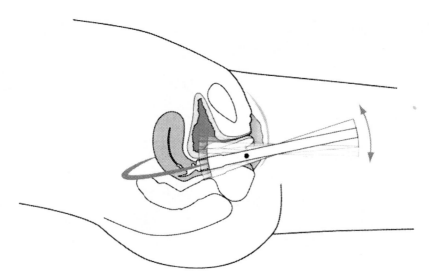

Figure 11–17. Probe position for the transvaginal coronal view. The marker dot is pointed toward the patient's right side.

Normal Early Pregnancy

Both transvaginal and transabdominal sonography can be used to detect an early intrauterine pregnancy. Transvaginal ultrasound can identify an intrauterine pregnancy at about 5 weeks gestational age (3 weeks postconception), about 7 to 10 days earlier than transabdominal ultrasound. The convention when referring to the age of a pregnancy is gestational age, which is the date from conception plus 2 weeks. An approximate correlation can be made between gestational age, β-hCG level, and pelvic ultrasound findings (Table 11–1).[2,24,47,57,94–100]

Transvaginal sonography is now the standard modality for evaluating early pregnancy. The following descriptions pertain to transvaginal sonography, except where specifically noted. The transvaginal technique is referred to as "endovaginal" sonography by some investigators. The first sonographic sign of early pregnancy, the intradecidual sign, can be seen at 4 to 5 weeks (Figure 11–18). The intradecidual sign is a small sac, only a few mm in diameter, which is completely embedded within the endometrium on one side of the uterine midline, not deforming the midline stripe.[24,94,101] There is a focal echogenic thickening of endometrium surrounding the sac. The intradecidual sign can only be seen using a high-resolution technique (5 MHz or higher) and is not an accurate indicator of intrauterine pregnancy.[101]

A gestational sac can be clearly identified at about 5 weeks. With transvaginal sonography, a gestational sac can be seen in most patients with β-hCG levels of 1000 to 2000 mIU/mL and in all patients with levels above 2000 mIU/mL.[95] A gestational sac is characterized by a sonolucent center (chorionic sac) surrounded by a thick symmetric echogenic ring, known as the chorionic rim. This finding is seen in most intrauterine pregnancies but can also be seen surrounding a pseudogestational sac associated with an ectopic pregnancy.[57] Doppler ultrasound can be used to measure peritrophoblastic flow to distinguish a true gestational sac from a pseudogestational sac.[102] However, since this is outside the realm of

▶ **TABLE 11–1.** CORRELATION OF GESTATIONAL AGE, β-HCG LEVEL, AND PELVIC ULTRASOUND FINDINGS

Gestational Age	β-hCG*†‡ (mIU/mL)	Transvaginal U.S. Findings	Transabdominal U.S. Findings
4–5 weeks	< 1,000	Intradecidual sac	N/A
5 weeks	1,000–2,000	Gestational sac (± DDS)	N/A
5–6 weeks	> 2,000	Yolk sac (± embryo)	Gestational sac (± DDS)
6 weeks	10,000–20,000	Embryo with cardiac activity	Yolk sac (± embryo)
7 weeks	> 20,000	Embryonic torso/head	Embryo with cardiac activity

* Significant individual variation in β-hCG levels at a given gestational age may occur.
† In multiple pregnancy (twins, triplets, etc.), β-hCG levels will be much higher at a given gestational age.
‡ β-hCG reference standard is the International Reference Preparation (IRP).

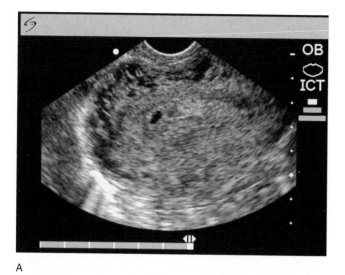

A

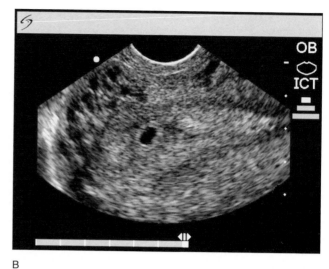

B

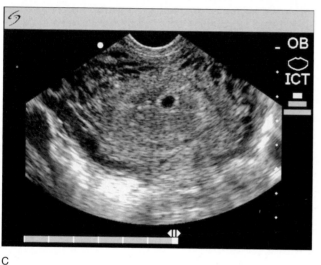

C

Figure 11–18. Intradecidual sign. Longitudinal transvaginal view of the uterus at 7.5 MHz (A). Magnified long axis view of the endometrium shows a 5-mm gestational sac within a slightly thickened endometrium (B). Transverse view of the same patient demonstrates the location within the upper portion of the endometrium and the lack of deformation of the midline stripe (C). All views show a prominent arcuate venous plexus (a variant of normal) within the myometrium of the uterus. *(Courtesy of James Mateer, MD.)*

bedside emergency sonography, identification of a simple gestational sac should not be used as definitive evidence of an intrauterine pregnancy.

Many investigators consider a clear double decidual sign as the first definitive evidence of an intrauterine pregnancy.[24,57,103] The double decidual sign is two concentric echogenic rings surrounding a gestational sac (Figure 11–19). The inner ring is the same structure as the chorionic ring and is called the decidua capsularis. The outer ring is called the decidua vera, derived from the stimulated endometrium of the uterus, while the thin hypoechoic layer between them is the endometrial canal.[24,103,104] A gestational sac with a vague or absent double decidual sign is not diagnostic of an intrauterine pregnancy and may be a pseudogestational sac. If two clear rings are seen, an intrauterine pregnancy is very likely. Unfortunately, the double decidual sign is present in only about half of all intrauterine pregnancies and is not 100% accurate.[105]

The yolk sac is the first structure that can be seen inside the gestational sac. Some investigators consider

the yolk sac the first definitive evidence of intrauterine pregnancy.[47,94] It is probably prudent for inexperienced sonographers to visualize the yolk sac before making a diagnosis of an intrauterine pregnancy, avoiding misinterpretation of more subtle findings like the double decidual sign. The yolk sac is a symmetric circular echogenic structure at the edge of the gestational sac (Figure 11–20). The yolk sac has a role in the transfer of nutrients to the embryo during the first trimester and early hematopoiesis takes place there. The yolk sac can first be seen by transvaginal sonography at about 5 to 6 weeks and then shrinks and disappears by about 12 weeks.[106]

The embryo appears as a thickening or small mass that is seen at the margin of the yolk sac between 5 and 6 weeks (Figure 11–21). The normal embryo will grow rapidly, about 1 mm per day. The embryo can first be seen when it is only 2 to 3 mm and cardiac activity may not be detectable initially. By 6 weeks, the embryo is a distinct structure separate from the yolk sac. Also, the tiny vitelline duct, which connects the yolk sac to the base of

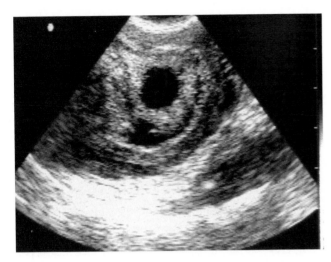

Figure 11–19. Double decidual sign surrounding an intrauterine gestational sac. Normal early pregnancy. Transvaginal image. This sign is often subtle and usually only noticeable along one side of the gestational sac but is very distinct in this example. *(Courtesy of James Mateer, MD.)*

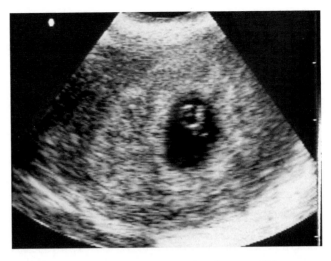

Figure 11–21. Small embryo and yolk sac within an intrauterine gestational sac. The 5-mm embryo is positioned along the right side of the yolk sac in this image and cardiac pulsations were visible during real time sonography. Transvaginal image at 7.5 MHz. *(Courtesy of James Mateer, MD.)*

the cord, can sometimes be seen between the yolk sac and the embryo.

Cardiac activity should be detected within the embryo at about 6 weeks. Any embryo measuring greater than 5 mm should have cardiac activity when transvaginal sonography is used At 7 weeks, the embryo will be about 12 mm and the head of the embryo will be clearly distinguished. At this age, the embryo's head contains a single, large cerebral ventricle and has an appearance similar to the yolk sac.[57] At 8 weeks, the head of the embryo is about the same size as the yolk sac and

limb buds begin to appear (Figure 11–22). Also, the physiologic midgut herniation can be visualized as an echogenic mass anterior to the trunk of the embryo. The bowel becomes intraabdominal and the hernia disappears by 12 weeks. At 8 weeks and beyond, a thin echogenic line, the amnionic sac, may be seen surrounding the embryo.

At 10 weeks, organogenesis is complete and the embryo is now referred to as a fetus (Figure 11–23). Between 10 weeks and the end of the first trimester, the contours of the fetus become much more obvious. The fingers and toes can be identified and counted. Limb movements can be observed and bones and joints can be recognized. In

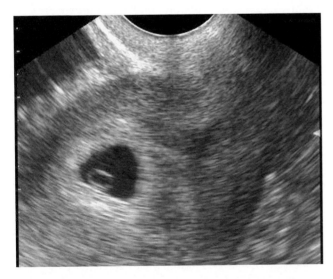

Figure 11–20. Yolk sac within an intrauterine gestational sac. Normal early pregnancy. Transvaginal image.

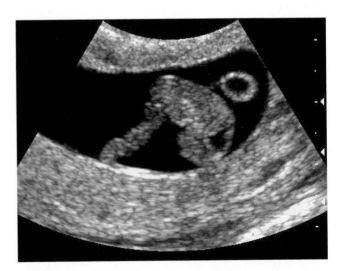

Figure 11–22. Intrauterine embryo and yolk sac. Normal pregnancy at 8 weeks. Transvaginal image.

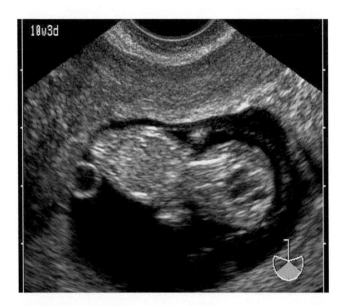

Figure 11–23. Intrauterine embryo and yolk sac with amnion surrounding the embryo. Normal pregnancy at 10 weeks. Transvaginal image.

the head, the falx cerebri becomes very distinct and the prominent choroid plexus can be seen in each of the lateral ventricles. The kidneys and bladder can be evaluated at 12 weeks. The heart and the stomach can also be identified inside the trunk and a four-chamber heart can be recognized by the end of the first trimester. Finally, the face and palate can be easily recognized late in the first trimester.

Routine screening for fetal abnormalities is not commonly performed during the first trimester; the optimal time for this is at 18 to 20 weeks. However, some obvious abnormalities may be identified and it is important to know which structures are usually seen during the first trimester. There is some utility to evaluating nuchal thickness with transvaginal sonography, between 11 and 14 weeks, as a screening test for exomphalos and trisomies 18 and 13, but this is outside the realm of emergency bedside sonography.

Pregnancy Dating
Measurements of both the gestational sac and the embryo are accurate in the first trimester. Tables and formulas are available for calculating the gestational age using these measurements.[2,107] However, modern ultrasound software automatically calculates gestational age when calipers are placed on the structures of interest.

The earliest measurement that can be used for pregnancy dating is mean sac diameter (MSD) of the gestational sac. MSD is the average of three orthogonal measurements of the gestational sac: (length + width + depth)/3. Pregnancy dating using MSD is only useful at 5 to 6 weeks, when the gestational sac is present but an embryo is not yet seen.

When an embryo is visible, at about 6 weeks, measurement of the crown–rump length (CRL) of the embryo should be used to date the pregnancy[47] (Figure 11–24). When measuring CRL, it is important to measure the maximal embryo length, excluding the yolk sac. Errors can occur when the calipers are not carefully placed at the margins of the embryo. Also, the embryo can flex and extend slightly, changing the measurement. Nevertheless, gestational age determination by CRL is accurate to within 5 to 7 d.[24]

Measurement of the biparietal diameter (BPD) of the fetal skull is used for pregnancy dating at the end of the first trimester and during the second trimester. The BPD is a transverse measurement of the diameter of the skull at the level of the thalamus. The calipers should be positioned from the leading edge of the skull (outer table) on the near side to the leading edge of the skull (inner table) on the far side (Figure 11–25A). Errors can be made by measuring the wrong part of the skull or if the image plane is not a true transaxial section through the fetal head. Pregnancy dating by BPD is also very accurate, especially prior to 20 weeks.[57] If the fetal skull is not in a position for measurement, a femur length is fairly easy to obtain and is also a commonly used measurement during the second trimester (Figure 11–25B and C).

Multiple Pregnancy
Early documentation of the chorionicity and amnionicity of a multiple pregnancy is important because it may be hard to determine later in pregnancy. The significance of these classifications are that dichorionic pregnancies have the lowest morbidity of twin pregnancies while monochorionic and/or monoamniotic gestations

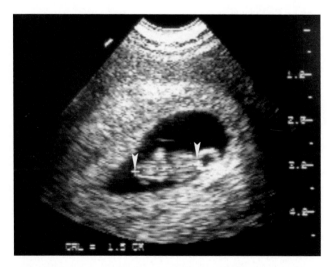

Figure 11–24. Crown rump length. Transvaginal ultrasound that shows proper placement of cursors for CRL measurement. Measure the maximal embryo length, excluding the yolk sac. *(Courtesy of James Mateer, MD).*

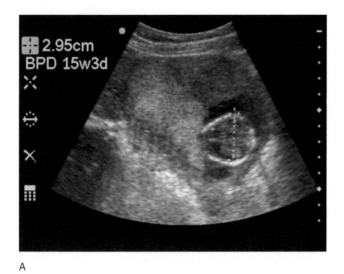

A

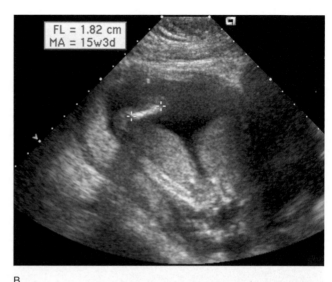

B

C

Figure 11–25. Gestational age measurements. The following measurements can be used for pregnancy dating during the early second trimester and were all obtained on a 15.5-week fetus: Biparietal diameter (A), femur length (B), and crown rump length (C). *(Courtesy of James Mateer, MD; Waukesha Memorial Hospital.)*

have an increasingly higher incidence of morbidity and fetal death.

There are several sonographic criteria that can be used to determine chorionicity and amnionicity in the first trimester. Two gestational (chorionic) sacs separated by deciduas may be seen as early as 6 weeks; this is good evidence of a dichorionic twins (Figure 11–26). Later in the first trimester, dichorionicity can be established by finding a thick septum separating the two chorionic sacs (Figure 11–27). If the septum separating the two pregnancies is thin, then it may be difficult to determine if it is the wall of a chorionic sac or an amnionic membrane. When the septum is thin, identification of a chorionic peak can confirm a dichorionic twin pregnancy. A chorionic peak is a triangular projection of tissue, of the same echogenicity as the placenta, emanating from the placenta and tapering to a point in the intertwin membrane.[24]

The amnionocity of a monochorionic pregnancy can also be determined by first trimester sonography. Count-ing the number of yolk sacs is the easiest way to determine amnionicity; if there are two yolk sacs, then there must be two amnions.[57] After about 8 weeks, amnionic membranes should be visible and diamnionic pregnancies should have a separate amnion surrounding each twin.

▶ COMMON AND EMERGENT ABNORMALITIES

Ectopic Pregnancy

Definite Ectopic Pregnancy

A live extrauterine embryo with cardiac activity can be seen with transvaginal sonography in about 15 to 20% of ectopic pregnancies (Figure 11–28).[51,53] An extrauterine gestational sac containing an embryo or yolk sac is also diagnostic and is seen in a significant percentage of ectopic pregnancies (Figure 11–29).[53]

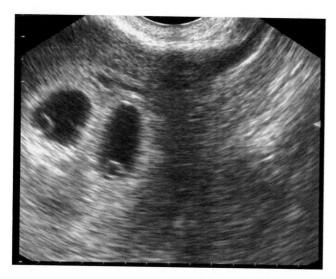

Figure 11–26. Dichorionic twins. Two chorionic sacs and two yolk sacs are clearly seen. Transvaginal image.

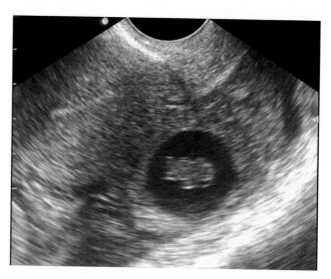

Figure 11–28. Ectopic pregnancy. Living embryo in the adnexa and empty uterus (endometrial echo is visible in the left upper portion of the image). Embryonic cardiac activity was present on real-time imaging. Transvaginal image.

NONSPECIFIC SIGNS OF ECTOPIC PREGNANCY: FREE FLUID, TUBAL RING, AND COMPLEX MASS.

There are several nonspecific sonographic findings that are not diagnostic but highly suggestive of an ectopic pregnancy in pregnant patients with an empty uterus (Table 11–2).[22,48,49,51–53,108–110] Some of these findings are subtle and can be easily missed, especially if transvaginal sonography is not available or an inexperienced sonographer performs the scan. Therefore, emergency physicians should obtain a "formal" ultrasound if no intrauterine pregnancy or ectopic pregnancy is identified with emergency bedside sonography.

FREE PELVIC OR INTRAPERITONEAL FLUID.

Free fluid in the posterior pelvic cul-de-sac or in other intraperitoneal sites is highly suggestive of ectopic pregnancy.[49,52,108] Transvaginal sonography is very sensitive for detecting free fluid in the posterior cul-de-sac (Figure 11–30).[24] Only about one-third of ectopic pregnancies have no free fluid in the cul-de-sac.[111] Also, free fluid is the only abnormal sonographic finding in about

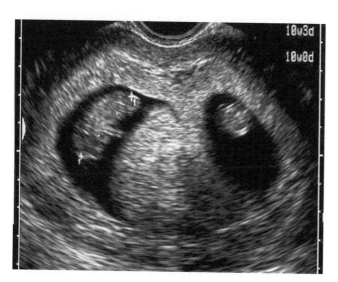

Figure 11–27. Dichorionic twins. Calipers mark the crown-rump length of one of the embryos. Gestational age is 10 weeks 0 days. Transvaginal image.

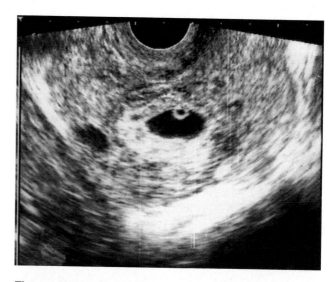

Figure 11–29. Ectopic pregnancy. Extrauterine gestational sac with a bright thick echogenic ring and a yolk sac within. A cursory exam could mistake the surrounding mid-level echoes as uterine tissue, but note the absence of any endometrial echo. Transvaginal image.

▶ **TABLE 11–2.** NONSPECIFIC SONOGRAPHIC SIGNS OF ECTOPIC PREGNANCY

Sonographic Findings	Likelihood of Ectopic Pregnancy (%)
Any free pelvic fluid	52
Complex pelvic mass	75
Moderate or large free pelvic fluid	86
Tubal ring	> 95
Mass and free fluid	97
Hepatorenal free fluid	~100

15% of ectopic pregnancies.[108] The greater the volume of free intraperitoneal fluid, the greater the likelihood of ectopic pregnancy (Figures 11–31, 11–32, and 11–33).[57] In fact, patients with a moderate to large amount of free pelvic fluid have about an 86% chance and those with hepatorenal free fluid have about a 100% chance of having an ectopic pregnancy.[52] Although a large amount of fluid predicts ectopic pregnancy, it is not a reliable indicator of tubal rupture. Only about 60% of those with a large amount of free fluid have a ruptured tube.[49,112] Free fluid may be due to leaking of blood from the end of the fallopian tube, which can occur slowly.

Echogenic fluid is more likely to represent blood and this also increases the chances of an ectopic pregnancy. If bleeding is brisk, clots may be seen in the pelvic cul-de-sac instead of fluid. Although a small amount of hypoechoic free pelvic fluid may be normal, it must be considered suspicious in the setting of a pregnant patient with an empty uterus.[48,49,52,108] The definition of "small amount" is fluid that is confined to the cul-de-sac

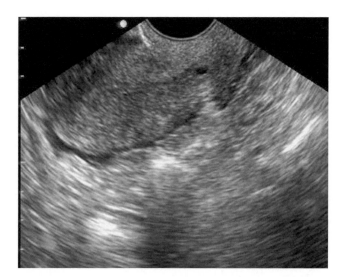

Figure 11–31. Ectopic pregnancy. Empty uterus. A rim of free fluid surrounds the uterus. Transvaginal image.

and covering less than one-third of the inferior posterior uterus. As stated above, anything more than a small amount is almost always associated with an ectopic pregnancy.[49,52,53]

Abdominal sonography of the hepatorenal space (Morison's pouch) should be performed on every patient with a possible ectopic pregnancy.[24,57] Free fluid in the hepatorenal space, or elsewhere outside the pelvis, is evidence of a large amount of intraperitoneal fluid[113] (Figure 11–34). In a pregnant woman with an empty uterus, this must be considered bleeding secondary to an ectopic pregnancy. Finding free fluid in the hepatorenal space with emergency bedside sonography reduces the

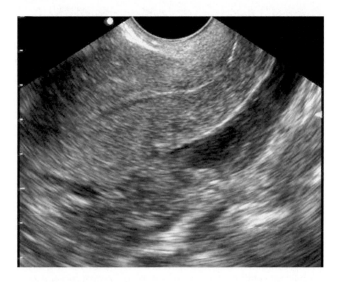

Figure 11–30. Ectopic pregnancy. Empty uterus and free fluid in the posterior cul-de-sac. Transvaginal sagittal image.

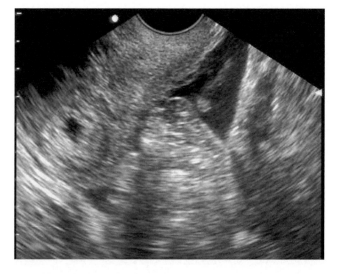

Figure 11–32. Ectopic pregnancy. Tubal ring (2 cm). Free pelvic fluid with floating bowel. Transvaginal image.

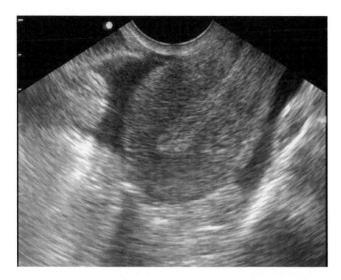

Figure 11–33. Ectopic pregnancy. Free fluid surrounding an empty uterus. Transvaginal image.

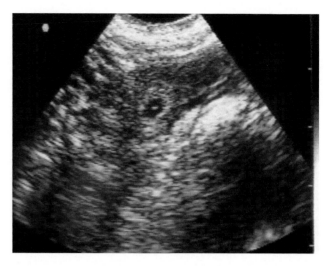

Figure 11–35. Tubal ring. Transvaginal view of the right adnexa shows a tiny (7-mm) brightly echogenic ring-like structure. This was determined to be a very early ectopic pregnancy. *(Courtesy of James Mateer, MD.)*

time to diagnosis and treatment of ectopic pregnancy.[4] A finding of hepatorenal free fluid "should give the surgeon a greater sense of urgency."[24]

TUBAL RING.
A tubal ring is nearly diagnostic of ectopic pregnancy.[51,53,108,109] A tubal ring is a concentric hypoechoic structure found in the adnexa (see Figure 11–32; and 11–35, 11–36). It is created by the trophoblast of the ectopic pregnancy surrounding the chorionic sac and is the equivalent to a gestational sac.[24] A tubal ring has a different sonographic appearance than a corpus luteum cyst or other ovarian cysts because it has a relatively thick and brightly echogenic, round, symmetric wall. Ovarian cysts have walls of varying thickness and are surrounded by

normal ovarian follicles. With transvaginal sonography, it may be possible to identify a tubal ring in more than 60% of ectopic pregnancies.[51,53] When a tubal ring is seen, the likelihood of ectopic pregnancy is greater than 95%.[53]

COMPLEX MASS.
The most common sonographic finding in ectopic pregnancy is a complex adnexal mass (Figures 11–37, 11–38, and 11–39).[44] A complex adnexal mass may represent a tubal hematoma, ectopic trophoblastic tissue, or distorted contents of an ectopic gestational sac.[51–53,57,108,110]

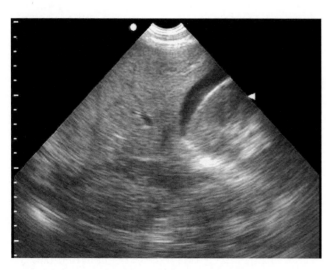

Figure 11–34. Ectopic pregnancy. Free fluid in the hepatorenal space. Transabdominal image.

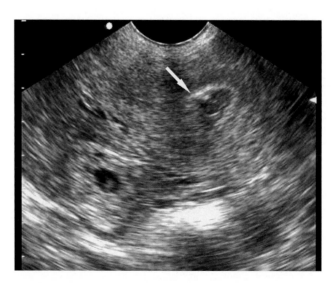

Figure 11–36. Ectopic pregnancy. Pseudogestational sac in the uterus (arrow) and 2.5-cm brightly echogenic tubal ring in the adnexa. Transvaginal image.

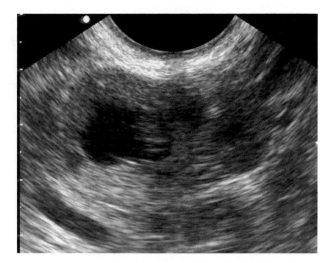

Figure 11–37. Ectopic pregnancy. Complex right adnexal mass located above the iliac vein on the image. Transvaginal technique.

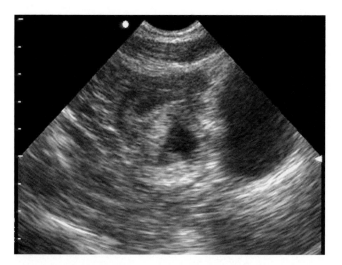

Figure 11–39. Ectopic pregnancy. A complex mass is adjacent to the bladder on this oblique trans-abdominal image.

A complex mass contains a mixture of cystic and solid components. This is a sensitive sonographic sign of ectopic pregnancy. When an experienced sonographer performs a transvaginal scan, it may be seen in up to 85% of cases.[53] However, a complex mass may be subtle and easily missed.[57] The mass may blend into adjacent structures with similar echogenicity and may have an appearance similar to the bowel or ovaries.

Several sonographic signs may help to differentiate a complex mass from the surrounding pelvic structures. Identifying the ovaries and then searching between the ovaries and the uterus is the best technique for locating an adnexal mass. To differentiate a mass from other pelvic

structures, examiners should press down on the patient's lower abdomen with the free hand during transvaginal scanning, in a manner similar to performing a bimanual pelvic examination. This will cause pelvic structures to move in relation to one another and examiners can recognize a mass as a separate structure, moving independently from the ovary and bowel. Also, if the transvaginal probe is held very still, peristalsis of the bowel can be seen, differentiating it from other pelvic structures.

Color Doppler has been used in an attempt to separate surrounding structures from an adnexal mass. High-velocity, low-impedance trophoblastic flow can sometimes be seen surrounding an ectopic sac; this is referred to as the "ring of fire."[114] However, color Doppler provides little additional information and is not more accurate than grayscale sonography for determining if an adnexal mass is an ectopic pregnancy.[24,82,115]

Pregnancy Loss

Embryonic Demise

There are several sonographic signs that can reliably predict embryonic demise. The earliest sign is a gestational sac without a yolk sac or embryo (Figure 11–40). With high-resolution transvaginal sonography (at or above 6.5 MHz), a yolk sac is usually seen within the gestational sac when MSD is 10 mm or greater and an embryo is usually seen when MSD is 16 mm or greater.[24,97,116,117] However, with a 5 MHz transvaginal probe or with transabdominal scanning, a yolk sac may not be seen until the MSD is 20 mm or larger.[57,118,119] For the purposes of emergency bedside transvaginal sonography, an empty gestational sac of 20 mm or larger is a good predictor of embryonic demise; this is commonly referred to as a blighted ovum but more accurately called early embryonic demise.

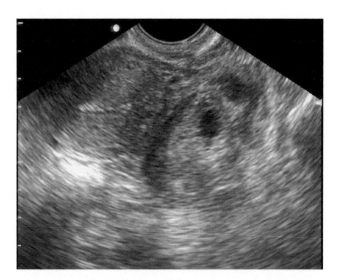

Figure 11–38. Ectopic pregnancy. An empty uterus is seen in transverse transvaginal view and is identified by the endometrial stripe. The complex mass is in the left adnexa and adjacent to the uterus.

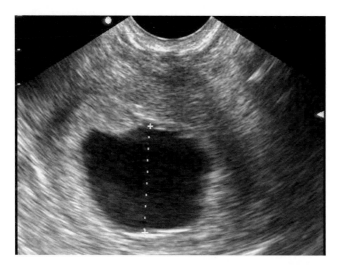

Figure 11–40. Early embryonic demise. Large (3-cm) empty intrauterine sac consistent with a "blighted ovum." Transvaginal image.

Another good indicator of embryonic demise is lack of embryonic cardiac activity (Figure 11–41). With transvaginal sonography, cardiac activity should be seen in all embryos greater than 5 mm long by crown–rump length.[24,57,74,120] With transabdominal sonography, cardiac activity should be seen in all embryos greater than 10 mm long.[57] When searching for embryonic cardiac activity it is important to be sure that the embryo is clearly seen. This is easier at 7 to 8 weeks when the embryonic head and torso can be identified. Also, it is essential to use a high-frame rate and turn off the frame-averaging mode when looking for cardiac activity.[24]

Several more subtle signs are also suggestive of embryonic demise or poor fetal outcome. Embryonic bradycardia predicts a poor prognosis.[121,122] The normal heart rate for an embryo longer than 5 mm by crown–rump length (6.3 weeks gestational age) is greater than 120 beats per min (bpm).[121] The lower the heart rate is below 120 bpm, the lower the survival rate of the embryo. Embryos longer than 5 mm with heart rates below 100 bpm have a survival rate of only 6%.[121] Very early pregnancies, with embryos less than 5 mm in length, normally have slower heart rates, but a rate less than 80 bpm is nearly always associated with embryonic demise.[121,122]

An abnormal yolk sac is another subtle sign of demise or abnormal pregnancy. A very small yolk sac (less than 2 mm diameter) between 8 and 12 weeks is usually associated with an abnormal pregnancy.[123] A very large yolk sac (more than 6 mm diameter) between 5 and 12 weeks is predictive of embryonic demise or a significant chromosomal abnormality.[24,124] Also, prior to 12 weeks, inability to visualize the yolk sac when an embryo is clearly present is strong evidence of impending embryonic demise.[124] Yolk sac shape is not associated with adverse

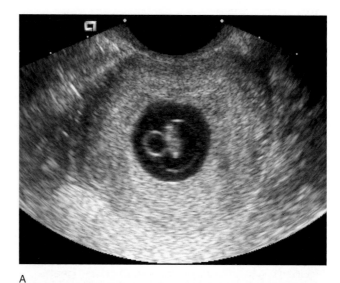

A

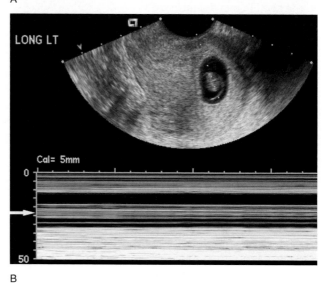

B

Figure 11–41. Embryonic demise. Transvaginal image of the fetal pole which measured 7 weeks via CRL (A). The yolk sac appears slightly enlarged and the amnion is clearly visible. There was no cardiac activity on real time sonography and this was documented by the M-mode exam (B). Note the lack of any motion in the fetal band (arrow). *(Courtesy of James Mateer, MD; Waukesha Memorial Hospital.)*

pregnancy outcome. Pregnancies with a normal size but irregularly shaped yolk sac have a normal outcome in nearly all cases.[24]

An odd-shaped or grossly distorted gestational sac is reportedly a good indicator of pregnancy failure, but this finding is subjective (Figure 11–42).[118] A gestational sac low in the uterus, with or without a yolk sac or embryo, is generally considered a sign of inevitable abortion (Figures 11–43 and 11–44). Also, a weakly echogenic or thin (less than 2 mm wide) trophoblastic reaction surrounding a gestational sac may indicate imminent demise.

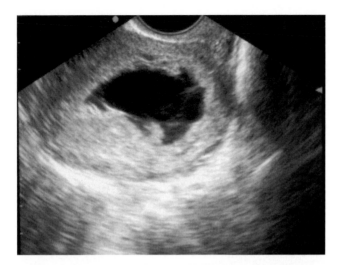

Figure 11–42. Embryonic demise. Distorted gestational sac. Transvaginal image.

Finally, a gestational sac, which is not more than 5 mm MSD larger than the crown–rump length of the embryo, is probably abnormal.[119,125]

Subchorionic hemorrhage is bleeding between the endometrium and chorionic membrane. This is a common finding late in the first trimester and is also known as an implantation hemorrhage as it is believed to occur during this process. Sonographically, part of the chorionic membrane and placenta are separated from the decidua vera (the endometrium) (Figure 11–45).[24] Acutely, the hemorrhage may appear hyperechoic or isoechoic relative to the placenta, with only slight elevation noted. Over the next week or two, the blood becomes hypoechoic. Patients who present with threatened abortion and have a subchorionic hemorrhage probably have a higher inci-

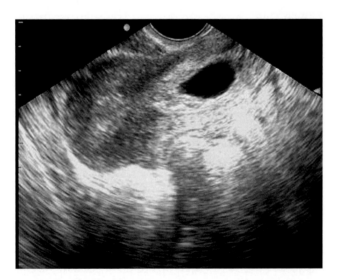

Figure 11–43. Inevitable abortion. The fundus is on the left of the image and the gestational sac is approaching the cervical portion of the uterus. Transvaginal image.

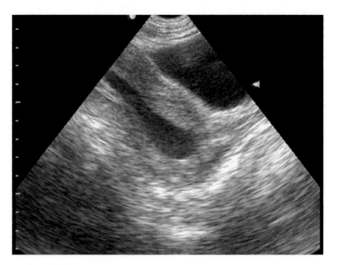

Figure 11–44. Embryonic demise with inevitable abortion. Large empty distorted intrauterine sac that is bulging toward the cervical canal. Transabdominal longitudinal view with the bladder and vaginal stripe along the right side of the image.

dence of embryonic demise.[126,127] Those with large subchorionic hemorrhages may have a much higher rate of pregnancy loss.[127]

Physicians should be conservative when interpreting findings of embryonic demise and give the pregnancy the benefit of the doubt in all cases. Ordering a "formal" ultrasound and obtaining an obstetrics consult is prudent when the diagnosis is unclear.

Completed Spontaneous Abortion

The uterus should be empty after a completed spontaneous abortion (Figure 11–46). A small amount of blood or clot may also be present.

RETAINED PRODUCTS OF CONCEPTION.

Patients with intrauterine echogenic material or a thickened midline stripe (10 mm wide or larger) after a spontaneous abortion probably have retained products of conception (Figure 11–47).[68,70,128] When curettage is performed in such cases, chorionic villi are identified in about 70%.[70] Many patients with retained products will do well with expectant management but they may require curettage and should be followed closely for bleeding and infection.[129]

► COMMON VARIANTS AND SELECTED ABNORMALITIES

Several normal anatomic variants may make transabdominal and transvaginal pelvic sonography more difficult. Retroversion of the uterus occurs in about 10% of women. It has little clinical significance but it makes transabdominal imaging difficult. Retroversion means that the body of

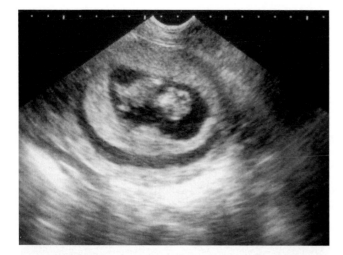

A

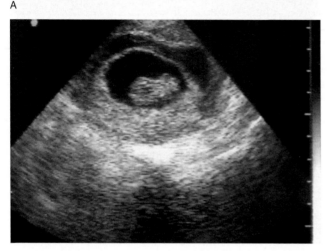

B

Figure 11–45. Subchorionic hemorrhage. (A, B) An echolucent crescent shaped stripe is located between the decidua capsularis and the decidual vera (endometrium) from implantation hemorrhage. Transvaginal images. *(Image B courtesy of James Mateer, MD.)*

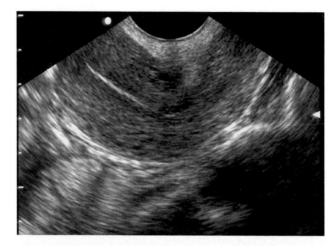

Figure 11–46. Empty uterus after a completed spontaneous abortion. Transvaginal image.

eral and coronal images may be helpful in this situation. When the uterus is deviated laterally, it may displace the ovary out of its usual location. The ovary may then be found superior to the uterus or in the posterior cul-de-sac.

Variation in the location of the ovaries can also make pelvic ultrasound difficult. Transvaginal sonography is needed to visualize most normal ovaries. Even with transvaginal scanning, however, they may be difficult to find. In women who have previously been pregnant, the ovaries may be found lateral, posterior, or superior to the uterus. In patients with an enlarged uterus, those who are pregnant or have uterine fibroids, the ovaries are often displaced superior to the uterus. When the ovaries are superior to the uterus, they are difficult to see with transvaginal sonography.

The fallopian tubes are not normally seen on pelvic ultrasound. If the tubes are filled with fluid secondary to

the uterus bends posterior toward the rectosigmoid colon instead of toward the anterior abdominal wall. The body of the uterus is then too far away from the transabdominal probe and resolution is poor (Figure 11–48A). Transvaginal sonography is much better for imaging a retroverted uterus because the probe can still be placed close to the body of the uterus (Figure 11–48B). When the uterus is retroverted the ovaries usually lie anterior and lateral to the body of the uterus.

Lateral deviation of the uterus is another normal variant that makes pelvic ultrasound difficult. When transabdominal or transvaginal scanning is performed and the uterus is not seen in the midline, then the probe should be aimed laterally, and sagittal oblique images obtained. It is not uncommon to find the body of the uterus bending toward the lateral pelvis. If this is the case, then the midline stripe may be difficult to see in just one plane. Lat-

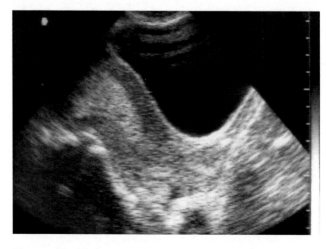

Figure 11–47. Intrauterine echogenic material (2–3 cm thick), consistent with retained products of conception. Transabdominal longitudinal image. *(Courtesy of James Mateer, MD.)*

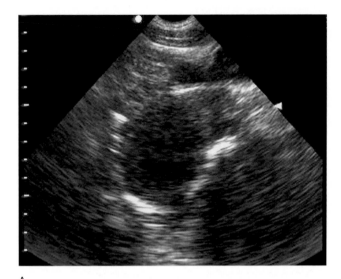

A

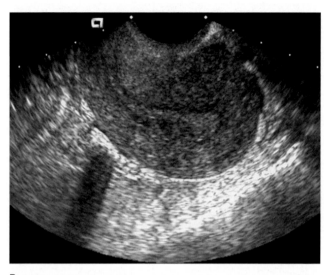

B

Figure 11–48. Transabdominal sagittal view of a retroverted uterus (A). The uterine body and fundus are not well visualized due to the uterine position and empty bladder. A transvaginal longitudinal view of the uterus (B) provides improved resolution. Note that with a retroverted uterus, the fundus is projected to the right side of the image and the cervix to the left. *(Courtesy of James Mateer, MD; Waukesha Memorial Hospital.)*

scarring or pelvic inflammatory disease, then they may be easily recognized. They will be found in the adnexa lateral to the uterine body. When imaged longitudinally, the fallopian tubes will appear as anechoic tubal structures; when imaged transversely, they will appear as cystic structures. If multiple redundant loops of the tube are adjacent to one another, then this may be misinterpreted as a large multicystic mass.

A small amount of fluid in the posterior cul-de-sac can be normal. This fluid may not be seen with transabdominal sonography but is easily visualized with transvaginal imaging (Figure 11–49).

Pelvic Masses

Corpus Luteum Cyst
Corpus luteum cysts are the most common pelvic masses found in early pregnancy. They are usually unilocular and have thin walls (Figures 11–50). Internal hemorrhage may result in internal septations and echogenic material (Figure 11–51).

Figure 11–49. Transvaginal sagittal view of the normal anteflexed uterus. Note that the fundus is displayed on the left side of the monitor. Minimal (physiologic) free fluid can be seen in the posterior cul-de-sac below the cervix. The patient has a moderately prominent arcuate venous plexus, which does not represent free fluid.

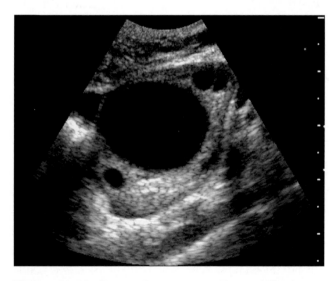

Figure 11–50. Corpus luteum cyst. Transvaginal image.

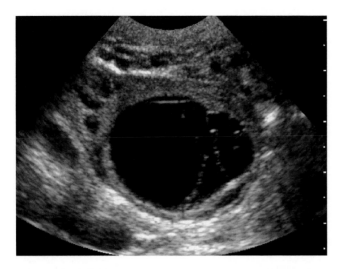

Figure 11–51. Corpus luteum cyst with fine septations from internal hemorrhage. Transvaginal image.

Leiomyomas

Uterine fibroids are very common and may grow during pregnancy. They are located in the uterine wall and have a variable sonographic appearance. They often cause dispersion of ultrasound and distortion of pelvic images (Figure 11–52). (Also see Chapter 13.)

Malignant Pelvic Masses

The most common tumors that enlarge during pregnancy are ovarian cystadenomas. Internal septations and papillary excrescences are suggestive of malignancy (Figure 11–53).

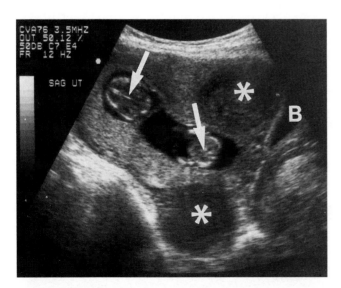

Figure 11–52. Uterine fibroids with pregnancy. Two uterine myomas (*), one posterior and one anterior, are seen in this 13-week pregnancy. Arrows point to fetal head and body. B = bladder. *(Reprinted with permission from Williams Obstetrics, 21st ed. New York: McGraw-Hill, 2001:929.)*

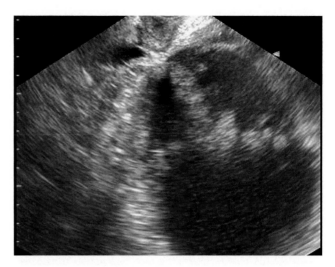

Figure 11–53. Large complex pelvic mass with papillary excrescences and septations. Possible malignancy. Transvaginal image.

Adnexal Torsion

Most cases of adnexal torsion occur in the presence of an enlarged ovary or an ovarian mass. Finding a normal ovary makes the diagnosis much less likely (see Chapter 13).

Gestational Trophoblastic Disease

Most cases of gestational trophoblastic disease present as a benign molar pregnancy. Those with an invasive mole or choriocarcinoma usually have a history of a molar pregnancy. The classic finding is the appearance of a cluster of "grapes," an intrauterine mass with diffuse hypoechoic vesicles (Figures 11–54). The appearance is not always classic in the first trimester and the diagnosis may be missed (Figure 11–55).

▶ PITFALLS

Ectopic Pregnancy

1. *Not performing pelvic sonography because of a recent last menstrual period or a low β-hCG.* Patients with a positive pregnancy test who present with abdominal pain or vaginal bleeding should undergo a pelvic ultrasound examination regardless of their reported last menstrual period or β-hCG level. Patients may misinterpret vaginal spotting during pregnancy for a menstrual period; thus, obtaining a menstrual history is not an accurate method for excluding ectopic pregnancy. Also, it is not uncommon for patients to have a low β-hCG level and a ruptured ectopic pregnancy.

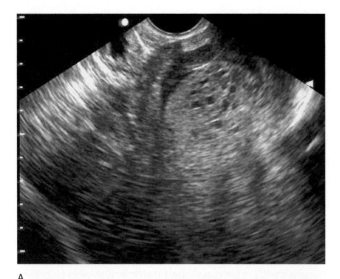

A

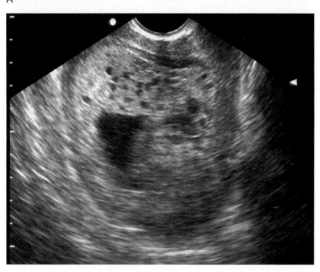

B

Figure 11-54. (A, B) Molar pregnancy. Transvaginal images.

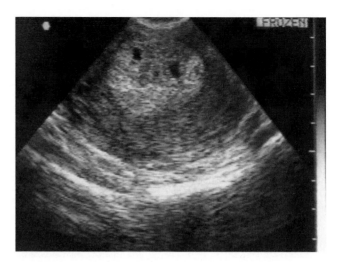

Figure 11-55. Early molar pregnancy. Transverse transvaginal image reveals a thick, echogenic endometrial echo with a few scattered irregular cystic areas in a patient with a high hCG level. *(Courtesy of James Mateer, MD.)*

nancy in most patients. The intradecidual sign and gestational sac are early signs of an intrauterine pregnancy, but neither is 100% reliable.[94,97,101] Sonographers should be careful not to mistake a pseudogestational sac associated with an ectopic pregnancy for a gestational sac.[24,57,102] A pseudo-gestational sac, also known as a decidual cast, is an intrauterine fluid collection surrounded by a single decidual layer (see Figures 11–36 and 11–56). A pseudogestational sac on transabdominal views occurs in up to 5 to 10% of ectopic pregnancies and appears as an elongated and odd-shaped sac in the center of the endometrial

2. *Attributing an empty uterus to a very early intrauterine pregnancy or a completed spontaneous abortion* (see Figure 11–31). More than 40% of ectopic pregnancies have a β-hCG level less than 1000mIU/mL; therefore, an empty uterus with a low β-hCG level should not be considered normal and the entire pelvis should be scanned for signs of an ectopic pregnancy.[55] Also, the only definitive evidence of a completed spontaneous abortion is passage of obvious products of conception or chorionic villi. Without definitive evidence of a completed abortion, the diagnosis of ectopic pregnancy must be ruled out.[40]

3. *Mistaking a pseudogestational sac for a gestational sac*. Visualizing an intrauterine pregnancy essentially excludes the diagnosis of ectopic preg-

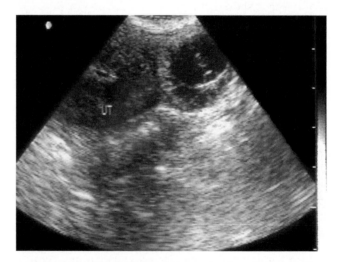

Figure 11-56. Interstitial ectopic. Transverse transvaginal ultrasound reveals a small fluid collection within the endometrium of the uterus. The round echogenic ectopic ring was partially imbedded within the uterine myometrium. *(Courtesy of James Mateer, MD.)*

cavity with inconsistent thickening of the endometrium.[57] A pseudogestational sac can usually be differentiated from a gestational sac using transvaginal sonography.[78] Also, Doppler ultrasound may help by finding high-velocity, low-impedance peritrophoblastic flow surrounding a true gestational sac.[102,114]

4. *Misidentifying an early intrauterine pregnancy.* Clinicians should avoid making the diagnosis of an intrauterine pregnancy when only a small gestational sac is visible. A clear double decidual sign is the first reliable evidence of an intrauterine pregnancy.[24,103] A yolk sac and embryo are obvious signs of an intrauterine pregnancy and should be seen when an inexperienced sonographer makes the diagnosis of an intrauterine pregnancy.[97] Cardiac activity should be seen in all embryos greater than 5 mm long, and this is regarded as the best evidence of an intrauterine pregnancy. It may be prudent for novice sonographers to see cardiac activity before diagnosing an intrauterine pregnancy.

5. *Overestimating the ability to identify subtle signs of ectopic pregnancy.* Although an empty uterus, free intraperitoneal fluid in the hepatorenal space, and free fluid in the pelvis are easy to identify, complex adnexal masses and tubal rings may be subtle. An experienced sonographer should repeat indeterminate bedside scans to look for these subtle signs.

6. *Performing a transvaginal ultrasound without a transabdominal scan.* The transabdominal pelvic view allows a broader view of the pelvis and may detect masses that are outside the field of view of the transvaginal probe. Also, the hepatorenal space should always be scanned to look for free intraperitoneal fluid.[57] Some patients may have minimal symptoms and normal vital signs despite a ruptured ectopic pregnancy with a large amount of intraperitoneal blood.

7. *Identifying a normal appearing pregnancy but not recognizing its location in relation to the uterus.* An ectopic pregnancy may appear to be an intrauterine pregnancy if its extrauterine location is not carefully noted (see Figure 11–29). Also, an interstitial ectopic pregnancy may appear to be intrauterine but careful imaging will reveal that it lies on the margin of the uterine wall and not in the intrauterine cavity. The entire endometrial echo of the uterus should be outlined to determine whether a gestational sac lies within its boundaries. Transabdominal sonography may help to clarify the big picture in cases of possible ectopic pregnancy.

8. *Mistaking an interstitial pregnancy for an intrauterine pregnancy.* An interstitial pregnancy may be mistaken for an intrauterine pregnancy. Interstitial pregnancies comprise about 2 to 5% of all ectopic pregnancies.[57] Most ectopic pregnancies occur in the ampullary segment of the fallopian tube but interstitial ectopic pregnancies occur within the portion of the tube that passes through the wall of the uterus (see Figure 11–56). They are partially enveloped by the myometrium. Because of the rich myometrial blood supply, an interstitial pregnancy can grow larger and rupture later than most ectopic pregnancies. When rupture occurs, intraperitoneal bleeding and vaginal bleeding may be brisk and profuse. Many of these patients exsanguinate and die before reaching the hospital. It may be difficult to identify an interstitial pregnancy because the gestational sac may initially appear to be completely surrounded by the uterus. However, on close inspection, an interstitial pregnancy will be located at the margin of the uterine wall rather than inside the endometrial echo of the uterine cavity. The eccentrically located gestational sac is surrounded by an asymmetric myometrial mantle with a free wall thickness usually less than 8 mm. The "interstitial line sign" is a fine echogenic line extending from the endometrial stripe to the interstitial gestational sac. This finding is diagnostic of an interstitial ectopic pregnancy. If the diagnosis is not made early, prior to rupture, up to 50% of patients may require a hysterectomy.[57]

9. *Failure to identify heterotopic pregnancy.* Failure to obtain a history of fertility medications or in vitro fertilization may lead to this pitfall. The risk of heterotopic pregnancy in such patients is as high as 1%, so finding an intrauterine pregnancy does not exclude the diagnosis of ectopic pregnancy. Also, patients without these risk factors may have a heterotopic pregnancy. Therefore, it is prudent to scan the entire pelvis looking for free pelvic fluid or an adnexal mass, even after an intrauterine pregnancy has been identified.

Other Pitfalls

1. *Fetal anomalies.* Failure to diagnose fetal anomalies by ultrasound has recently become a significant source of malpractice litigation. To avoid this problem, patients should be informed that emergency bedside sonography is a screening examination only and is not designed to detect most embryonic abnormalities.

2. *Embryonic demise.* Many potential pitfalls are associated with the diagnosis of embryonic demise. When poor resolution or poor quality scans are obtained, normal structures may not be visualized,

leading to the errant diagnosis of a blighted ovum. Also, inability to identify embryonic cardiac activity can occur secondary to mistaking another structure for the embryo or using a frame-averaging ultrasound mode. These pitfalls can be avoided by positively identifying the embryo and by using a high-frame rate setting when searching for embryonic cardiac activity. Before the diagnosis of embryonic demise is made, the pregnancy should be given the benefit of the doubt. Sonography by an experienced operator and consultation with obstetrics may be prudent before the patient is informed of the definitive diagnosis.

3. *Multiple pregnancy.* When twins are identified by bedside ultrasound, it is important to inform the patient that about 25% of twin pregnancies diagnosed in the first trimester will become singleton pregnancies by the second trimester.

4. *Pelvic masses.* The most common pitfall when identifying a pelvic mass is neglecting to arrange close follow-up and informing the patient of the finding. Pelvic masses may enlarge during pregnancy and are usually incidental findings on pelvic sonography. Ovarian malignancy may rarely present during pregnancy.

5. *Pelvic pain.* Pelvic pain is a common complaint in early pregnancy. A common pitfall of using pelvic ultrasound in these patients is that the finding of an intrauterine pregnancy often ends the work-up for the etiology of the patient's symptoms. Once ectopic pregnancy is excluded, the patient's pelvic pain may be attributed to the pregnancy and diagnoses such as appendicitis or adnexal torsion may not be considered. Physicians should remember that appendicitis is relatively common in pregnancy and 20% of adnexal torsion occurs during pregnancy.

6. *Gestational trophoblastic disease (GTD).* Advanced molar pregnancy is usually obvious on pelvic ultrasound. However, early in pregnancy, the findings may be subtle. Serum β-hCG will always be very high in GTD. A potential pitfall is assuming that this diagnosis is excluded because it is not seen on bedside ultrasound. Such patients need close follow-up and repeat ultrasound examinations.

► CASE STUDIES

Case 1

Patient Presentation

A 21-year-old woman presented to the emergency department with complaints of vaginal spotting. She reported that her last menstrual period was 5 weeks ago. She denied any abdominal or pelvic pain or urinary symptoms. She stated that she had an ectopic pregnancy treated with methotrexate 1 year ago and that she had not been taking any fertility medications.

On physical examination, her blood pressure was 122/68 mm Hg, heart rate was 88 beats per min, respirations 18 per min; and temperature was 37.2°C. She was resting comfortably. Her head, neck, pulmonary, cardiovascular, and back examinations were unremarkable. Abdominal examination revealed a soft, nontender, scaphoid abdomen. Genitourinary examination revealed a closed cervical os with a trace amount of dark blood in the vaginal vault. No uterine, adnexal, or ovarian masses were noted. There was no cervical motion tenderness or adnexal tenderness.

Management Course

Her urine pregnancy test was positive. Transabdominal ultrasound examination revealed a small intrauterine sac without a double decidual sac sign and the hepatorenal view was normal. Transvaginal sonography revealed an intrauterine pregnancy with a gestational sac and a double decidual sac sign. A yolk sac was also seen within the gestational sac (see Figure 11–20). Also, normal appearing ovaries were identified bilaterally and there was no fluid in the pelvis. A blood type was ordered and subsequently found to be A negative. The patient was given 50 μg of intramuscular Rh immune globulin. The risk of spontaneous abortion was explained to the patient. Obstetrical follow up was arranged in 1 week and she was instructed to return for increased vaginal bleeding or passage of fetal tissue.

Commentary

Case 1 was an example of a patient with an intrauterine pregnancy that was identified with transvaginal ultrasound. She had a significant risk factor for an ectopic pregnancy so this diagnosis needed to be evaluated. An intrauterine sac was seen with transabdominal sonography but this was not diagnostic of an intrauterine pregnancy and did not exclude ectopic pregnancy. Transvaginal sonography allowed a more detailed view of the intrauterine structures and a definitive diagnosis of intrauterine pregnancy, which essentially ruled out an ectopic pregnancy.

Case 2

Patient Presentation

A 32-year-old woman presented to the emergency department with complaints of syncope, weakness, and nausea. She was confused and could not remember when her last menstrual period was. She denied any significant pain.

On physical examination, her blood pressure was 80/42 mm Hg, heart rate was 88 beats per min, respirations were 24 per min, and temperature was 37°C. The patient was diaphoretic and appeared uncomfortable.

Her head, neck, pulmonary, and back examinations were unremarkable. Cardiac examination revealed a grade I/VI systolic murmur. Abdominal examination was significant for mild bilateral lower quadrant tenderness with no rebound or guarding. Genitourinary examination revealed a closed cervical os and no bleeding. She had mild cervical motion and bilateral adnexal tenderness.

Management Course

Prior to obtaining a urine pregnancy test, the emergency physician performed a transabdominal ultrasound examination, which revealed a hypoechoic sac in the uterus, a tubal ring in the left adnexa, and a small amount of free pelvic fluid (Figure 11–57). A scan of the upper abdomen revealed free fluid in the hepatorenal space (Figure 11–58). A urine pregnancy test was positive. After 2 L of intravenous normal saline, the patient's blood pressure was 92/54 mm Hg with a heart rate of 86 beats per min; infusion of O-negative packed red blood cells was initiated. The on-call obstetrician was immediately contacted and the operating room was set up. While the obstetrician was en route, an emergency bedside transvaginal ultrasound examination confirmed an obvious ectopic pregnancy with a yolk sac in the left adnexa (Figure 11–59). The patient was taken directly to the operating room when the obstetrician arrived. A ruptured ectopic pregnancy and 2 to 3 L of free intraperitoneal blood were found at surgery. The patient required a left salpingectomy. Her serum β-hCG level was 917 mIU/mL.

Commentary

Case 2 illustrated a patient with a ruptured ectopic pregnancy. She was in shock and required immediate resuscitation. She could not provide a reliable history and was not aware that she was pregnant. She had relatively mild abdominal symptoms and was not tachycardic, which is

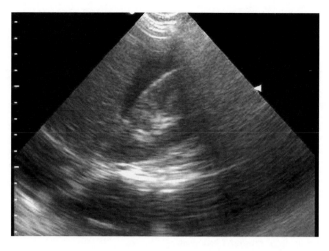

Figure 11–58. Free fluid in the hepatorenal space. Transabdominal right upper quadrant image.

not uncommon with acute intraperitoneal blood loss. Transabdominal sonography revealed hepatorenal free fluid and a tubal ring. Hepatorenal free fluid alone, in a young pregnant woman with nontraumatic hypotension, is nearly diagnostic of a ruptured ectopic pregnancy and was enough evidence to proceed to surgery. In addition, this patient had a tubal ring, which was also nearly diagnostic of an ectopic pregnancy. Transvaginal scanning allowed a more detailed view of the mass and revealed the definite ectopic pregnancy, a picture of which the emergency physician showed to the obstetrician on arrival in the emergency department.

Case 3

Patient Presentation

A 19-year-old woman presented to the emergency department with complaints of right lower quadrant abdominal

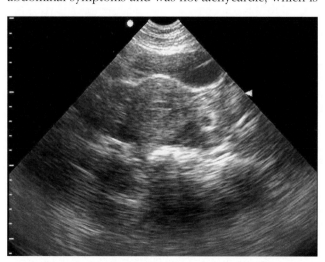

Figure 11–57. Pseudogestational sac within the uterus and tubal ring in the left adnexa. Transabdominal transverse image.

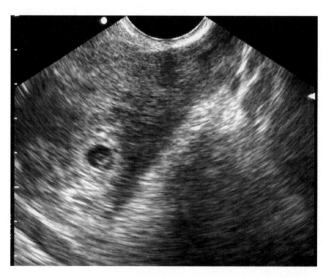

Figure 11–59. Ectopic gestation with yolk sac located in the adnexa, near the iliac vein. Transvaginal image.

pain and vaginal bleeding for 2 d. The patient was un-
sure of her last menstrual period. She denied any fever,
vomiting, diarrhea, or urinary symptoms.

On physical examination, her blood pressure was
132/62 mm Hg, pulse was 92 beats per min, respirations
were 16 per min, and temperature was 36.8°C. The patient
was well appearing and in no apparent distress. Her head,
neck, pulmonary, cardiovascular, and back examinations
were unremarkable. Her abdomen was soft with minimal
right lower quadrant tenderness and no rebound or guarding. A genitourinary examination revealed a closed cervical os, blood in the vaginal vault, and mild cervical motion
and right adnexal tenderness.

Management Course

A urine sample sent by the nurse revealed a negative
urinalysis and a positive pregnancy test. Transabdominal sonography revealed an empty uterus. Transvaginal
sonography revealed a small amount of fluid within the
uterus but no evidence of an intrauterine pregnancy or
ectopic pregnancy (Figure 11–60). A blood type and
quantitative serum β-hCG level were sent and a "formal"
pelvic ultrasound examination was ordered. The formal
pelvic ultrasound examination performed in the medical
imaging department identified a complex mass in the
right adnexa (Figure 11–61). The radiologist's interpretation was a probable ectopic pregnancy. Her blood type
was AB+ and serum β-hCG level was 780 mIU/mL. The
on-call obstetrician was consulted. After examination
and review of the ultrasound examinations, the obstetrician decided to administer intramuscular methotrexate.
The patient agreed after a discussion of the pertinent
risks and benefits of medical management of an ectopic
pregnancy. Follow-up was arranged for the next day in
the obstetrician's office. The patient was instructed to expect some pain but to return sooner if she had severe abdominal pain, significant vaginal bleeding, or syncope.

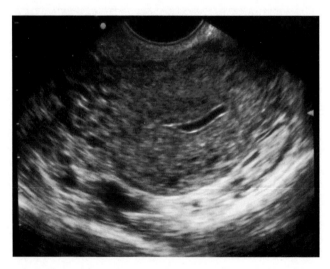

Figure 11–60. Intrauterine fluid without evidence of a
gestational sac. Transvaginal image.

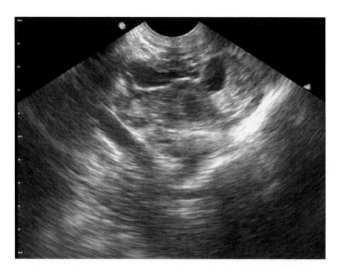

Figure 11–61. Complex adnexal mass. Transvaginal
image.

Commentary

Case 3 was an example of a stable patient with an ectopic
pregnancy that had not ruptured. The clinical history
was suspicious for an ectopic pregnancy. The emergency
bedside ultrasound examination was indeterminate. The
serum β-hCG level was low but this should not have dis-
suaded the emergency physician from ordering a "formal"
ultrasound examination. The formal ultrasound examination revealed a complex adnexal mass, which had a very
high likelihood of being an ectopic pregnancy. Had the
emergency physician been reassured by the low β-hCG
and discharged the patient, the opportunity to treat the
patient medically may have been lost and the patient may
have suffered serious morbidity or mortality.

REFERENCES

1. ACEP. Clinical policy for the initial approach to patients
   presenting with a chief complaint of vaginal bleeding.
   Ann Emerg Med 1997;29:435–458.
2. Reardon R, Jehle D. Pelvic ultrasonography. In: Tintinalli
   J, ed. Emergency medicine: a comprehensive study
   guide. New York: McGraw-Hill, 2000:737–748.
3. Brennan DF. Ectopic pregnancy—part II: diagnostic procedures and imaging. Acad Emerg Med 1995;2:1090–1097.
4. Rodgerson J, Heegaard W, Plummer D. Emergency department right upper quadrant ultrasound is associated
   with a reduced time to diagnosis and treatment of ruptured ectopic pregnancies. Acad Emerg Med 2001;8:331.
5. Cartwright P. Performance of a new enzyme linked im-
   munoassay for the detection of ectopic gestation. Ann
   Emerg Med 1986;15:1198.
6. Marill KA, Ingmire TE, Nelson BK. Utility of a single
   beta HCG measurement to evaluate for absence of
   ectopic pregnancy. J Emerg Med 1999;17:419–426.
7. Stovall TG, Kellerman AL, Ling FW, Buster JE. Emergency
   department diagnosis of ectopic pregnancy. Ann Emerg
   Med 1990;19:1098–1103.

8. Stovall TG, Ling FW, Andersen RN, Buster JE. Improved sensitivity and specificity of a single measurement of serum progesterone over serial quantitative beta-human chorionic gonadotrophin in screening for ectopic pregnancy. Hum Reprod 1992;7:723–725.

9. Valley VT, Mateer JR, Aiman EJ, et al. Serum progesterone and endovaginal sonography by emergency physicians in the evaluation of ectopic pregnancy. Acad Emerg Med 1998;5:309–313.

10. Vermesh M, Graczykowski J, Sauer M. Revaluation of the role of culdocentesis in the management of ectopic pregnancy. Am J Obstet Gynecol 1990;162:411.

11. Lipscomb GH, Stovall TG, Ling FW. Primary care: non-surgical treatment of ectopic pregnancy. N Engl J Med 2000;343:1325–1329.

12. Krause R, Janicke D. Ectopic pregnancy. In: Tintinalli J, ed. Emergency medicine: a comprehensive study guide. New York: McGraw-Hill, 2000:686.

13. Krol L, Abbott T. The current role of culdocentesis. Am J Emerg Med 1992;10:354.

14. Brennan DF. Diagnosis of ectopic pregnancy. J Fla Med Assoc 1997;84:549–556.

15. Pelsang RE. Diagnostic imaging modalities during pregnancy. Obstet Gynecol Clin North Am 1998;25:287–300.

16. Kaplan BC, Dart RG, Moskos M, et al. Ectopic pregnancy: prospective study with improved diagnostic accuracy. Ann Emerg Med 1996;28:10–17.

17. Peterson HB, Xia Z, Hughes JM, et al. The risk of ectopic pregnancy after tubal sterilization. U.S. collaborative review of sterilization working group. N Engl J Med 1997;336:762–767.

18. Loffredo A. EM residents can perform bedside ultrasound with a high degree of sensitivity and specificity of detect intra-uterine pregnancy with cardiac activity. Acad Emerg Med 2001;8:213–215.

19. Durham B, Lane B, Burbridge L, Balasubramaniam S. Pelvic ultrasound performed by emergency physicians for the detection of ectopic pregnancy in complicated first-trimester pregnancies. Ann Emerg Med 1997;29:338–347.

20. Cashner K, Christopher C, Dysert G. Spontaneous fetal loss after demonstration of a live fetus in the first trimester. Obstet Gynecol 1987;70:827–830.

21. Wilson R, Kendrick V, Wittmann B. Spontaneous abortion and pregnancy outcome after normal first-trimester ultrasound examination. Obstet Gynecol 1986;67:352–355.

22. Mateer JR, Valley VT, Aiman EJ, et al. Outcome analysis of a protocol including bedside endovaginal sonography in patients at risk for ectopic pregnancy. Ann Emerg Med 1996;27:283–289.

23. Braen R, Krause R. Ectopic pregnancy. In: Harwood-Nuss A, ed. The clinical practice of emergency medicine. Philadelphia: Lippincott Williams & Wilkins, 2001:334–340.

24. Lyons E, Levi C, Dashefsky S. The first trimester. In: Rumack C, Wilson S, Carboneau J, eds. Diagnostic ultrasound, vol. 2. St. Louis: Mosby-Year Book, 1998:975–1011.

25. DeVoe R, Pratt J. Simultaneous intrauterine and extrauterine pregnancy. Am J Obstet Gynecol 1984;56:1119–1125.

26. Richards SR, Stempel LE, Carlton BD. Heterotopic pregnancy: reappraisal of incidence. Am J Obstet Gynecol 1982;142:928–930.

27. Richards SR, Stempel LE, Carlton BD. Heterotopic pregnancy. Am J Obstet Gynecol 1984;148:227–228.

28. Reece EA, Petrie RH, Sirmans MF, et al. Combined intrauterine and extrauterine gestations: a review. Am J Obstet Gynecol 1983;146:323–330.

29. Bright DA, Gaupp FB. Heterotopic pregnancy: a reevaluation. J Am Board Fam Pract 1990;3:125–128.

30. Jerrard D, Tso E, Salik R, Barish RA. Unsuspected heterotopic pregnancy in a woman without risk factors. Am J Emerg Med 1992;10:58–60.

31. Berger M, Taymor M. Simultaneous intrauterine and tubal pregnancies following ovulation induction. Am J Obstet Gynecol 1972;113:812–813.

32. Gamberoella F, Marrs R. Heterotopic pregnancy associated with assisted reproductive technology. Am J Obstet Gynecol 1999;160:1520–1523.

33. Control CfD. Ectopic pregnancy-United States, 1987. MMWR 1990;39:401–403.

34. Lipscomb GH, McCord ML, Stovall TG, et al. Predictors of success of methotrexate treatment in women with tubal ectopic pregnancies. N Engl J Med 1999;341:1974–1978.

35. Schlager D, Whitten D, Tolan K. Emergency department ultrasound: impact on ED stay times. Am J Emerg Med 1997;15:216–217.

36. Shih CH. Effect of emergency physician-performed pelvic sonography on length of stay in the emergency department. Ann Emerg Med 1997;29:348–351.

37. Burgher SW, Tandy TK, Dawdy MR. Transvaginal ultrasonography by emergency physicians decreases patient time in the emergency department. Acad Emerg Med 1998;5:802–807.

38. Durston WE, Carl ML, Guerra W, et al. Ultrasound availability in the evaluation of ectopic pregnancy in the ED: comparison of quality and cost-effectiveness with different approaches. Am J Emerg Med 2000;18:408–417.

39. Mateer JR, Aiman EJ, Brown MH, Olson DW. Ultrasonographic examination by emergency physicians of patients at risk for ectopic pregnancy. Acad Emerg Med 1995;2:867–873.

40. Abbott J, Emmans LS, Lowenstein SR. Ectopic pregnancy: ten common pitfalls in diagnosis. Am J Emerg Med 1990;8:515–522.

41. Barnhart K, Mennuti MIB. Prompt diagnosis of ectopic pregnancy in an emergency department setting. Obstet Gynecol 1994;84:1010–1015.

42. Trautlein J, Lambert R, Miller J. Malpractice in the emergency department-review of 200 cases. Ann Emerg Med 1984;13:709–711.

43. Holbrook J, Aghababian R. A computerized audit of 15,009 emergency department records. Ann Emerg Med 1984;13:709–711.

44. Braffman BH, Coleman BG, Ramchandani P, et al. Emergency department screening for ectopic pregnancy: a prospective US study. Radiology 1994;190:797–802.

45. Barnhart K. Diagnostic accuracy of ultrasound above and below the beta-hCG discriminatory zone. Obstet Gynecol 1999;94:583–587.

46. Barnhart K, Coutifaris C. Diagnosis of ectopic pregnancy. Ann Emerg Med 1997;29:295–296.

47. Timor-Tritsch I. Sonoembryology. In: Bronshtein M, Zimmer E, eds. Transvaginal sonography of the normal and abnormal fetus. New York: Parthenon, 2001:7–34.

48. Shalev E, Yarom I, Bustan M, et al. Transvaginal sonography as the ultimate diagnostic tool for the management of ectopic pregnancy: experience with 840 cases. Fertil Steril 1998;69:62–65.

49. Sadek AL, Schiotz HA. Transvaginal sonography in the management of ectopic pregnancy. Acta Obstet Gynecol Scand 1995;74:293–296.

50. Nyberg DA, Filly RA, Laing FC, et al. Ectopic pregnancy. Diagnosis by sonography correlated with quantitative HCG levels. J Ultrasound Med 1987;6:145–150.

51. Cacciatore B. Can the status of tubal pregnancy be predicted with transvaginal sonography? A prospective comparison of sonographic, surgical, and serum hCG findings. Radiology 1990;177:481–484.

52. Mahony BS, Filly RA, Nyberg DA, Callen PW. Sonographic evaluation of ectopic pregnancy. J Ultrasound Med 4:1985;221–228.

53. Brown DL, Doubilet PM. Transvaginal sonography for diagnosing ectopic pregnancy: positivity criteria and performance characteristics. J Ultrasound Med 1994;13:259–266.

54. Stovall T, Ling F. Ectopic pregnancy diagnostic and therapeutic algorithms minimizing surgical interventions. J Reprod Med 1993;38:807–812.

55. Dart RG, Kaplan B, Cox C. Transvaginal ultrasound in patients with low beta-human chorionic gonadotropin values: how often is the study diagnostic? Ann Emerg Med 1997;30:135–140.

56. Counselman FL, Shaar GS, Heller RA, King DK. Quantitative B-hCG levels less than 1000 mIU/mL in patients with ectopic pregnancy: pelvic ultrasound still useful. J Emerg Med 1998;16:699–703.

57. Weston M. The first trimester. In: Dewbury K, Meire H, Cosgrove D, eds. Clinical ultrasound: a comprehensive text, vol. 3. London: Churchill Livingstone, 2001:151–187.

58. Dart R, Howard K. Subclassification of indeterminate pelvic ultrasonograms: stratifying the risk of ectopic pregnancy. Acad Emerg Med 1998;5:313–319.

59. Parvey R, Maklad N. Pitfalls in the diagnosis of ectopic pregnancy. J Ultrasound Med 1993;3:139.

60. Hammer R, Milad M. Overview of the management of tubal pregnancy. In: Sciarra J, ed. Gynecology and obstetrics, vol. 1. Philadelphia: Lippincott Williams & Wilkins, 2000:1–14.

61. Shalev E, Peleg D, Tsabari A. Spontaneous resolution of ectopic tubal pregnancy: natural history. Fertil Steril 1995;63:15–19.

62. Cacciatore B, Korhonen J, Stenman U. Transvaginal sonography and serum hCG in monitoring of presumed ectopic pregnancies selected for expectant management. Ultrasound Obstet Gynecol 1995;5:297.

63. Everett C. Incidence and outcome of bleeding before the 20th week of pregnancy: prospective study from general practice. BMJ 1997;315:32.

64. Wilcox A, Weinberg C, O'Connor J. Incidence of early loss of pregnancy. N Engl J Med 1988;319:189–194.

65. Filly R. Ultrasound evaluation during the first trimester. In: Callen P, ed. Ultrasonography in obstetrics and gynecology. Philadelphia: Saunders, 1994:63–85.

66. Scott J. Early pregnancy loss. In: Scott J, DiSaia P, Hammond C, eds. *Danforth's obstetrics and gynecology.* Philadelphia: Lippincott, 1994:175.

67. Falco P, Milano V, Pilu G. Sonography of pregnancies with first trimester bleeding and a viable embryo: a study of prognostic indicators by logistic regression analysis. Ultrasound Obstet Gynecol 1996;7:165–169.

68. Cetin A, Cetin M. Diagnostic and therapeutic decision-making with transvaginal sonography for first trimester spontaneous abortion, clinically thought to be incomplete or complete. Contraception 1998;57:393–397.

69. Mansur MM. Ultrasound diagnosis of complete abortion can reduce need for curettage. Eur J Obstet Gynecol Reprod Biol 1992;44:65–69.

70. Rulin M, Bornstein S, Cambell J. The reliability of ultrasonography in the management of spontaneous abortion, clinically thought to be complete. Am J Obstet Gynecol 1993;168:12–15.

71. Jurkovic D, Ross JA, Nicolaides KH. Expectant management of missed miscarriage. Br J Obstet Gynaecol 1998;105:670–671.

72. Goldstein S. Embryonic death in early pregnancy: a new look at the first trimester. Obstet Gynecol 1994;84:294.

73. Goldstein SR. Early detection of pathologic pregnancy by transvaginal sonography. J Clin Ultrasound 1990;18:262–273.

74. Levi C, Lyons E, Zheng X. Endovaginal ultrasound: demonstration of cardiac activity in embryos of less that 5.0 mm in crown-rump length. Radiology 1990;176:71–74.

75. Landy H, Weiner S, Corson S. The "vanishing twin": ultrasonographic assessment of fetal disappearance in the first trimester. Am J Obstet Gynecol 1986;155:14–19.

76. Sampson A, de Crespigny L. Vanishing twins: the frequency of spontaneous fetal reduction of a twin pregnancy. Ultrasound Obstet Gynecol 1992;2:107–109.

77. Whitecar MP, Turner S, Higby MK. Adnexal masses in pregnancy: a review of 130 cases undergoing surgical management. Am J Obstet Gynecol 1999;181:19–24.

78. Fleischer AC, Shah DM, Entman SS. Sonographic evaluation of maternal disorders during pregnancy. Radiol Clin North Am 1990;28:51–58.

79. Lev-Toaff A, Coleman B, Arger P. Leiomyomas in pregnancy: sonographic study. Radiology 1985;164:375.

80. Beischer N, Buttery B, Fortune D. Growth and malignancy of ovarian tumors in pregnancy. Aust NZ J Obstet Gynecol 1971;11:208.

81. Bider D, Mashiach S, Dulitzky M, et al. Clinical, surgical and pathologic findings of adnexal torsion in pregnant and nonpregnant women. Surg Gynecol Obstet 1991:173:363–366.

82. Fleischer A. Sonographic evaluation of first-trimester pain and/or bleeding. In: Bluth E, Arger P, Benson C, et al., eds. Ultrasound: a practical approach to clinical problems. New York: Thieme, 2000:273–280.

83. Grendys EC, Jr., Barnes WA. Ovarian cancer in pregnancy. Surg Clin North Am 1995;75:1–14.

84. Pena JE, Ufberg D, Cooney N, Denis AL. Usefulness of Doppler sonography in the diagnosis of ovarian torsion. Fertil Steril 2000;73:1047–1050.

85. Albayram F, Hamper UM. Ovarian and adnexal torsion: spectrum of sonographic findings with pathologic correlation. J Ultrasound Med 2001;20:1083–1089.

86. Warner M, Fleischer A, Bundy A. Adnexal torsion: sonographic findings and clinical implications. Radiology 1985;154:773.

87. Houry D, Abbott JT. Ovarian torsion: a fifteen-year review. Ann Emerg Med 2001;38:156–159.

88. Abbott J, Thickman D. Vaginal bleeding and pelvic pain. In: Rosen P, ed. Diagnostic radiology in emergency medicine. St. Louis: Mosby-Year Book, 1992: 581–589.

89. Freedman RS, Tortolero-Luna G, Pandey DK, et al. Gestational trophoblastic disease. Obstet Gynecol Clin North Am 1996;23:545–571.

90. Teng FY, Magarelli PC, Montz FJ. Transvaginal probe ultrasonography. Diagnostic or outcome advantages in women with molar pregnancies. J Reprod Med 1995;40:427–430.

91. Zimmer E, Bronshtein M. Transvaginal scanning in pregnancy. In: Bronshtein M, Zimmer E, eds. Transvaginal sonography of the normal and abnormal fetus. New York: Parthenon, 2001:48–50.

92. Disantis D, Scatarige J, Kemp G. A prospective evaluation of transvaginal sonography for detection of ovarian disease. AJR 1993;161:91.

93. Rottem S, Thaler I, Goldstein SR, et al. Transvaginal sonographic technique: targeted organ scanning without resorting to "planes". J Clin Ultrasound 1990;18: 243–247.

94. Yeh H, Goodman J, Carr L. Intradecidual sign: a US criterion of early pelvic intrauterine pregnancy. Radiology 1986;161:463–467.

95. Sengoku K, Tamate K, Ishikawa M. Transvaginal ultrasonographic findings and hCG levels in early intrauterine pregnancies. Nippon-Sanka-Fujinka-Gakkai-Zasshi 1991;43:535–540.

96. Pellicer A, Calatayud C, Miro F. Comparison of implantation and early developement of human embryos fertilized in vitro versus in vivo using transvaginal ultrasound. J Ultrasound Med 1991;10:31–35.

97. Nyberg DA, Mack LA, Harvey D, Wang K. Value of the yolk sac in evaluating early pregnancies. J Ultrasound Med 1988;7:129–135.

98. Fossum GT, Davajan V, Kletzky OA. Early detection of pregnancy with transvaginal ultrasound. Fertil Steril 1988;49:788–791.

99. Filly R. The first trimester. In: Callen P, ed. Ultrasonography in obstetrics and gynecology. Philadelphia: Saunders, 1988:19–46.

100. Keith S, O'Brien T, London S. Serial transvaginal ultrasound scans and B-human chorionic gonadotropin levels in early singleton and multiple pregnancies. Fertil Steril 1993;59:1007–1010.

101. Laing F, Brown D, Price J. Intradecidual sign: is it effective in diagnosis of an early intrauterine pregnancy? Radiology 1997;204:655–660.

102. Dillon E, Feycock A, Taylor K. Pseudogestational sacs: Doppler ultrasound differentiation from normal and abnormal intrauterine pregnancies. Radiology 1990;176:359.

103. Nyberg DA, Laing FC, Filly RA, et al. Ultrasonographic differentiation of the gestational sac of early intrauterine pregnancy from the pseudogestational sac of ectopic pregnancy. Radiology 1983;146:755–759.

104. Bradley WG, Fiske CE, Filly RA. The double sac sign of early intrauterine pregnancy: use in exclusion of ectopic pregnancy. Radiology 1982;143:223–226.

105. Parvey R, Dubinsky T, Johnson D. The chorionic rim and low-impedance intrauterine arterial flow in the diagnosis of early intrauterine pregnancy: evaluation of efficacy. AJR 1996;167:1479–1485.

106. Stampone C, Nicotra M, Muttinelli C. Transvaginal sonography of the yolk sac in normal and abnormal pregnancy. JCU 1996;24:3–9.

107. Kurtz A. Estimating gestational age. In: Benson C, Arger P, Bluth E, eds. Ultrasonography in obstetrics and gynecology: a practical approach. New York: Thieme, 2000:112–121.

108. Nyberg DA, Hughes MP, Mack LA, Wang KY. Extra-uterine findings of ectopic pregnancy of transvaginal US: importance of echogenic fluid. Radiology 1991; 178:823–826.

109. Fleischer A, Pennell R, McKee M. Ectopic pregnancy: features at transvaginal sonography. Radiology 1990;174:375.

110. Nyberg D, Mack L, Jeffery R. Endovaginal sonographic evaluation of ectopic pregnancy: a prospective study. AJR 1987;149:1181.

111. Russell S, Filly R, Damato N. Sonographic diagnosis of ectopic pregnancy with endovaginal probes: what really has changed? J Ultrasound Med 1993;3:145.

112. Frates M, Brown D, Doubilet P. Tubal rupture in patients with ectopic pregnancy: diagnosis with transvaginal US. Radiology 1994;191:769.

113. Abrams BJ, Sukumvanich P, Seibel R, et al. Ultrasound for the detection of intraperitoneal fluid: the role of Trendelenburg positioning. Am J Emerg Med 1999; 17:117–120.

114. Taylor K, Ramos I, Feycock A. Ectopic pregnancy: duplex Doppler evaluation. Radiology 1989;173:93–97.

115. Achiron R, Goldenberg M, Lipitz S. Transvaginal Doppler sonography for detecting ectopic pregnancy: is it really necessary? Isr J Med Sci 1994;30:820.

116. Kobayashi F, Sagawa N, Konishi I, et al. Spontaneous conception and intrauterine pregnancy in a symptomatic missed abortion of ectopic pregnancy conceived in the previous cycle. Hum Reprod 1996;11: 1347–1349.

117. Levi C, Lyons E, Lindsay D. Early diagnosis of nonviable pregnancy with endovaginal US. Radiology 1988;167:383.

118. Nyberg D, Laing F, Filly R. Threatened abortion: sonographic distinction of normal and abnormal gestational sacs. Radiology 1986;158:397–400.

119. Rowling S, Coleman B, Langer J. First-trimester US parameters of failed pregnancy. Radiology 1997;203:211.

120. Pennell R. Prospective comparison of vaginal and abdominal sonography in normal early pregnancy. J Ultrasound Med 1990;10:63.

121. Doubilet PM, Benson CB, Chow JS. Long-term prognosis of pregnancies complicated by slow embryonic heart

rates in the early first trimester. J Ultrasound Med 1999;18:537–541.

122. Doubilet P, Benson C. Embryonic heart rate in the first trimester: What rate is normal? J Ultrasound Med 1995;14:431–434.

123. Green J, Hobbins J. Abdominal ultrasound examination of the first trimester fetus. Am J Obstet Gynecol 1988; 159:165.

124. Lindsay D, Lovett I, Lyons E. Yolk sac diameter and shape at endovaginal US: predictors of pregnancy outcome in the first trimester. Radiology 1992;183: 115–118.

125. Bromley B, Harlow B, Laboda L. Small sac size in the first trimester: a predictor of poor fetal outcome. Radiology 1991;178:375.

126. Nyberg D, Cyr D, Mack L. Sonographic spectrum of placental abruption. AJR 1987;148:161–164.

127. Bennet G, Bromley B, Lieberman E. Subchorionic hemorrhage in first trimester pregnancies: prediction of pregnancy outcome with sonography. Radiology 1996;200:803–806.

128. Kurtz AB, Shlansky-Goldberg RD, Choi HY, et al. Detection of retained products of conception following spontaneous abortion in the first trimester. J Ultrasound Med 1991;10:387–395.

129. Nielsen S, Hahlin M, Platz-Christensen J. Randomised trial comparing expectant with medical management for first trimester miscarriages. Br J Obstet Gynaecol 1999;106:804–807.

CHAPTER 12

Second and Third Trimester Pregnancy

Bradley W. Frazee, Katie Bakes, and Eric Snoey

Over the last 30 years, ultrasound has played an essential role in the care of the obstetric patient. The body of knowledge and expertise in obstetric sonography is now enormous. Ultrasound is the primary imaging modality for the evaluation of uterine, cervical, and amniotic fluid abnormalities; placental and umbilical cord problems; and determination of gestational age, fetal congenital abnormalities, multiple gestation, and fetal presentation.[1] While some of these applications are of limited relevance in the emergency setting, certain information can be rapidly obtained with bedside ultrasound that is potentially critical to the emergency care of an obstetric patient.

This chapter discusses the use of emergency ultrasound to evaluate pregnant patients in the second and third trimester. During this time period, the major indications for its use are the initial assessment of the pregnant trauma patient, evaluation of vaginal bleeding and preterm labor, and evaluation of abdominal pain. Emphasis will be placed on a focused or goal-directed ultrasound examination to rapidly measure fetal cardiac activity, estimate gestational age, and exclude placenta previa. Additional applications include assessment of amniotic fluid volume, cervical length and fetal position, and the evaluation of non-obstetric causes of abdominal pain.

► CLINICAL CONSIDERATIONS

Confirming the presence of an intrauterine pregnancy when symptoms arise in the first trimester is now considered a standard application of emergency ultrasound. The clinical indications for performing the examination, the limited information sought, and the recommended techniques are all widely agreed upon and well described. In contrast, the role of emergency ultrasound in the second and third trimester of pregnancy is not well established. Yet, emergency and acute care physicians are frequently faced with evaluating women in the latter part of pregnancy. Pregnant women may present to the emergency department because of trauma, profuse vaginal bleeding, or severe abdominal pain. Depending on the practice setting, obstetric consultation may not be rapidly available and patients may have had no prior prenatal care. Increasingly, ultrasound is immediately available in the emergency setting and clinicians are adept in its use. Clearly, there are a number of clinical situations during the second and third trimester of pregnancy where a rapid, goal-directed ultrasound examination can both expedite diagnosis and improve the overall care of mother and fetus.

A discussion of the use of emergency ultrasound in the second and third trimester of pregnancy must begin by addressing the following questions:

1. What are the standard clinical indications for emergency ultrasound in the second and third trimester of pregnancy? In what clinical situations should emergency ultrasound be routinely employed?
2. What focused ultrasound applications are reasonable uses for the clinician?
3. For the major clinical indications, what are the goals of the ultrasound examination?
4. Are there alternative imaging modalities to ultrasound that should be considered?

Standard Clinical Indications for Emergency Ultrasound in the Second and Third Trimester of Pregnancy

The concept that emergency ultrasound should remain focused, or goal-directed, helps to define its appropriate use in the latter part of pregnancy. In this setting, the focused concept takes on particular importance for the following reasons. First of all, because the scope and quantity of information potentially available through ultrasound in late pregnancy is enormous, the physician performing ultrasound in the emergency setting must have a distinct, clinically relevant scanning goal in mind before placing the probe on the abdomen. It would be inappropriate, for example, to assess fetal cardiac morphology. Similarly, the idea of performing a screening ultrasound examination on a clinically stable patient with established pregnancy, simply to confirm gestational age or fetal well being, may not be an appropriate indication for emergency ultrasound. Even in the hands of obstetric ultrasound specialists, the impact of screening ultrasound on perinatal outcome remains debatable.[2] Secondly, the medicolegal ramifications of basing clinical decisions on emergency ultrasound in the obstetric patient mandate caution. In one analysis of malpractice claims involving diagnostic ultrasound, obstetric ultrasound constituted 75% of the cases.[3] Not only should the information sought with each application be carefully limited, but ultrasound should be used only for emergency indications where the immediate benefit of the information outweighs the possibility of a missed diagnosis.

Major clinical indications for the use of emergency ultrasound that seem to satisfy these constraints include the initial evaluation of a pregnant trauma patient, mid- and late-trimester vaginal bleeding, preterm labor, and abdominal pain of unclear etiology in a pregnant patient.

Focused Ultrasound Applications with Reasonable Uses for the Clinician

Several standard emergency ultrasound applications are indicated in late pregnancy and are considered safe and accurate in this setting. These include the focused assessment with sonography for trauma (FAST) examination to exclude hemoperitoneum, a right upper quadrant ultrasound examination to assess for gallstones and signs of cholecystitis, and a renal ultrasound examination to evaluate for severe hydronephrosis. In addition, the following focused applications are unique to the obstetric setting. Ultrasound may be used to rapidly visualize fetal cardiac activity. The fetal heart rate can be measured using M-mode scanning. In the second and third trimesters, gestational age may be estimated by measuring biparietal diameter or femur length. Transabdominal scanning can be used to evaluate for possible placental abruption, to exclude placenta previa, to assess amniotic fluid volume, and to ascertain the position of the fetus. Transvaginal or translabial scanning may be used to clarify the relationship of the placenta to the internal os and to measure cervical length.

Major Clinical Indications: The Goals of the Ultrasound Examination

In other words, given the patient's clinical problem, what clinically important question(s) can be answered rapidly with a focused ultrasound examination? For example, in a trauma patient who is comatose and appears to be possibly pregnant, the following questions could be answered with emergency ultrasound: Is the patient pregnant? Is there evidence of free intraperitoneal fluid (from hemoperitoneum or uterine rupture)? Is the fetus alive? What is the gestational age of the fetus (and might it survive in the extrauterine environment)? Is there obvious retroplacental hematoma? Figure 12–1 presents a goal-directed approach to emergency ultrasound in the second or third trimester of pregnancy based on the patient's clinical problem.

Alternative Imaging Modalities to Ultrasound that Should Be Considered

The emergence of ultrasound as the main imaging modality in pregnancy is based in part on its being considered extremely safe for the fetus. Human organogenesis largely takes place before the 10th week of gestation, when diagnostic ultrasound is often used. The absence of an association between ultrasound and fetal structural anomalies supports its safety in early pregnancy.[4] The critical period of brain development is during the 14th to 22nd week of gestation. The theoretical adverse affect of ultrasound on the fetal brain, due to production of thermal energy and cavitation, has been the topic of several important epidemiologic studies, all of which have found no deleterious effects on cognitive development.[1,5,6] By contrast, the risk to the fetus associated with exposure to ionizing radiation, particularly from abdominal computed tomography (CT), is considered significant.

For assessment of fetal well being, alternatives to sonography include the hand-held Doppler stethoscope for measurement of fetal heart tones and cardiotocography to continuously monitor fetal heart rate and uterine activity. Cardiotocography is a form of fetal assessment that simultaneously records fetal heart rate, fetal movements, and uterine contractions to investigate hypoxia. Cardiotocography is a sensitive, although indirect, test for the diagnosis of placental abruption after trauma, and remains the cornerstone of that evaluation. In the absence of a reliable menstrual history, a very rough estimate of gestational age can be obtained by measuring fundal height. This crude test represents the only alternative to sonography for estimating the age of the fetus if the history is not available.

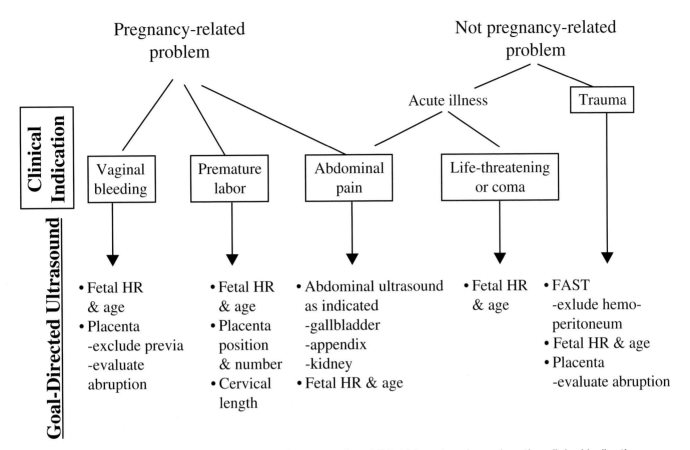

Figure 12–1. Goal-directed ultrasound in the second and third trimesters based on the clinical indication.

For the evaluation of vaginal bleeding in late pregnancy, sonography has supplanted the traditional double set-up examination as a means of excluding placenta previa. Placental abruption is usually diagnosed on clinical grounds, with the assistance of cardiotocography. Use of magnetic resonance imaging has been described in the work-up of relatively stable patients with unexplained vaginal bleeding, but it has not been widely adopted.[7]

Ultrasound frequently plays a complementary role to the physical examination and cardiotocography in the evaluation and management of preterm or precipitous labor. Ultrasound is the only imaging modality used in this setting to assess cervical length, amniotic fluid volume, and fetal position.

Abdominal pain of unclear etiology is the single major clinical indication for use of emergency ultrasound in late pregnancy where alternative imaging modalities, such as plain radiography, CT, and pyelography, are commonly employed in the nonpregnant patient.

► CLINICAL INDICATIONS

The clinical indications for performing emergency ultrasound in the second and third trimesters of pregnancy are:

- Trauma
- Vaginal bleeding
- Premature labor
- Abdominal pain

Trauma

Trauma occurs in 6% of pregnant patients[8] and is a leading cause of nonobstetrical mortality.[9] Furthermore, fetal loss as a result of trauma far exceeds maternal mortality.[10] Emergency ultrasound has the potential to play a critical role in the initial evaluation of obstetrical trauma. Use of the FAST examination to evaluate maternal intraabdominal hemorrhage has been shown to be beneficial.[11] Because fetal well-being is dependent on adequate maternal circulation, a tenet of trauma care is that resuscitation of the mother and assessment of maternal injuries is the initial priority. Besides maternal shock, processes that contribute to fetal loss include direct fetal injury, uterine rupture, placental abruption, ruptured membranes, and premature labor. Of these, placental abruption is the most common and may occur after relatively minor trauma and in the absence of other injuries.[12] While cardiotocography and observation for the occurrence of frequent contractions remains the cornerstone of the evaluation,[8] ultrasound may rapidly confirm the presence of significant abruption, usually in the setting of a high clinical suspicion.[12] In addition, and perhaps more importantly, emergency ultrasound can be used to rapidly demonstrate fetal cardiac activity and determine gestational age.[11]

Fetal Cardiac Activity in Trauma

Fetal assessment begins with measurement of fetal cardiac activity to establish fetal viability. This step is recommended early, not only in evaluation of the pregnant trauma patient,[12] but in patients with vaginal bleeding[13] and preterm labor as well.[14] The normal fetal heart rate following the first trimester is 120 to 160 beats per min. Sustained bradycardia is associated with fetal hypoxia and acidemia. Historically, in emergency medicine, fetal cardiac activity was established by measuring fetal heart tones with a hand-held Doppler stethoscope.

Bedside ultrasound is an attractive alternative to the hand-held Doppler stethoscope for initial detection of fetal cardiac activity. Using B-mode scanning of the gravid uterus, locating the fetal heart and assessing the presence of cardiac motion is relatively straightforward. Using M-mode scanning, the waveform produced by cardiac motion can be recorded. Fetal heart rate is then determined rapidly and accurately with the aid of obstetrics software, contained in most ultrasound machines. In the setting of significant trauma, assessment of fetal cardiac activity can be done as an adjunct to the FAST examination. Furthermore, sonography should be used to confirm fetal cardiac activity whenever cardiotocography is not immediately available, or if a fetal heart rate signal cannot be detected by the Doppler probe on this device.[8]

Estimation of Gestational Age in Trauma

Knowledge of gestational age is critical in this setting since decisions need to be made for emergency cesarean section, such as in the setting of maternal cardiac arrest.[15] In a stable trauma patient, gestational age may influence the decision to proceed to exploratory laparotomy.[11] Additionally, the gestational age and fetal maturity influence the management of placenta previa, preterm labor, rupture of membranes, eclampsia, and other severe medical illnesses in late pregnancy. In the setting of trauma, sonographic assessment of gestational age, along with fetal heart rate, can be done as an adjunct to the initial FAST examination.

When assessing gestational age, the following general points should be born in mind. By current convention, obstetric dating begins with the first day of the last normal menstrual period, referred to as gestational age or menstrual age, and is equal to the fetal or conceptual age plus 14 d. The ability of the fetus to survive outside the uterine environment is assumed when the gestational age is greater than 24 weeks. The pregnancy is considered term at 38 weeks. Sonographic estimates of gestational age are progressively less accurate (less predictive validity) the later in pregnancy they are obtained, due to increasing variation in biological size of the fetus (Table 12–1). A sim-

▶ **TABLE 12-1.** VARIABILITY OF GESTATIONAL AGE ESTIMATES*

Parameter Measured	Gestational Age Interval (weeks)			
	14–20	20–26	26–38	32–42
BPD	1.4	2.1	3.8	4.1
HC	1.2	1.9	3.4	3.8
FL	1.4	2.5	3.1	3.5

*Two standard deviations, in weeks.
BPD = biparietal diameter; FL = femur length; HC = head circumference.
Source: Adopted with permission from Benson CB, Doubilet PM. Sonographic prediction of gestational age: accuracy of 2nd and 3rd trimester measurements. Am J Radiol 1991;157:1275–1277.

ple rule that reinforces this principle is that the variability (2 standard deviations from the mean) of a gestational age estimate is equal to approximately 8% of the predicted age.[16] An ultrasound measurement of biparietal diameter that yields a gestational age of 32 weeks has a variability of ±19 d. Nevertheless, estimates based on biparietal diameter, obtained as late as 20 weeks, still outperform menstrual history for predicting onset of labor.[17] If possible, gestational age should be based on results of a formal ultrasound examination performed prior to 20 weeks, or on a reliable menstrual history. Beyond 20 weeks, use of emergency ultrasound to estimate gestational age may be necessary if there has been no prenatal care, menstrual dates seem unreliable, or when the mother has an altered mental status.

In the first trimester, crown–rump length is the preferred biometric measurement for establishing gestational age. In the second and third trimester, measurements that are commonly used and well validated to estimate gestational age include biparietal diameter (BPD), head circumference (HC), and femur length (FL). Modern ultrasound machines generally come equipped with software that will automatically calculate gestational age based on any one of these parameters. In choosing which biometric parameter to measure, the established predictive validity of the parameter (see Table 12–1) should be considered, and the ease and speed with which it can be obtained. A parameter that has excellent predictive validity according to the obstetric literature, but is difficult to measure and therefore prone to error, may not be well suited to the emergency setting.

In the second trimester, BPD and HC are the most widely used measurements.[16,18] Although in expert hands, HC has a somewhat better predictive validity than BPD, measurement of BPD is preferable in the emergency setting because of the relative ease and, therefore, accuracy with which it is obtained. Whereas HC must be calculated in a particular plane, BPD can be measured in any plane, provided the line of measurement intersects the thalamus and third ventricle.[16,19] Of particular relevance to the emergency setting is a study that directly correlated neonatal survival in premature infants with various biometric measurements obtained by ultrasound shortly before birth. Based on analysis of receiver operator curves, a BPD of greater than 54 mm was the single best predictor of survival.[20]

In the third trimester, FL is a frequently used alternative to BPD for estimating gestational age.[16,21] In late pregnancy, measurement of BPD may be difficult because the fetal skull is frequently located within the maternal pelvis and obscured by acoustic shadowing. The predictive validity of FL is slightly better than BPD at this stage.[18] Femur length is relatively easy to measure because the transducer need only be parallel to the femoral long axis.[16,22]

In late third trimester, identification of ossified epiphyses around the knee represents a potentially very rapid means of estimating gestational age, and is therefore attractive in the emergency setting. Appearance of the distal femoral epiphyseal ossification center indicates a gestational age of 29 weeks or greater, whereas its absence means the gestational age is less than 34 weeks.[23] Similarly, appearance of an ossified proximal tibial epiphysis suggests a gestational age of at least 35 weeks and that the fetus is at or very near term.[16]

Abruption from Trauma

The term placental abruption refers to the separation of a normally implanted placenta prior to the birth of the fetus. Any significant trauma occurring beyond the first trimester may potentially result in placental abruption, but particular attention must be given to victims of motor vehicle crashes, falls from height, and domestic violence.[8,24,25] When trauma results in major maternal injuries, the reported incidence of abruption is as high as 35%. Abruption requiring emergent delivery is possible even when the maternal physical examination is normal.[12] A heightened index of suspicion is made even more critical given the variable and sometimes subtle presentation of abruption. Although the classic presentation is the triad of vaginal bleeding, uterine tenderness, and labor, patients may manifest few if any signs or symptoms early in their course. The evaluation may be further complicated by the presence of distracting injuries, drawing attention away from early clues to the diagnosis. Finally, abruption is a dynamic process demanding close observation and ongoing monitoring for fetal-maternal effects. A trauma-induced abruption may be self-limited or continue to evolve up to 24 h after the inciting event.[8]

The diagnosis of abruption following trauma remains largely clinical, beginning with a meticulous search for evidence of vaginal bleeding, uterine tenderness, labor or fetal distress, the latter being the key to diagnosis. Uterine contractions are present in nearly all cases of abruption, although they may be difficult to appreciate by either the physician or patient. Contractions are characteristic of high frequency but low amplitude. Pearlman and colleagues demonstrated that 6 h of cardiotocographic mon-

itoring after trauma was 100% sensitive for predicting all subsequent complications.[12] A similar study confirmed that even rare cases of late onset abruption or fetal distress after trauma were heralded in each instance by early abnormalities on cardiotocography.[25] Hence, an absence of signs of uterine irritability or fetal distress remains an excellent indicator of maternal–placental well-being, suggesting that abruption is either absent or clinically insignificant. Cardiotocography should be a routine part of the initial evaluation of every pregnant trauma patient, even those who are asymptomatic. The stable patient without evidence of uterine irritability for 6 h may be discharged home with appropriate follow-up and instructions. If the patient demonstrates any degree of uterine irritability during the 6-h observation period, it is recommend that monitoring be continued for 24 h.

As stated previously, the role of ultrasound in the pregnant trauma patient remains first and foremost the assessment of free intraperitoneal fluid, fetal viability, and gestational age. Ultrasound has a limited role in the diagnosis and management of placental abruption. Fewer than 50% of sonographic studies are positive in the setting of known abruption.[26] Although it is reasonable to include a rapid assessment of the placenta as part of the FAST examination, the examiner must interpret the findings in the context of other supporting evidence for abruption. Given the poor sensitivity and specificity of sonography for abruption, any result that contradicts other clinical or cardiotocographic evidence for or against abruption must be viewed with skepticism. One scenario where the diagnostic utility of ultrasound is enhanced is that of the pregnant trauma patient with vaginal bleeding originating from the cervix, where the main considerations are placenta previa or abruption. In this setting, ultrasound can effectively diagnose abruption by excluding previa as the cause of the bleeding.[27]

Several laboratory markers are available to assist in the evaluation of potential abruption. Coagulation tests indirectly implicate abruption by showing evidence of fibrinolysis and disseminated intravascular coagulation. These markers, however, are neither specific nor sensitive for the diagnosis of abruption. The Kleihauer–Betke test, which assesses the presence of fetal hemoglobin in the maternal circulation, has been suggested as another screening test for abruption because, on average, abruption causes 15 mL of fetal blood to be mixed into the maternal circulation. Drawbacks of this test include the long processing time and general lack of prognostic value.[28] Multiple studies have shown the Kleihauer–Betke test to be of little clinical value in the overall management of placental abruption.[8,28]

Uterine Rupture

Uterine rupture is a rare complication of blunt trauma in pregnancy, occurring in only about 0.6% of cases,[8] and is much more common as a complication of labor.

Traumatic uterine rupture usually results from a high-energy mechanism. Uterine rupture invariably results in fetal demise; accompanying maternal mortality is approximately 10%.[8] Traumatic uterine rupture is likely to be diagnosed by emergency ultrasound during the initial FAST examination or while attempting to establish fetal viability.[11]

During labor, uterine rupture and uterine dehiscence usually occur at the site of a previous uterine incision, such as for cesarean section or myomectomy. Uterine rupture is defined as complete disruption of the fetal membranes, causing communication between the uterine and peritoneal cavities, and usually involves extensive tearing of the uterine scar and severe hemorrhage.[29] The clinical presentation of uterine rupture is variable, but often dramatic. It may include pain described as "tearing," vaginal hemorrhage, maternal shock, and loss of station of the fetus. Uterine dehiscence, by definition, leaves the uterine serosa and fetal membranes intact. It often involves only a small rent in an old myometrial scar and may cause only minor additional symptoms during labor. The overall incidence of uterine rupture and dehiscence is approximately 0.05% of pregnancies, rising to 0.8% of those involving labor after prior cesarean section.[29]

Vaginal Bleeding

Vaginal bleeding beyond 20 weeks of gestation complicates 5% of pregnancies. It is caused by placental abruption 13% of the time and by placenta previa 7% of the time.[30,31] Placenta previa and abruption account for the vast majority of cases requiring transfusion or cesarean section, as opposed to the approximately 80% of vaginal bleeding cases that are due to early labor or lower genital lesions or remain undiagnosed. Overall, vaginal bleeding in the second and third trimester is associated with fetal mortality or adverse outcome in nearly one-third of all cases.[32–34]

Placenta Previa

In placenta previa, the placenta is implanted in the lower pole of the uterus instead of high up in the fundus; it is located either over or very near the internal os. Placenta previa has traditionally been subdivided into complete, meaning the entire os is covered by placenta, and partial, meaning that, when dilated, the os is partially covered. This distinction, however, is usually irrelevant to the sonographic evaluation prior to the onset of labor.

Placenta previa is present at term in only approximately 0.5% of pregnancies. Yet, routine ultrasound in early second trimester has found low-lying placenta in up to 45% of patients and an apparent placenta previa in 5%.[35–37] This paradox is widely referred to as placental migration. In fact, it is due not to reimplantation of the placenta at a more superior location on the uterus, but rather to the relatively rapid elongation of the lower uterine segment, effectively drawing the placenta away from the os.[24]

Maternal risk factors for placenta previa include advanced age, multiparity, non-Caucasian race, previous cesarean section, and prior history of placenta previa.[24] Placenta previa usually presents as painless vaginal bleeding. However, pain from contractions sometimes accompanies the hemorrhage. The first episode of bleeding typically occurs in the third trimester, but may not occur until after the 36th week in up to one-third of cases.[24]

The evaluation of possible placenta previa begins with transabdominal scanning since it is rapid, noninvasive, and reliable in locating a non-low-lying placenta. Also, a digital vaginal examination can precipitate severe hemorrhage in the presence of placenta previa. Ultrasound can be used to locate the placenta and exclude placenta previa prior to vaginal examination, obviating the traditional "double set-up" examination. Because its sensitivity for diagnosing placenta previa is 92 to 98%,[38,39] a placenta seen to be located at or near the fundus by transabdominal ultrasound effectively excludes previa. After excluding the diagnosis of placenta previa, the clinician can then proceed to evaluate the patient for placenta abruption. On the other hand, if the placenta is clearly seen to cover the entire os, particularly in the third trimester, the diagnosis of placenta previa is generally confirmed. However, when the placenta appears on transabdominal ultrasound to be low lying or partially covering the os, or if an adequate view cannot be obtained, further evaluation with transvaginal or translabial scanning is generally indicated. With the transabdominal approach, the relationship of the inferior edge of the cervix to the internal os is frequently obscured by patient obesity, an overdistended bladder, myometrial contractions, a posterior placenta, or the ossified fetal skull.[40,41] In one study of patients with suspected previa, assessment of the placenta–os relationship was impossible in 31% of transabdominal scans.[42] Diagnosis of placenta previa by transabdominal scanning has a high false-positive rate, up to 17% in one large study.[43] Nevertheless, in the case of severe hemorrhage, if findings on transabdominal ultrasound appear consistent with previa, the patient should proceed directly to the operating room. A double set-up examination may then be performed in the operating room at the obstetrician's discretion.

Transvaginal sonography is a widely accepted modality for further evaluation of possible placenta previa when transabdominal scanning reveals a low-lying placenta or is nondiagnostic.[24,30] Since the late 1980s, numerous studies have documented that it is safe and more accurate than transabdominal scanning.[38,43–46] Optimal imaging is usually obtained with the endovaginal probe no closer than 3 cm to the cervix,[42] and there have been no reported cases of the procedure precipitating or worsening hemorrhage. In all but one study, sensitivity for the diagnosis of placenta previa has been 100%, where an internal os-placenta distance of less than 2 cm is taken as positive. Transvaginal scanning is able to image the internal os–placenta relationship and eliminates the majority of false positive transabdominal scans.[43] In a study that is particularly relevant to the emergency setting, Oppenheimer and associates demonstrated that when the distance from the placenta edge to the internal os was greater than 2 cm, vaginal delivery was possible in every case. Cesarean section for vaginal bleeding was required in seven of eight cases in which the distance was less than or equal to 2 cm.[44] Transvaginal scanning also has the technical advantage over transabdominal scanning that the bladder need not be fully distended.

Translabial, or transperineal, sonography is an increasingly accepted alternative to transvaginal scanning.[24,47] As with transvaginal scanning, the os–placenta relationship is almost always well visualized, thereby clarifying the findings of transabdominal scanning[40,48] and a full bladder is not required. The advantages of translabial scanning over transvaginal scanning are that it is noninvasive, theoretically safer, and does not require an endovaginal probe. Translabial scanning can be performed immediately after an apparently positive or nondiagnostic transabdominal scan without changing probes. It, therefore, may be particularly well suited to the emergency setting.

The approach to management of placenta previa depends largely on the sonographic assessment of fetal well-being and gestational age. Although cesarean section is the definitive treatment, vaginal bleeding due to confirmed placenta previa is frequently managed in an expectant fashion. The rationales for expectant management are: (1) bleeding prior to the third trimester is often self-limited and can be treated by transfusion, if necessary; (2) vaginal bleeding represents little direct risk to the fetus in the absence of significant abruption or maternal shock; and (3) delaying delivery, to maximize fetal maturity, improves perinatal outcome.[24] Obviously, confirmation of fetal well-being is a prerequisite to expectant management. A rapid initial measurement of fetal cardiac activity can be performed in the emergency setting with transabdominal ultrasound, although cardiotocography is then required for ongoing fetal monitoring. Other measures of fetal well-being, such as amniotic fluid volume and biophysical profile, also may have an impact on management.

A determination of gestational age also is required to guide treatment decisions.[13] The following general guidelines have been proposed with regard to management of previa based on gestational age. When gestational age is less than 24 weeks, delivery is only indicated for hemorrhage which is life-threatening to the mother. Between 24 and 34 weeks, fetal distress and life-threatening hemorrhage are indications for delivery. Beyond 34 to 37 weeks, delivery is indicated for significant bleeding or labor.[24]

Placental Abruption

Any abnormal separation of the placenta occurring after 20 weeks of gestation is defined as a placental abruption. Prior to this date, placental separation is considered part of the overall process of spontaneous abortion. While it affects less than 1% of all pregnancies, abruption accounts for more than a quarter of all perinatal mortality.[13,24] The epidemiology of placental abruption suggests a variety of risk factors contribute to its development, many of which relate to more general microvascular disease. One of the strongest associations is with maternal hypertension, both chronic and pregnancy-induced.[49] Cigarette smoking and cocaine abuse have also been linked to higher rates of abruption.[50,51] Trauma is an uncommon but important cause of abruption.

Hemorrhage begins at the point of separation between the placenta and the uterus, or the placenta and the amnion. The timing and degree of subsequent bleeding from the cervix is dependent on the size of the hemorrhage and its location relative to the placenta. The amount of vaginal bleeding is not a reliable guide to the degree of placental abruption or the severity of hemorrhage. In 20% of cases, patients may experience no vaginal bleeding despite significant placental separation. The amount of vaginal bleeding must never be taken as a guide to degree of internal hemorrhage. Similarly, the presence of abdominal pain, considered a hallmark symptom for abruption, will be absent in nearly half of all cases.[13,24] It follows, therefore, that any evaluation of painless vaginal bleeding in pregnancy must consider the possibility of abruption.[12,24,29] The most consistent finding in abruption will be the presence of uterine irritability and contractions.[12] These may be unappreciated by both patient and physician without the aid of cardiotocography.

Because neither the character of the bleeding nor the presence of pain can be relied upon to differentiate placental abruption from previa, it is recommended that the evaluation of vaginal bleeding in the second and third trimester always begin with an ultrasound examination to exclude placenta previa. Once previa is excluded sonographically, abruption becomes the major diagnostic consideration. The diagnosis of abruption is usually made clinically, rather than with imaging, and rests on cardiotocographic findings of uterine irritability and fetal distress. Although ultrasound will show evidence of placental hemorrhage in up to 50% of cases, it lacks sufficient sensitivity and specificity to serve as a reliable diagnostic standard. Use of magnetic resonance imaging has been described in the work-up of relatively stable patients with unexplained vaginal bleeding, but it has not been widely adopted.[7]

Once diagnosed, immediate cesarean section remains the definitive treatment for placental abruption. Decisions regarding the manner and timing of any intervention will necessarily reflect an overall assessment of maternal–fetal well-being. If the fetus is immature and the abruption is judged to be mild, an expectant approach may be attempted. Signs of preterm labor may be difficult to distinguish from mild abruption.[24] If there is no evidence of fetal distress, a cautious trial of tocolytic or magnesium therapy may be considered. The evidence suggests that such pregnancies can be successfully prolonged without serious consequence to the fetus. A term fetus or evidence of uterine irritability refractory to tocolytic therapy should prompt expedited delivery. Similarly, fetal distress or maternal signs of abruption indicate a need for immediate cesarean section.[24,30]

Premature Labor

Approximately 7% of newborns are premature at birth, resulting in both mental and physical impairment.[52] Preterm labor is defined as regular uterine contractions accompanied by characteristic changes in the cervix, occurring prior to 37 weeks of gestation. The main goal of the emergency evaluation of preterm labor is assessment of the potential for premature delivery. Ultrasound plays a pivotal role in this setting, as it is a safe, rapid, and accurate method of imaging the cervix for signs of labor. In addition, ultrasound can be used to estimate gestational age and confirm the presence of a fetal heart rate. Fetal well-being may be further assessed sonographically through the biophysical profile and measurement of amniotic fluid volume. Amniotic fluid volume and biophysical profile are of potential utility in the setting of any severe maternal illness, when expectant versus active management depends on fetal well-being. Finally, when the clinician is faced with a patient in active labor, ultrasound can be invaluable in rapidly identifying fetal lie or the presence of multiple gestations.

Cervical Effacement

The primary indication for assessing the cervix in late pregnancy is to confirm the onset of labor in the setting of regular contractions prior to 37 weeks. As labor begins, the cervix undergoes effacement followed by dilation. Although the digital examination has traditionally been used to evaluate such cervical change, ultrasound has emerged as a safer, more accurate means to do so.[53] Sonographic measurement of cervical length represents an objective way to quantify effacement.

There are several justifications for using an ultrasound examination rather than the digital examination in this setting. First, a direct contraindication to digital examination may exist, such as placenta previa or ruptured membranes. Digital examination in these settings can produce life-threatening bleeding or chorioamnionitis, respectively. A transabdominal or translabial ultrasound examination obviates the need for an invasive examination. Second, an ultrasound examination has been shown in numerous studies to be more accurate than digital examination in estimating cervical length and predicting preterm labor. This accuracy is, in part, because the anterior to superior portion of the cervix is located beneath the bladder, inaccessible to the examining finger.[53] Funneling (dilatation of the internal os) occurs when amniotic contents begin to protrude into the cervical canal and is one of the earliest signs of labor. Because the internal os cannot be palpated manually, this sign is assessed strictly by sonography.[53–57]

There are three methods for imaging the cervix with ultrasound: transabdominal, transvaginal, and translabial (transperineal). The transabdominal and the translabial approaches have the advantage of being noninvasive. The transabdominal approach is the least reliable, successfully imaging the cervix in only 46% of patients without, and 86% with, a full bladder.[58] Presenting fetal parts and a large maternal habitus may obscure the cervix. The transvaginal technique produces the most consistent findings, touted to result in visualization of the cervix in up to 100% of patients.[54] The limitations of this technique lie in its invasive nature and need for an endocavitary probe. It carries a theoretical risk of chorioamnionitis if rupture of membranes has occurred. Translabial (or transperineal) ultrasound is considered the most technically difficult method. In the hands of a skilled sonographer, however, this approach provides an adequate view of the cervix in up to 95% of patients.[54,59] In the emergency setting, a reasonable approach is to begin with transabdominal scanning and proceed to translabial scanning with the same probe if the cervix is poorly visualized.

From studies involving all three techniques, it has become clear that cervical measurements can predict the risk of preterm delivery. In a seminal study of nearly 3000 women at 24 to 28 weeks of gestation, Iams and associates demonstrated a positive correlation between short cervical length (less than 30 mm) and risk for preterm birth before 35 weeks[55] (Figure 12–2). Another study of patients between 16 and 28 weeks of gestation found a 79% rate of preterm delivery in those with cervical funneling of greater than 50%.[60] Subsequent studies have confirmed the predictive value of both short cervical length and the presence of funneling, and have extended the findings to twin pregnancies.[54,57,61] For the most part, subjects in these studies were asymptomatic outpatient patients, limiting applicability to the emergency setting. Moreover, the impact of such findings on clinical management, such as the need for cervical cerclage, remains uncertain.

The utility of cervical sonography has also been demonstrated in the setting of symptomatic preterm labor. A study in patients presenting at 20 to 35 weeks of gestation with contractions but no ruptured membranes found that the presence of funneling or short cervical length successfully predicted the need for preterm delivery. The mean cervical length in patients requiring preterm deliveries was 16.9 mm, compared to 31.9 in those proceeding to term.[56]

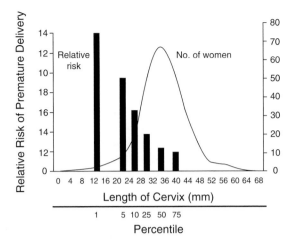

Figure 12–2. Relative risk of premature delivery (solid bars) versus cervical length, measured by transvaginal ultrasound at 24 weeks. Cervical length is expressed both in millimeters and percentiles of the normal distribution. The number of subjects versus cervical length is also shown (solid curve). *(Reprinted, with permission, from Iams JE, Goldenberg RL, Meis PJ, et al. The length of the cervix and the risk of spontaneous premature delivery. N Engl J Med 1996;334:567.)*

Using ultrasound to determine the presence or absence of cervical changes can help the emergency physician risk stratify patients with symptoms suggestive of labor. The critical cervical length, less than which preterm delivery becomes likely, appears to be 30 mm. Cervical sonography should be used in conjunction with clinical variables, such as results of the biophysical profile, gestational age, and history of preterm births, to influence management decisions. The goal of such an evaluation is to identify patients that would benefit from

admission and tocolysis versus candidates for outpatient follow-up. The utility of cervical sonography in preterm labor was retrospectively evaluated at one facility. Women were hospitalized only if they had a cervical length less than 30 mm. This protocol produced a decrease in hospital days of 48% without affecting the rate of preterm births.[62]

Fetal Position and Number

Lie refers to the relationship of the fetus to the long axis of the uterus. Presentation describes what fetal part is nearest the cervix. In normal deliveries, the fetal lie is longitudinal and the presentation is cephalic. Transverse lie and breech presentation (where the fetal sacrum or feet, respectively, are engaged in the pelvis) are referred to as malpresentations. The classification of breech presentations is presented in Figure 12–3.

In the emergency setting, it is absolutely essential to know the presenting fetal part. Even with good prenatal care, fetal presentation is often unknown because prior to 25 weeks the fetus frequently changes position. Breech presentations, which account for some 3 to 4% of all deliveries, are fraught with complications such as asphyxia, cord prolapse, and spinal cord injuries to the fetus.[63] Knowledge of the presentation allows the emergency physician to mobilize the appropriate equipment and support staff needed for delivery. In an emergency vaginal delivery, the presenting part is discovered easily by physical examination of the vagina or perineum. Prior to this point, determining fetal position by palpation may be difficult, particularly for a nonobstetrician. Moreover, when preterm labor is accompanied by vaginal bleeding or premature rupture of membranes, vaginal examination is contraindicated. In such cases, an ultrasound examination can be used to establish fetal position.

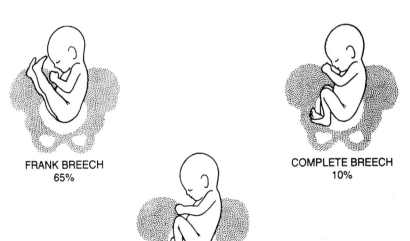

FRANK BREECH
65%

COMPLETE BREECH
10%

FOOTLING BREECH (Single or Double)
25%

Figure 12–3. Types of breech presentation. In a frank breech presentation (the most common), the thighs are flexed at the hips with the legs and knees extended. In complete breech (the least common), the thighs are flexed at the hips, and there is flexion of the knees as well. One or both hips and knees are extended in the footling breech. The risk of cord prolapse is greatest with a footling breech and least with a frank breech. *(Reprinted with permission from Callen PW. The obstetric ultrasound examination. In: Callen PW, ed. Ultrasonography in obstetrics and gynecology, 4th ed. Philadelphia: WB Saunders, 2000:13.)*

As important as the fetal position is determination of fetal number. Ultrasound is invaluable in identifying the "surprise twin" prior to labor and delivery.[64,65] Perinatal death occurs seven times more frequently in twin deliveries as compared to singletons.[66] Like breech presentations, delivery of twins requires additional expertise, support, and equipment.

Amniotic Fluid Volume

Besides providing a perfect acoustic window for the sonographer, amniotic fluid serves multiple functions for the developing fetus. It cushions, regulates temperature, helps prevent infection, and provides fluid and nutrients to the developing embryo. Late in pregnancy, the main source of amniotic fluid is the kidney. Thus, a normal amount of amniotic fluid is considered a sign of at least one functioning kidney. Fetal swallowing and intramembranous absorption are the main sources of elimination.[67,68]

In addition to being an important, measurable component of the biophysical profile, amniotic fluid volume is often used by itself to monitor maternal–fetal well-being. Alterations in amniotic fluid volume have been found to correlate with numerous maternal and fetal problems. Hence, some familiarity with amniotic fluid volume measurement is essential for the emergency sonographer. Like the full biophysical profile, measurement of amniotic fluid volume is most likely to be done in the emergency setting when sonographic indicators of maternal–fetal health might influence the course of management.

A number of semiquantitative methods for assessing amniotic fluid volume by ultrasound have been proposed, including the amniotic fluid index, largest vertical pocket, and two-diameter pocket. A seasoned sonographer can often accurately assess amniotic fluid volume subjectively.[69] Amniotic fluid index is considered by many investigators to be the most accurate measurement technique, but also the most time-consuming. It is also the most widely used by many obstetricians. For a more rapid assessment, either the largest vertical pocket or the two-diameter pocket techniques can be used. Compared to the largest vertical pocket, the two-diameter pocket technique is more sensitive in detecting oligohydramnios. In the case of multiple gestations, the largest vertical pocket may be superior in quantifying amniotic fluid volume associated with each fetus.[68] In the emergency setting, any one of these techniques is reasonable and the choice will depend on the clinician's experience.

Although its significance is controversial, oligohydramnios is defined as less than 300 mL of amniotic fluid volume and can be divided into acute and chronic presentations. Acute oligohydramnios is usually due to premature rupture of membranes. The emergency provider should be aware that in these patients, a low amniotic fluid volume is associated with a shorter latency time from rupture to delivery.[68] Chronic oligohydramnios is commonly associated with post-date pregnancies, as the

fetus outgrows the placenta. Uteroplacental insufficiency, often from maternal hypertension or autoimmune disorders, causes shunting of blood away from the kidneys towards more vital organs such as the brain. This results in oligohydramnios. Common fetal anomalies, pulmonary hypoplasia, low Apgar scores, and need for cesarean section have all been associated with oligohydramnios. Despite these associations, some investigators have found no correlation with fetal morbidity or mortality. They argue that more aggressive and unnecessary interventions, such as cesarean sections, are undertaken solely due to low amniotic fluid volumes, leading to higher fetal and maternal morbidity.[67,68]

Present in up to 1.7% of pregnancies, polyhydramnios (more than 2000 mL) is usually found at prenatal evaluation of a "large-for-dates" pregnancy. Polyhydramnios can also be divided into acute and chronic presentations. The acute form usually occurs in the second trimester and is found when the mother or fetus is very ill. Chronic presentations outnumber acute presentations 50 to 1, and can be divided into maternal (15%), fetal (13%), and unknown (67%) causes. The most common maternal cause is glucose intolerance, which leads to fetal macrosomia. Other causes are infection (syphilis, rubella, cytomegalovirus, toxoplasmosis, and parvovirus) and fetal central nervous system and gastrointestinal malformations. For the obstetrician, polyhydramnios prompts a more thorough workup, including amniocentesis for chromosome analysis, antibody screening, glucose screening and the drawing of TORCH [toxoplasmosis, other (syphilis), rubella, cytomegalovirus, herpes simplex] titers.[68] In the emergency setting, chronic polyhydramnios is of little significance in an otherwise well-appearing patient.[68]

Biophysical Profile

There are multiple non-invasive measures to evaluate the health of the unborn child. Traditionally, nonstress testing and amniotic fluid volume measurement have been used. The biophysical profile was first described by Manning in 1980.[69-71] It is a more sophisticated instrument that combines nonstress testing and amniotic fluid volume with three additional sonographic parameters, fetal tone, movement and breathing, to derive an objective score that reflects overall fetal well-being (Table 12–2).[72] The idea behind the biophysical profile is that the central nervous system, which is very sensitive to hypoxia, controls all of the measured parameters. Thus, a low biophysical profile score may indicate either acute or chronic fetal hypoxia.[73,74] Investigators have found a strong direct correlation of the biophysical profile score with Apgar scores as well as cord blood pH.[75] Although the validity of the relationship of biophysical profile to hypoxia, and actual utility of the biophysical profile, remain controversial, prominence of the biophysical profile in the practice of high-risk obstetrics requires that the emergency physician be familiar with its use. Results of

▶ **TABLE 12–2.** CRITERIA FOR FIVE COMPONENTS OF THE FETAL BIOPHYSICAL PROFILE*

Biophysical Variable	Normal (score = 2)	Abnormal (score = 0)
Fetal breathing movements	One or more episode of ≥20 s duration in 30 min	Absent or no episode of ≥20 s in 30 min
Gross body movements	Two or more discrete body/limb movements in 30 min (episodes of active continuous movement considered as single movement)	Less than two episodes of body/limb movements in 30 min
Fetal tone	One or more episode of active extension with return to flexion of fetal limb(s) or trunk (opening and closing of hand considered normal tone)	Slow extension with return to partial flexion, movement of limb in full extension, absent fetal movement, or partially open fetal hand
Reactive fetal heart rate	Two or more episodes of acceleration of ≥15 bpm and of >15 s associated with fetal movement in 20 min	One or no episode of acceleration of fetal heart rate or acceleration of <15 bpm in 20 min
Qualitative amniotic fluid volume	One or more pockets of fluid measuring ≤2 cm in vertical axis	Either no pockets or largest pocket <2 cm in vertical axis

*A score of 8 or more is considered normal.
Source: Manning FA. Fetal biophysical profile. Obstet Gynecol Clin North Am 1999:26(4):557.

the biophysical profile are always considered together with gestational age and maternal and fetal comorbidities[72-79] (Table 12–3).

Abdominal Pain

Abdominal pain arising in the second and third trimester of pregnancy represents a significant challenge for the clinician. Besides the usual complement of etiologies, obstetric causes of pain must be added to the list. The impact of any diagnostic or management decisions on both mother and fetus must also be weighed. The anatomic and physiologic changes of pregnancy may alter the traditional presentation of many disorders. The symptomatology of pregnancy itself may overlap with that of early abdominal pathology. Concerns over ionizing radiation or medication teratogenicity may limit choices of diagnostic imaging or therapy. All of these elements conspire to confuse the clinical picture, delay definitive diagnosis, and alter therapy, which risk higher morbidity for both mother and fetus. Ultrasound offers the safest and most effective means of deciphering these complex anatomic and pathophysiologic relationships.

Nonobstetric causes of abdominal pain in pregnancy occur at rates similar to that of the non-pregnant population. Similarly, the need for urgent abdominal surgery appears to parallel that of the general population, once ectopic pregnancy and cesarean section are excluded.[80,81] However, the morbidity associated with virtually every abdominal emergency remains higher in the pregnant patient due in large part to the challenge of early diagnosis.[82]

The evaluation of abdominal pain in the second and third trimester demands maintaining a broad differential and an awareness of the altered presentation of various abdominal disorders common to the emergency setting. Table 12–4 lists the more common obstetrical and nonobstetrical causes of abdominal pain, including several extrauterine etiologies specific to pregnancy. Every workup begins with a careful history and physical examination that should significantly narrow the differential. Laboratory tests must be interpreted in the context of pregnancy-induced changes (e.g., leukocytosis and relative anemia) and are frequently of limited diagnostic value.

Sonography is the next diagnostic step in most cases and stands to substantially narrow the differential diagnosis, if not confirm the diagnosis. As an example, right upper quadrant pain in the third trimester engenders a broad differential that should include gallstone disease, pyelonephritis, nephrolithiasis, appendicitis, and liver disorders. Normal laboratory tests and urinalysis would quickly reduce the list of likely possibilities to gallstone-related and appendicitis (although up to 15% of patients with renal colic may present without hematuria). Ultrasound would then be used to confirm or exclude both of these disorders while providing additional information on the pregnancy itself.

Ultrasound is the traditional first-line imaging modality for abdominal pain in pregnancy because it offers excellent anatomic and functional information about the mother and fetus without exposing either to the effects of ionizing radiation. Intrauterine exposure to radiation may have both oncogenic and teratogenic effects. Case-controlled studies of childhood cancer show a slight but significant increase in relative risk among the children of female radiologists exposed to 1000 mrems of radiation.[81] The potential for teratogenicity and carcinogenesis appears to be greatest in the period of 2 to 15 weeks and decreases proportionally as the fetus nears term. In the first trimester, in-utero radiation exposure is graded as low,

► **TABLE 12–3.** INTERPRETATION OF BIOPHYSICAL PROFILE SCORE*

Result	Interpretation	Percent Risk of Asphyxia (umbilical venous blood pH < 7.25)	Risk of Fetal Death (per 1000/week)	Recommended Management
10/10	Nonasphyxiated	0	0.565	Conservative management
8/10 (normal AFV)	Nonasphyxiated	0	0.565	Conservative management
8/8 (NST not done)	Nonasphyxiated	0	0.565	Conservative management
8/10 (decreased AFV)	Chronic compensated asphyxia	5–10 (estimate)	20–30	If mature (≥37 weeks), deliver; serial testing (twice weekly) in the immature fetus
6/10 (normal AFV)	Acute asphyxia possible	0	50	If mature (≥37 weeks), deliver; repeat test in 24 hours in immature fetus; if ≤6/10, deliver
6/10 (decreased AFV)	Chronic asphyxia with possible acute asphyxia	> 10	> 50	Factor in gestational age; if ≥32 weeks, deliver; if <32 weeks, test daily
4/10 (normal AFV)	Acute asphyxia likely	36	115	Factor in gestational age; if ≥32 weeks, deliver; if ≤32 weeks, test daily
4/10 (decreased AFV)	Chronic asphyxia with acute asphyxia likely	> 36	> 115	If ≥26 weeks, deliver
2/10 (normal AFV)	Acute asphyxia nearly certain	73	220	If ≥26 weeks, deliver
0/10	Gross severe asphyxia	100	550	If ≥26 weeks, deliver

*Also shown are estimates of fetal morbidity, mortality, and recommended management based on score.
AFV = amniotic fluid volume; NST = nonstress test.
Source: Manning FA. Fetal biophysical profile. Obstet Gynecol Clin North Am 1999;26(4):557.

▶ **TABLE 12–4.** DIFFERENTIAL DIAGNOSIS OF ABDOMINAL PAIN IN THE SECOND AND THIRD TRIMESTER

Obstetric causes
  Labor
  Placental abruption
  Placental previa
  Chorioamnionitis
  Pre-eclampsia/HELLP
Nonobstetric causes
  Appendicitis
  Cholecystitis
  Peylonephritis
  Nephrolithiasis
  Hepatitis
  Peptic ulcer disease and reflux

moderate, and high as a function of total dose, with the clearest evidence for harm above a threshold level of 150 mGy (Table 12–5).[83] Significant variability exists, however, depending on gestational age, body habitus, and type of study. Exposure in the second and third trimester is less critical with an estimated relative increase in cancer risk of 64% per rad (10 mGy), which corresponds to a 0.05 % relative increase in rate of childhood malignancies. Fortunately, the majority of abdominal radiographic tests fall well below these threshold levels and plain radiography and CT remain viable diagnostic tools in the gravid patient with abdominal pain.[83] That said, the decision to use radiography in the pregnant patient must take into account a number of competing elements: the risk of radiation to the developing fetus, the risk of delayed diagnosis if available imaging techniques are not used, and the relative suitability of alternative imaging or management strategies. There are also the intangible concerns of mother and physician about radiation exposure that, while not supported by data, nevertheless push toward alternative imaging. The use of diagnostic radiography in the preg-

▶ **TABLE 12–5.** QUALITATIVE RADIATION RISK CATEGORIES AND ESTIMATED FETAL DOSE BY TYPE OF RADIOGRAPH

Qualitative radiation risk categories	
Risk Category	Dose Range (mGy)*
Low	< 10
Intermediate	10–250
High	> 250
Fetal dose estimation by type of radiograph	
Diagnostic Procedure	Estimated Dose (mGy)*
Conventional radiograph	2 mGy/exposure
CT (abdomen or pelvis)	5 mGy/slice
Fluoroscopy (pelvis or abdomen)	10 mGy/min

*10 mGy = 1 rad.
Source: Mann F, Nathens A, Langer S, et al. Communicating with the family the risks of medical radiation to conceptuses in victims of major blunt-force trauma. J Trauma 2000;48(2), 354.

nant patient is often appropriate provided the risks and benefits are weighed in a manner that assures the best outcome for the mother and fetus. Nevertheless, ultrasound assumes a position of primacy in the evaluation of the pregnant patient with abdominal pain given its safety and unique ability to assess fetal well-being.

As pregnancy advances into the second and third trimester, a number of anatomic and physiologic changes occur. These changes in turn alter the way a variety of common disease processes may present. The primary sonographic approach to these disorders must change accordingly. As the uterus develops, the intestinal tract is displaced upward, backward, and to the sides. Correspondingly, the appendix moves to the right upper quadrant and away from the omentum (Figure 12–4). Increased intraabdominal pressure leads to increased esophageal reflux while the gravid uterus compresses the ureters, vena cava, and bladder.[80,81] The pregnant woman commonly experiences varying degrees of anorexia, nausea, vomiting, and back and flank pain, which are all related to the compressive and postural effects of the gravid uterus. These same symptoms, likely to be dismissed as "normal," may in fact herald a serious intraabdominal process. Alternative presentations, masked signs and symptoms, and distorted anatomy all serve to prevent timely diagnosis and treatment in the pregnant patient.

Obstetric Causes of Abdominal Pain

The primary obstetric causes of abdominal pain in the second and third trimester are preterm labor, placental abruption, and chorioamnionitis.[80–85] Preterm labor can often be diagnosed by history alone with its characteristic periodicity and crescendo and decrescendo pain. It is important to remember that while preterm labor is usually idiopathic, it may be in response to any general abdominal or systemic disorder. The diagnosis is confirmed with tocodynamometry. Ultrasound may play an important role in determining gestational age, fetal position, state of the cervix, and fetal well-being, all of which will help define patient management. Similar to preterm labor, mild placental abruption may present only with signs of early labor. Contractions are typically high frequency but low amplitude. Vaginal bleeding is common but may be absent in 20% of cases. Pain and tenderness range from mild to severe, crampy to constant, but also will be absent in over half of all patients. Ultrasound lacks sufficient sensitivity to confirm or exclude the diagnosis of abruption. Diagnosis and management decisions are based largely on clinical information in conjunction with cardiotocography. Chorioamnionitis refers to an infection of the amniotic fluid, typically following a rupture of membranes. In rare cases, infection may occur without membrane rupture causing pain, preterm labor, and systemic signs of infection. Diagnosis can be made by ultrasound-guided amniocentesis.[80–85]

There are several disorders unique to pregnancy that may cause abdominal pain in rare situations. Severe

Figure 12–4. Location of the appendix during succeeding months of pregnancy. *(Adapted from Baer JL, Reis RA, Arens RA. JAMA 98:1359, 1932.)*

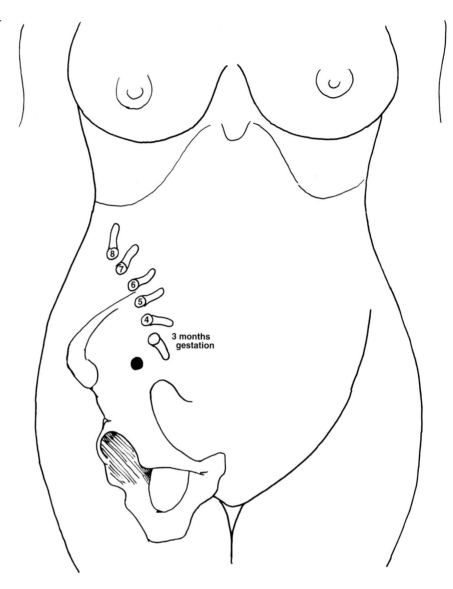

3 months gestation

pregnancy-induced hypertension is complicated by the HELLP syndrome in 5–10% of cases, which is characterized by hemolysis, low platelets, and elevations in liver function tests. Midepigastric or right upper quadrant pain may be present in 25% of cases. Spontaneous liver or spleen subcapsular hematomas can also develop, usually, but not always, in association with pregnancy-induced hypertension. Patients may experience right or left upper quadrant pain, mild coagulopathy, but normal liver function tests. Hematoma rupture results in diffuse peritonitis and hemorrhagic shock. The diagnosis is often difficult since, early, this condition may resemble uterine rupture or abruption. Ultrasound can be useful in differentiating these conditions.[81,86]

Appendicitis

Appendicitis is the most common surgical emergency in pregnancy, accounting for two-thirds of all laparotomies.[86,87] In the first half of pregnancy, the clinical presentation of appendicitis remains similar to that of non-pregnant patients. Thereafter, the clinical picture becomes more atypical.[87] As mentioned previously, early constitutional symptoms are often subtle or dismissed as pregnancy-related. The abdominal pain is predominantly right-sided and corresponds to the right upper quadrant location of the appendix. Leukocytosis is a common but inconsistent finding and 20% of patients demonstrate a sterile pyuria. The differential diagnosis includes other sources of right upper quadrant pain, specifically cholecystitis, pyelonephritis, or hepatitis.[80,81,88]

Once suspected on clinical grounds, the diagnosis may be confirmed by graded compression ultrasound, reported to be highly accurate for the diagnosis of appendicitis during pregnancy. In one study of 45 pregnant women, graded compression ultrasound demonstrated a sensitivity of 100% and specificity of 96% for the diagnosis of appendicitis.[89] However, earlier studies found a considerably lower sensitivity of 75 to 89%, although with similar specificities.[90,91] These results, along with its well-established diagnostic performance in nonpregnant patients, would suggest that ultrasound for appendicitis in pregnancy should be regarded as a diagnostic test that is specific, but of limited sensitivity. A negative ultrasound examination in the setting of an intermediate- or high-pretest probability would demand further testing.

The sonographic evaluation of appendicitis is challenging and highly operator-dependent. During pregnancy, this assessment is further complicated by the upward and outward displacement of the appendix by the growing uterus. A graded compression test is performed with additional attention paid to overall appendiceal diameter, wall thickening, or the presence of surrounding fluid and debris. The specific sonographic findings of appendicitis are discussed in Chapter 8. In the third trimester, the sheer size of the uterus may preclude adequate visualization, despite a proper high-lateral approach.[89] Placing the patient in the left lateral decubitus position may resolve this obstacle.

As an alternative, abdominal CT can be considered. Although increasingly common in the evaluation of nonpregnant patients with suspected appendicitis, there are no studies describing its reliability during pregnancy. Concerns over fetal radiation exposure make any large comparison studies unlikely. Finally, laparoscopy or laparotomy may be indicated. It has been recommended that surgeons maintain a lower threshold for surgical exploration in the setting of pregnancy and possible appendicitis, given the variability of clinical signs and the increased morbidity associated with diagnostic delay. Negative exploration rates as high as 40% in the third trimester are commonplace and considered acceptable.[91] The functional absence of the omentum in pregnancy means that a ruptured appendix is less likely to be walled off, resulting in earlier peritonitis. Perinatal mortality rises from 4.8% in unperforated appendicitis to 27.8% when the appendix ruptures.[87]

Cholelithiasis and Cholecystitis

Acute gallbladder disease appears to be slightly more common in pregnancy than in the non-gravid population, which is a fact that reflects a higher prevalence of gallstones in fertile women (3.5 to 11%).[92,93] Signs and symptoms are essentially the same as the general population: abrupt onset of stabbing or colicky right upper quadrant abdominal pain accompanied by nausea and vomiting. While the presence of fever and a Murphy's sign suggest acute cholecystitis, mild elevations in the white blood cell count, amylase, and alkaline phosphatase can be normal during pregnancy. The differential diagnosis includes appendicitis, pyelonephritis, nephrolithiasis, and rare entities such as the HELLP syndrome or subcapsular hematoma. The pregnant patient with right upper quadrant pain should invariably undergo imaging tests in order to secure the diagnosis.

As in the non-pregnant population, sonography is the imaging modality of choice; its technique and diagnostic performance are essentially unaltered by pregnancy. Oral cholecystograms and HIDA scans are effective but less attractive options in the pregnant patient due to the attendant risks of radiation exposure. Ultrasound will identify virtually all gallstones.[93] The presence of gallbladder wall thickening or pericholecystic fluid is a strong sonographic indicator of gallbladder inflammation. Most patients with acute cholecystitis can be managed conservatively with IV hydration, analgesia, and antibiotics. The risk of fetal loss with cholecystectomy approaches 5% but appears to be lowest when performed in the second trimester. However, surgery must not be delayed if the patient becomes toxic or develops pancreatitis since the fetal loss rate may reach 50% in such cases.[93]

Urinary Tract Disorders

The anatomy and physiology of the urinary tract are altered in pregnancy, affecting both the incidence of urinary tract infections and the sonographic appearance of the collecting system. The unifying theory appears to be increased urinary stasis due to mechanical pressure on the bladder and ureters, incomplete emptying of the bladder, and progesterone-induced relaxation of ureteral peristalsis.[94] Due to the compressive effects of the gravid uterus, asymptomatic dilatation of one or more of the collecting systems may be seen in 41 to 93% of patients.[95] The right ureter is often slightly more dilated than the left. This obstructive effect may occur at as early as 15 to 20 weeks of gestation and persist throughout pregnancy. By 6 weeks post partum, the collecting systems have reverted to normal.[95]

Because of increased stasis, the incidence of urinary tract infection rises during pregnancy. This affects between 1 and 2% of all pregnant women. Pregnant women with cystitis complain of urinary urgency and frequency and suprapubic discomfort, all symptoms common to pregnancy without infection. Dysuria is less often encountered in normal pregnancy and is perhaps a more specific indicator of lower tract infections. If undiscovered, a third of cases of cystitis may progress to pyelonephritis, which present with typical symptoms of fever, chills, nausea, vomiting, and flank pain. Diagnosis is based on the clinical picture together with urine demonstrating an infection. Pyuria is present in 20% of appendicitis cases, but bacteriuria will be absent.[85,94]

Despite the higher incidence of urinary stasis and infection, there is no apparent increased risk of nephrolithiasis during pregnancy. Patients present with the usual abrupt onset of unilateral flank pain, nausea, and hematuria. It is estimated that up to 15% of nephrolithiasis will not exhibit hematuria, making this a challenging diagnosis.

Traditional imaging modalities, such as intravenous pyelogram (IVP) and spiral CT, do not lend themselves well to the pregnant patient due to concerns over ionizing radiation. Hydronephrosis revealed on sonography, normally taken as strong indirect evidence of a ureteral stone, must be interpreted cautiously. Similarly, a urinary tract infection in the setting of hydroureter should not necessarily imply infection with obstruction. On the other hand, pregnancy alone rarely causes marked ureteral distention (over 1 cm) and such a finding on the same side as the pain would strongly suggest the presence of an obstructing stone.[80,84,95] Ultrasound may occasionally allow direct visualization of a calyceal or uretovesicular junction stone. Patient management should be directed at relief of symptoms and a meticulous search for infection and alternative causes of pain. Most patients with nephrolithiasis can be managed successfully with IV fluids and analgesia with the eventual spontaneous passage of the stone. Rarely, ureteral stenting or basket retrieval will be needed.

Acid Peptic Disease

Reflux esophagitis is a common complication of pregnancy and may mimic a number of the more serious abdominal disorders. The increased intraabdominal pressure and compressive effects of the gravid uterus on gastric emptying make reflux symptoms pervasive during the latter stages of pregnancy. Women will complain of episodic pain in the epigastrium, nausea, vomiting, and early satiety. Changing dietary patterns, patient positioning, and adding antacid therapy may mitigate these symptoms. In contrast, peptic ulcer disease is an infrequent occurrence in pregnancy. A reduction in gastric acid secretion and intestinal motility combined with increased mucus production during pregnancy explain this phenomenon.[80,84]

▶ ANATOMIC CONSIDERATIONS

By the 13th week, or the beginning of the second trimester, the fundus of the gravid uterus is easily palpable above the pelvic brim and, by 20 weeks, it normally reaches the level of the umbilicus. Beyond 20 weeks, the distance in centimeters from the pubic symphysis to the fundus approximates gestational age in weeks (Figure 12–5). As the uterus and developing fetus grow, the intestines are displaced posteriorly, superiorly, and toward the flanks. As a result, by the third trimester, the appendix is normally found in the right upper quadrant (see Figure 12–4). The growing uterus also compresses the ureters, frequently resulting in asymptomatic hydroureter, which occurs more often on the right side.

A thorough familiarity with the anatomy of the lower uterine segment, the cervix, and surrounding pelvic structures is essential for sonographic evaluation of placenta previa and cervical length (Figure 12–6). The normal cervix is a 3- to 5-cm long, mouth-like structure at the uterine

opening. In late pregnancy, the inner one-third of the cervix, or isthmus, elongates to form the lower uterine segment. The long axis of the cervix is defined by the endocervical canal. Normally, it lies at a right angle to the vagina. An area of glandular tissue, which may be hypoechoic or hyperechoic, surrounds the endocervical canal. This glandular zone disappears after 31 weeks of gestation, indicative of cervical ripening, making the canal difficult to locate sonographically.[54,64] The bladder, with its echogenic wall and anechoic urine, lies anterior to the vagina and cervix. As the bladder distends, it impinges on the anterior wall of the lower uterine segment. The rectum and sacral promontory lie posterior to the cervix and lower uterus.

Understanding the sonographic appearance of placental abruption in its various forms requires familiarity with the underlying uterine and placental anatomy. The placenta is primarily a fetal organ, with its size, thickness, and texture reflecting the health and gestational age of the developing fetus. By the early phase of the second trimester, the placenta is easily visible sonographically as a homogeneous, hyperechoic rim of tissue around the gestational sac.[96] The thickness of the placenta in millimeters will approximate the gestational age in weeks and rarely exceeds 4 cm.[97] By the latter part of the second trimester, the relevant anatomic segments of the placenta become more established. These include (from outside in) the myometrium, decidua basalis (endometrial–placental interface), intervillous space (area of maternal–fetal exchange), chorion (membrane that envelopes the fetal vessels), and amnion (membrane that overlies the placenta, separating it from amniotic fluid) (Figure 12–7). Fetal (umbilical) vessels course within the chorion whereas maternal (endometrial) vessels are located within the decidua.

The sonographic appearance of these layers is variable. Prominent endometrial arteries and veins within the decidua may appear as hypoechoic bands of tissue separating the myometrium from the fetal placenta, which is termed the retroplacental hypoechoic complex.[96] In the intervillous space, sonolucent pools of maternal blood, called villous lakes, can lend a heterogeneous appearance to this middle layer. The addition of Doppler in both of these cases may help to determine the vascular nature of a sonolucent area. Lastly, the subchorionic segment may undergo cystic changes associated with fibrin deposition in up to 20% of patients. These echogenic, cyst-like lesions can grow to 1 cm in size but are of no clinical significance.[96,97] The normal occurrence of these lesions conspire to limit the specificity of the ultrasound in the evaluation of possible abruption.

A discussion of fetal anatomy and development is beyond the scope of this chapter and has limited relevance to emergency ultrasound. Fetal anatomic landmarks that must be recognized for the biparietal diameter

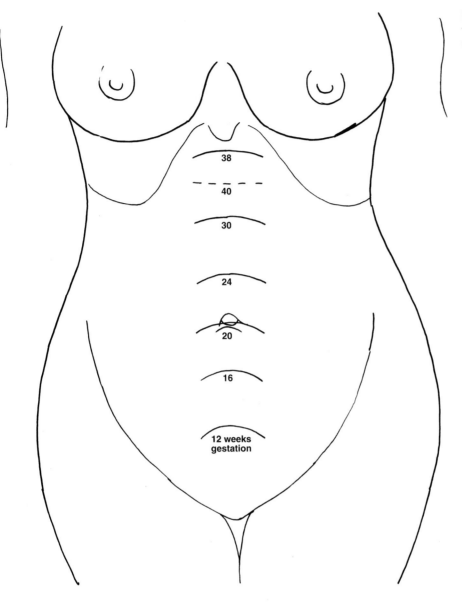

Figure 12-5. Estimation of gestational age of a singleton pregnancy by height of the fundus.

and femur length measurements are described in the "Technique and Normal Ultrasound Findings" section.

▶ TECHNIQUE AND NORMAL ULTRASOUND FINDINGS

Fetal Heart Rate Determination

Fetal heart rate should be determined by transabdominal scanning using a 3.5 MHz probe. The ultrasound machine should be set for simultaneous B-mode and M-mode recording and obstetric measurements. Scan plane is unimportant, although fanning the probe in a plane transverse to the fetal spine is one method of rapidly locating the heart. The cursor on the B-mode image should be positioned over a clearly oscillating portion of the heart, such as the mitral valve, for several cycles. Once

a continuous waveform is evident on the M-mode tracing at a depth corresponding to the heart, the image should be frozen. Finally, with the ultrasound machine set for fetal heart rate determination, the distance of one or two cycle lengths should be measured (depending on the ultrasound machine's software) and fetal heart rate should be automatically displayed (Figure 12–8).

Sonographic Determination of Gestational Age

Biparietal Diameter

Because of its good predictive validity and relative ease of measurement, BPD is the biometric measurement of choice for estimating gestational age after 14 weeks, when it supplants crown–rump length. Determinations of gestational age during the second and third trimester should be performed by transabdominal scanning using

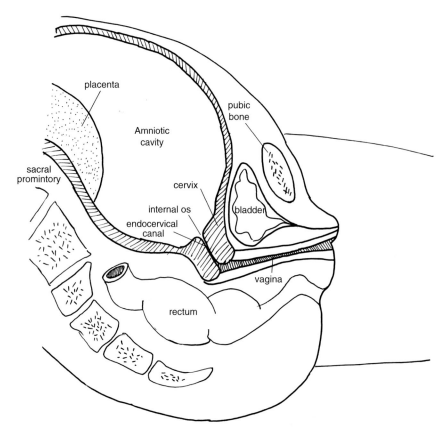

Figure 12–6. Diagram of cervix and surrounding structures, sagittal view.

a 3.5 to 5 MHz transducer. By widely accepted convention, the BPD should be measured at the level of the third ventricle, paired thalami, quadrigeminal cistern, and cavum septi pelucidi.[18,21] Although counterintuitive, the fetal ventricles and subarachnoid space are echogenic compared to brain due to the relative prominence of the choroid plexus and pia-arachnoid matter. The junction of the hyperechoic third ventricle and quadrigeminal cistern forms an easily recognizable sonographic landmark, referred sometimes to as the arrow sign (Figure 12–9). It has been proposed that BPD be measured in any plane as long as the line of measurement crosses the thalami and the third ventricle.[19] The endpoints of measurement should be either from outer edge of the near calvarial wall to the inner edge of the far wall, or from the middle of the near calvarial wall to the middle of the far wall. The near and far calvarial walls should appear symmetric. Care should be taken not to include overlying soft tissue and scalp in the measurement (Figure 12–10).[19]

Femur Length

Beyond 26 to 32 weeks of gestation, femur length (FL) is an alternative to BPD, and may be easier to measure. Femur length is actually a measurement of the ossified portion of the diaphysis and metaphysis only, and does

not include the cartilaginous portions of the bone. The endpoints of measurement are the junction of the ossified metaphysis with the cartilaginous segments at either end. The distal femoral epiphysis, a secondary ossification center, is not included. Femur length can be measured in any plane as long as it is parallel to the long axis of the bone and includes the accepted endpoints. To avoid an oblique, falsely short measurement, the plane of the section should include the femoral head or greater trochanter and the distal femoral condyle, all of which are cartilaginous (Figure 12–11).[22] Although not included in the FL measurement, the distal femoral and proximal tibial epiphyses should be sought, whether or not they are ossified (Figure 12–12).

Location of the Placenta

Transabdominal Approach

To exclude placenta previa, the sonographic evaluation of vaginal bleeding should begin with transabdominal scanning using a 3.5 to 5.0 MHz transducer. The placenta should be located and scanned in a sagittal plane to determine if it extends into the lower uterine segment (Figure 12–13). If so, transverse and oblique scans should be performed to determine if it is centrally or laterally located. When the placenta is low-lying, measurement of

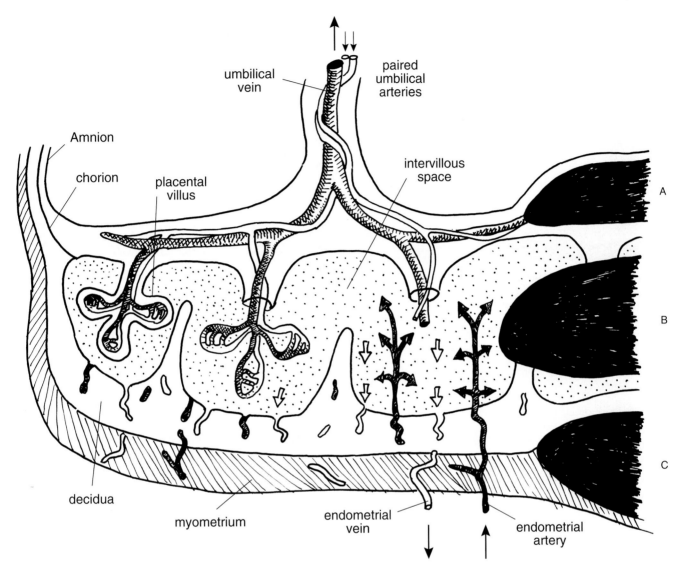

Figure 12–7. Diagram of the anatomy of the third trimester placenta. The location of three types of placental abruption is also shown: A, preplacental, B, subchorionic, C, retroplacental. *(Adapted from Moore KL, Persaud TVN. The developing human, 6th ed. Philadelphia: WB Saunders, 1999.)*

the os placenta distance by transabdominal ultrasound is often difficult because the endocervical and inferior placental edge are not in the same sagittal plane.[98]

The bladder should be full to best visualize the lower uterine segment and internal os. However, if the placenta appears to approach the os with the bladder full, scanning should be repeated after the patient has voided. A full bladder may create a false impression of placenta previa by pushing the anterior wall of the lower uterus against the posterior wall, thereby shortening the distance between the artificially long cervix and the placenta (Figure 12–14). Myometrial contractions, which in the second trimester may not be felt by the mother, also may result in a false positive diagnosis of previa. A myometrial thickness of greater than 2 cm

is suggestive of a contraction.[96] Repeat scanning in 20 to 30 min has been suggested to avoid a false positive diagnosis of previa due to contractions; however, this option may be unrealistic in the emergency setting. In cases where the fetal presenting part obscures the region of the internal os, an attempt can be made to manually elevate the fetus by placing the patient in the Trendelenburg position and applying sustained pressure on the lower abdominal segment on either side of the midline.

Transvaginal Approach

Transvaginal or translabial sonography should be employed to clarify the internal os-placenta relationship when transabdominal scanning is nondiagnostic. The

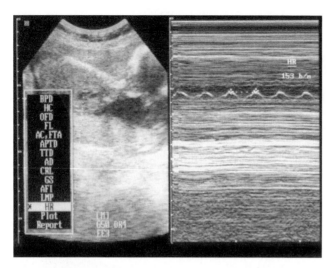

Figure 12–8. Fetal heart rate determination. B-mode image and M-mode tracing are simultaneously displayed. Doppler cursor passes through fetal heart. Cardiac oscillations are evident on M-mode tracing. With image frozen, a cardiac cycle length is automatically calculated and displayed with obstetrics measurement software.

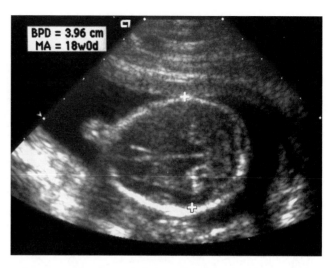

Figure 12–10. Biparietal diameter to estimate gestational age. Measurement is taken form outer wall of calvarium to inner wall (see marker cursors), in a line that crosses the paired thalami and third ventricle. In the plane shown, the cavum septi pellucidi is seen.

main contraindication to these techniques is ruptured or bulging membranes.[96] Transvaginal ultrasound is considered safe in the setting of second and third trimester bleeding because optimal images usually are obtained with the probe inserted only about 2.5 cm beyond the introitus and no closer than 3 cm to the cervix.[44,45] Also,

the angle between the probe and the cervix is usually sufficient to prevent the probe from inadvertently slipping into the cervix. The technique should be performed using a 5.0 to 7.5 MHz endovaginal probe covered by scanning medium and a sterile condom. The examination should begin with sagittal scanning and the probe subsequently can be rotated and its angle changed to gain a longitudinal view of the placenta and fully image its inferior edge. Care should be taken to thoroughly investigate the lateral walls of the uterus. If the inferior

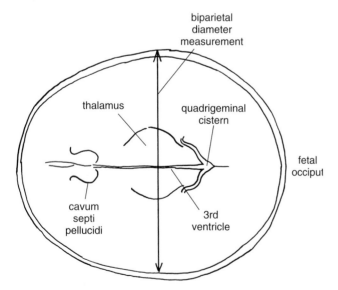

Figure 12–9. Schematic diagram of fetal anatomic landmarks used to locate the correct plane for biparietal diameter measurement. The "arrow sign" arises from the junction of third ventricle (shaft of the "arrow") and quadrigeminal cistern (forms the "arrowhead"), which points toward the fetal occiput.

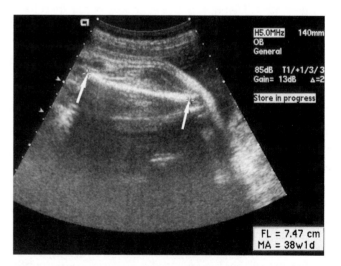

Figure 12–11. Femur length to estimate gestational age. Inclusion of cartilaginous greater trochanter and lateral condyle in the image assures proper long axis plane. However, measurement includes only the ossified (Brightly hyperechoic) portion of bone (arrows).

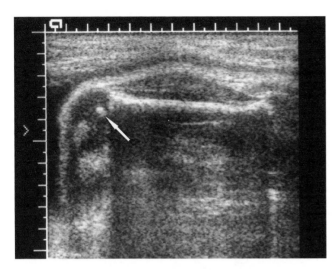

Figure 12–12. Distal femoral epiphesis. Longitudinal view of the femoral shaft with bent knee on the left. Appearance of a distal femoral epiphesis (arrow) indicates that the gestational age is at least 29 weeks.

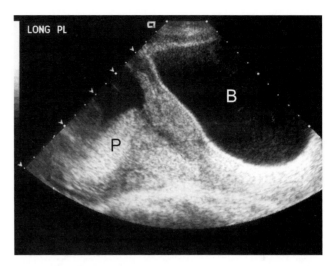

Figure 12–14. Posterior marginal placenta previa (P). Transabdominal approach, sagittal plane. In this case, an overdistended bladder (B) may be compressing the lower uterine segment, causing a false positive impression of previa.

placental edge appears near the internal os, the os to placental distance should be measured. To do so, the endocervical canal, which appears sonographically as a faint, hyperechoic or hypoechoic line, must first be located. The internal os is assumed to be located at the junction of endocervical canal and the anterior cervical wall. The probe should be angled and rotated until the imaging plane contains both the os and the lowest part of the placenta, at which point the image should be frozen and a measurement taken (Figure 12–15).

Imaging may be enhanced with the bladder empty. It has been proposed that in cases where image quality

is suboptimal, instillation of water into the vagina may enhance image quality while allowing a greater distance to be maintained between probe and cervix.[99]

Translabial Approach

A translabial (or transperineal) ultrasound examination is performed using a 3.5 to 5.0 MHz transducer to which scanning medium is applied, then a sterile cover, and, finally, a thin layer of sterile jelly over the cover. If available, a phased array transducer with a small footprint is preferable. The bladder should be empty. The probe should be placed over or between the labia majora, posterior to the urethra and anterior to the vaginal introitus. Scanning should be performed in a sagittal plane, with the bladder to the left on the monitor (Figures 12–16 and 12–17). Once the cervical os and placenta are visualized, the transducer should be angled laterally to image the entire surface of the cervix and lateral walls of the lower uterine segment.

When a low-lying placenta is encountered by translabial scanning, the os to placenta distance should be measured. In addition, it has been proposed that previa can be excluded by translabial scanning when a fetal part is visualized directly adjacent to the cervix or when the cervix is separated from a fetal part only by amniotic fluid without intervening placental tissue.[43]

Cervical Length Assessment

The three scanning approaches available for measuring cervical length, transabdominal, transvaginal, and translabial, are essentially identical to those just described for assessing placenta previa. The transabdominal approach tends to suffer from various impediments to visualizing

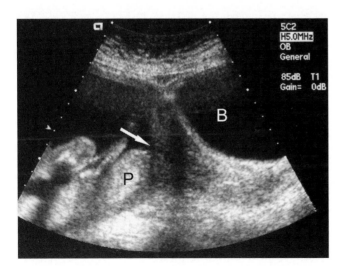

Figure 12–13. Posterior marginal placenta previa (P). Transabdominal approach, sagittal plane. The endocervical canal (arrow) is obscured by edge artifact emanating from the bladder (B).

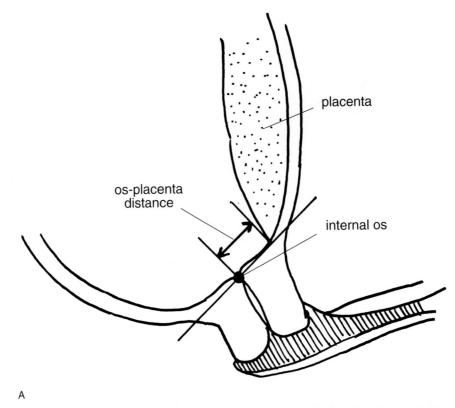

A

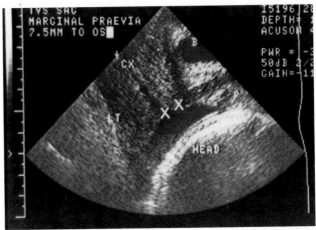

B

Figure 12-15. (A) Diagram of measurement of os-placental distance. (B) Transvaginal ultrasound of os-placental distance. *(Reprinted with permission from Cunningham et al. Williams Obstetrics, 21st ed. New York: McGraw-Hill, 2001.)*

the entire cervix, such as large maternal habitus, an intervening presenting part, or a shadow from the bony pubis. A distended bladder provides an advantageous acoustic window (Figure 12–18), but may also create an artificially lengthened cervix by pushing the anterior wall of the lower uterine segment against the posterior wall. If transabdominal scanning fails to provide an adequate view of the cervix, transvaginal or translabial scanning is required.

The translabial approach to measuring cervical length generally requires more experience to perform because proper image acquisition and interpretation are somewhat difficult. With the presenting part toward the left

on the monitor, the imaging plane should be adjusted so that the vagina courses directly away from the transducer between the bladder and the rectum. The cervical canal is normally at a right angle to the vagina (Figure 12–19).[59] In translabial scanning, rectal gas can obscure the distal cervix and the pubic symphysis may obscure the proximal cervix.[54,64] A left-side down decubitus position and partially full bladder may facilitate imaging. Transla-bial scanning of the cervix is particularly difficult prior to 20 weeks or with a posteriorly directed cervix.[54]

Regardless of the approach employed, cervical measurements are made in a sagittal plane, from internal os

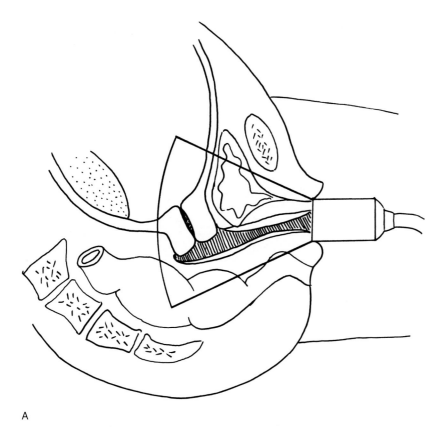

A

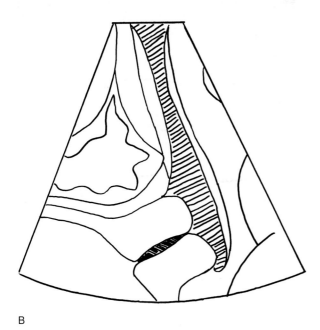

B

Figure 12-16. Diagram of translabial ultrasound of the cervix and placenta previa (A). Image acquisition in the sagittal plane and standard image projection are shown (B). *(Adapted from Hertzberg SB, Bowie JD, Carroll BA, et al. Diagnosis of placenta previa during the third trimester: role of transperineal sonography. AJR 1992;159:83–87.)*

to external os. The first task should be to locate the endocervical canal, which may appear hypo- or hyperechoic. The internal os is located at the junction of the endocervical canal and the anterior cervical wall. To locate the external os, the anterior and posterior lips of the cervix should be visualized (see Figure 12–18). The cervix is a dynamic organ, and thus should be observed for 3 to 5 min before any measurements are made.[54,64] In general, the shortest cervical length should be recorded. This measurement will provide a conservative estimate of risk of preterm delivery. The normal cervix measures between 2.9 and 5 cm in length.[100] At the same time, as cervical length is measured, an assessment of any cervical funneling should be made.

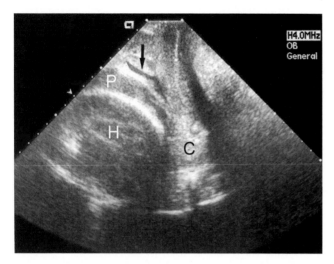

Figure 12–17. Translabial ultrasound showing the fetal head (H) overlying internal os and a low lying placenta (P). The bladder is collapsed (arrow) and the vaginal stripe is seen between the transducer and cervix (black C).

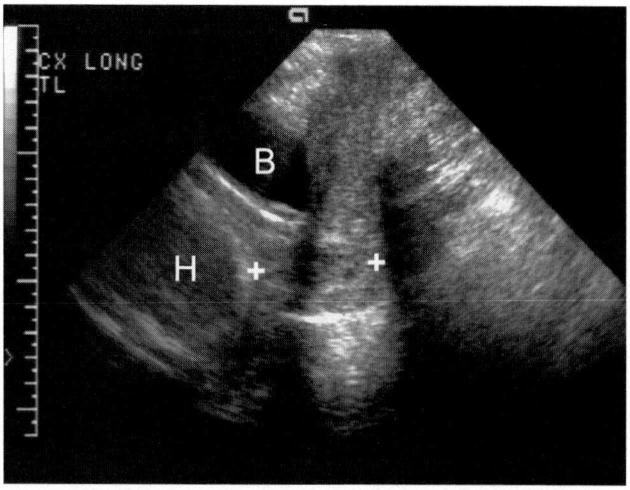

Figure 12–19. Normal cervical length measurement (5 cm by cursors), translabial approach, sagittal plane. The vaginal canal is visualized in the near field and the cervix lies at right angle to the vaginal canal. B = bladder; H = fetal head.

Fetal Position and Number

Although usually straightforward, assessment of fetal number and position by bedside sonography should be performed systematically and carefully. Not only does the recognition of breech presentation or twins have important management ramifications, but also correctly interpreting sonographic images of a moving, near term fetus can be difficult. Position should be documented using the maternal bladder as the reference point.[64] The presenting part should be scrutinized in multiple imaging planes to confirm cephalic or breech presentation versus transverse lie. It may be helpful to deliberately scan the fetal spine in both a long axis and transverse plane (Figure 12–20). In the case of an established breech presentation, an attempt should be made to characterize it as frank, complete, or footling breech (see Figure 12–3). To avoid missing a multiple gestation, the clinician should systematically interrogate the entire uterine cavity, making sure to image the attachment of the fetal head to the fetal body in view.[65]

Assessment of Amniotic Fluid Volume

There are three techniques for measuring amniotic fluid volume. A 3.5 to 5.0 MHz sector, convex, or linear transducer is recommended for making these measurements.[101]

To obtain an amniotic fluid index, the uterus is divided into four quadrants using the umbilicus and the linea nigra as external landmarks (Figure 12–21). Fluid should be measured vertically in each quadrant, with the transducer parallel to the maternal sagittal plane. The sum of the largest pocket measured in each quadrant should be between 5 and 20 cm. A sum value below or above this range is considered oligohydramnios or polyhydramnios, respectively. If the amniotic fluid index measures less than 8 cm, the examination should be repeated three times and the results averaged. Of note, fetal movements should not effect amniotic fluid index.[96] In twin pregnancies, a separate amniotic fluid index can be calculated for each amniotic sac and the normal range is the same as for singleton gestations.[102]

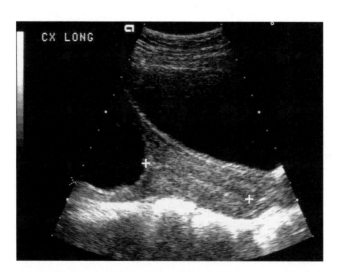

Figure 12–18. Normal cervical length measurement, taken from external os to internal os (see cursors). Transabdominal approach, sagittal plane.

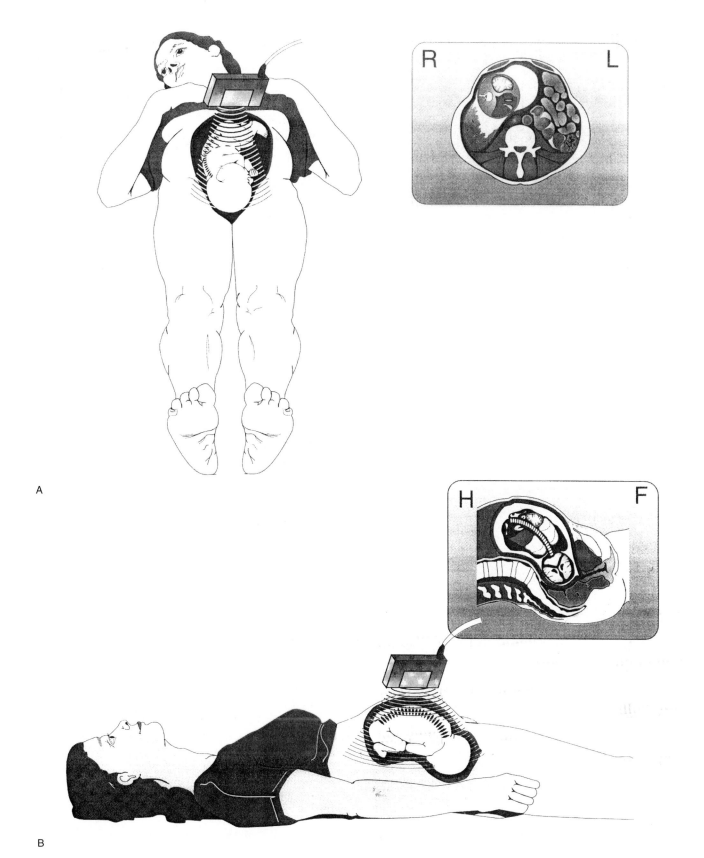

Figure 12–20. Sonographic technique for determining fetal position: (A) Transverse scan of longitudinal lie, vertex presentation; (B) Sagittal scan of longitudinal lie, vertex presentation.

Transverse Lie
Head, Maternal Right

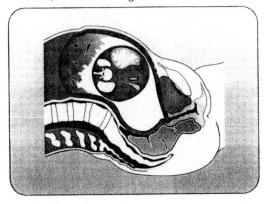

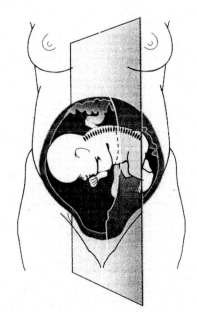

C

Figure 12–20. *(continued)* (C) Sagittal scan of transverse lie. *(Reprinted with permission from Callen PW. The obstetric ultrasound examination. In: Callen PW, ed. Ultrasonography in obstetrics and gynecology, 4th ed. Philadelphia: WB Saunders, 2000:10.)*

For the largest vertical pocket technique, the single deepest pocket should be measured in the vertical plane (Figure 12–22). A value between 2 and 8 cm is considered to be normal. Both largest vertical pocket and amniotic fluid index are prone to overestimate amniotic fluid volume if the pocket measured is long but narrow (Figure 12–23).[69] Like largest vertical pocket, in the two-diameter pocket method, the single deepest pocket of fluid should be sought, but should be measured both vertically and horizontally. The product of these measurements should be between 15 and 50 cm².

Compared to the largest vertical pocket, this technique is felt to be more sensitive and have a lower false negative rate in detecting oligohydramnios.[103]

Biophysical Profile

As mentioned previously, the biophysical profile involves assessment of the following five parameters, four of which are purely sonographic: amniotic fluid volume, fetal breathing, fetal movement, fetal tone, and a nonstress test. The assessment of each sonographic component is detailed in Table 12–2. In scoring the biophysical profile, each variable is assigned a maximum value of 2, giving a maximum overall score of 10. A score of 8/10 or greater is considered normal, provided the amniotic fluid volume component is normal.[70,104] Taking advantage of this scoring system, many obstetricians will eliminate the nonstress test portion because it is the most time-consuming part of the assessment, requiring 30 min to conduct, and longer if the fetus is asleep. Eliminating the nonstress test makes the biophysical profile a fairly rapid, purely sonographic test. The nonstress test is included only if another parameter is abnormal (i.e., without it the score would be less than 8). Further modifications of biophysical profile scoring have been proposed based on the amniotic fluid volume component. For each type of amniotic fluid volume measurement, two normal criteria have been proposed: a two-diameter pocket at least 2 × 2 cm versus a two-diameter pocket 1 × 1 cm, and largest vertical pocket of at least 1 cm versus largest vertical pocket of at least 2 cm.[64,104,105]

▶ COMMON AND EMERGENT ABNORMALITIES

Placenta Previa

The term placenta previa refers to a placenta that completely covers the internal cervical os. Some clinicians use the term partial previa to describe a placenta that does not completely cover the os. When the placental edge is located within 3 cm of the internal os, it is termed marginal placenta previa. The term low-lying placenta is useful for describing the case of a placenta located in the lower portion of the uterus in which the exact os-placenta relationship cannot be defined, or for describing an apparent placenta previa when seen in the second trimester (Figures 12–13 and 12–24).

Transabdominal scanning can occasionally diagnose or exclude placenta previa when the placenta and cervix are clearly visualized. When the placenta appears low-lying by transabdominal scanning, translabial or transvaginal scanning are often required to clarify the os-placenta relationship (see Figures 12–15B and 12–17).

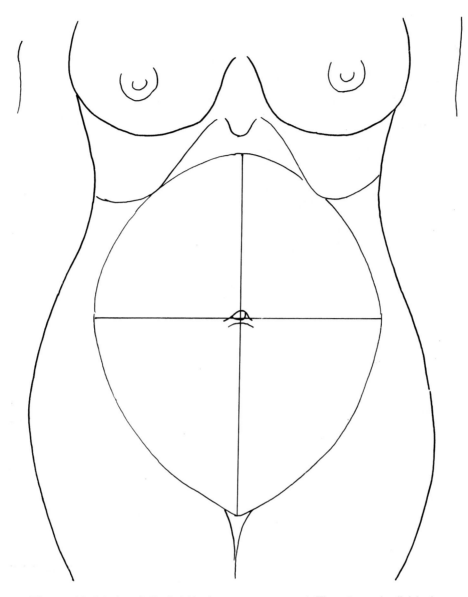

Figure 12–21. Amniotic fluid index measurement. The uterus is divided into four quadrants, using the linea nigra and umbilicus as landmarks. Measure the deepest pocket in each quadrant, scanning in the sagittal plane. Add these four values to obtain the amniotic fluid index. *(Adapted from Gabbe et al. Obstetrics: normal and problem pregnancies, 2nd ed. New York: Churchill Livingstone, 1991.)*

Placental Abruption

During placental abruption, a hemorrhage occurs within a layer of the placenta causing separation from the adjacent uterine wall.[106] This separation and hemorrhage may remain partial and self-limited or progress on to complete abruption. The clinical manifestations of abruption and its prognosis are directly determined by the extent to which placental circulation is compromised, which in turn depends both on its size and location. Hemorrhage confined to the edge of the placenta is referred to as marginal. The degree or size of placental-

uterine separation is graded as mild (grade 1), partial (grade 2), or complete (grade 3) (Figure 12–25).[27,32] These categories correlate reasonably well with the clinical presentation and prognosis. Grade 1 separations are usually marginal, involve less than a few cm of the placental border, and are usually not clinically significant In contrast, grade 3 abruption can be fatal to both the fetus and mother.

Abruption is further categorized by the anatomic location of the hematoma relative to the placenta: retroplacental (in the decidua basalis, between placenta and uterine wall), subchorionic (between decidua and the

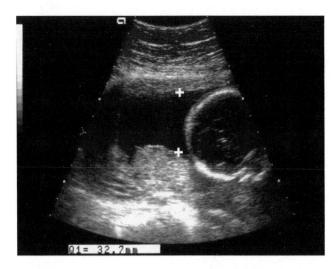

Figure 12–22. Largest vertical pocket measurement to estimate amniotic fluid volume. The pocket shown is 3.27 cm deep; 2 to 8 cm is considered normal.

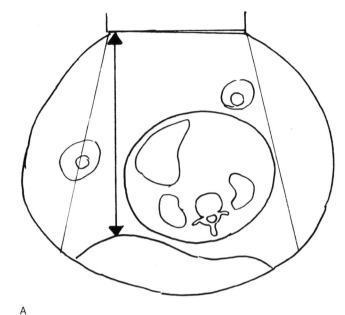

A

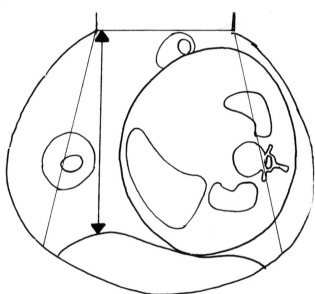

B

Figure 12–23. Diagram illustrating how vertical measurements of amniotic fluid pockets, as done in the amniotic fluid index and largest vertical pocket, can lead to overestimation of amniotic fluid volume if the pocket is long but thin.

membranes), and preplacental (between placenta and amniotic fluid, immediately beneath the amnionic membrane) (see Figure 12–7).[107] These distinctions also have significant prognostic implications, but primarily for fetal outcome. While retroplacental hemorrhage of 60 mL or more carry a 50% fetal mortality rate, similar sized subchorionic hemorrhage translate to only a 10% rate of fetal demise. Preplacental hemorrhage is often self-limited and clinically silent, with 30% detected only after delivery.[32,107] They appear sonographically as an irregular bulge along the inner border of the placenta. Rupture of these hematomas results in the classic "port-wine" staining of the amniotic fluid.

Although vaginal bleeding is considered a hallmark for abruption, its overall reliability as a diagnostic indicator is poor since it depends on the anatomic location of the hemorrhage and its proximity to the edge of the placenta (see Figure 12–25). Abruption in which the hemorrhage does not communicate with the external os is referred to as concealed.

The most consistent sonographic finding in abruption is hemorrhage and hematoma, the appearance of which will depend not only on its quantity and location but also on the timing of the ultrasound in relation to the onset of hemorrhage. Acute hemorrhage appears isoechoic to slightly hyperechoic relative to the highly vascular normal placenta (Figure 12–26).[108,109] This is analogous to the situation of splenic hematomas where subcapsular and intraparenchymal hemorrhage may be indistinguishable from the adjacent normal spleen. Gradually, over 1 to 2 weeks, the hematoma becomes sonolucent and more easily distinguished from the adjacent placenta. Hence, sonograms obtained 1 to 2 weeks after the onset of abruption may identify sonolucent hematoma not apparent on an initial study. Isoechoic hematomas may be suspected if

a portion of the placenta appears unusually thick or heterogeneous in texture. For this same reason, hematomas of abruption are occasionally mistaken for uterine leiomyomas. Another obstacle to sonographic diagnosis is that acute hemorrhage may spontaneously decompress to an adjacent area or out through the vagina, such that the amount of retroplacental blood remaining is inadequate for visualization by ultrasound examination.[16,30,32]

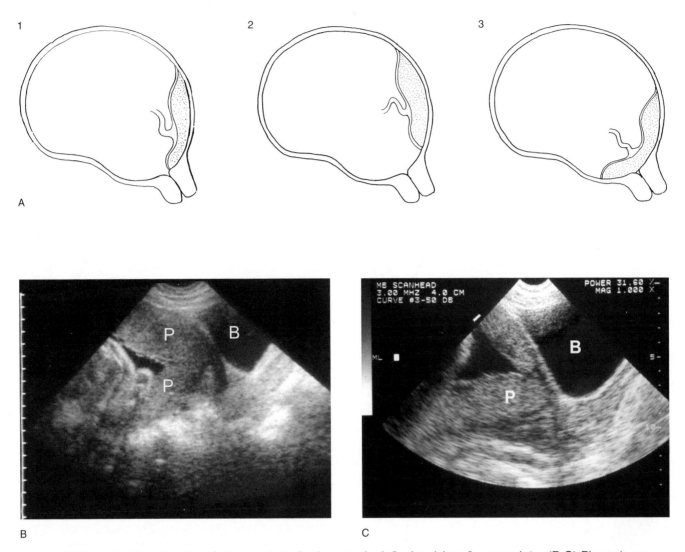

Figure 12–24. (A) Classification of placenta previa: 1 = marginal; 2 = low lying; 3 = complete. (B,C) Placenta previa. Transabdominal longitudinal ultrasound demonstrates complete previa (B) and partial previa (C). B = bladder; P = placenta. *(Sonograms courtesy of L. Sens and L. Green, Gulfcoast Ultrasound.)*

Cervical Changes in Labor

Labor is heralded by regular contractions associated with cervical change. Cervical change consists of effacement of the cervix followed by dilation of the external os. The degree of effacement can be quantified sonographically by assessment of cervical length and the presence or absence of funneling. As a general guideline, a cervical length of 1.5 cm and 1 cm represents 50% and 75% effacement, respectively. Funneling is a phenomenon that occurs during the beginning stage of cervical effacement, where dilatation of the internal os results in protrusion of amniotic contents into the cervical canal. Funneling can be described by its appearance as the letters Y, V, and U (Figure 12–27).[54] As effacement progresses, the contour of the internal os progresses from a Y-shape to a V, and then to a U. Several criteria have been established that attempt to further quantify the degree of funneling, including funnel length, width, and residual cervical length. The most often utilized value is the percentage of funneling, which is the ratio of the funnel length to total cervical length expressed as a percentage (Figure 12–28).[54]

Nonobstetrical Abdominal Emergencies

The ultrasound findings associated with cholecystitis, appendicitis, and renal colic are discussed in Chapters 7, 8, and 9, respectively.

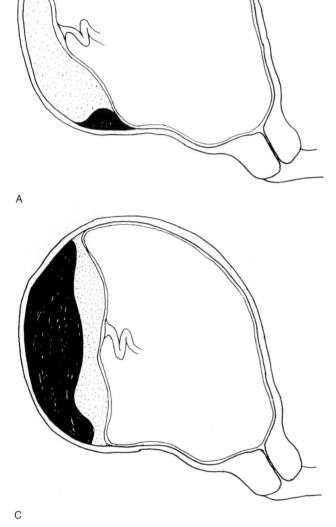

A

B

C

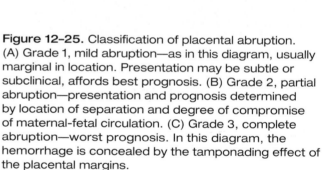

Figure 12–25. Classification of placental abruption. (A) Grade 1, mild abruption—as in this diagram, usually marginal in location. Presentation may be subtle or subclinical, affords best prognosis. (B) Grade 2, partial abruption—presentation and prognosis determined by location of separation and degree of compromise of maternal-fetal circulation. (C) Grade 3, complete abruption—worst prognosis. In this diagram, the hemorrhage is concealed by the tamponading effect of the placental margins.

▶ COMMON VARIANTS AND SELECTED ABNORMALITIES

Uterine Rupture

Uterine rupture is most likely to be diagnosed by ultrasound when it occurs in the setting of trauma.[11,29] Sonographic findings associated with uterine rupture include free intraperitoneal fluid, which may represent amniotic fluid or blood, and lack of fetal cardiac activity. Additionally, the uterus may be empty, with the fetus discovered in the peritoneal cavity. There are numerous case reports describing use of sonography to diagnose uterine dehiscence during labor.[110,111] Sonographic findings include a visible defect in the uterine wall, fetal membranes intact

and ballooning through the uterine wall, subchorionic hematoma adjacent to scar in the lower uterine segment, or evidence of blood layering within amniotic fluid. When uterine rupture during labor is strongly suspected on clinical grounds, an ultrasound examination is discouraged, as it may delay cesarean section.[15]

▶ PITFALLS

Placenta Previa

1. *Full bladder.* Although it provides an acoustic window, a full bladder may create a false impression of placenta previa by pushing the ante-

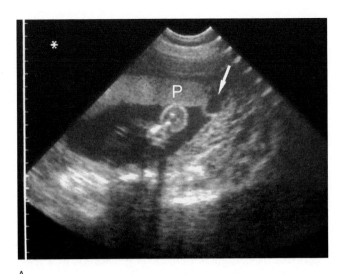

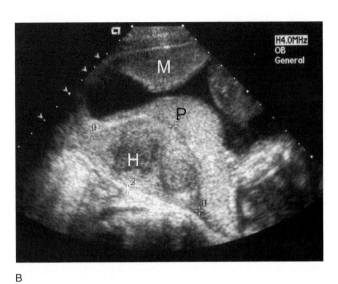

A   B

Figure 12–26. (A) Placental abruption. Transabdominal long axis scan shows an anterior placenta with a contained marginal abruption (arrow). *(Courtesy of L. Sens and L. Green, Gulfcoast Ultrasound.)* (B) Placental abruption. Transabdominal scan, sagittal plane, demonstrating retroplacental hematoma (H) in an 18-week pregnancy. The placenta (P) is located on the posterior wall. A myometrial contraction (M) of the anterior wall is evident.

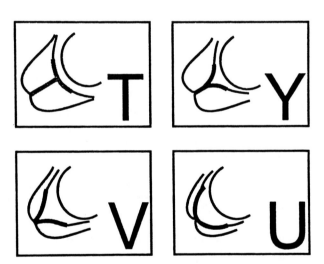

Figure 12–27. Diagram of funnel shapes described as T, Y V, U. As the cervix becomes progressively more effaced, funnel shape progresses from Y to V to U and cervical length decreases. *(Reprinted with permission from Zilanti ZM, Azuaga A, Calderon F, et al. Monitoring the effacement of the uterine cervix by transperineal sonography: a new perspective. J Ultrasound Med 1995;14:719.)*

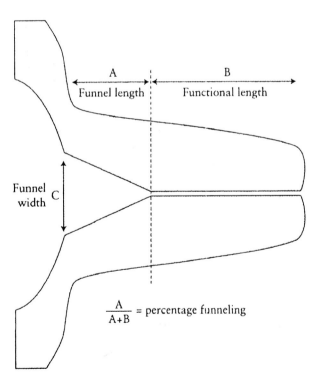

Figure 12–28. Percentage of funneling. Funnel length (A) divided by total cervical length (A+B) × 100. *(Reprinted with permission from Berghella V, Tolosa JE, Kuhlman K, et al. Cervical ultrasonography compared with manual examination as a predictor of preterm delivery. Am J Obstet Gynecol 1997;177:723.)*

rior wall of the lower uterine segment against the posterior wall, thereby shortening the distance between the artificially long cervix and the placenta (see Figure 12–14).

2. *Myometrial contractions.* These contractions may lead to a false positive diagnosis of placenta previa by thickening and shortening the lower uterine wall.

3. *Incomplete examination.* A false negative diagnosis may result from failure to sweep the sonographic beam across the entire lower segment, thereby overlooking placental tissue that encroaches on the lateral aspect of the internal os.

Placental Abruption

The diagnosis of abruption cannot be excluded solely by an ultrasound examination. The specificity of ultrasound is hampered by the common occurrence of prominent endometrial vessels, subchorionic cysts, and villous lakes. These are sonolucent or hyperechoic structures that may mimic the appearance of abruption but are of no clinical significance. Cardiotocographic monitoring is required for all patients when this diagnosis is considered.

Cervical Length Assessment

1. *Full bladder.* A full bladder may create an artificially lengthened cervix by pushing the anterior wall of the lower uterine segment against the posterior wall (see Figure 12–14).

2. *Pseudodilatation of the cervix.* A contracting lower uterine segment can produce pseudodilatation of the cervix. This can be distinguished from true dilatation by the following findings: length of the cervix is greater than 5 cm; the distal cervix is normal; there is thickened myometrium adjacent to the cervix; and the dilatation passes after the contraction ceases.[54]

3. *Other pitfalls.* Advanced dilatation is difficult to distinguish from total effacement. In the translabial examination, the bladder wall can be mistaken for the lower uterine segment.[59]

Amniotic Fluid Volume

1. *Measurement errors.* Measurements may be deceptive if vertically long, but very narrow pockets are present (see Figure 12–23).[69] Excessive pressure on the maternal abdomen may result in falsely low measurements of fluid depth.

2. *Improper gain settings.* Measuring a pocket containing mainly umbilical cord should be avoided. This can look like fluid, particularly when the gain is low or in an obese patient. Adjusting the gain upward or using Doppler may help identify the cord, particularly in an obese patient.

Gestational Age Estimate

The main pitfalls for gestational age estimation are: failure to carefully follow guidelines for gestational age estimation; failure to recognize the inherent variability of estimates; and measurement of femur length in an oblique plane relative to the long axis of the bone, which may result in a falsely short measurement.

▶ CASE STUDIES

Case 1

Patient Presentation

A 25-year-old woman was brought to the emergency department by paramedics after being involved in a high-speed motor vehicle crash. The patient was a restrained passenger and, according to other occupants, had been drinking alcohol and was pregnant. The patient complained to paramedics of abdominal pain. Out-of-hospital vital signs were stable. On arrival, the patient complained of abdominal pain, but was uncooperative with further history.

On physical examination, she was a young, obviously pregnant woman, laying supine on a backboard, with the odor of alcohol on her breath. Her blood pressure was 100/60 mm Hg, pulse was 130 beats per min, respirations 25 per min, and pulse oximetry was 100% on high flow oxygen. The head, neck, and chest examinations were normal. Abdominal examination revealed an obviously gravid uterus and lower abdominal tenderness. Moderate vaginal bleeding was noted on inspection. The patient was confused and unable to follow commands.

Management Course

Two L of normal saline were rapidly infused. In conjunction with obtaining plain radiographs of the chest and cervical spine, an emergency ultrasound examination was performed. The FAST examination revealed no free intraperitoneal fluid. A singleton pregnancy was identified with a fetal heart rate of 160 beats per min. Biparietal diameter was measured at 75 mm, consistent with 28 weeks of gestation. The placenta was located at the fundus and no retroplacental hematoma was evident. Bedside cardiotocography was immediately ordered.

The patient continued to complain of abdominal pain. Her pulse decreased to 110 beats per min and her blood pressure rose to 110/70 mm Hg. Chest and cervical spine radiographs were normal. Her hematocrit was 35. Urinalysis was normal. Cardiotocography revealed uterine contractions occurring approximately every 10 min, which were accompanied by late fetal heart rate decelerations. A head CT was normal. The patient was then taken to the operating room for urgent cesarean section based on the clinical diagnosis of placental abruption. A

30-week boy was delivered and intubated after an initial Apgar score of 3. Following delivery, an exploratory laparotomy revealed no maternal abdominal injuries. Evidence of severe abruption was evident upon examination of the placenta.

Commentary

Case 1 was an example of a woman in the early third trimester of pregnancy that sustained significant blunt trauma resulting in a closed head injury and placental abruption. The prominent complaint of abdominal pain and initial evidence of hemodynamic compromise made maternal abdominal injuries an important initial possibility. The finding of vaginal bleeding made traumatic placental abruption an early consideration, but exclusion of placenta previa as the cause was also required. The mother's altered level of consciousness made determination of gestational age by dates impossible.

Emergency ultrasound played a critical role in this case in several ways. The possibility of hemoperitoneum as the cause of abdominal pain and shock was greatly reduced by the negative FAST examination, as was the possibility of traumatic uterine rupture. Ultrasound measurement of fetal heart rate and biparietal diameter rapidly confirmed fetal life and established the extrauterine viability of the infant. Placenta previa as the cause of vaginal bleeding was easily excluded by the clearly fundal location of the placenta; however, abruption remained likely despite no sonographic evidence of hematoma. As is usually the case, the diagnosis of abruption was made clinically with the aid of cardiotocography demonstrating frequent contractions and fetal bradycardia.

Case 2

Patient Presentation

A 30-year-old woman presented to the emergency department complaining of contractions. She was gravida 2 para 3, and stated she was 30-weeks pregnant and had yet to establish prenatal care. She did not believe her membranes had ruptured, and denied vaginal bleeding or other complaints.

On physical examination, she was well-appearing and experiencing infrequent abdominal pain. Her blood pressure was 120/70 mm Hg, pulse was 110 beats per min, and respirations 24 per min. The head, neck, and chest examinations were normal. Her abdomen was nontender and fundal height was measured at 28 cm above the symphysis pubis. The fetal position could not be determined by palpation. There was a small amount of blood at the introitus and a vaginal examination was not performed.

Management Course

An IV line was established and cardiotocographic monitoring was initiated. Contractions occurred irregularly at 3- to 8-min intervals, but fetal heart tones could not be detected. A bedside ultrasound examination was per-

formed, which revealed a singleton pregnancy and fetal cardiac activity at 150 beats/min. The fetal position was breech and fetal head circumference was measured at 78 mm, consistent with 31 weeks of gestation. The placenta was located at the fundus and appeared normal. The cervix was obscured by the presenting part, so a translabial scan was performed that revealed 40%, Y-shaped funneling of the internal os. The cervical length was measured at 30 mm.

The patient was admitted to the obstetric service for preterm labor and breech presentation. Cardiotocography subsequently showed normal heart rate reactivity. The score on a formal ultrasound biophysical profile was 10. With bedrest, IV hydration, and tocolysis, labor was stopped. The patient eventually delivered a healthy baby at 35 weeks by cesarean section.

Commentary

Case 2 was an example of a woman presenting in apparent preterm labor, having had no prior prenatal care. The finding of vaginal bleeding and uncertainty about possible rupture of membranes precluded a digital vaginal examination. On initial cardiotocography, the Doppler probe did not pick up fetal heart tones. Emergency ultrasound rapidly revealed several critical features of this case. First, viability of a single fetus was established by finding a normal cardiac activity and a gestational age of approximately 31 weeks. Secondly, a breech presentation was discovered. If labor had progressed rapidly, the emergency provider would have been prepared for a difficult delivery and the likely need for cesarean section. Finally, in the setting of irregular contractions, the diagnosis of preterm labor and a significant likelihood of preterm delivery were confirmed by sonographic evidence of cervical effacement. If labor had stopped soon after presentation and cervical shortening and funneling had been absent, the obstetric consultant might have elected for outpatient management.

Case 3

Patient Presentation

A 37-year-old woman presented to the emergency department with an 8-h history of mid and right upper quadrant abdominal pain. The pain was initially intermittent and crampy, then became constant and more severe in the past h. She admitted to mild nausea but no vomiting, diarrhea, vaginal discharge, or urinary symptoms. Her last menstrual period was 6 months earlier and she believed she might be pregnant.

On physical examination, she was an obese, obviously pregnant woman in moderate distress. Her blood pressure was 130/95 mm Hg, pulse was 110 beats per min, respirations 20 per min, and temperature was 98.4°F. The pulmonary and cardiac examinations were normal. Abdominal examination was notable for a gravid abdomen and an estimated gestational age of 30 weeks by fundal height. She had marked tenderness to palpation of the midepigastric and right upper quadrant regions. No costovertebral angle tenderness or uterine tenderness was noted. Stool was guaiac negative. The pelvic examination revealed a normal white discharge and no blood. Extremity examination was notable for trace pedal edema and normal reflexes.

Management Course

The patient was placed on oxygen and a normal saline infusion was begun. She was administered morphine and ondansetron (Zofran) IV for symptom relief. Laboratory studies revealed a white blood cell count of 15.7, and normal liver function tests, platelet count, lipase, and urinalysis. An emergency ultrasound examination revealed a singleton pregnancy with a gestational age by femur length of 32 weeks. The placenta appeared to be located in the fundus without evidence of hematoma. Right upper quadrant sonography revealed an enlarged gallbladder containing two hyperechoic stones; a sonographic Murphy's sign was present. There was no evidence of gallbladder wall thickening or pericholecystic fluid. The common bile duct was of normal caliber. The liver appeared homogenous. Ultrasound examination of the kidneys revealed mild right-sided hydronephrosis and a similar degree of hydronephrosis on the left. Cardiotocography was initiated immediately and maintained continuously for 4 h without evidence of uterine irritability or fetal distress. The patient experienced complete relief of pain and tenderness after the initial medications and observation, and later tolerated oral intake. Blood pressure prior to discharge was 110/70 mm Hg. She was discharged home with a presumptive diagnosis of cholelithiasis, biliary colic, and intrauterine pregnancy, and instructed to follow up with a general surgeon.

Commentary

Case 3 was an example of a woman who presented with an unexpected pregnancy and new onset right upper quadrant abdominal pain. The differential diagnosis in this case was necessarily broad and included typical causes of right upper quadrant pain (biliary colic, pyelonephritis, and nephrolithiasis), abruption, displaced appendicitis due to the gravid uterus, as well as unusual causes such as HELLP syndrome and liver hematoma. The patient's elevated blood pressure and pedal edema suggest possible pregnancy-induced hypertension/HELLP syndrome, which was effectively excluded by a negative urinalysis, normal liver enzymes, platelet count, and stable cardiotocography. Similarly, right-side hydronephrosis suggested a possible ureteral stone with obstruction until similar dilatation was confirmed on the contralateral side. Appendicitis was a chief consideration in this case; however, the presence of gallstones and a sonographic Murphy's sign were compelling evidence for the diagnosis of biliary colic or cholecystitis. Leukocytosis was non-

specific in the setting of pregnancy and may be a normal variant. More reliable predictors for cholecystitis would have been gallbladder wall thickening, pericholecystic fluid, and a failed response to simple pain control. The management of gallstones in pregnancy is supportive, with cholecystectomy scheduled after delivery. If surgery is deemed unavoidable, it preferably is performed in the second trimester.

REFERENCES

1. Callen PW. The obstetric ultrasound examination. In: Callen PW, ed. Ultrasonography in obstetrics and gynecology, 4th ed. Philadelphia: WB Saunders, 2000;3.
2. Ewigman BG, Crane JP, Frigoletto FD, et al. Effect of prenatal ultrasound screening on perinatal outcome. N Eng J Med 1993;329:821–827.
3. Sanders RC. Legal problems related to obstetrical ultrasound. Ann NY Acad Sci 1998;847:220–227.
4. Bioeffects report subcommittee. Bioeffects considerations for the safety of diagnostic ultrasound. J Ultrasound Med 1998;7:s1–s38.
5. Stark CR, Orleans M, Haverkamp AD, et al. Short and long-term risks after exposure to diagnostic ultrasound in utero. Obstet Gyncecol 1984;63:194–200.
6. Salvensen KA, Bakketeig IS, Elk-Nes SH, et al. Routine ultrasonography in utero and school performance at age 8–9 years. Lancet 1992;62:339–342.
7. Kay HH, Spritzer CE. Preliminary experience with magnetic resonance imaging in patients with third trimester bleeding. Obstet Gynecol 1991;78:424.
8. Pearlman MD, Tintinalli JE, Lorenz RP. Blunt trauma in pregnancy. N Eng J Med 1990;323:1609–1613.
9. Varner MW. Maternal mortality in Iowa from 1952–1986. Surg Gynecol Obstet 1989;168:555–562.
10. Agran PF, Dunkle DE, Winn DG, et al. Fetal death in motor vehicle accidents. Ann Emerg Med 1987;16:1355–1358.
11. Ma OJ, Mateer JR, DeBehnke DJ. Use of ultrasonography for the evaluation of pregnant trauma patients. J Trauma 1996;40:665–668.
12. Pearlman MD, Tintinalli JE, Lorenz RP. A prospective controlled study of outcome after trauma during pregnancy. Am J Obstet Gynecol 1990;162:1502–1510.
13. Van De Kerkhove K, Johnson TRB. Bleeding in the second half of pregnancy: maternal and fetal assessment. In: Pearlman MD, Tintinalli JE, eds. Emergency care of the woman. New York: McGraw-Hill, 1998:77–98.
14. Anderson HF. Emergency management of preterm labor. In: Pearlman MD, Tintinalli JE, eds. Emergency care of the woman. New York: McGraw-Hill, 1998:13.
15. Katz VL, Dotters DJ, Droegemueller W. Perimortem cesarean delivery. Obstet Gynecol 1986;68:571–576.
16. Filly RA, Hadlock FP. Sonographic determination of menstrual age. In: Callen PW, ed. Ultrasonography in obstetrics and gynecology, 4th ed. Philadelphia: Saunders, 2000;146–169.

17. Waldenstrom U, Axelsson O, Nilsson S. A comparison of the ability of a sonographically measured biparietal diameter and the last menstrual period to predict the spontaneous onset of labor. Obstet Gynecol 1990;76: 336–338.

18. Benson CB, Doubilet PM. Sonographic prediction of gestational age: accuracy of second and third trimester fetal measurements. AJR 1991;157:1275–1277.

19. Shepard M, Filly RA. A standardized plane for biparietal diameter measurement. J Ultrasound Med 1982;1: 145–150.

20. Smith RS, Bottoms SF. Ultrasound prediction of neonatal survival in extremely low birth weight infants. Am J Obstet Gynecol 1993;169:490–493.

21. Wolfson RN, Peisner DB, Chik LL, et al. Comparison of biparietal diameter and femur length in the third trimester: effects of gestational age and variation in fetal growth. J Ultrasound Med 1986;5:145–149.

22. Goldstein RB, Filly RA, Simpson G. Pitfalls in femur length measurements. J Ultrasound Med 1987;6:203–207.

23. Mahony BS, Callen PW, Filly RA. The distal femoral epiphyseal ossification center in the assessment of third-trimester menstrual age: sonographic identification and measurement. Radiology 1985;155:201–204.

24. Clark S. Placenta previa and abruptio placentae. In: Creasy F, Resnick S, eds. Maternal–fetal medicine, 4th ed. Philadelphia: WB Saunders, 2000:616.

25. Curet MJ, Schermer CR, et al. Predictors of outcome in trauma during pregnancy: identification of patients who can be monitored for less than 6 h. J Trauma 2000;49:18.

26. Pearlman MD. Trauma in pregnancy. In: Pearlman MD, Tintinalli JE, eds. Emergency care of the woman. New York: McGraw-Hill, 1998;69–76.

27. Kuhlman RS, Warsof S. Ultrasound of the placenta. Clin Obstet Gynecol 1996;39:519.

28. Towery R, English TP, Wisner D. Evaluation of the pregnant women after blunt injury. J Trauma 1993; 35:731.

29. Ripley D. Uterine emergencies: atony, inversion and rupture. Obstet Gynecol Clin 1999;26:419—434.

30. Scott J. Placenta previa and abruption. In: Dansforth J, ed. Obstetrics and gynecology, 8th ed. Philadelphia: Lippincott, Williams & Wilkins, 1999:407.

31. Baron F, Hill WH. Placenta previa, placenta abruptio. Clin Obstet Gynecol 1998;41:527–532.

32. Ananth CV, Savitz DA, Luther ER. Maternal cigarette smoking as a risk factor for placental abruption, placenta previa and uterine bleeding in pregnancy. Am J Epidemiol 1996;144:881–889.

33. Ajayi RA, Soothill PW, Campbell S, et al. Antenatal testing to predict outcome in pregnancies with unexplained antepartum hemorrhage. Br J Obstet Gynaecol 1992;99:122–125.

34. Lipitz S, Admon D, Menczer J, et al. Midtrimester bleeding–variables which affect the outcome of pregnancy. Gynecol Obstet Invest 1991;32:24–27.

35. Wexler P, Gottesfeld K. Early diagnosis of placenta previa. Obstet Gynecol 1979;54:231–234.

36. Rizos N, Doran TA, Miskin M, et al. Natural history of placenta previa ascertained by diagnostic ultrasound. Am J Obstet Gynecol 1979;133:287–291.

37. Iyasu, S, Saftlas AK, Rowley DL, et al. The epidemiology of placenta previa in the United States, 1979 through 1987. Am J Obstet Gynecol 1993;168:1424–1429.

38. Leerentveld RA, Gilberts EC, Marinua JCW, et al. Accuracy and safety of transvaginal sonographic placental localization. Obstet Gynecol 1990;76:759–762.

39. Harris RD, Alexander RD. Ultrasound of the placenta and umbilical cord. In: Callen PW, ed. Ultrasonography in obstetrics and gynecology, 4th ed. Philadelphia: WB Saunders, 2000:607–613.

40. Hertzberg BS, Bowie JD, Carroll BA, et al. Diagnosis of placenta previa during the third trimester: role of transperineal sonography. AJR 1992;159:83–87.

41. Brown JE, Thieme GA, Shah DM, et al. Transabdominal and transvaginal endosonography: evaluation of the cervix and lower uterine segment in pregnancy. Am J Obstet Gynecol 1986;155:721–726.

42. Farine D, Fox HE, Jakobson S, et al. Vaginal ultrasound for diagnosis of placenta previa. Am J Obstet Gynecol 1988;159:566–569.

43. Tan NH, Abu M, Woo JL, et al. The role of transvaginal sonography in the diagnosis of placenta praevia. Aust NZ J Obstet Gynaecol 1995;35:42–45.

44. Oppenheimer LW, Farine D, Ritchie K, et al. What is a low-lying placenta? Am J Obstet Gynecol 1991;165: 1036–1038.

45. Taipale P, Hiilesmaa V, Ylostalo P, et al. Diagnosis of placenta previa by transvaginal sonographic screening at 12–16 weeks in a nonselected population. Obstet Gynecol 1997;89:364–367.

46. Laurie MR, Smith RS, Treadwell CH, et al. The use of second-trimester transvaginal sonography to predict placenta previa. Ultrasound Obstet Gynecol 1996;337–340.

47. Doubilet PM, Benson CB. Emergency obstetrical ultrasonography. Semin Roentgenol 1998;33:339–350.

48. Dawson WB, Dumas MD, Romano WM, et al. Translabial ultrasonography and placenta previa: does measurement of the os-placenta distance predict outcome? J Ultrasound Med 1996;15:441–446.

49. Pritchard J, Mason R, Coley M, et al. Genesis of severe placental abruption. Am J Obstet Gynecol 1970;108:22.

50. Landy HJ, Hinson K. Placenta abruption associated with cocaine use. Reprod Toxicol 1987;1:203.

51. Ananth, CV, Smulian JC, Vintileos AM. Incidence of placental abruption in relation to cigarette smoking and hypertensive disorders during pregnancy: a meta analysis of observational studies. Obstet Gynecol 1999;93:622.

52. Cunningham FG, MacDonald PC, Leveno KJ, et al. Parturition: biomolecular and physiologic processes. In: Williams obstetrics, 19th ed. Norwalk, CT: Appleton & Lange, 1993:297.

53. Berghella V, Tolosa JE, Kuhlman K, et al. Cervical ultrasonography compared with manual examinations a predictor of preterm delivery. Am J Obstet Gynecol 1997;177:723.

54. Scheerer LJ and Bartolucci L. Ultrasound evaluation of the cervix. In: Callen PW, ed. Ultrasonography in obstetrics and gynecology, 4th ed. Philadelphia: WB Saunders, 2000:557.

55. Iams JE, Goldenberg RL, Meis PJ, et al. The length of the cervix and the risk of spontaneous premature delivery. N Engl J Med 1996;334:567.

56. Timor-Tritsch LE, Boozarjomehri F, Masakowski Y, et al. Can a "snapshot" sagittal view of the cervix by transvaginal ultrasonography predict active preterm labor? Am J Obsete Gynecol 1996;174:990.

57. Crane JM, Van Den Hof M, Armson BA, et al. Transvaginal ultrasound in the prediction of preterm delivery: singleton and twin gestations. Obstet Gynecol 1997;90:357.

58. Anderson HF. Transvaginal and transabdominal ultrasonography of the uterine cervix during pregnancy. J Clin Ultrasound 1991;19:77.

59. Mahony BS, Nyberg DA, Luthy DA, et al. Translabial ultrasound of the third-trimester uterine cervix. J Ultrasound Med 1990;9:717.

60. Berghella V, Kuhlman K, Weiner S, et al. Cervical funneling: sonographic criteria predictive of preterm delivery. Ultrsound Obstet Gynecol 1997;10:161.

61. Mercer BM, Goldenberg RL, Meis PJ, et al. The preterm prediction study: prediction of preterm premature rupture of membranes through clinical findings and ancillary testing. The national institute of child health and human development maternal-fetal medicine units network. Am J Obstet Gynecol 2000;183:738.

62. Rageth JC, Kernen B, Saurenmann E, et al. Premature contractions: possible influence of sonographic measurement of cervical length on clinical management. Ultrasound Obstet Gynecol 1997;9:183.

63. Fontenot T, Compbell B, Mitchell-Tutt E, et al. Radiographic evaluation of breech presentation: is it necessary? Ultrasound Obstet Gynecol 1997;10:338.

64. Sanders RC, Miner NS. Uncertain dates. In: Sanders RC, Miner NS, eds. Clinical sonography: a practical guide, 3rd ed. Philadelphia: Lippincott, 1998:92.

65. Callen PW. The obstetric ultrasound examination. In: Callen PW, ed. Ultrasonography in obstetrics and gynecology, 4th ed. Philadelphia: WB Saunders, 2000:8.

66. Benson CB, Doubilet PM. Sonography of multiple gestations. Radiol Clin North Am 1990;28:149.

67. Magann EF, Martin JN. Amniotic fluid volume assessment in singleton and twin pregnancies. Obstet Gynecol Clin North Am 1999;26:579.

68. Larmon JE, Ross BS. Clinical utility of amniotic fluid volume assessment. Obstet Gynecol Clin North Am 1998;25:639.

69. McGrath-Ling M. Fetal well-being and fetal death. In: Sanders RC, Miner NS, eds. Clinical sonography: a practical guide, 3rd ed. Philadelphia: Lippincott, 1998:173.

70. Manning FA, Platt LD, Sipos L. Antepartum fetal evaluation: Development of fetal biophysical profile. Am J Obstet Gynecol 1980;136:787.

71. Manning FA. Dynamic ultrasound-based fetal assessment: the fetal biophysical profile score. Clin Obstet Gynecol 1995;38:26.

72. Walkinshaw SA. Fetal biophysical profile scoring. Br J Hosp Med 1992;47:444.

73. Manning FA. Fetal biophysical profile. Obstet Gynecol Clin North Am 1999;26:557.

74. Babbitt NE. Antepartum fetal surveillance. SD J Med 1996;49:403.

75. Garmel SH, D'Alton ME. Diagnostic ultrasound in pregnancy: an overview. Seminars Perinatol 1994;18:117.

76. Manning FA, Morrison I, Harman CR, et al. Fetal assessment by fetal BPS: experience in 19,221 referred high-risk pregnancies. The false negative rate by frequency and etiology. Am J Obstet Gynecol 1987;157:880.

77. Alfirevic Z, Neilson JP. Biophysical profile for fetal assessment in high-risk pregnancies. Cochrane Database Syst Rev 2000;2:CD000038.

78. Ghidine A, Salafia CM, Kirn V, et al. Biophysical profile in predicting acute ascending infection in preterm rupture of membranes before 32 weeks. Obstet Gynecol 2000;96:201.

79. Lewis DF, Adair CD, Weeks JW, et al. A randomized clinical trial of daily nonstress testing versus biophysical profile in the management of preterm premature rupture of membranes. Am J Obstet Gynecol 1999; 181:1495.

80. Nathan L, Huddleston J. Acute abdominal pain in pregnancy. Obstet Gynecol Clin North Am 1995;22:55.

81. Morrison LJ. Unique concerns of pregnancy. In: Rosen P, Barken R, eds. Emergency medicine: concepts and clinical practice, 3rd ed. St. Louis: Mosby, 1998:2327–2340.

82. Cunningham F, McCubbin J. Appendicitis complicating pregnancy. Obstet Gynecol 1975;45:415.

83. Mann F, Nathens A, Langer S, et al. Communicating with the family the risks of medical radiation to conceptuses in victims of major blunt-force trauma. J Trauma 2000;48:354.

84. Abbott JT: Acute complications related to pregnancy. In: Rosen P, Barken R, eds. Emergency medicine: concepts and clinical practice, 3rd ed. St Louis: Mosby, 1998:2342–2364.

85. Manas KJ. Hepatic hemorrhage without rupture in preeclampsia. N Engl J Med 1985;312:424.

86. Weingold AB. Appendicitis in pregnancy. Clin Obstet Gynecol 1983;26:801.

87. Varner M. General medical and surgical diseases in pregnancy. In: Dansforth J, ed. Obstetrics and gynecology, 8th ed. Philadelphia: Lippincott Williams & Wilkins, 1999:427.

88. Lim HK, Bae SH, Seo GS. Diagnosis of acute appendicitis in pregnant women: value of sonography. AJR 1992;159:539.

89. Abu-Yousef MM, Bleichen JJ, Maher JW, et al. High-resolution sonography of acute appendicitis. AJR 1987;149:53.

90. Gomez A, Wood M. Acute appendicitis during pregnancy. Am J Surg 1979;137:180.

91. Mahmoodian S. Appendicitis complicating pregnancy. South Med J 1992;85:19.

92. Williamson S, Williamson M. Cholecystosonography in pregnancy. J Ultrasound 1984;3:329.

93. Simon JA. Biliary tract disease and related surgical disorders during pregnancy. Clin Obstet Gynecol 1983;26:810.

94. Duff P. Pyelonephritis in pregnancy. Clin Obstet Gynecol 1984;29:17.

95. Fried A, Woodring J, Thompson D. Hydronephrosis of pregnancy: a prospective sequential study of the course of dilatation. J Ultrasound Med 1983;2:255.

96. Harris RD, Alexander RD. Ultrasound of the placenta and umbilical cord. In: Callen PW, ed. Ultrasonography in obstetrics and gynecology, 4th ed. Philadelphia: WB Saunders, 2000:597–615.

97. Hoddick W, Mahoney B, Collen P, et al. Placental thickness. J Ultrasound Med 1985;4:479.

98. Gilllieson MS, Winer-Muram HT, Muram D. Low-lying placenta. Radiology 1982;144:577–580.

99. Devevec C, Adair CD, Veille JC. Letter to the editor. J Ultrasound Med 1995;14:804.

100. Sanders RC, Miner NS. Uncertain dates. In: Sanders RC, Miner NS, eds. Clinical sonography: a practical guide, 3rd ed. Philadelphia: Lippincott, 1998:108.

101. Del Valle GO, Bateman L, Gaudier FL, et al. Comparison of three types of ultrasound transducers in evaluating the amniotic fluid index. J Reprod Med 1994;39:869.

102. Hill LM, Krohn M, Lazebnik N, et al. The amniotic fluid index in normal twin pregnancies. Am J Obstet Gynecol 2000;182:950.

103. Larmon JE, Ross BS. Clinical utility of amniotic fluid volume assessment. Obstet Gynecol Clin North Am 1998;25:639.

104. Walkinshaw SA. Fetal biophysical profile scoring. Br J Hosp Med 1992;47:444.

105. Finberg HJ, Kurtz AB, Johnson RL, et al. The biophysical profile: a literature review and reassessment of its usefulness in the evaluation of fetal well-being. J Ultrasound Med 1990;9:583.

106. Gant N. Obstetrical hemorrhage. In: Cunningham FG, MacDonald PC, Gant NF, et al, eds. Williams obstetrics, 20th ed. Stamford, CT: Appleton & Lange, 1997:760.

107. Ananth CV, Berkowitz G, Savitz D, et al. Placental abruption and adverse outcomes. JAMA 1999;282:1646.

108. Nyberg DA, Mack LA, Benedetti TJ. Placental abruption and placental hemorrhage: correlation of sonographic findings with fetal outcome. Radiology 1987;358:357.

109. Nyberg DA, Cyr DR, Mack L. Sonographic spectrum of placental abruption. AJR 1987;148:161.

110. Shrout AB, Kopelman JN. Ultrasonographic diagnosis of uterine dehiscence during pregnancy. J Ultrasound Med 1995;14:399–402.

111. Gale JT, Mahony BS, Bowie JD. Sonographic features of rupture of the pregnant uterus. J Ultrasound Med 1996;5:713–714.

CHAPTER 13

Gynecologic Applications

J. Christian Fox and Michael J. Lambert

Female patients presenting to the emergency department or urgent care setting with lower abdominal pain may present a diagnostic challenge to the physician. Faced with a large differential diagnosis (Table 13–1), their clinical work-up is often time-and-resource consuming. Bedside endovaginal ultrasonography provides a great deal of diagnostic information that helps expedite patient care.

While the spectrum of gynecologic pathology visualized by ultrasound is presented in this chapter, the focus will be on ovarian torsion, tubo-ovarian abscess (TOA), and ovarian cysts. The rationale is that there are only two life- or organ-threatening gynecologic emergencies identifiable by pelvic ultrasound: ovarian torsion and ruptured TOA. Likewise, identification of an ovarian cyst frequently abates further time-consuming diagnostic studies.

▶ CLINICAL CONSIDERATIONS

Imaging the pelvis is a crucial step in the evaluation of women with lower abdominal pain or pelvic pain. Accurate management is predicated on choosing the most effective diagnostic tool. Four diagnostic modalities are available for evaluating the pelvis: laparoscopy, computed tomography (CT), magnetic resonance imaging (MRI), and ultrasonography. Several clinical entities are considered with regard to the advantages and disadvantages of each modality.

CT is generally considered a second-line imaging modality to ultrasound in the evaluation of pelvic pain. It is used routinely for the preoperative evaluation of masses that are suspicious for malignancy. The advantage of CT is the ability to image the full extent of a large adnexal lesion that cannot be visualized in its entirety with sonog-

raphy alone. Another advantage of CT is its usefulness in diagnosing other disease entities, such as appendicitis and diverticulitis. Disadvantages of CT stem from the availability and cost involved in obtaining these readings. CT is not portable and is not immediately available at the bedside for serial examinations. Patients must be transported to the radiology suite, which expends personnel resources. CT exposes patients to radiation and, if IV contrast is used, can be harmful to the kidneys. Finally, the direct cost to the patient for image acquisition, printing film, and radiologist interpretation is substantially more than a bedside ultrasound examination.

MRI is also considered a second-line imaging modality. It has several advantages over CT. MRI does not expose the patient to radiation and provides more detailed information necessary to detect the subtle tissue differentiation of pelvic organs. Since MRI has better tissue resolution than ultrasound, MRI is more accurate in diagnosing pelvic inflammatory disease (PID) and pelvic masses. In 1999, Tukeva and co-workers compared MRI to endovaginal ultrasound for the diagnosis of laparoscopy-proven PID. Of the 21 patients proven to have PID, MRI diagnosed 20 (95%) patients while endovaginal ultrasound correctly diagnosed 17 (81%) patients.[1] However, several of the disadvantages of CT apply to MRI as well. Since MRI is not portable, the test cannot be performed at the bedside. Also, the availability and cost of MRI are problematic.

While laparoscopy remains the gold standard for the diagnosis of PID and pelvic masses, its use may not be readily available or justified in patients with vague symptoms. Laparoscopy is invasive, costly, time-consuming, and requires the small but measurable risk of general anesthesia. Furthermore, laparoscopy does not detect subtle signs of inflammation within fallopian tubes or any

▶ **TABLE 13–1.** DIFFERENTIAL DIAGNOSIS OF LOWER ABDOMINAL PAIN IN FEMALE PATIENTS

Gastrointestinal
   Appendicitis
   Inflammatory bowel disease
   Irritable bowel syndrome
   Constipation
  Gastroenteritis
   Diverticulitis
Urinary tract
   Cystitis
   Pyelonephritis
   Nephrolithiasis
Reproductive
   Ectopic pregnancy
   Intrauterine pregnancy
   Pelvic inflammatory disease
   Tubo-ovarian abscess
   Ovarian cyst
   Hemorrhagic functional cysts
   Ovarian torsion
   Mittelschmerz
Dysmenorrhea
Endometriosis

findings consistent with endometritis.[2] The advantage of laparoscopy, however, is the ability to reveal other pathologic conditions that have been misdiagnosed as PID. In one study, 12% of patients diagnosed with PID revealed other pathologic findings during laparoscopy, such as appendicitis or endometriosis.[3] Another advantage of laparoscopy is the ability to intraoperatively intervene in a pathologic process, such as the untwisting or resection of a torsed ovary or the drainage of an abscess.

Ultrasound has proven to be a rapid, noninvasive, portable, repeatable, inexpensive, and accurate method for visualizing and diagnosing pathology within the pelvis. These advantages over CT, MRI, and laparoscopy have made ultrasound the first-line diagnostic tool in patients with acute pelvic pain, PID, or pelvic masses. Ultrasound is immediately available to the physician at the bedside during the initial physical examination. This accessibility has far-reaching benefits to patient care by curtailing other diagnostic tests and serving to focus the differential diagnosis. Ultrasound has no exposure radiation. Since the clinician is at the bedside performing the ultrasound examination, patients perceive this as more time spent with their physician. This serves to improve patient satisfaction, provides them with more time to ask questions, and ultimately increases their confidence in their physician. Another advantage is the ability of color flow Doppler sonography to evaluate structures for adequacy of blood flow.

The main disadvantage of ultrasound with respect to the other imaging modalities is its limited scope. Other imaging modalities, such as CT and MRI, may yield valuable information about other organ system pathology and the extent to which a disease process may have progressed. Another disadvantage of ultrasonography is the inability of sound waves to penetrate structures filled with air. When sound waves becomes scattered by bowel gas, information distal to the bowel is generally unobtainable by ultrasonography and an alternate imaging modality must then be utilized.

▶ CLINICAL INDICATIONS

Clinical indications for performing a pelvic ultrasound examination include:

- Acute pelvic pain
- Acute pelvic inflammatory disease
- Evaluation of pelvic or adnexal masses

Acute Pelvic Pain

Acute pelvic pain in women is a common complaint in the emergency or ambulatory care setting. The differential diagnosis includes possible etiologies from multiple organ systems: gastrointestinal, urologic, gynecologic, musculoskeletal, neurologic, and vascular. Although life-threatening conditions, such as appendicitis or ectopic pregnancy, are in the differential, the majority of patients can be treated and discharged home. For most of these conditions, management typically consists of pain control and observation. While the definitive evaluation of these patients ultimately may involve CT scan, pelvic sonography is the diagnostic imaging modality indicated in the initial evaluation.

Ovarian Torsion

This entity should be considered in the differential diagnosis of any woman with lower abdominal pain (Table 13–2). Ovarian torsion is a surgical emergency that can result in both reproductive and hormonal compromise if not promptly diagnosed. Because the diagnosis is often elusive and sufficiently delayed, detorsion of the ovary is rarely an option. A twisting of the ovarian attachments through the utero-ovarian ligament to the uterus and

▶ **TABLE 13–2.** DIFFERENTIAL DIAGNOSIS OF OVARIAN TORSION

Appendicitis
Adnexal mass
Pelvic mass
  Myoma
  Ectopic pregnancy
  Tubo-ovarian abscess
Ruptured viscus

through the infundibulopelvic ligament to the pelvic side-wall causes this condition. This results in congestion of the ovarian parenchyma and eventual hemorrhagic infarction from decreased ovarian blood supply.[4] The "classic" symptoms of acute, severe, unilateral lower abdominal or pelvic pain are present in approximately one-third of the patients with confirmed ovarian torsion. Ovarian torsion is frequently missed on the preoperative diagnosis; the two incorrect preoperative diagnoses that are most commonly made instead are tubo-ovarian abscess and ruptured corpus luteal cyst.[5]

Torsion can occur in normal ovaries, although the incidence is more common in ovaries containing cysts or tumors. These masses are thought to act as a fulcrum by which torsion can propagate. One study demonstrated that ovarian torsion was associated with palpable adnexal masses in over 90% of adults compared with only 50% of children.[6] Other researchers reported that a unilaterally enlarged ovary with small peripherally located cysts (1 to 6 mm) was the most common finding (56%) in young and adolescent girls.[7] In 1985, it was reported that ovarian masses were associated with cases of torsion in only 50% of patients. Pregnancy appears to be a risk factor as well; 20% of all cases can been found to occur during pregnancy.[8]

Abnormal blood flow detected by Doppler sonography is highly predictive of ovarian torsion and is therefore useful in the diagnosis of ovarian torsion. However, when normal flow is detected by Doppler sonography, it does not necessarily exclude ovarian torsion. In fact, ovarian torsion is missed in 60% of these cases, and time to diagnosis is therefore delayed. In patients undergoing hormonal therapy for ovarian stimulation, the sensitivity of Doppler for ovarian torsion increases to 75%.[9] Despite being intuitively similar to other organs, such as the testicle, lack of blood supply to the ovary cannot be adequately excluded using Doppler. The reason for this is twofold. First, Doppler flow may be present in one part of the ovary (peripheral or central) but not in the other due to the fact that the ovary has a dual blood supply. Second, thrombosis of venous structures produces the symptoms of ovarian torsion before the arterial system becomes occluded. While some investigators have suggested that absent blood flow on pulsed Doppler and color Doppler is specific for torsion,[10,11] others suggest that observing blood flow to the ovary should not be relied upon to definitively exclude this diagnosis.[12] Stark and Siegel reported that the presence of a Doppler signal was present in 9 of 14 patients ultimately proven to have ovarian torsion.[13]

Grayscale findings may be useful in diagnosing ovarian torsion by identifying a large ovary with enlarged follicles or an enlarged complex cystic adnexal mass. Conversely, it has been suggested that normal ovarian size and texture may be helpful in excluding this diagnosis. Graif and colleagues studied 41 patients suspected of having ovarian torsion who had transabdominal ultrasound performed. Eleven patients had ovarian torsion proven at surgery, and 7 of the 11 patients were correctly diagnosed by ultrasound. Ovarian enlargement was detected in all 11 patients. This study (albeit a very small sample size) yielded a positive predictive value of 87.5%. In the other 28 patients, sonography correctly excluded the diagnosis, yielding a specificity of 93%. All patients were followed for 63 months on an outpatient basis.[14]

Vaginal Conditions

Some gynecologic procedures involve instrumentation that result in postoperative complications. These patients may present to the emergency department with vaginal bleeding, acute pelvic pain, and unstable vital signs. Ultrasound can play a crucial role in the timely diagnosis and management of these patients. For example, ultrasound can localize and diagnose a vaginal hematoma in a hypotensive patient who recently underwent a dilatation and curettage procedure. Typically, the ultrasound examination is performed transabdominally in an attempt to localize the hematoma within the vaginal tissue planes.

Acute Pelvic Inflammatory Disease

Acute PID, defined as an infection in the upper genital tract, represents a spectrum of disease entities, including any combination of endometritis, salpingitis, oophoritis, pelvic peritonitis, and TOA.[15] More than 1 million women are diagnosed with PID annually and 25% of them proceed to suffer at least one sequela of PID, which include infertility, ectopic pregnancy, or chronic abdominal pain.[16] The severity of its clinical presentation corresponds poorly with the damage to the fallopian tubes. Many young women with PID have mild and vague symptoms.[17] Therefore, the diagnosis of PID on clinical grounds has been notoriously difficult and was shown to be only 66% accurate in one study.[18] Endovaginal ultrasound was demonstrated to be superior to bimanual examination alone in the diagnosis of findings consistent with PID.[19]

Early sonographic signs of PID are increased adnexal volume and periovarian inflammation with fluid collections. On ultrasound, this appears as structures that lack the distinct margins that are normally identified. Another sonographic sign of PID is the decreased ability of the ovary to slide smoothly in the adnexa (sliding organ sign) when the ultrasound probe is inserted and withdrawn from the vagina. This sign suggests that the ovary has been tethered to the fallopian tube by inflammatory adhesions. These sonographic findings were correlated with laparoscopic evidence of periovarian exudates and adhesions by Patten in 1990.[20] In 1992, it was demonstrated that sonographic evidence of free fluid had a sensitivity of 77% and specificity of 79% in culture-proven PID. Finally, the presence of "polycystic-like" ovaries containing increased stroma with several follicles scattered throughout the stroma has been found to be indicative of

PID; Cacciatore demonstrated a sensitivity of 100% and a specificity of 71% for this finding.[21]

In another study evaluating the role of ultrasound in diagnosing PID, Boardman and co-workers studied four ultrasound markers to suggest evidence of PID: free fluid in the cul-de-sac, multicystic ovaries, visualization of fallopian tube or tubal fluid, and presence of an adnexal mass or TOA. These investigators found that in patient populations that have a high prevalence of PID, an endovaginal ultrasound examination positive for these markers is useful for suggesting the diagnosis of PID in patients, and thus helping to avoid laparoscopy. A negative ultrasound examination, however, should not be viewed by the clinician as being reliable for excluding the diagnosis of PID in a patient who appears clinically ill. In this subset of patients, laparoscopy may be required to make the diagnosis.[22]

Pelvic and Adnexal Masses

Tubo-Ovarian Abscess

Women who present with a pelvic mass may have a TOA, tubo-ovarian complex, uterine fibroid, hydrosalpinx, ovarian cyst, or a variety of other complex adnexal masses. Clinicians cannot rely solely on their bimanual examination to accurately detect pelvic masses; 70% of pelvic masses found on ultrasound examination were initially missed during the bimanual examination.[23] A pelvic mass detected on physical examination is an indication for a pelvic ultrasound examination. If a cystic structure is found within the ovary, this provides a hard finding for the clinician to explain the patient's symptoms and a clear disposition that often negates further work-up during that visit. The presence of a cystic structure on the ovary, however, is very common and does not exclude the presence of other concomitant pathology.

Pelvic ultrasonography is indicated in cases of severe, recurrent PID with or without the presence of a mass on physical examination. It is critically important that a distinction be made between PID and TOA in order to direct specific treatment regimens. Since the same clinical diagnostic difficulties of PID apply to TOA, ultrasonography plays a crucial role in the diagnosis. Understanding that the development of a TOA occurs through a stepwise fashion will aid the sonologist with the ultrasound examination. The first stage involves inflammation of the tubal mucosa. The wall eventually thickens and purulent material fills the lumen and spills into the cul-de-sac. If either end of the fallopian tube becomes blocked by pus, a pyosalpinx can occur. As the pressure within the lumen increases, the walls are stretched thin and the tube becomes distended. In some patients, the process stops at this stage, resulting in chronic hydrosalpinx. When the remnants of the endosalpingeal folds become fibrotic, they appear as spokes outlined by anechoic fluid ("cogwheel sign"). As the acute inflammatory process continues to proceed, it erodes through the distended wall. If the ovary has a recent defect from the ruptured corpus luteum, it becomes exposed to this inflammation and purulent material enters this space. The final stage of abscess formation occurs when the pus walls itself off, fusing the tube and ovary together.

The incidence of PID developing into TOA has been reported to be between 4%[24] and 30%.[25] TOA requires a different treatment regimen than PID since it forms an abscess, tends to be polymicrobial, and consists of anaerobes.[26] Since the mid-1970s, ultrasonography has been shown to be an accurate, sensitive, and noninvasive imaging technique for diagnosing TOA.[27,28] Furthermore, serial ultrasound examinations have proven to be useful in following TOAs that are managed nonoperatively. Pelvic ultrasonography also assists in the selection of the most effective treatment regimen.[29,30] In a study of 106 patients with clinically suspected PID, ultrasound findings demonstrated 19 patients with pyosalpinx and 4 patients with hydrosalpinx. These 23 patients had their medical therapy directly altered as a result of the endovaginal ultrasound.[31]

Uterine Fibroids

Uterine fibroids represent the most common gynecologic tumor. Leiomyomas start as a mass of smooth muscle proliferation in a whorled spherical configuration. Atrophy and vascular compromise eventually ensue, which result in necrosis and calcification. Clinically, the patient presents with dysuria, dysmenorrhea, constipation, or low back pain (from compression of lumbar plexus).

▶ ANATOMIC CONSIDERATIONS

To understand the pelvic anatomy, it may be helpful to think of the pelvis as two separate areas: the true pelvis and false pelvis. The true pelvis has a basin-shaped contour and is bounded anteriorly by the pubic symphysis and pubic rami. It is bounded posteriorly by the sacrum and coccyx and inferiorly by the perineal musculature. The false pelvis is located superior to the true pelvis. The abdominal wall represents its anterior border, the iliac bones define its lateral border, and the sacral promontory outlines its posterior border. The empty bladder lies within the true pelvis and, when distended, enters the false pelvis (Figure 13–1).

The uterus is a thick-walled, muscular structure with a shape that can vary with cyclical menstrual changes and distention of the bladder and rectum. Typically, the uterus is found in the anteverted position in its relationship with the bladder; in 25% of women, it is retroflexed. During the reproductive years, the uterus measures up to 7 cm × 4 cm × 5 cm. The postmenopausal uterus mea-

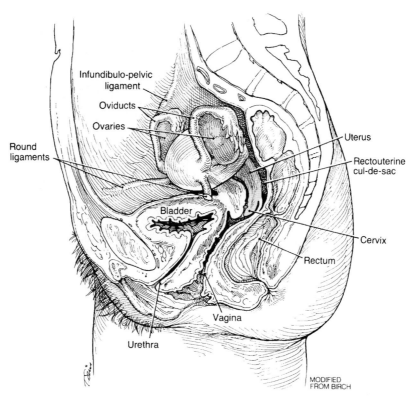

Figure 13–1. Normal pelvic anatomy. *(Reprinted with permission from Cunningham et al: Williams obstetrics, 21st ed. New York: McGraw-Hill, 2001, p. 36.)*

sures 7 cm in length and 1 to 2 cm in transverse. The endometrial thickness varies with the menstrual cycle from 6 mm to less than 1 mm following menstruation.

The ovaries are elliptical-shaped structures and are found in a range of positions in the parous woman. In the nulliparous woman, the ovaries are located more reliably on the posterolateral wall of the true pelvis, adjacent to the internal iliac vessels. The menstrual cycle is categorized into two phases: the proliferative phase, which culminates in ovulation, followed by the secretory phase, which ends in menstruation. Cystic follicles regularly occur during the proliferative phase and are not officially termed a "cyst" until they reach a diameter of 2.5 cm. A corpus luteum then forms at the site of ovulation during the secretory phase, but rarely exists for more than 6 wk in the non-pregnant patient. Therefore, in the absence of ovulation, these cysts cannot occur. Once ruptured, the only evidence of their existence may be the presence of free fluid in the posterior cul-de-sac.[32]

The pouch of Douglas is a term that refers to the potential space in the posterior cul-de-sac of the pelvis. It consists of the peritoneal reflection posterior to the uterus and anterior to the rectosigmoid colon. Because this is the most dependent portion of the supine woman, a trace of free fluid is normally seen here, especially in

the 5 d prior to menstruation.[33] The anterior cul-de-sac lies between the bladder (anterior) and the uterus (posterior). Since this potential space is not dependent, it only contains free fluid when a significant amount is present in the pelvis (see Figure 13–1).

▶ TECHNIQUE AND NORMAL ULTRASOUND FINDINGS

Transabdominal

The advantage of the transabdominal approach is that it is rapid, noninvasive, and provides a good overall view of the pelvis. The disadvantage is that the pelvic organs are several cm away from the ultrasound transducer head and a lower frequency probe must be utilized.

With the transabdominal technique, the ultrasound probe should be placed on the lower aspect of the abdominal wall just above the pubic symphysis. While scanning the pelvic organs from a transabdominal approach, transducer frequency and bladder filling both play a significant role in image quality. To best visualize pelvic organs, a transducer in the 3.5 to 5.0 MHz range should be utilized. Filling the bladder will enhance the quality of sonographic images by displacing the air-filled bowel out of the true pelvis and aligning the solid organs perpendicular to the transducer.

The pelvic structures are scanned in two planes: longitudinal and transverse. To scan in the longitudinal plane, the probe should be placed in the up and down position with the indicator toward the patient's head. In this plane, the bladder takes on a triangular, or "tear drop," appearance. The uterus is pear shaped and typically measures 5 to 7 cm in length in the menstruating female (Figure 13–2). The examiner may need to angle the probe in an oblique fashion since the uterus may not be located in the midline or central axis. The endometrial stripe is a thin, hyperechoic line running down the center of the uterus along its length, and it fluctuates with the menstrual cycle. It appears thin and less echogenic just following menses in the proliferative phase, and becomes thick and more echogenic following ovulation during the secretory phase. In this longitudinal plane, the endometrial stripe is visualized as the probe is fanned from left to right. The vaginal stripe that is unique to the transabdominal approach can be visualized in the longitudinal plane. It appears as a thin echo bright stripe seen posterior to the bladder. The cervix is visualized between the uterus and vagina.

The majority of women have an anteverted uterus found angulated 90° to the midline vaginal stripe when the bladder is empty. Filling the bladder straightens out the uterus so that it comes to lie in a more parallel alignment to the vaginal stripe. A retroverted uterus can be seen extending in an opposite direction to the bladder and appears linear when the bladder is full.

In the transverse view, the probe should be oriented in the left to right fashion with the indicator pointed toward the patient's right side. The ovaries are best viewed in this plane and are typically found posterior and lateral to the uterus (Figure 13–3). The ovaries are typically lo-

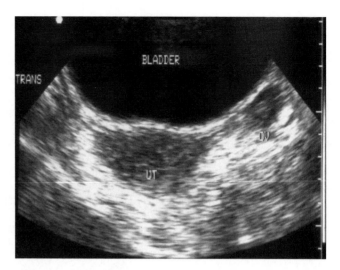

Figure 13–3. Transabdominal transverse view of the uterus and left ovary. *(Courtesy of James Mateer, MD.)*

cated anterior and medial to the iliac vessels. In the multiparous patient, ovaries may be found in a variety of positions, from as posterior as the pouch of Douglas to as anterior as the uterine fundus. Normal ovaries measure 2 cm × 2 cm × 3 cm in adults and are characterized by hypoechoic follicular structures in the periphery (cortex).

The uterus appears as a circular structure in the transverse plane (see Figure 13–3). It is important to scan the uterus from the fundus to the cervix by fanning the beam in a top to bottom fashion. In this plane, the ovaries can be identified on either side of the uterus. Normal fallopian tubes generally cannot be visualized unless surrounded by fluid.

Endovaginal

The advantage of the endovaginal approach is that the endovaginal probe is closer to the organs of interest and so a higher frequency probe, usually in the 5.0 to 7.5 MHz range, can be utilized. These higher frequency probes have enhanced axial and lateral resolution that results in superior image quality. Most women report that the endovaginal technique is less uncomfortable than the transabdominal technique. Even among adolescent patients undergoing evaluation for PID, 28% preferred the endovaginal route.[34] The advantage of not requiring patients to have a full bladder helps make the experience less uncomfortable.

This technique initially involves disinfecting the probe with standard bactericidal agents between each usage. A proper acoustic medium should be applied on both sides of the condom. Any air bubbles within the condom should be displaced in order to avoid beam scattering artifacts. In patients undergoing infertility therapy, the ultrasound gel should not contain any spermicidal agent; in these cases, tepid sterile water is suitable for lubrication.

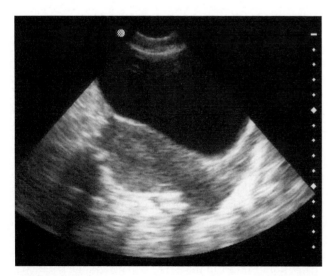

Figure 13–2. Transabdominal sagittal view of bladder, uterus, and cervix. *(Courtesy of James Mateer, MD.)*

In a systematic fashion, the entire pelvis should be scanned in both sagittal and coronal planes. The patient should be placed in the lithotomy position. With the handle of the endovaginal probe being held in a "pistol-grip" fashion, the endovaginal probe should be carefully inserted with the indicator pointed toward the ceiling. While inserting the probe, it is important to document the bladder as a landmark anterior to the uterus. It should be clearly discerned from any fluid collection in the anterior cul-de-sac. In a midline sagittal view of the uterus, the endometrial stripe should be clearly identified (Figure 13–4). Maintaining this sagittal plane, the entire uterus is evaluated. By extending into both lateral projections, the boundaries of the uterus should be defined. To scan patients with a retroverted uterus, it may be necessary to slightly remove the probe and then severely angle the probe face posteriorly (handle towards the ceiling). This allows the beam to be directed in a posterior fashion, which permits sound waves to access the fundus. If the fundus still lies beyond the angle of the beam, the probe may be inverted 180°, reversing the on-screen direction of fundal image but allowing for adequate (and more comfortable) uterus evaluation.

From the midline sagittal plane, the probe is then rotated 90° in a counter-clockwise fashion (indicator toward patient's right) to view structures in the coronal plane. The coronal plane can also be thought of as axial, or transverse, and simply refers to the cross-sectional view of the uterus. Views are obtained by fanning through the entire uterus from cervix to fundus. The uterus and endometrial stripes assume a round appearance in this projection.

Ovaries are typically identified by the presence of circular hypoechoic follicles. These follicles can be confused with cross-sectional uterine vessels that become tubular when the probe is rotated. Normal ovaries are mobile and may be found in different positions during the same examination. To view the left ovary, the examiner should start in the coronal plane with the top of the probe pointed toward the patient's left. Starting at the fundus, the examiner should scan until the uterine origin of the left fallopian tube is identified. Then, this structure should be followed into the patient's left adnexa until the characteristic follicles of the left ovary are identified. The right ovary is similarly identified, except the probe is turned toward the patient's right into the coronal plane. Ovaries may also be found in the sagittal plane by fanning laterally until an iliac vessel in a transverse plane is identified. From here, fine adjustments to bring the iliac vessel into a longitudinal plane should be made, which typically reveal the ovary anterior and medial to this structure (Figure 13–5).

The fallopian tube is a poor sonic reflector, which makes it virtually impossible to scan in a transabdominal approach. Even utilizing an endovaginal approach, healthy fallopian tubes are not typically visualized. Changing patient positioning or optimizing scanning techniques can occasionally enable visualization of the fallopian tube. For example, placing patients in reverse-Trendelenburg takes full advantage of any physiologic fluid that may be present in the pelvis. After ovulation, up to 10 cc of free fluid may be released from a functional ovarian cyst. Blood, ascites, or an exudative/infectious process producing free fluid in the pelvis will similarly enhance image acquisition. In addition, when the endovaginal probe is gently inserted further or removed slightly, it has the benefit of a third scanning plane along its own axis. This effectively moves the adnexa into various positions to enhance imaging. As a general rule, if the lumen of the fallopian tube is identifiable, the suspicion of a pathologic process is heightened. Normally, the tubal lumen is not visualized unless it is filled with fluid. Once the entire tubal lumen is filled, the fimbriae may then be

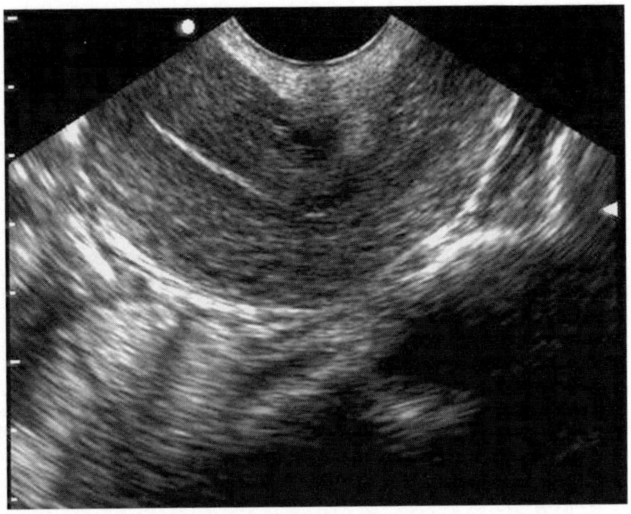

Figure 13–4. The endometrial stripe in a midline sagittal view of the uterus.

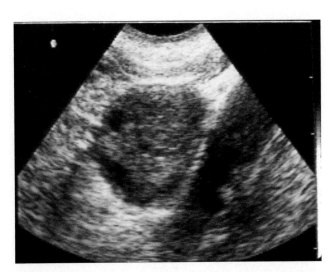

Figure 13–5. In a longitudinal plane, the ovaries can be located anterior and medial to the external iliac vessels. *(Courtesy of James Mateer, MD.)*

identified. In the longitudinal axis, the tortuous fallopian tube varies in length. Similarly, the transverse axis may vary in width depending on the plane in which it is cut. The width typically approximates 1 cm in normal individuals. The proximal (myometrial) portion of the fallopian tube occasionally may be visualized as a hyperechoic line as it enters the uterus.

► COMMON AND EMERGENT ABNORMALITIES

Functional Simple Cysts

These cysts are the most common ovarian masses in non-pregnant young women. Sonographically, they appear as thin-walled, unilocular anechoic spheres. Using specific criteria, a thin-walled, anechoic structure within the ovary is a physiologic cyst until it reaches a diameter greater than 2.5 cm. Follicular cysts can range from 2.5 cm to over 14 cm (Figure 13–6). As opposed to the anechoic structure of a simple cyst, cysts containing heterogenic variable echoes are considered hemorrhagic (Figure 13–7). Typically unilateral, they may be found in both ovaries, as seen in polycystic ovarian disease.[35] Not all cystic structures within the pelvis are simple ovarian cysts. Ovarian cysts contain heterogeneous tissue, with peripheral follicles frequently identified along its border. It is not uncommon for these simple ovarian cysts to rupture. This event, however, is a clinical diagnosis and not a sonographic one. Regardless, clinical suspicion for a ruptured cyst should remain high in any patient who presents with severe lower abdominal pain and free fluid in the pelvis, with or without an ovarian cyst (Figure 13–8).

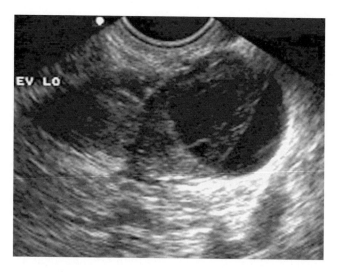

Figure 13–7. Hemorrhagic ovarian cyst.

Corpus Luteum Cyst

A corpus luteum cyst begins to form within the follicle following ovulation. When a patient becomes pregnant, a corpus luteal cyst can persist up to 16 weeks gestation and reach a diameter of up to 13 cm. If intermittent bleeding occurs within this cystic structure, it often appears heterogeneous and can be mistaken for an ectopic pregnancy.[36] A corpus luteum cyst can also persist and develop internal hemorrhage during a dysfunctional (nonpregnant) menstrual cycle. These corpus luteum cysts can have a variety of appearances (Figures 13–9 and 13–10). Similar to a functional simple cyst of the ovary, corpus luteal cysts may also rupture resulting in severe abdominal pain[37] (Figure 13–11).

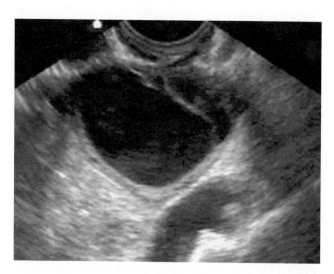

Figure 13–6. Follicular cyst. A 4-cm cyst as seen with endovaginal sonography.

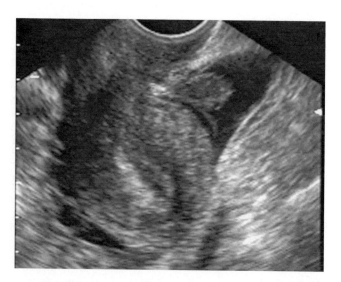

Figure 13–8. Retroverted uterus with free fluid in the cul-de-sac.

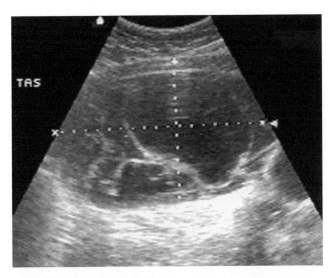

Figure 13–9. Transabdominal image. Large, echogenic, scalloped corpus luteum cyst.

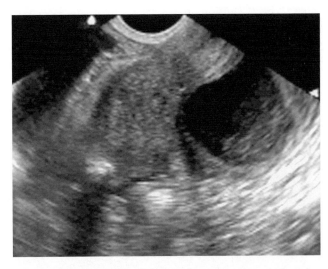

Figure 13–10. Longitudinal endovaginal view reveals a hemorrhagic cyst in the cul-de-sac and a small calcified fibroid in the uterine fundus.

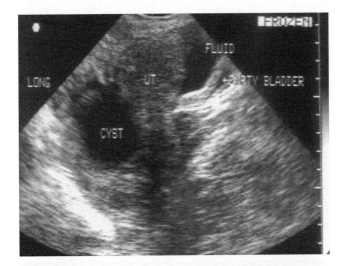

A

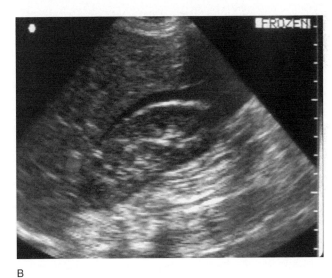

B

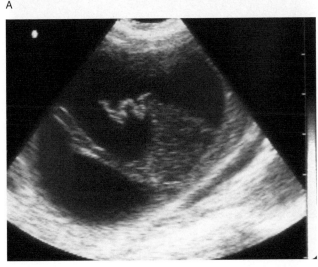

C

Figure 13–11. Ruptured corpus luteum cyst. (A) Long axis transabdominal image shows a collapsed bladder with fluid in the anterior cul-de-sac and a large cyst in the posterior cul-de-sac. (B) A small stripe of free fluid was noted in Morison's pouch. (C) Endovaginal ultrasound reveals a hemorrhagic cyst that has not fully ruptured. *(Courtesy of James Mateer, MD.)*

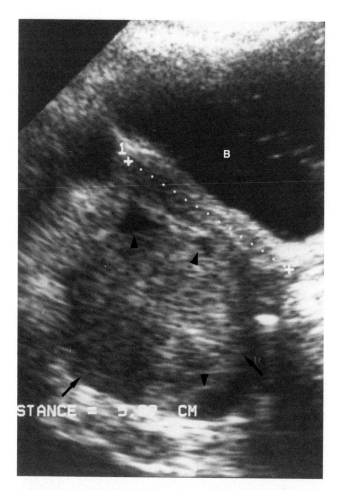

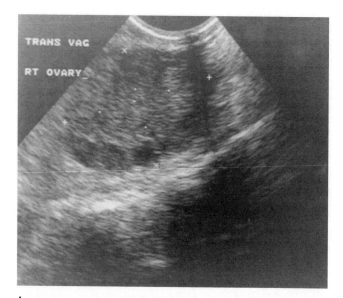

A

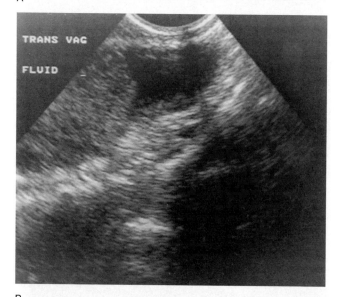

B

Figure 13–12. Ovarian torsion. Pelvis. Longitudinal plane. The uterus is marked off by measurement points. It is 5 cm in length. Posterior to it is a large solid mass (*arrows*) with a few peripheral cysts (*arrowheads*). This is a relatively classic image for ovarian torsion, although the echogenicity of the ultrasound image is related to the variable internal contents of the torsed ovary. This mass, which is the patient's torsed left adnexa, was much larger than the patient's normal right adnexa. B = bladder. *(Reproduced from Cohen HL, Sivit CJ: Fetal and pediatric ultrasound. New York: McGraw-Hill, 2001;516.)*

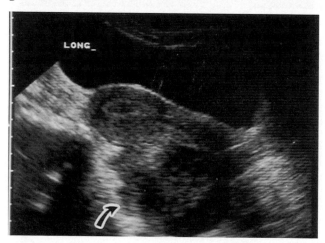

C

Figure 13–13. Adnexal (ovarian) torsion. (A) Transvaginal sonogram showing enlarged right ovary *(between +'s)* with mildly echogenic area resulting from internal hemorrhage. (B) Cul-de-sac fluid adjacent to left side of uterus in same patient. (C) Two days later, ovary has enlarged secondary to retorsion. On transabdominal sonography (TAS), enlarged size of ovary relative to uterus can be better appreciated. *(Reproduced from Fleischer et al: Sonography in obstetrics and gynecology, 6/e. New York: McGraw-Hill, 2001;899.)*

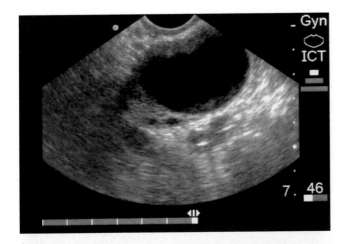

A

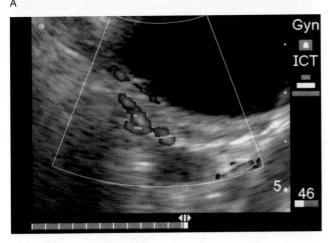

B

Figure 13–14. Ovarian cyst. Endovaginal view of a 3 × 4 cm cyst demonstrates a peripheral rim of ovarian tissue that helps to identify the etiology of the cyst (A). Color Doppler revealed normal flow within the ovarian tissue. *(Courtesy of James Mateer, MD.)*

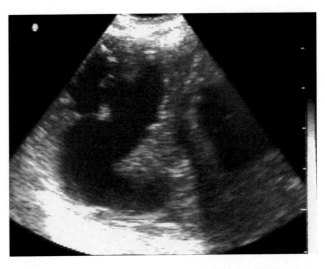

Figure 13–15. Hydrosalpinx. A serpiginous fluid-filled structure is noted in the adnexa. *(Courtesy of James Mateer, MD.)*

Ovarian Torsion

The only specific sonographic sign of ovarian torsion is demonstration of multiple follicles in the cortical part of a unilaterally enlarged ovary. Transudative fluid flows into the multiple follicles as the ovary becomes congested from circulatory impairment. Ovarian enlargement, when present, is relatively obvious. It has been reported that a torsed ovary is at least 34 times larger than the average *prepubescent* ovary and 8 times larger than the average *adult* ovary[38] (Figures 13–12 and 13–13A–C).

Doppler can be helpful in making the diagnosis of ovarian torsion when there is complete absence of blood flow to one ovary. Comparing the blood flow between the involved ovary and the unaffected ovary is useful. It is important to scan in several different planes when examining the ovary for presence of blood flow (Figure 13–14). By changing the scanning angle, the sonographer decreases the likelihood that the finding of absent blood flow is due to the angle at which the blood was moving in relation to the ultrasound beam.[39]

Tubo-Ovarian Abscess

Imaging the TOA has several caveats. First, the process of TOA formation usually occurs bilaterally, but not necessarily in step; therefore, bilateral TOA may appear "out of phase" with one another. Second, there often is absence of the sliding organ sign. Third, organisms producing gas result in highly echogenic reflectors within the abscess. Finally, the fallopian tube surrounds the ovary causing it to lose the typical appearance of anechoic follicles in the periphery. This appears sonographically as an ovary connected to, or embraced by, the fluid-filled serpiginous fallopian tube[40,41] (Figures 13–15 through 13–19).

Uterine Fibroids

On ultrasound, the uterus appears heterogeneous and globular, with discrete masses embedded in the uterine wall. They can be hyper or hypoechoic (see Figure 13–10). Fibrotic changes and calcifications cause sonographic attenuation and loss of definite margins, which make size estimations problematic. Color Doppler can identify those fibroids containing a vascular supply, which may be responsive to hormonal therapy.[42] Because fibroids tend to reflect the sound waves, there is usually significant shadowing distal to the mass. In fact, the shadowing is often dense enough that it interferes with high frequency imaging with the endovaginal technique (Figure 13–20). For

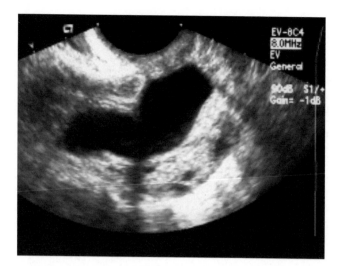

Figure 13–16. Hydrosalpinx. A fluid-filled tubular structure is adjacent to the ovary. There was no color flow detected within this structure.

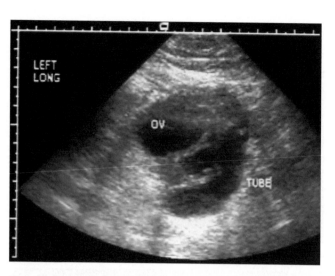

Figure 13–18. Tubo-ovarian complex. Endovaginal image of the left adnexa shows a distorted ovary (OV) partially encircled by a fluid filled hydrosalpinx (TUBE).

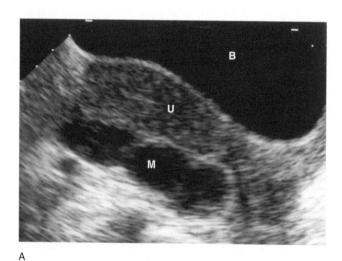

A

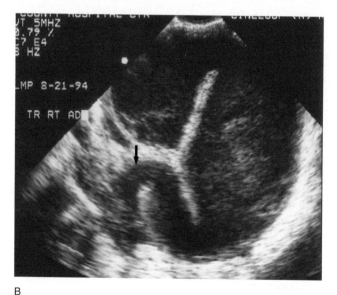

B

Figure 13–17. Pyosalpinx. Pelvic ultrasound. (A) Midline longitudinal plane. The uterus (U) is posterior to the bladder on this magnified image. Posterior to the uterus, in the cul de sac, is a tubular cystic mass (M) with some contained echogenicity. In this teenager with symptoms of pelvic inflammatory disease, this is at least a hydrosalpinx. The contained echoes point to the greater but not exclusive possibility of pyosalpinx. (B) Transvaginal exam. Region of right adnexa. This pyosalpinx was better imaged by higher-frequency transvaginal scanning, performed with the transducer very near the object of interest. The tubular nature of this relatively echoless, debris-filled mass can be readily recognized. An arrow points to a turn in the less dilated proximal end of the fallopian tube. This tube was noted on other views to extend from the uterine cornu. Its contained echogenicity suggests but does not confirm the presence of infected material, i.e., pus. *(Reproduced from Cohen HL, Sivit CJ: Fetal and pediatric ultrasound. New York: McGraw-Hill, 2001;524.)*

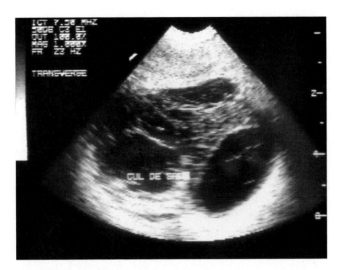

Figure 13–19. Tubo-ovarian abscess. Endovaginal transverse view of the cul-de-sac area shows a complex septated cystic mass 4 × 6 cm in size which proved to be a TOA. *(Courtesy of James Mateer, MD.)*

this reason, patients with large or multiple fibroids may require a transabdominal, full-bladder technique to obtain adequate images of the pelvic structures.

▶ COMMON VARIANTS AND SELECTED ABNORMALITIES

Uterine Conditions

Bicornuate Uterus
One relatively common anatomic variant is the bicornuate uterus (Figure 13–21). As the sonographer fans the ultrasound beam from left to right, the uterine fundus

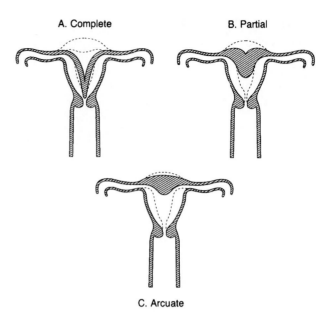

Figure 13–21. Class IV: Bicornuate uterus in which the septum is complete down to the internal os (A), partial (B), or arcuate (C). *(Reproduced from Cunningham et al: Williams obstetrics, 21/e. New York: McGraw-Hill, 2001;920.)*

will appear to "re-grow." It is important to note that in this longitudinal plane both fundi will not be visualized simultaneously, but rather in succession. On transverse views, the separated endometrial echoes may be visible (Figures 13–22 and 13–23).

Intrauterine Device
Occasionally, patients present to the emergency department or acute care clinic because of concerns that an intrauterine device (IUD) has been dislodged during

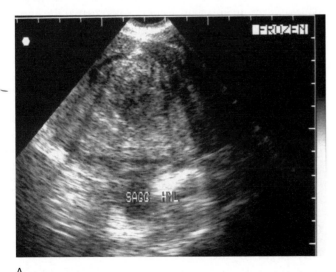

A

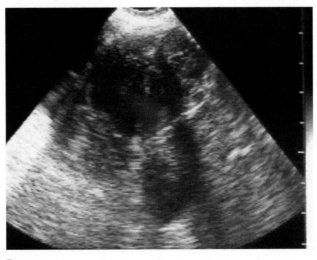

B

Figure 13–20. Uterine fibroids. (A) Endovaginal views demonstrate a slightly hyperechoic fibroid with faint lines of posterior shadowing. (B) A large hypoechoic fibroid is located in the lower uterine segment. These often interfere with adequate endovaginal imaging. *(Courtesy of James Mateer, MD.)*

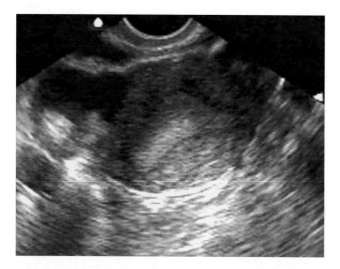

Figure 13–22. Transverse (coronal) endovaginal view of the endometrium shows an Y shape consistent with an arcuate pattern of bicornuate uterus.

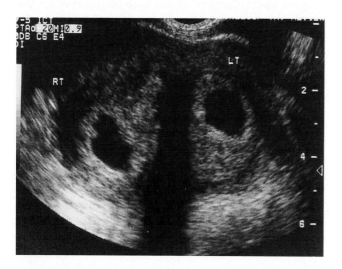

Figure 13–23. Bicornuate uterus. The separate uterine horns are well visualized in this transverse endovaginal ultrasound. The uterine cavity has been filled with fluid to enhance imaging of the endometrium (sonohysterography). *(Reprinted with permission from Fleischer et al: Sonography in obstetrics and gynecology, 6/e. New York: McGraw-Hill, 2001,1151.)*

vigorous vaginal intercourse. This becomes further complicated when the string normally attached to the IUD has broken off or is missing. Sonographically, the IUD is strongly reflective and easily identified on endovaginal views unless located outside the uterus (Figure 13–24).[43] It is important to note that even though they represent a highly echoic structure, IUDs may not be distinguishable from the endometrial stripe using the transabdominal approach.

Endometritis

Endometritis is most often seen with PID, during postpartum or after instrumentation. The endometrial stripe appears prominent or irregularly shaped. Fluid, gas, or debris can often be visualized.

Endometriosis

Ectopic endometrial tissue is usually found in the cul-de-sac, ovaries, and fallopian tubes. During menses, this tissues hemorrhages, resulting in multiple small fluid collections (endometriomas) that generally are not easily visualized by ultrasound. An enlarged endometrioma (termed "chocolate cyst") appears on ultrasound as a cystic structures with thickened walls and containing mid-level echogenic centers.[44] The viscous-fluid center can be mistaken for a solid ultrasound mass, but is identified as a cyst by posterior acoustic enhancement distal to the structure.

Uterine Polyps

Uterine polyps, found in 10% of women, are pedunculated sections of endometrial tissue that can occur as a single lesion or as multiple lesions. They may become so large that they protrude through the cervical os. The endometrium is thickened with areas of focal echogenicity or endocavitary masses surrounded by fluid.

Endometrial Hyperplasia

Endometrial hyperplasia results from the unopposed estrogen stimulation of endometrial proliferation without the shedding effects of progesterone. The sonographic findings are nonspecific but do suggest a thickened endometrial stripe often greater than 5 mm. Post-menopausal patients with greater than 1 cm of endometrial thickness usually indicates hyperplasia or carcinoma.[45]

Endometrial Neoplasm

Tumors range in echogenicity from hyper- to hypoechoic. Some tumors may simply stretch the endometrium without directly invading it, making them difficult to visualize on ultrasound. Tumors greater than 1 cm in anterior to posterior dimension or ones greater than 10 cc in volume may warrant endometrial biopsy. Hyperplasia in general is a known precursor to carcinoma.[46]

Cervical Conditions

Nabothian Cysts

Nabothian cysts occur when the endocervical glands becomes obstructed and dilated. This is a benign condition that commonly occurs without symptoms and has no

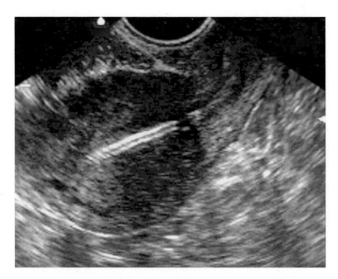

Figure 13–24. An IUD is strongly reflective and easily identified on endovaginal views.

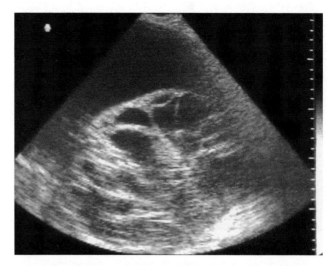

Figure 13–25. Mucinous cystadenoma. The transabdominal ultrasound is at maximum viewing depth for a 3.5-MHz probe. A-38 pound seromucinous cystadenoma was confirmed at laparotomy. *(Courtesy of James Mateer, MD.)*

clinical or pathologic significance. They appear sonographically within the cervix as a thin-walled, anechoic cystic structure up to 1 cm in diameter.

Cervical Malignancy

The majority (90%) of cervical malignancies is squamous cell and appears as bulky heterogeneous material within the cervix. This entity is seen best in the sagittal view.

Ovarian Conditions

Ovarian cysts are common in all age groups, but especially in women of menstrual age. There exists a great deal of overlap in the sonographic appearances of the various masses found in the ovary and the adnexa. Their sonographic characteristics become even more similar when the subset of masses with a complex morphology is considered. It is the task of the clinician to sort through which findings require immediate diagnostic evaluation and which can be monitored on an outpatient basis.

Mucinous Cystadenomas.

Mucinous cystadenomas are benign masses that represent the largest of the ovarian neoplasms. They are capable of growing to occupy the entire abdominal cavity such that patients appear gravid. They contain mucinous material, which appear sonographically as multiple fine, low-level echoes[47] (Figure 13–25).

Serous Cystadenomas

Serous cystadenomas, constituting approximately 20% of all benign neoplasms of the ovary, appear sono-

graphically as a multilocular cystic mass containing few or no internal echoes. Septations are sufficiently thin so as to undulate with gentle transducer palpation. In the benign form, nodularity is typically absent; therefore, any solid tissue noted should raise concern for malignancy.

Cystadenocarcinoma

Ultrasound distinction between benign cystadenomas and malignant cystadenocarcinoma is difficult. Biopsy of the ovary has borderline histology 15% of the time.[48] Sonographic characteristics that suggest malignant histology include thick septa, increased mural nodularity, presence of solid tissue, and ascites. The presence of ascites was noted in over 50% of malignant epithelial neoplasms of the ovary and is completely absent with benign disease.[49]

Dermoid Cysts

Dermoid cysts, the second most common cause of ovarian masses, may contain areas of hair and fat, both of which produce strong echogenic reflectors. Calcified structures, such as teeth, produce strong shadows and are easily identified on plain films[46] (Figures 13–26, 13–27).

Paraovarian Cysts

Arising from remnants of the Wolffian duct within the broad ligament, a paraovarian cyst accounts for 10% of all adnexal masses. These generally have the character-

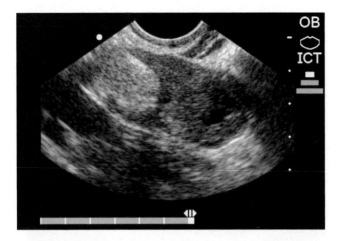

Figure 13–26. Early dermoid. Endovaginal view of the right ovary reveals a small (2-cm) echogenic mass within the borders of the ovary. *(Courtesy of James Mateer, MD.)*

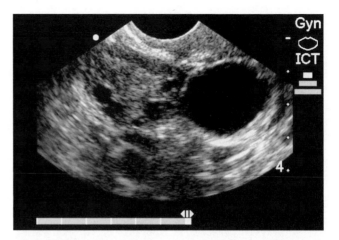

Figure 13–28. Paraovarian cyst. Transverse view of the ovary demonstrates a small (2-cm) paraovarian cyst. *(Courtesy of James Mateer, MD.)*

istics of a simple cyst and range from 1.5 to 19 cm in size. A paraovarian cyst should be suspected when the ovary can be identified as a separate structure (Figure 13–28).

Polycystic Ovaries

Represented as multiple immature follicles less than 1 cm packed along the periphery. Sometimes described as "beads on a string" morphology.[47] When stimulated with hormones, they have an exaggerated appearance resembling a stained glass window.

Vaginal Conditions

Vaginal Hematoma

Ultrasound can be used to localize and diagnose a vaginal hematoma. Typically, the ultrasound examina-

tion is performed transabdominally in an attempt to localize the hematoma within the vaginal tissue planes (Figure 13–29).

▶ PITFALLS

1. *Presence of blood flow in the involved ovary does not necessarily exclude the diagnosis of ovarian torsion.* Absence of ovarian blood flow is helpful in diagnosing ovarian torsion. The converse has not been shown to be reliable for excluding ovarian torsion. In other words, in the correct clinical setting, the index of suspicion for ovarian torsion should be maintained even if blood flow is present in the involved ovary.

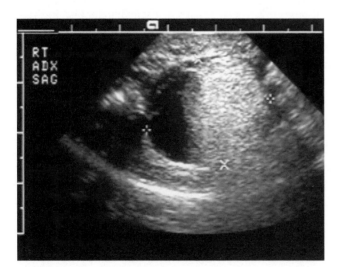

Figure 13–27. Dermoid. Endovaginal image of the right adnexa shows the typical appearance of a dermoid demonstrating the echogenic solid component and a cystic portion.

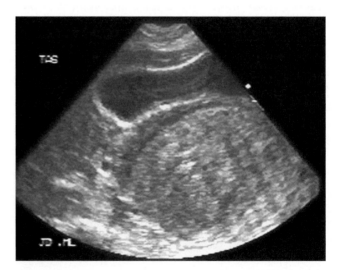

Figure 13–29. Vaginal hematoma. Transabdominal ultrasound view of a vaginal hematoma in patient who recently underwent a dilatation and curettage procedure.

2. *The uterine vasculature may appear cystic on cross-sectional image planes and are commonly mistaken for follicles within an ovary.* The ovary can be confirmed by these cystic structures lacking blood flow. These structures should remain cystic in different scanning planes. Vascular structures contain blood flow and lengthen out when viewed in alternate scanning planes.

3. *Large ovarian follicles may be mistaken for fallopian tubes.* These ovarian follicles will change during the cycle and be localized within the ovary.

4. *Small ovarian cysts can falsely appear as a thin-walled hydrosalpinx.* The finding of ovarian tissue in the periphery helps to exclude this diagnosis.

5. *Retained mucous secretions can imitate tumors by appearing to have endometrial thickening.*

6. *Other disease processes, such as tuberculosis and various gynecologic malignancies, can cause peritoneal implantation to the uterine serosa.* These disease entities are easily identified sonographically when surrounded by fluid.

7. *Imaging the shrunken postmenopausal ovary is difficult due to its lack of follicles, decreased pelvic fluid, and decreased vaginal elasticity inhibiting probe movement.*

▶ CASE STUDIES

Case 1

Patient Presentation

A 22-year-old nulliparous woman presented to the emergency department with a 1-d history of severe right lower quadrant abdominal pain and scant vaginal discharge. The patient was seen by her primary care physician 4 d previously and was treated for a urinary tract infection. She reported having unprotected sex with one sexual partner for the past several months. Her past medical history and past surgical history was unremarkable. Review of systems was significant for tactile fever and decreased oral intake.

On physical examination, the patient had a blood pressure, 110/70 mm Hg; heart rate, 123 beats per min; respiratory rate, 18 per min; and temperature, 39.8°C. She appeared toxic. The abdominal examination revealed severe right lower quadrant tenderness slightly inferior to McBurney's point, no rebound or guarding, normoactive bowel sounds, and no costovertebral angle tenderness. The rectal examination lateralized tenderness to the right and the stool was guaiac negative. Sterile speculum examination revealed a friable cervix with scant purulent discharge. Bimanual examination revealed right adnexal tenderness, cervical motion tenderness, but no evidence of fullness or masses. A urinalysis specimen was unremarkable, and the urine pregnancy

test was negative. The white blood cell count was 15,000 with a left shift.

Management Course

At this stage in the work-up, acute appendicitis was suspected. A general surgeon ordered a CT scan of the abdomen and pelvis with triple contrast. This test was read as negative for appendicitis but did reveal a complex structure associated with the right ovary. A bedside endovaginal ultrasound revealed a cogwheel formation of the right ovary, absence of the sliding ovary sign, and heterogenic material within the right fallopian tube. A diagnosis of TOA was made, triple antibiotic therapy was initiated, and the gynecologist was consulted. The patient was taken to the operating room for laparoscopy with abscess drainage.

Commentary

Case 1 illustrated the diagnostic role that ultrasonography can have in the work-up of a young woman with lower abdominal pain. Ectopic pregnancy and urinary tract disease had been excluded by the urine sample. Appendicitis initially was at the top of the differential diagnosis. A negative CT scan, however, is not 100% accurate for excluding appendicitis, and the general surgeon continued to entertain thoughts of taking the patient to the operating room to perform an appendectomy. The pelvic ultrasound examination confirmed the diagnosis of TOA and the patient's care was expedited by having the gynecologist perform the laparoscopic procedure for abscess drainage.

Case 2

Patient Presentation

A 16-year-old nulliparous woman presented to the emergency department with the sudden onset of severe left lower quadrant abdominal pain. The symptoms started 30 min prior to arrival and were associated with nausea, three episodes of vomiting, and chills. The patient denied vaginal bleeding or discharge and any prior history of sexual intercourse. Past medical history and past surgical history were unremarkable.

On physical examination, the patient had a blood pressure, 120/70 mm Hg; heart rate, 118 beats per min; respiratory rate, 20 per min; and temperature, 37.8°C. She appeared in severe distress secondary to the pain and nausea. Abdominal examination revealed moderate tenderness in left lower quadrant without rebound or guarding. Bowel sounds were normal. There were no masses or costovertebral tenderness. Rectal examination was nontender and stool was guaiac negative. Sterile speculum examination was unremarkable and bimanual examination revealed left adnexal tenderness, cervical motion tenderness, normal right adnexa, and no masses or fullness. The white blood count was normal, and the urinalysis and urine pregnancy test were negative.

Management Course

The emergency physician's differential diagnosis included ovarian torsion, ruptured ovarian cyst with chemical peritonitis, and TOA. The physician's bedside endovaginal ultrasound examination showed no evidence of free fluid, ovarian mass, or TOA. There was, however, an enlarged left ovary with complete absence of any discernible blood flow despite evaluation in multiple planes. The right ovary had normal-appearing blood flow. A gynecologist was immediately called to the bedside for suspected ovarian torsion and she took the patient to the operating room for laparoscopy. Her ovary was immediately detorsed with intraoperative visual evidence of good perfusion.

Commentary

Case 2 was an example of a young woman who presented with acute ovarian torsion. This case illustrated that the pelvic ultrasound examination could be performed rapidly at the patient's bedside, which is one of the main advantages of ultrasonography. The emergency physician was able to expedite the patient's disposition to the operating room. This helped the gynecologist salvage the young woman's left ovary.

▶ Case 3

Patient Presentation

A 32-year-old, gravida 4, para 4 woman presented to the emergency department with worsening right lower quadrant abdominal pain over the past several days. She admitted that this pain felt like the same pain she has had in the past with her ovarian cysts. She denied vaginal discharge, vaginal bleeding, fever, chills, nausea, or vomiting. She had no past medical history or past surgical history.

On physical examination, the patient had a blood pressure, 110/70 mm Hg; heart rate, 92 beats per min; respiratory rate, 16 per min; and temperature, 37.2°C. She appeared in mild distress secondary to abdominal pain. Abdominal examination revealed moderate tenderness to deep palpation in her right lower quadrant. No rebound or guarding was appreciated and there were no masses or costovertebral tenderness. Rectal examination was nontender and the stool was guaiac negative. Sterile speculum examination was unremarkable; however, bimanual examination revealed adnexal fullness on the right side with moderate tenderness. No cervical motion tenderness was elicited and the left adnexa was normal. The white blood count was normal, and the urinalysis and urine pregnancy test were negative.

Management Course

The differential diagnosis included appendicitis, ovarian torsion, PID, and TOA. The emergency physician performed a screening bedside endovaginal ultrasound examination that revealed a 4-cm right ovarian cyst and evidence of normal appearing blood flow to the surrounding ovarian tissue and trace free fluid in the posterior cul-de-sac (see Figure 13–6). The patient's symptoms were alleviated with oral ibuprofen and she was discharged home. Arrangements were made with her gynecologist to schedule a repeat ultrasound examination later that week in her office. This follow-up ultrasound examination revealed resolution of the cyst with a moderate amount of free fluid in the posterior cul-de-sac.

Commentary

Case 3 demonstrated how utilization of bedside emergency ultrasound allowed the physician to avoid ordering expensive, time-consuming diagnostic tests for the evaluation of the patient's complaint. While the patient's differential diagnosis included several worrisome disease entities, the physician was able to match the patient's clinical picture to a finding on the ultrasound examination, and then initiated the appropriate therapy.

REFERENCES

1. Tukeva TA, Aronen HJ, Karjalainen PT, et al. MR imaging in pelvic inflammatory disease: comparison with laparoscopy and ultrasound. Radiology 1999;210:209–216.
2. Centers for Disease Control and Prevention. 1998 guidelines for treatment of sexually transmitted diseases. MMWR 1998;47:79.
3. Jacobson L. Objectivized diagnosis of acute PID. Am J Obstet Gynecol 1969;105:1088–1098.
4. Graif M, Itzchak Y. Sonographic evaluation of ovarian torsion in childhood and adolescence. Am J Radiol 1988;50:647–649.
5. Hibbard L. Adnexal torsion. Am J Obstet Gynecol 1985;152:456–460.
6. Schultz LR, Newton WA, Clatoworthy HW. Torsion of previously normal tube and ovary in children. N Engl J Med 1963;268:343–346.
7. Stark J, Siegel M. Ovarian torsion in prepubertal and pubertal girls: sonographic findings. AJR 1994;163:1479–1482.
8. Hibbard L. Adnexal torsion. Am J Obstet Gynecol 1985;152:456–460.
9. Pena JE. Usefulness of Doppler sonography in the diagnosis of ovarian torsion. Fertil Steril 2000;73:1047–1050.

10. Surratt J, Siegel J. Imaging of pediatric ovarian masses. RadioGraphics 1991;11:533–548.

11. Van Hoorhis B, Schwaiger J, Syrop C, et al. Early diagnosis of ovarian torsion by color Doppler sonography. Fertil Steril 1992;58:215–217.

12. Rosado W, Trambert M, Gosink B, et al. Adnexal torsion: diagnosis by using Doppler sonography. Am J Radiol 1992;159:1251–1253.

13. Stark J, Siegel M. Ovarian torsion in prepubertal and pubertal girls: sonographic findings. Am J Radiol 1994;163:1479–1482.

14. Graif M, Itzchak Y. Sonographic evaluation of ovarian torsion in childhood and adolescence. Am J Radiol 1988;150:647–649.

15. Centers for Disease Control and Prevention. 1998 guidelines for treatment of sexually transmitted diseases. MMWR 1998;47:79.

16. Washington AE, Katz P. Cost of and payment source for pelvic inflammatory disease: trends and projections, 1983 through 2000. JAMA 1991;226:2565.

17. Lawson MA, Blythe MJ. Pelvic inflammatory disease in adolescents. Pediatr Clin North Am 1999;46:4.

18. Jacobson L. Objectivized diagnosis of acute PID. Am J Obstet Gynecol 1969;105:1088–1098.

19. Arbel–DeRowe Y, Tepper R, Rosn DJ, et al. The contribution of pelvic ultrasonography to the diagnostic process in pediatric and adolescent gynecology. J Pediatr Adolesc Gynecol 1997;10:3.

20. Patten RM. PID. Endovaginal sonography and laparoscopic correlation. J Ultrasound Med 1990;9:681–689.

21. Cacciatore B, Leminen A, et al. Transvaginal sonographic findings in ambulatory patients with suspected pelvic inflammatory disease. Obstet Gynecol 1992;6:912–916.

22. Boardman L, Peipert J, Brody J, et al. Endovaginal sonography for the diagnosis of upper genital tract infection. Endovaginal Sonography 1997;90:54–57.

23. Teisala K, Heinonen PK, Punnonen R, et al. Transvaginal ultrasound in the diagnosis and treatment of tubo-ovarian abscess. Br J Obstet Gynecol 1990;77:178–180.

24. Roberts W, Dockery JL. Management of tubo-ovarian abscess due to pelvic inflammatory disease. South Med J 1984;77:7.

25. Reed S, Landers D, Sweet RL. Antibiotic treatment of tuboovarian abscess: comparison of broad-spectrum beta-lactam agents versus clindamycin-containing regimens. Am J Obstet Gynecol 1991;164:1556–1562.

26. Landers DV. Tubo-ovarian abscess complicating pelvic inflammatory disease. In: Landers DV, Sweet RL, eds. Pelvic inflammatory disease. New York: Springer Verlag, 1996:94.

27. Taylor KJW, et al. Accuracy of grey-scale ultrasound diagnosis of abdominal and pelvic abscesses in 220 patients. Lancet 1978;1:83–84.

28. Uhrich PC, Sanders RC. Ultrasound characteristics of pelvic inflammatory masses. Clin Ultrasound 1976;4:199–204.

29. Landers DV. Tubo-ovarian abscess complicating pelvic inflammatory disease. In: Landers DV, Sweet RL, eds. Pelvic inflammatory disease. New York: Springer Verlag, 1996:94.

30. McNeeley SG. Medically sound, cost-effective treatment for pelvic inflammatory disease and tuboovarian abscess. Am J Obstet Gynecol 1988;178:1272–1278.

31. Bulas DI, Ahlstrom PA, Sivit CJ, et al. Pelvic inflammatory disease in the adolescent: comparison of transabdominal and transvaginal sonographic evaluation. Radiology 1992;183:435–439.

32. Holt SC, Levi CS, Lyons EA, et al. Normal anatomy of the female pelvis. In: Callen P, ed. Ultrasonography in obstetrics and gynecology. St. Louis: WB Saunders, 1993:550–551.

33. Davis JA, Gosnick BB. Fluid in the female pelvis: cyclic patterns. J Ultrasound Med 1986;5:75–79.

34. Bulas DI, Ahlstrom PA, Sivit CJ, et al. Pelvic inflammatory disease in the adolescent: comparison of transabdominal and transvaginal sonographic evaluation. Radiology 1992;183:435–439.

35. Holt SC, Levi CS, Lyons EA, et al. Normal anatomy of the female pelvis. In: Callen P, ed. Ultrasonography in obstetrics and gynecology. St. Louis: WB Saunders, 1993:555.

36. Holt SC, Levi CS, Lyons EA, et al. Normal anatomy of the female pelvis. In: Callen P, ed. Ultrasonography in obstetrics and gynecology. St. Louis: WB Saunders, 1993:561–562.

37. Rottem S, Timor-Tritsch I. Ovarian pathology. In: Timor-Trisch I, Rottem S, eds. Transvaginal sonography. New York: Elsevier, 1991:156.

38. Graif M, Itzchak Y. Sonographic evaluation of ovarian torsion in childhood and adolescence. AJR 1988;150:647–649.

39. Zagebski J. Doppler instrumentation. In: Essentials of ultrasound physics. St. Louis: Mosby, 1996:90.

40. Rottem S, Timor-Tritsch I. Ovarian pathology. In: Timor-Trisch I, Rottem S, eds. Transvaginal sonography. New York: Elsevier, 1991:155

41. Cacciatore B, Leminen A, et al. Transvaginal sonographic findings in ambulatory patients with suspected pelvic inflammatory disease. Obstet Gynecol 1992;80:912–916.

42. Rottem S, Timor-Tritsch I. Ovarian pathology. In: Timor-Trisch I, Rottem S, eds. Transvaginal sonography. New York: Elsevier, 1991:155.

43. Comstock, C. Ultrasonography of gynecologic disorders. In: Pearlman M, Tintinalli J, eds. Emergency care of the woman. New York: McGraw Hill, 1998:669.

44. Rottem S, Timor-Tritsch I. Ovarian pathology. In: Timor-Trisch I, Rottem S, eds. Transvaginal sonography. New York: Elsevier, 1991:157.

45. Fleischer A, Kepple D, Entman A. Transvaginal sonography of uterine disorders. In: Timor-Tritsch I, Rottem S, eds. Transvaginal sonography. New York: Elsevier, 1991:119.

46. Comstock, C. Ultrasonography of gynecologic disorders. In: Pearlman M, Tintinalli J, eds. Emergency care of the woman. New York: McGraw Hill, 1998:671.

47. Rottem S, Timor-Tritsch I. Ovarian pathology. In: Timor-Trisch I, Rottem S, eds. Transvaginal sonography. New York: Elsevier, 1991:155.

48. Mendelson EB, Bohm-Velez M, Joseph N, Neiman HL. Gynecologic imaging: comparison of transabdominal and transvaginal sonography. Radiology 1988;166:321–324.

49. Cramer DW, Welch WR. Determinants of ovarian cancer risk. Inferences regarding pathogenesis. J Natl Cancer Inst 1983;71:717.

CHAPTER 14

Lower Extremity Deep Venous Thrombosis

Michael Blaivas

In recent years, medicine has seen the spread of bedside ultrasonography beyond the traditional scope of practice employed by early emergency sonologists.[1-4] Many of the new applications adopted by emergency sonologists have resulted from a clinical need to improve efficiency of patient care. One such application has been ultrasonography for the detection of deep venous thrombosis (DVT).[5,6]

Approximately 260,000 cases of lower extremity DVT are diagnosed each year in the United States.[7] These, in turn, are thought to lead to as many as 50,000 pulmonary embolism deaths per year.[7] To combat the potentially deadly side effects of lower extremity DVT, physicians in the United States order almost 500,000 lower extremity duplex ultrasound examinations per year.[8] Many vascular laboratories, however, find it difficult to maintain 24 h coverage, 7 d per week, for emergency evaluation.[9] This has resulted largely from lack of funding and trained personnel. Many hospitals now have an absence of vascular laboratory services during off-hours. The result is the emergency or primary physician has to empirically treat and usually admit patients that may have a lower extremity DVT.

▶ CLINICAL CONSIDERATIONS

The high incidence and considerable morbidity and mortality resulting from DVT, coupled with the occasional difficulty encountered in trying to diagnose it, has made this a disease of considerable importance.[10] With the addition of low-weight-heparin to the medical arsenal it is now possible to send some patients home without obtaining a diagnostic study. The patient can then undergo an outpatient study the following day, which if negative, would lead to termination of anticoagulation therapy.[11,12] However, there are some drawbacks to this strategy. Patients who are sent home require training in self-administration of low-molecular-weight heparin. This may be difficult to accomplish in a busy emergency department or outpatient setting. Further, despite the relatively low incidence of bleeding with low-molecular-weight heparin, complications are occasionally encountered and can be severe. Another reality is that many primary physicians still elect to admit their patients with actual or suspected DVT.

It is not surprising that physicians have long sought a means of more accurately diagnosing or excluding lower extremity DVT at the bedside. This is reflected by the many clinical decision rules developed over the years and attempts to integrate laboratory tests such as the D-dimer assay, which differs from one facility to another and is not specific for the presence of DVT.[13,14] Considering the consequences of missing a diagnosis of DVT, the various rules are generally not accurate enough.

Emergency ultrasound can, within minutes, diagnose or exclude lower extremity DVT. With such rapid diagnosis available, lower extremity ultrasound examinations could be utilized routinely for bedside diagnosis.

▶ CLINICAL INDICATIONS

The clinical indication for performing a lower extremity duplex examination is:

- Suspicion of lower extremity DVT.

Suspicion of Deep Vein Thrombosis

An examination of the deep veins in the lower extremity is indicated whenever a proximal DVT is suspected. Proximal DVT is loosely defined as a clot in the popliteal vessel or higher in the leg. Its significance is that it is associated with a greater risk of embolization than a calf vein DVT.[15]

The complete duplex examination performed by imaging specialists is somewhat lengthy, with one leg taking up to 37 min in one study.[16] In addition, it may or may not include an evaluation of the veins below the trifurcation of the popliteal vein, distal to the knee. The complete study involves a slow, painstaking evaluation of each vein roughly one-probe width at a time. Each small segment of vein is visualized and checked for complete collapse under pressure from the transducer. Multiple blood flow measurements are taken using color and spectral Doppler.

In recent years, a number of studies have shown the traditional complete examination may not be necessary and an abbreviated approach still maintains high accuracy and patient safety while decreasing the time required for an examination. The abbreviated approach argues for spot checks of vein compressibility, usually at the common femoral and popliteal vein. This allows for considerable time saving and increases patient comfort. Some imaging specialists have expressed concerns regarding this approach. There is considerable evidence, however, that this method is safe and effective.

Lensing and co-workers studied a group of 204 consecutive patients who had undergone elective, major lower extremity surgery.[17] These patients were part of a general screening for lower extremity DVT and were not specifically referred for testing. The researchers found that simply compressing the vein to assess its patency produced a sensitivity of 60% and a specificity of 96%. The addition of color Doppler did not improve the study results. In these patients, venous compression was performed over the entire leg, a time-consuming task. Perhaps the most important point here is that color Doppler did little to improve detection of proximal DVT. This is in sharp contrast to the general beliefs held by many imaging specialists.

In 1989, a group of investigators published their findings on a head-to-head comparison of contrast venography with B-mode ultrasonography in 220 consecutive patients.[18] The only criterion used to detect DVT with ultrasound was lack of compression in either the common femoral or popliteal veins. For proximal vein thrombosis, the study yielded a sensitivity of 100%. When patients with calf vein thrombi (located on venogram) were included, the sensitivity and specificity were 91% and 99%, respectively. The study showed that, in comparison to the gold standard, this simple method of DVT detection was highly accurate.

A number of other studies also confirmed high sensitivity and specificity for the detection of proximal lower extremity DVT without the utilization of color Doppler.[7,8,16,17] The studies also noted considerable time-savings when segmental checks were performed. Thus, the necessity of compressing every inch of vein in the proximal venous system should also be questioned. The most frequent argument from imaging specialist sources is the potential for occurrence of segmental DVTs. These are venous thrombi that are limited to only one section of the deep venous system. For example, the popliteal vein may be without thrombus as well as most of the superficial femoral vein; however, a 3-in. section of the superficial femoral vein in the mid-thigh could contain thrombus. This is the reason some investigators argue that every cm of the venous system should be evaluated.

Lund and associates examined the incidence of a small, isolated thrombus segment, such as in the iliac and popliteal veins, and found an incidence of zero out of 195 legs studied.[19] Thus, the chance of missing evidence of segmental thrombi is very small. Poppiti and co-workers prospectively studied 72 patients for DVT using an abbreviated technique with only two compression sites per leg.[16] The two sites used were the saphenofemoral junction and the lower popliteal vein. For proximal DVT, the sensitivity and specificity of simple compression in these two sites were 100% and 98%, respectively. The investigators addressed potential criticism of their abbreviated technique by noting that in a study of 491 patients found to be without DVT by compression ultrasonography, only 1.5% had a proximal DVT during the 6-month follow-up evaluation.[20]

In 1996, a radiology group prepared a study on the safety of abbreviated studies for DVT. Frederick and associates studied 721 patients, on whom 755 examinations were performed.[21] All patients were referred to a vascular laboratory for suspicion of DVT. A complete examination was performed on each patient and the investigators attempted to make retrospective inferences from the results. They declared that DVT limited to a single vein occurs with enough frequency that the ultrasound survey for thrombosis should not be limited. However, the investigators failed to note that even the isolated thrombus segments in their study were usually within the area interrogated by the abbreviated approach and would have been detected.

In 1998, a large study evaluated the abbreviated compression approach in 405 consecutive outpatients suspected of having a first-time lower extremity DVT.[8] Each patient had his or her common femoral and popliteal veins assessed for compressibility. In those with normal results, testing was repeated in 5 to 7 d. Regardless of symptoms, patients with negative results on compression ultrasound did not receive anticoagulation. Follow-up was performed on all patients at 3 months after the initial negative. Of the patients studied, 63 had DVT detected on initial ultrasound examination. Repeat ultrasound studies picked up 7 proximal DVTs that were not present on initial examination and may have propagated proximally from veins in the calf. None of the patients with normal results died of pulmonary embolism during the follow-up period.

The patency of lower extremity veins should be checked in any patient that a clinician suspects of having a lower extremity DVT. Patients with symptoms suggestive of DVT typically have calf swelling and pain posteriorly.[22] Redness of the posterior calf can also be suggestive. Although a number of studies have suggested that DVT is unlikely to be present without a minimum of a 2 cm difference in calf diameter between and affected and contralateral sides, in practice this is not always the case.[23] Further, there may be considerable medicolegal pressure to exclude DVT during the initial evaluation.

The risk factors commonly described for the development of DVT include smoking, abdominal surgery, lower extremity injury, venous stasis, previous history of DVT, and congestive heart failure, among others.[24–26] Thus, any person who has a risk factor and presents with calf pain and swelling is a candidate for undergoing a study to exclude DVT. Despite a number of studies that have suggested at least several risk factors must be present to warrant emergency evaluation for DVT, many physicians may feel obligated to exclude the presence of the disease for marginal indications.[24–26] Anecdotal experience in several environments has shown that the pressure from referring and consulting physicians can be so great that a large number of unnecessary lower extremity duplex examinations may be ordered.

Bedside emergency ultrasound examination of lower extremity veins is of greatest use in facilities that lack vascular laboratory access at night and/or on weekends. Emergency or primary physicians often find themselves having to empirically treat patients they suspect of having a DVT. This typically involves either admission for heparin therapy or discharge on low-molecular-weight heparin therapy. The latter can be made difficult if expeditious follow up cannot be arranged or if the local medical culture frowns on outpatient treatment of uncomplicated DVTs. The high accuracy that can be achieved with a modified lower extremity duplex will allow discharge without anticoagulant therapy of those patients found to have a negative study. It is imperative to keep in mind that all patients who require a lower extremity duplex to exclude a DVT should have a repeat scan in 5 to 7 d. This will allow for diagnosis of distal DVT (those in the calf itself) if they progress proximally. This is expected to occur in up to 20% of distal DVT cases.[8]

In general, bedside emergency ultrasonography is not recommended for diagnosing DVTs limited to the calf or ankle. Success rates can be as low as 40%, even for experienced vascular sonographers; if complicated by edema or large body habitus, success rates will be even lower.[27] Many vascular laboratories no longer scan below the calf and prefer to rescan patients or perform venography if high suspicion of a calf DVT exists.

▶ ANATOMIC CONSIDERATIONS

The venous system of the lower extremity is quite simple until the calf is reached in a proximal to distal examination. Although many clinicians may feel they have a "sixth sense" for the location of the femoral vein and artery after several years of practice and the placement of numerous central lines, few clinicians are truly aware of the variations that exist even at that level of the thigh. While physicians are taught that the femoral vein is located just medial to the pulse from the femoral artery, the novice sonographer quickly discovers that vein and artery may often lie on top of one another rather than side by side. When this happens, a typical arrangement is for the femoral artery to lie on top of the femoral vein.

The femoral vein flows into the iliac vein. Proceeding distal from proximal, the first segment is the common femoral vein. The common femoral vein then diverges into the deep femoral and superficial femoral veins (Figure 14–1). The nomenclature used here is deceptive and there have even been efforts to change the name of the superficial femoral vein as inexperienced clinicians have sometimes mistaken reports of thrombus in the superficial femoral vein as being outside of the deep venous system. The deep femoral vein proceeds deep into the thigh. The superficial femoral vein proceeds distally until it dives into the obturator canal. In this region, the vein is difficult to access until it emerges behind the knee as the popliteal vein.

▶ TECHNIQUE AND NORMAL ULTRASOUND FINDINGS

To perform a lower extremity venous ultrasound examination, a high-resolution linear array is required. Not all basic ultrasound systems have this capability but with recent improvements in technology, more and more ultrasound units in emergency and urgent care settings are capable of performing the examination. Color Doppler can be extremely helpful, especially if vascular structures are difficult to distinguish due to poor visualization of tissue. Power Doppler, a more sensitive but nondirectional version of color Doppler, can be used as well and is even more likely to detect very slow blood flow, such as in veins.

Ideally, a patient is positioned as needed to maximally distend the leg veins. Many full-length protocols include having the patient dangle his or her leg over the edge of a bed or table (Figure 14–2). This kind of manipulation is not realistic for many clinicians, especially when dealing with acutely ill patients. That said, distended veins do make better targets and it is best to have the head of the patient's bed up at least 30°, with 45° being preferable (Figure 14–3). This allows for blood to

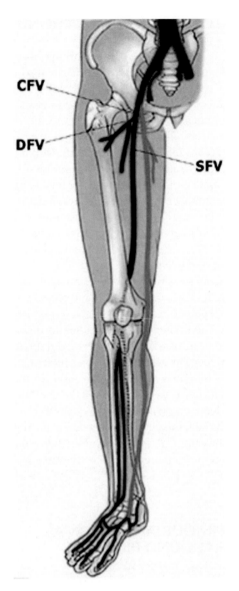

Figure 14–1. The deep femoral and superficial femoral veins are seen to come together, forming the common femoral vein. CFV = common femoral vein; DFV = deep femoral vein; SFV = superficial femoral vein.

pool in the lower extremities and may make evaluation of the vein in question much easier.

An ultrasound transducer with appropriate resolution should be used. Thin patients may require a 7.5 to 10 MHz transducer. Larger patients may need the increased penetration of a 5 MHz probe. All of these frequencies can be obtained in a single broadband probe available on many new ultrasound systems. A probe should be utilized that will allow for adequate compression of underlying vascular structures (Figure 14–4). Transducers with a curved face can make it difficult to achieve adequate compression of soft tissue to ensure collapse of a patent's vein or veins. If challenged by lack of adequate equipment, enterprising physicians can make due with a wide range of transduc-

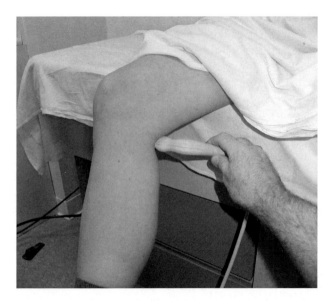

Figure 14–2. The leg is allowed to hang over the edge of the bed with the probe positioned in the popliteal fossa.

ers, even an endovaginal probe, although the compression achieved may be poor.

The patient's leg may be bent at the knee and turned outward (Figure 14–5). This allows for greater access to the femoral vessels in the proximal thigh and the popliteal vein. The proximal inner thigh and popliteal fossa should be well exposed. The femoral vein and artery are easiest to find, with the transducer placed transverse to the long axis of the vessels (Figure 14–6).

An adequate amount of ultrasound gel should be placed on the area of skin where the transducer will be located. The examination should start as proximally as possible; generally at this location the common femoral vein and artery are visualized. The transducer slowly should be moved distally, while keeping it transverse to the vessels. Once the junction of common femoral, superficial femoral, and deep femoral veins is encountered, a firm compression should be applied to visualize the collapse of the vein (Figure 14–7). The normal vein should collapse easily while the artery should remain largely intact (Figure 14–8). If there is any difficulty distinguishing artery from vein, color Doppler may be helpful. While both vein and artery may show color flow, the flow in the artery will usually appear more pulsatile than in the vein. The pulse repetition frequency (PRF) can be adjusted so that slower, and presumably venous, flow will not be picked up. The most reliable method to differentiate venous from arterial flow would be to activate spectral Doppler and compare waveforms between the vessels. The waveform seen in veins will tend to be continuous, with flow still noted in diastole. Arterial waveforms should have a peak and trough quality or a frank triphasic flow pattern.

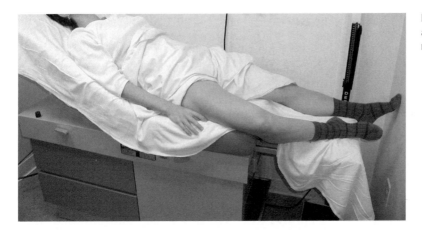

Figure 14–3. A bed angle of 30° to 45° allows lower extremity veins to fill and make them easier to locate.

After assuring patency of the femoral vein junction, the simplified approach then calls for continuing on to the popliteal fossa. The probe is placed behind the knee and the popliteal artery and vein are located (Figure 14–9). Again, firm pressure is applied to collapse popliteal vein. Applying counterpressure with the non-scanning hand on the outside of the knee will facilitate compression of the popliteal vein. Duplication of the popliteal vein is possible and, if present, both should collapse completely. Complete collapse of the vein's lumen should be visualized, as described above for the femoral vein (see Fig-

ure 14–8). Partial collapse can indicate the presence of a clot in the vein; however, poor collapse of the lumen may also be caused by inadequate compression of the vein. This can be improved by transducer adjustment or patient manipulation.

Opinions vary on whether or not the contralateral leg should be scanned on a routine basis. Two studies that studied a combined 3202 patients concluded that in

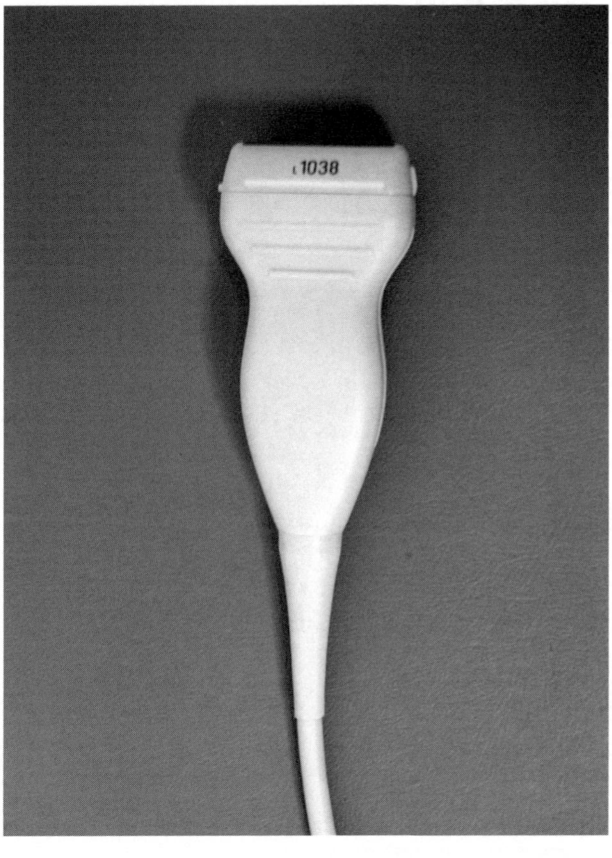

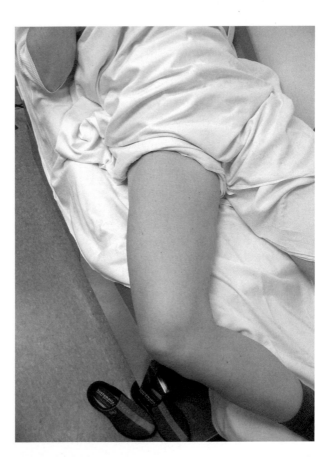

Figure 14–5. The leg is bent at the knee and rotated outward to allow best exposure of popliteal fossa as well as the junction of the common, deep, and superficial femoral veins.

Figure 14–4. A linear array transducer is shown.

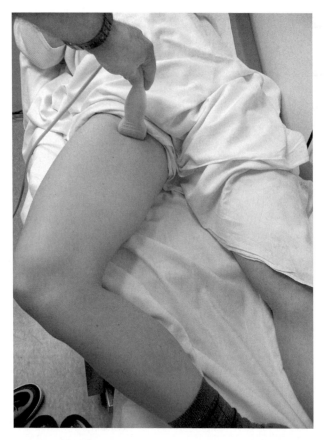

Figure 14–6. The approximate position of the linear probe is shown transversely over the common femoral vein. The probe handle is being held near the cord for demonstration.

patients with unilateral leg symptoms, scanning the contralateral leg was neither indicated nor cost-effective.[28,29] Others have argued that bilateral DVTs are not uncommon and scanning the contralateral leg is indicated.[30] However, this view fails to account for the fact that treatment for unilateral DVT is usually identical to treatment for bilateral DVT. Novice sonologists may find it helpful to compare the anatomy of the contralateral leg when it appears confusing on the extremity being investigated.

Otherwise, routinely scanning the asymptomatic leg appears to be unnecessary.

When a DVT is diagnosed, locating the most proximal end of the thrombus may be helpful. Hence, if examination of the femoral vein is normal, but a DVT is found in the popliteal fossa, the clot should continue to be tracked proximally. Identifying the proximal end of the thrombus and noting it in the patient's chart may facilitate patient follow-up, especially if a repeat examination after anticoagulation identifies continued presence of thrombus. Longitudinal views of the vein may be helpful in outlining the shape and extent of the thrombus. Comparison with the position of the proximal end of the thrombus at the time of diagnosis will allow the patient's primary physician to decide if treatment is failing or if disease progression has occurred, either of which may result in more invasive interventions to safeguard the patient from embolization.

► COMMON AND EMERGENT ABNORMALITIES

The inability to collapse a vein on ultrasound indicates the presence of thrombus within the vein (Figure 14–10). The same does not apply to arteries, which can be difficult to collapse. It is imperative to recognize that the examiner must have adequate access to the vein to test collapsibility. Applying pressure at an angle or in an area where overlying structures may distribute pressure away from the vessel lumen may result in false positive findings.

Acute Deep Vein Thrombosis

The clot itself may be seen as an echogenicity within the lumen, and the vein will not collapse completely with compression (Figure 14–11). Longitudinal views of a vein may be helpful in outlining the shape and extent of thrombus (Figure 14–12). In many instances, especially with lower end equipment, the only evidence of a DVT is the inability to compress the vein. Almost complete compression of the vein is not sufficient for excluding DVT (see Figure 14–10). The lumen of the vessel must

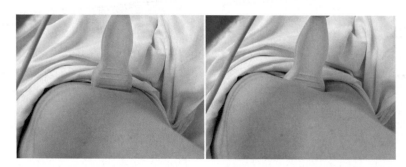

Figure 14–7. A moderate amount of pressure is applied to the leg as shown on the right in this figure. Inadequate pressure can lead to incomplete collapse of the vein.

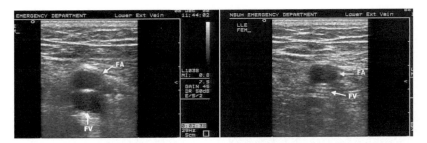

Figure 14–8. Pressure applied to the transducer results in complete collapse of the femoral vein. FA = femoral artery; FV = femoral vein.

disappear completely to exclude the presence of a clot (see Figure 14–8).

Chronic Deep Venous Thrombosis

This condition refers to the presence of an old clot within a vein that has recannulated and allowed venous flow around or through the clot. Complete collapse of the venous lumen will not be possible. However, acute DVT may have a similar appearance and occlude only part

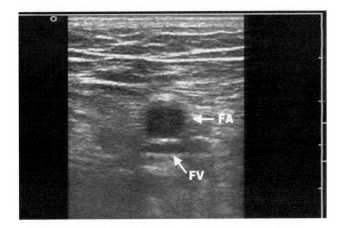

Figure 14–10. The femoral vein is not completely collapsed. If adequate pressure has been applied a thrombus is likely present. FA = femoral artery; FV = femoral vein.

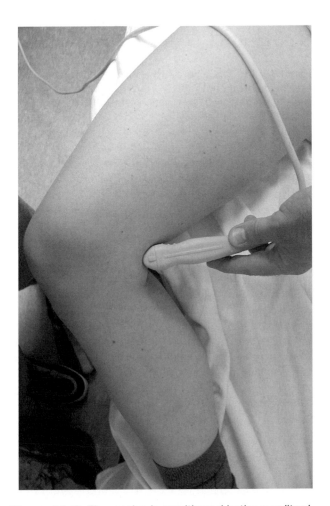

Figure 14–9. The probe is positioned in the popliteal fossa for visualization of the popliteal artery and vein.

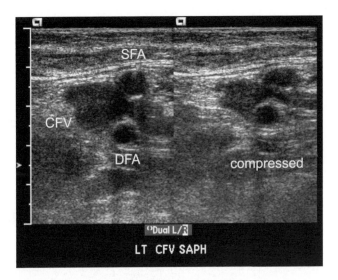

Figure 14–11. Split-screen image of left common femoral vein (CFV) near saphenous junction. The superficial and deep branches of the femoral artery are labeled (DFA, SFA). The CFV contains echoes that represent clot, and does not fully collapse with compression (right image). *(Courtesy of James Mateer, MD, Waukesha Memorial Hospital.)*

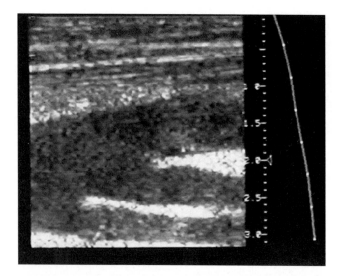

Figure 14–12. Longitudinal view of the common femoral vein reveals intralumenal clot also involving all of the branching vessels. *(Courtesy of Lori Green, Gulfcoast Ultrasound.)*

of the vein. Acute clots tend to be less echogenic than chronic ones; however, this is not always reliable (Figure 14–13). Further, clots tend to recanalize centrally and thus may leave a channel of blood flow through the central area of the clot (Figure 14–14). Despite the fact that there may be historical indications that a clot is chronic, as well as echogenicity differences between acute and chronic clot, it may still be difficult to differentiate between the two in a newly diagnosed patient. Review of

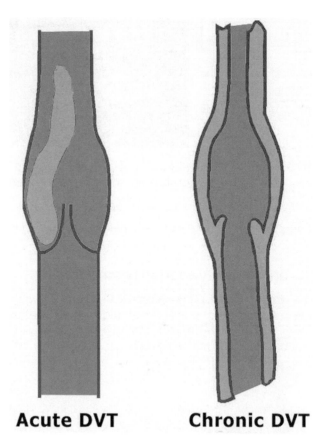

Acute DVT   **Chronic DVT**

Figure 14–14. The illustration on the right shows a re-canalized, old thrombus. The left image demonstrates an early acute thrombus, which can enlarge and obstruct flow completely.

prior ultrasound studies is helpful when available. If the diagnosis remains uncertain at this point, it would be prudent to treat the patient for an acute DVT on an inpatient or outpatient basis, with a complete ultrasound examination performed within 24 h.

Superficial Venous Clot

The physician evaluating the source of focal leg pain and swelling may encounter a superficial venous clot. It is not uncommon to find a clot limited to the saphenous vein when investigating DVT in the thigh. Although recommendations for treatment of superficial clot, such as in the saphenous vein, differ from source to source, superficial venous thrombosis clearly does not pose the same degree of danger in most patients unless it is propagating into the saphenofemoral junction.

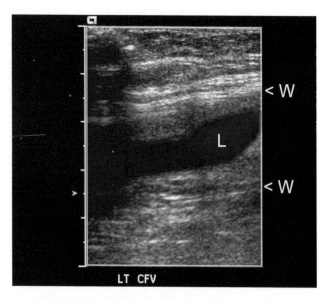

Figure 14–13. Longitudinal view of the common femoral vein shows chronic echogenic clot along the walls (W) with central recanulation of the lumen (L). *(Courtesy of James Mateer, MD, Waukesha Memorial Hospital.)*

► COMMON VARIANTS AND SELECTED ABNORMALITIES

When evaluating the lower extremity venous system, other cystic structures may be mistaken for normal and pathologic findings. Lymph nodes may be encountered while

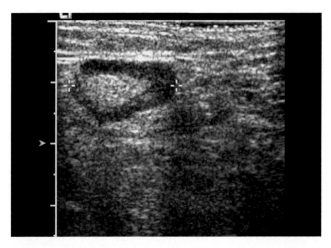

Figure 14–15. Typical appearance of an enlarged inguinal lymph node (2 cm). The thickened capsule is hypoechoic while the central hilum is echogenic. *(Courtesy of James Mateer, MD, Waukesha Memorial Hospital.)*

studying the common femoral and femoral vein junction, especially in ill patients (Figure 14–15). An inflamed lymph node can be initially mistaken for a non-collapsing vein due to similar echogenicity and cross-sectional structure. The use of color Doppler will help identify the lymph node. The blood flow pattern of a lymph node will differ from a vein. Furthermore, careful ultrasonographic evaluation of the structure will show its true shape. Duplication of vessels can also occur, especially venous structures in the calf. It is important to identify any extra vessels and ensure their patency as well.

Findings in the popliteal fossa include Baker's cysts, which can be confusing when small in size (Figure 14–16A). Careful examination of the structure should lead to its discrimination from the popliteal vein (Figure 14–16B). Rupture of a Baker's cyst should be considered in any patient with calf swelling who has a prior history of chronic arthritis or knee effusion. These can present with impressive swelling and pain and may reveal subcutaneous fluid below the knee on ultrasound (Figure 14–17). Popliteal artery aneurysms are occasionally encountered and may make it harder to compress the popliteal vein in one location. Aneurysms over 2 cm can cause complications and should be followed closely.

▶ PITFALLS

1. *Contraindication.* There are no absolute contraindications to evaluating the deep venous system of the lower extremities. Patient comfort or level of cooperation may limit the examination. There are no documented cases of embolization as a result of DVT evaluation in a patient.

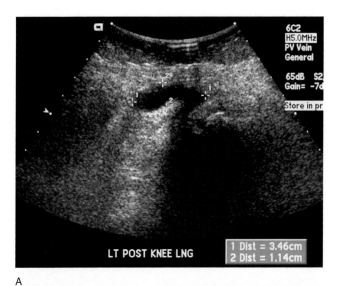

A

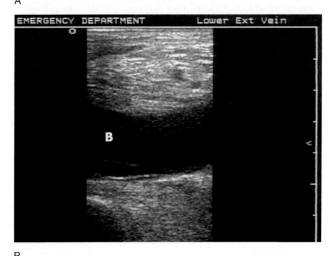

B

Figure 14–16. (A) Longitudinal view of the posterior knee reveals a small Baker's cyst. *(Courtesy of James Mateer, MD, Waukesha Memorial Hospital.)* (B) A longitudinal section of a large Baker's cyst is shown. B = Baker's cyst.

2. *Imaging challenging subjects.* Some physical limitations exist on the technology and patients who are morbidly obese or have severe lower extremity edema may be very difficult to image. The ultrasound beam greatly deteriorates with increased fat as well as distance. Newer technology, such as tissue harmonics, allow improved visualization at greater depths. Tissue harmonic imaging has been tested for improved visualization of small, poorly visualized superficial lesions, such as breast masses. To date, however, no studies regarding deep vein recognition on difficult patients have been published. The extent of the difficulty was underlined in the Frazee study, which encountered an indeterminate rate of almost 18%.[5]

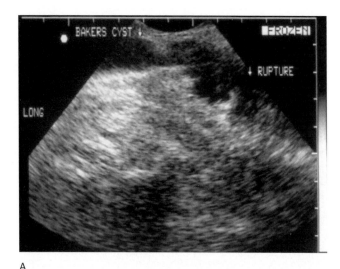

A

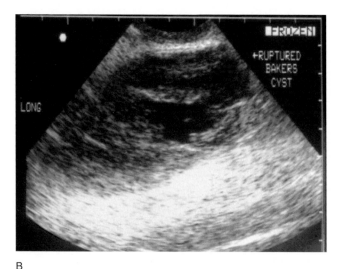

B

Figure 14–17. (A) Ruptured Bakers's cyst. Longitudinal view of the posterior knee shows a Baker's cyst (left upper image) communicating with subcutaneous fluid in the upper calf. (B) Longitudinal view over the mid calf of the same patient shows a significant amount of subcutaneous fluid dissecting inferiorly. *(Courtesy of James Mateer, MD.)*

This number could have been slightly reduced if the investigators had color Doppler available.[9]

3. *Elusive segmental DVT.* One concern of this examination is the possibility of segmental DVT; for instance, a DVT potentially may span several cm of the femoral vein mid thigh but cannot be found anywhere else. The true incidence of such an occurrence is not known but evidence suggests that it is very rare. However, as is recommended for all lower extremity ultrasound studies to exclude DVT, a repeat ultrasound examination should be performed in 5 to 7 d to exclude propagation of an undetected calf thrombosis. Such a repeat examination would also catch a propagating segmental clot.

4. *Misunderstanding the limitations of ultrasonography.* Although ultrasound is now the method of choice for detecting the presence of lower extremity thrombosis, the test is not 100% accurate. Practitioners should understand the limitation of this examination, especially when considering that the method proposed in this chapter does not attempt to evaluate veins in the calf. When faced with overwhelming clinical suspicion for a DVT and a negative ultrasound result, it would be reasonable to continue on to more definite testing. For example, a patient with a known malignancy and recent hip surgery who now has unilateral calf pain and swelling, who cannot be anticoagulated as a result of a recently diagnosed chronic subdural hematoma, should probably undergo a venogram for a definitive diagnosis.

5. *Mistaking artery for vein.* This is not a common pitfall but novice sonographers should be aware that

in some cases an artery can be pliable enough to collapse under moderate transducer pressure while the vein lumen is held open by the presence of clot. If available, color Doppler techniques may help to simplify the identification of blood vessels.

6. *Femoral lymph nodes mistaken for a DVT.* Occasionally, lymph nodes encountered in the groin can be mistaken for an incompressible deep vein. This is especially true for inflamed lymph nodes and less experienced sonologists. Figure 14–18 shows an example of a large lymph node that was mistaken by a resident physician for a femoral DVT. The lymph node is a finite structure and moving the transducer proximally or distally will allow the sonologist to identify the edges of the

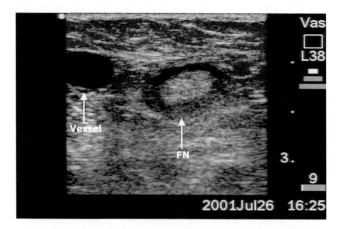

Figure 14–18. The femoral node next to the actual vein has an uncanny resemblance to a lumen filled with thrombus. FN = Femoral lymph node.

lymph node. Rotating the probe will also frequently show the boundaries of the lymph node as well as its atypical appearance for a blood vessel.

▶ CASE STUDIES

Case 1

Patient Presentation

A 25-year-old woman presents to the emergency department with a complaint of right calf swelling and pain. The patient is a graduate student who is studying for final examinations at law school. She denies any strenuous activity and notes spending most of the last week sitting in the library. The patient in normally athletic and rides a stationary bicycle daily. She has an unremarkable medical history and does not smoke. She states that she thinks her older sister had a "blood clot" several years ago.

Physical examination reveals a healthy young woman with normal vital signs, including an oxygen saturation of 98% on room air. She has a moderately tender right calf without any visible erythema or palpable cord. The patient has moderate discomfort on manipulation of her foot at the ankle. Her right calf measures approximately 1.5 cm larger than the left, a fact the patient attributes to a left knee injury while playing soccer in college.

Management Course

The vascular laboratory is not open on Saturday and the on-call radiologist recommends the patient be anticoagulated and admitted into the hospital until she can be imaged as the first case on Monday morning. The patient is originally from another state and does not have a primary care physician in the area. She insists that she must study for her law school finals and, unless medically necessary, she would prefer to go home. She does voice concern regarding the possibility of a DVT as she notes her sister was "very sick" from her blood clot. The emergency physician performed an ultrasound examination of the patient's right leg. The common femoral vein junction, with the deep femoral and superficial femoral veins, is located and complete obliteration of the lumen is seen with moderate compression. The popliteal vein is visualized behind the knee and also compresses normally. The patient is given appropriate instructions and is requested to follow up with the university's clinic Monday after her examinations. She is told that she should have a follow-up ultrasound evaluation in 5 to 7 d.

Commentary

Case 1 represents an example of a fairly low-risk patient who can still inspire considerable angst for the treating physician. With her symptoms and suggestive family history, the patient may present a medicolegal risk if she was discharged home without definitive diagnostic imaging. Conversely, if the patient were to be admitted to await an imaging study, she would spend the weekend in the hospital and miss her law school examinations. This scenario is quite realistic in many facilities. Staffing a vascular laboratory 24 h a day, 7 days a week, can be too expensive, especially when coupled with a shortage of sonographers. Treating the patient with low-molecular-weight heparin as an outpatient may seem attractive, but has some limitations. The patient must be trained to administer the injections. Further, while the risk of bleeding is low, it is present and could once again be a medicolegal issue for some physicians. In this case, the emergency physician was able to confidently exclude a proximal DVT and promptly discharge the patient. She could follow up in 2 d with the school's clinic and have a repeat ultrasound examination arranged to exclude propagation of a calf vein thrombosis.

Case 2

Patient Presentation

A 60-year-old gentleman with a history of chronic obstructive pulmonary disease, arthritis, coronary artery disease, and hypertension presents to the ED with complaints of vague pain in his left lower extremity. The patient notes that he typically has pain in either or both legs and requests a prescription for rofecoxib, which has helped with the pain in the past. He denies any new leg swelling and states that they are both a little swollen all the time. The patient further denies chest pain or shortness of breath and gives no history of thrombosis in the past.

Physical examination reveals a comfortable-appearing man. The patient's vital signs are within normal limits with an oxygen saturation of 96% on room air. The cardiac and lung examination are remarkable for distant heart sounds and coarse breath sounds. The lower extremity examination reveals venous stasis changes on both lower legs as well as tenderness at both knees and ankles on range of motion. The patient appears to complain of calf pain on both sides but more so on the left. There is mild non-pitting edema. No palpable cord is felt and no erythema is seen posteriorly.

Management Course

The vascular laboratory is contacted but is unable to perform the examination for several hours due to a backlog from the floor. The patient asks to be discharged, stating this is just his arthritis and he will see his own physician when he is back from vacation next week. A bedside ultrasound examination is performed and shows a normally collapsing femoral vein. However, the popliteal vein does not collapse completely with compression (Figure 14–19). The partner covering the patient's primary physician was contacted and agreed to see the patient in the office the next morning if a low-molecular-weight heparin injection

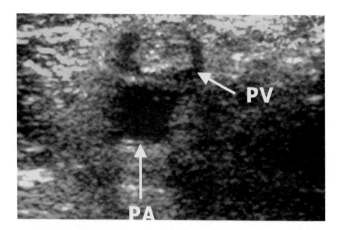

Figure 14-19. The popliteal vein is visualized above the popliteal artery and has a distinct echogenic central thrombus within it. PA = popliteal artery; PV = popliteal vein.

could be administered to the patient. The patient receives an injection and is discharged to been seen approximately 12 h later by his physician.

Commentary
Case 2 illustrates the utility of limited compression venous ultrasound. The patient had several confounding issues, such a chronic arthritic pain and lower extremity swelling. However, he deserved an ultrasound evaluation to exclude thrombosis. The vascular laboratory, busy as most are, was not able to perform the examination for several hours. A rapid examination of the proximal deep veins in the affected leg revealed a popliteal DVT. The patient was able to be treated with an injection of low-molecular-weight heparin and was discharged to follow up with his physician. The care of the patient was simplified and saved a considerable amount of time.

Case 3
Patient Presentation
A 22-year-old woman with a history of sickle cell disease presents with a complaint of left lower-leg swelling and pain. The patient states she first began to notice discomfort in the leg 4 d ago and today notices swelling, redness, and increased pain. She denies any history of trauma and states her typical sickle cell pain is higher in the leg and different from this episode.

Physical examination reveals normal vital signs with a temperature of 100°F. The examination is within normal limits except for the patient's lower left leg. She has erythema and increased temperature of the anterior shin as well as non-pitting edema. The area is sensitive to the touch. The calf is mildly tender and may be slightly swollen. The patient's ankle is also swollen but no deformity is noted. She has diffuse pain in the ankle and ante-

rior shin with flexion and extension of the foot. Distal pulses are present and equal to the contralateral side.

Management Course
The patient is seen at night and no vascular laboratory testing is available. A bedside ultrasound examination of the left leg is performed and shows normally collapsing femoral and popliteal veins. With no proximal clot detected, the patient is given a dose of parenteral first-generation cephalosporin and is discharged on oral antibiotics. The patient is scheduled for follow-up the next day with the primary care physician, who is advised to obtain a follow-up lower extremity Doppler examination in 5 to 7 d to rule out propagation of an undetectable distal venous clot.

Commentary
In case 3, the patient is once again low risk, but cellulitis must be differentiated from a possible DVT. The clinician's ability to perform a bedside ultrasound examination provided accurate diagnosis and rapid disposition of the patient.

REFERENCES

1. Blaivas M, Sierzenski P, Lambert M. Emergency evaluation of patients presenting with acute scrotum using bedside ultrasonography. Acad Emerg Med 2001;8:90–93.
2. Blaivas M. Bedside emergency department ultrasonography in the evaluation of ocular pathology. Acad Emerg Med 2000;7:947–950.
3. Roy S, Dewitz A, Paul I. Ultrasound-assisted ankle arthrocentesis. Am J Emerg Med 1999;17:300–301.
4. Hilty WM, Hudson PA, Levitt MA, Hall JB. Real-time ultrasound-guided femoral vein catheterization during cardiopulmonary resuscitation. Ann Emerg Med 1997;29:331–337.
5. Frazee BW, Snoey ER, Levitt A. Emergency department compression ultrasound to diagnose proximal deep vein thrombosis. J Emerg Med 2001;20:107–112.
6. Jolly BT, Massarin E, Pigman EC. Color Doppler ultrasonography by emergency physicians for the diagnosis of acute deep venous thrombosis. Acad Emerg Med 1997;4:129–132.
7. Trottier SJ, Todi S, Veremakis C. Validation of an inexpensive B-mode ultrasound device for detection of deep vein thrombosis. Chest 1996;110:1547–1550.
8. Birdwell BG, Raskob GE, Whitsett TL, et al. The clinical validity of normal compression ultrasonography in outpatients suspected of having deep venous thrombosis. Ann Intern Med 1998;128:1–7.
9. Blaivas M, Lambert M, Harwood R, et al. Lower extremity Doppler for deep venous thrombosis: can emergency physicians be accurate and fast? Acad Emerg Med 2000;7:120–126.

10. Chance JF, Abbitt PL, Tegtmeyer CJ, Powers RD. Real-time ultrasound for the detection of deep venous thrombosis. Ann Emerg Med 1991;20:494–496.

11. Rydberg EJ, Westfall JM, Nicholas RA. Low-molecular-weight heparin in preventing and treating DVT. Am Fam Physician 1999;59:1607–1612.

12. Vinson DR, Berman DA. Outpatient treatment of deep venous thrombosis: a clinical care pathway managed by the emergency department. Ann Emerg Med 2001;37:251–258.

13. Bates SM, Grand'Maison A, Johnston M, et al. A latex D-dimer reliably excludes venous thromboembolism. Arch Intern Med 2001;161:447–453.

14. Anderson DR, Wells PS, Stiell I, et al. Management of patients with suspected deep vein thrombosis in the emergency department: combining use of a clinical diagnosis model with D-dimer testing. J Emerg Med 2000;19:225–230.

15. Philbrick JT, Becker DM. Calf deep venous thrombosis. A wolf in sheep's clothing? Arch Intern Med 1988;148:2131–2138.

16. Poppiti R, Papanicolaou G, Perese S, Weaver FA. Limited B-mode venous imaging versus complete color-flow duplex venous scanning for detection of proximal deep venous thrombosis. J Vasc Surg 1995;22:553–557.

17. Lensing AWA, Doris CI, McGrath FP, et al. A comparison of compression ultrasound with color Doppler ultrasound for the diagnosis of symptomless postoperative deep vein thrombosis. Arch Intern Med 1997;157:765–768.

18. Lensing AWA, Prandoni P, Brandjes D, et al. Detection of deep-vein thrombosis by real-time B-mode ultrasonography. N Engl J Med 1989;320:342–345.

19. Lund F, Diener L, Ericsson JLE. Postmortem intraosseous phlebography as an aid in studies of venous thromboembolism. Angiology 1969;20:155–176.

20. Heijboer H, Buller HR, Lensing AWA, et al. A comparison of real-time compression ultrasonography with impedance plethysmography for the diagnosis of deep-vein thrombosis in symptomatic outpatients. N Engl J Med 1993;329:1365–1369.

21. Frederick MG, Hertzber BS, Kliewer MA, et al. Can the US examination for lower extremity deep venous thrombosis be abbreviated? A prospective study of 755 examinations. Radiology 1996;199:45–47.

22. Lennox AF, Delis KT, Serunkuma S, et al. Combination of a clinical risk assessment score and rapid whole blood D-dimer testing in the diagnosis of deep vein thrombosis in symptomatic patients. J Vasc Surg 1999;30:794–803.

23. Swarczinski C, Dijkers M. The value of serial leg measurements for monitoring deep vein thrombosis in spinal cord injury. J Neurosci Nurs 1991;23:306–314.

24. Sellman JS, Holman RL. Thromboembolism during pregnancy. Risks, challenges, and recommendations. Postgrad Med 2000;108:71–84.

25. Motykie GD, Caprini JA, Arcelus JI, et al. Risk factor assessment in the management of patients with suspected deep venous thrombosis. Int Angiol 2000;19:47–51.

26. Diamond PT, Macciocchi SN. Predictive power of clinical symptoms in patients with presumptive deep venous thrombosis. Am J Phys Med Rehabil 1997;76:49–51.

27. Eskandari MK, Sugimoto H, Richardson T, et al. Is color-flow duplex a good diagnostic test for detection of isolated calf vein thrombosis in high-risk patients? Angiology 2000;51:705–710.

28. Sheiman RG, McArdle CR. Bilateral lower extremity US in the patient with unilateral symptoms of deep venous thrombosis: assessment of need. Radiology 1995;194:171–173.

29. Strothman G, Blebea J, Fowl RJ, Rosenthal G. Contralateral duplex scanning for deep venous thrombosis is unnecessary in patients with symptoms. J Vasc Surg 1995;22:543–547.

30. Naidich JB, Torre JR, Pellerito JS, et al. Suspected deep venous thrombosis: is US of both legs necessary. Radiology 1996;200:429–431.

CHAPTER 15

Vascular Access

John S. Rose and Aaron E. Bair

Establishing reliable vascular access in an emergency situation is of critical importance. Many factors, including body habitus, volume depletion, shock, history of intravenous drug abuse, congenital deformity, and cardiac arrest, can make obtaining vascular access in the critically ill or injured patient extremely difficult. The introduction of real-time bedside 6 into emergency and acute care settings has been an important advance for facilitating rapid and successful vascular access. This chapter discusses the use of ultrasound for both central and peripheral emergency vascular access.

► CLINICAL CONSIDERATIONS

For central access, the use of an anatomic landmark-guided approach is the traditional practice. Internal jugular vein location traditionally relies on the sternocleidomastoid muscle and clavicular landmarks; the femoral vein relies on the inguinal ligament and femoral artery pulsation landmarks; and the subclavian vein relies on clavicular landmarks. In many patients, however, these landmarks may be distorted, obscured, or non-existent. In addition, normal variations in the anatomic relationship of the internal jugular vein may make cannulation difficult.[1] In the emergent situation, attempting central vascular access with poor external landmarks is frequently approached using a "best guess" estimate of the vessel location. This may lead to multiple needle passes to locate the vessel. Excessive bleeding, inadvertent arterial puncture, vessel laceration, pneumothorax, and hemothorax are some of the potential complications of central vascular access. The incidence of complications increases when multiple attempts are required for cannulation.[2–5] In patients with an underlying coagulopathy (pathologic or therapeutic), multiple attempts can carry significant morbidity due to hemorrhage.[6,7]

The introduction of portable bedside ultrasound has been very effective in assisting with the placement of central venous access catheters. For internal jugular vein cannulation, ultrasound use has been described by numerous disciplines, including emergency medicine, critical care medicine, anesthesiology, obstetrics/gynecology, nephrology, surgery, and radiology.[2,3,8–10] When compared to the external landmark approach, ultrasound-guided internal jugular vein cannulation results in fewer complications and is more effective in time-to-cannulation and first-attempt success.[2,6,11–14] For femoral vein cannulation, the ultrasound-guided approach was found to be more successful than the landmark approach in patients presenting in cardiac arrest.[15]

Peripheral venous access is used more commonly in the emergency setting than central access. The inability to find an adequate peripheral vein, however, requires that the clinician consider central venous access. Traditionally, successful peripheral venous cannulation requires that a vein first be visualized or palpated. Some peripheral veins that are not readily apparent on the skin surface can be clearly visualized with the use of ultrasound. This obviates the need for central access.[16–18] The basilic and cephalic veins of the arm are superficial veins that are not generally visible but are readily cannulated using ultrasound guidance. Cannulation of the basilic vein has been shown to be very successful in the emergency setting in patients for whom it was difficult to obtain other peripheral vascular access.[18] Additionally, the basilic vein has been cannulated using ultrasound in patients requiring prolonged outpatient intravenous access.[17]

► CLINICAL INDICATIONS

Indications for ultrasound guidance for vascular access are:

- *To confirm vessel location prior to landmark-based approach.*
  This is termed the *static approach* and is the most common application of ultrasound for intravenous access. The patient is positioned and the ultrasound transducer is placed on the patient to confirm the predicted landmark-based anatomy. The transducer is then removed and the patient is prepped for vascular access via the standard landmark-based technique. It can be done with a single operator and does not require additional adjunctive equipment such as a sterile transducer sleeve. This approach is particularly useful when the patient is unable to assume the standard position for cannulation and the operator wishes to confirm vessel location.
- *To assist in real-time cannulation under direct ultrasound visualization.*
  This is termed the *dynamic approach*. The ultrasound transducer is inserted into a sterile sleeve and placed on the patient after the sterile preparation. The operator can visualize the needle enter the vessel under real-time ultrasound guidance. The disadvantage of this technique is that this frequently requires two people to perform. This technique is particularly useful in patients without apparent landmarks. Although this method may require more preparation time, it can save precious minutes when no routine landmarks are evident in the critically ill or injured patient.
- *To minimize number of vascular access attempts.*
  In certain clinical situations, definitive access is needed in patients at risk for significant complications from multiple vascular attempts. Patients with therapeutic anticoagulation, disseminated intravascular coagulation, thrombocytopenia, hemophilia, or any condition that adds significant risk to vascular access attempts, can benefit from the higher first-attempt success rate afforded by ultrasound.
- *To assist in alternative peripheral access.*
  Alternative peripheral vascular access is important in many patients. Either static or dynamic ultrasound techniques can be used to locate and facilitate cannulation of peripheral vessels. Saphenous, basilic, and cephalic veins are all easily located with ultrasound but difficult to locate with surface visualization. Some clinical situations require vascular access but choosing a central approach may add unwarranted risk. Ultrasound-guided approach to peripheral veins allows for reliable access without the need for central venous access.
- *To facilitate arterial puncture or cannulation.*
  Ultrasound can be used to locate arteries for puncture or cannulation. Radial, brachial, and femoral arteries are easily located with ultrasound. Both dynamic and static techniques can be used to facilitate arterial puncture.

► ANATOMIC CONSIDERATIONS

At times, it may not be easy to distinguish veins from arteries with B-mode ultrasound. Recognition of key sonographic characteristics can help distinguish veins from arteries. In comparison to arteries, veins have several distinct sonographic features: (1) they are more easily compressed, (2) have thinner walls, and (3) have no arterial pulsation. Additionally, central veins possess characteristic triphasic venous pulsations that can be distinguished from arteries.

Central Venous Cannulation

Ultrasound-assisted central venous cannulation can improve vessel localization by permitting visualization of the vessel of interest. This is in contrast to the external landmark-based approach that relies exclusively on surface relationships. As described previously, two general approaches are used during vascular access: *static* and *dynamic*. Ultrasound is used to verify the vessel location prior to using external standard landmark-based approach (static technique) or it is used for real-time imaging of the venipuncture (dynamic technique). The primary indications for central venous catheter placement using ultrasound are largely unchanged from those for standard technique.

Cannulation of the Internal Jugular Vein
Ultrasound allows for easy localization of the internal jugular vein (Figure 15–1). Additionally, the carotid artery can be distinguished from the adjacent internal jugular vein. The internal jugular vein lies deep to the sternocleidomastoid muscle and is lateral and superficial to the carotid artery. Using the sternocleidomastoid muscle as the external landmark, the internal jugular vein sits below the bifurcation of the sternal and clavicular heads of the muscle. It is important to note that the relative relationship of the carotid artery to the internal jugular vein may change with head position. Specific technical details of internal jugular vein cannulation are provided as follows.

Cannulation of the Subclavian Vein Using a Supraclavicular Approach
Placement of a central venous catheter into the subclavian vein at the take-off of the internal jugular vein is possible using ultrasound guidance (see Figure 15–1). The use of ultrasound with the infraclavicular approach to subclavian vein catheter placement is limited by the large acoustic shadow created by the clavicle. In contrast, the supraclavicular approach allows for adequate sonographic visualization of the proximal subclavian

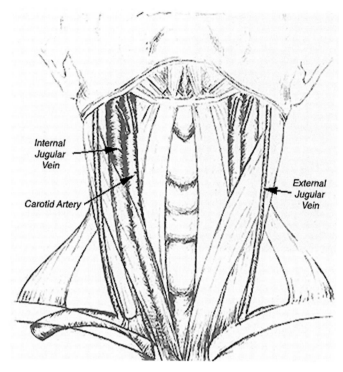

Figure 15-1. The anterior superficial structures of the neck. *(Courtesy of John S. Rose, MD, and Aaron E. Bair, MD.)*

vein anatomy. This technique is described in more detail in a subsequent section.

Cannulation of the Femoral Vein

The initial vascular survey is initiated by placing the transducer in a transverse position just below the mid-portion of the inguinal ligament. Identification of the key vascular structures begins just below the inguinal ligament and medial to the femoral arterial pulsation. The compression technique can be used to distinguish the readily compressible vein from the less compressible artery (Figure 15–2). Additionally, patient positioning can be optimized by appreciating the variable relationships of the vascular structures with respect to limb position (Figure 15–3). Either the static or dynamic technique can be utilized for femoral vein cannulation.

Peripheral Venous Cannulation

Ultrasound will permit localization of veins that often do not have consistent anatomic relationships or are too deep to be readily palpable. Of note, the superficial venous structures are easily collapsed with even slight pressure of the transducer on the skin. This feature of collapsibility is useful for distinguishing between veins and arteries. Superficial veins may not be identified, however, if they are collapsed by inadvertent excessive pressure on the transducer. Once a suitable vein is identified, the process of intravenous catheter placement is largely unchanged from standard practice using routinely avail-

able venous catheters. With respect to ultrasound guidance in peripheral venous access, either the static or dynamic technique may be successfully utilized.

Cannulation of the External Jugular Vein

Since the external jugular vein is superficial, it is often readily identified by visualization and palpation without

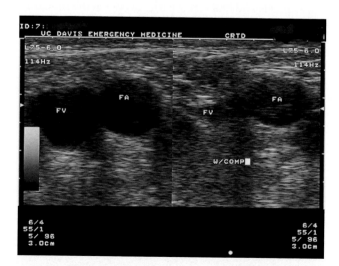

Figure 15-2. Gentle pressure is applied to the transducer to identify venous structures by their easy compressibility. Femoral vein (FV) collapses with compression, the femoral artery (FA) retains its shape even with compression.

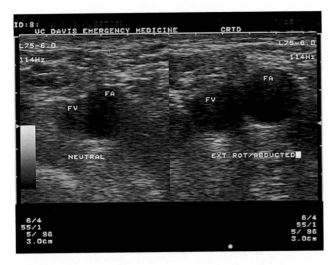

Figure 15–3. Femoral vein (FV) position is seen to vary with hip abduction and external rotation. In neutral position (left frame), the vein is closely opposed to the femoral artery (FA); however, when the hip is abducted and rotated the vein is displaced from the artery (right frame).

ultrasound assistance (see Figure 15–1). However, limited range of motion (i.e., cervical spine precautions) or adiposity may make this vessel difficult to cannulate without ultrasound guidance (Figure 15–4).

Cannulation of the Brachial and Cephalic Veins of the Upper Extremity

The antecubital veins of the arms are commonly used for venous access in the emergency setting, as are the more proximal cephalic and brachial veins (Figure 15–5A and B). The cephalic and brachial veins lie deeper in the structures

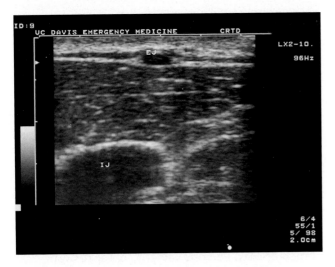

Figure 15–4. Transverse orientation of the external and internal jugular veins.

of the upper arm and are not readily palpable; consequently, these veins are not generally used for intravenous catheter placement in the absence of ultrasound guidance. Caution should be used with the more proximal brachial vein since it lies immediately adjacent to the ulnar and median nerves. Of note, in most patients, the depth of these vessels and angle required for cannulation mandates that a longer catheter (1.75 to 2.0 in.) be used. An example of probe placement and vessel visualization for proximal vein cannulation is demonstrated in Figure 15–6.

Arterial Cannulation

In the absence of color-flow Doppler, real-time arterial pulsation, thickness of arterial wall, and lack of arterial compressibility are all sonographic features that help distinguish arterial from venous anatomy. The mechanics of placing an arterial catheter or simple arterial puncture can proceed along traditional technical guidelines once the pertinent anatomy has been recognized.

▶ TECHNIQUE AND NORMAL ULTRASOUND FINDINGS

Ultrasound-Guided Internal Jugular Vein Cannulation

With the patient in the Trendelenburg position, the transducer is placed on the patient's anterior to lateral neck in anticipation of using a central approach for internal jugular vein cannulation. A 7.5 or 10 MHz, linear array transducer is positioned in a transverse plane and is angled cephalad in to survey the vascular structures of interest (Figure 15–7). The pulsatile internal carotid artery and larger internal jugular vein are identified (Figure 15–8). At this point, either the static or dynamic technique can be used to proceed with venipuncture. The static technique option may involve marking the skin with either ink or a dimple impression using a blunt device (e.g., pen cap) to serve as a guide for skin entry with the operating needle. To proceed with the dynamic technique, the patient is then prepared for a sterile procedure in the usual fashion. Careful application of coupling gel to the transducer probe prior to placement in a sterile sleeve is necessary to avoid entrapment of air bubbles. Sterile coupling gel is then applied to the outside of the transducer sleeve prior to further imaging. With the sterile barrier in place, the transducer is used to localize the anatomy of interest. In this case, the internal jugular vein is brought into view and centered in the middle of the monitor screen. By centering the vessel on the monitor screen, the center of the probe becomes the directional guide for the operator performing the venipuncture (Figure 15–9). Tissue motion during

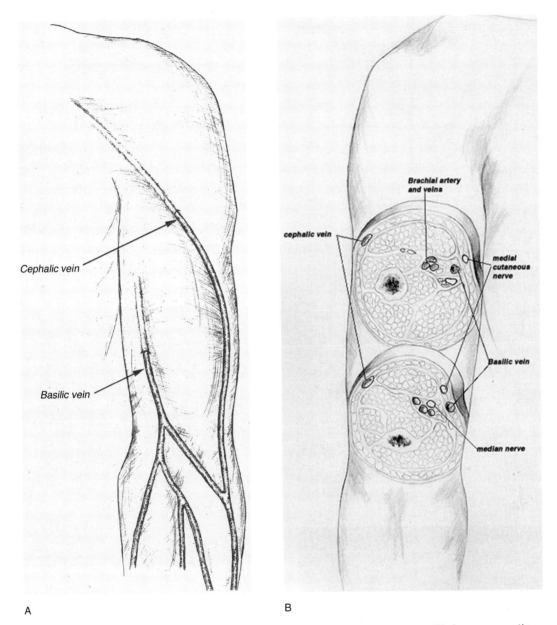

A

B

Figure 15–5. (A) The superficial veins of the proximal upper extremity. (B) A cross section of the neuro-vascular structures of the proximal upper extremity. *(Courtesy of John S. Rose, MD, and Aaron E. Bair, MD.)*

real-time imaging of the procedure can help direct the advancing needle prior to visualization of the needle itself. The needle will subsequently be detectable through ring-down artifact (Figure 15–10). The needle is directed toward the vessel while using the monitor display to locate the needle tip. Prior to successful cannulation, the vein will be seen to deform with the pressure of the advancing needle (Figure 15–11). Confirmation of successful venipuncture proceeds as usual with a flush of venous blood into the syringe. With either the static or dynamic technique, the mechanics of catheter placement (i.e., using guide-wire based Seldinger technique) proceeds

unchanged from the standard after venous cannulation is verified by demonstration of venous blood flow into the operating syringe.

Ultrasound-Guided Subclavian Vein Cannulation Using the Supraclavicular Approach

The primary skin puncture site for catheter placement will be approximately 1 cm lateral to the sternal notch and 1 cm superior to the clavicle. For ultrasound guidance, the transducer is located inferiorly from the anticipated needle entry site and angled caudally (Figure 15–12).

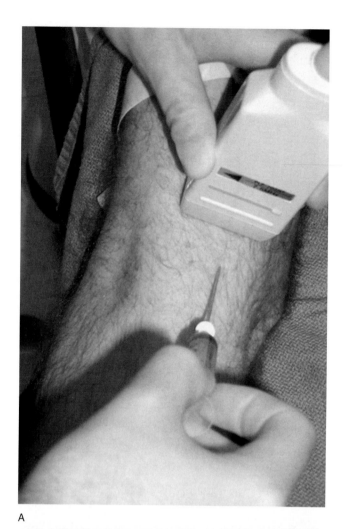

A

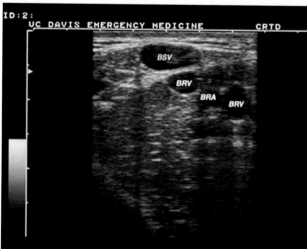

B

Figure 15–6. (A) Demonstration of probe placement for cannulation of the basilic vein. (B) An image demonstrating transverse orientation of the relatively superficial basilic vein (BSV) with deeper-lying brachial artery and veins (BRA, BRV). Note the proximity of the brachial artery to its venous counterpart makes inadvertent arterial puncture a possibility.

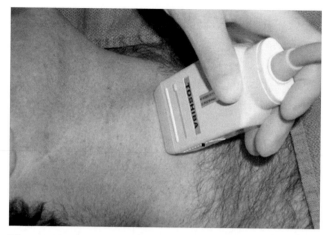

Figure 15–7. Initial probe position for survey of jugular vein.

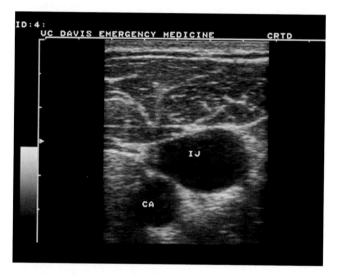

Figure 15–8. Transverse orientation of right internal jugular vein (IJ) and right carotid artery (CA).

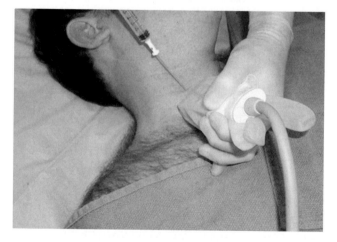

Figure 15–9. The center of the transducer is used as a directional guide for the skin puncture.

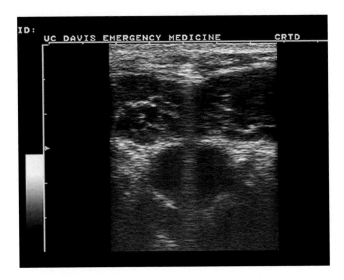

Figure 15–10. Ring-down artifact overlying the internal jugular vein.

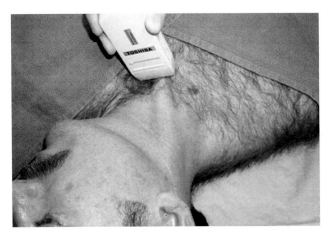

Figure 15–12. Placement of the transducer to facilitate visualization of the internal jugular/subclavian vein junction using a supraclavicular approach.

After identification of the venous anatomy (Figure 15–13), cannulation can proceed with direction by either the static or dynamic technique.

Transducer Orientation: Longitudinal versus Transverse

Variations of probe positioning will yield different information relative to vessel and needle placement. Transverse probe positioning provides information related to lateral orientation. The longitudinal probe position gives depth and slope information (Figure 15–14). The authors generally rely primarily on transverse imaging to assist with venous cannulation. The transverse orientation is

most helpful with demonstrating relationships to other adjacent anatomy. The longitudinal orientation will help with needle orientation in the long axis of the vessel of interest (Figures 15–15 and 15–16).

Static versus Dynamic Placement Technique

Techniques utilizing ultrasound-assisted venous cannulation may vary depending on the clinical scenario and the availability of assistance, as well as the necessity of strict sterile technique. The use of ultrasound to survey the vascular anatomy and then mark the skin for subsequent attempts at venipuncture is referred to here as "static" technique (Figures 15–17 and 15–18). This is in contrast to the "dynamic" technique that maintains a sterile probe in the operating field while attempts at venipuncture proceed. The advantage of dynamic technique is that it

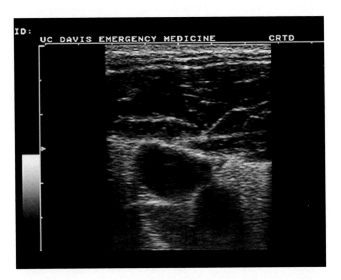

Figure 15–11. Internal jugular vein demonstrating slight deformation as introducer needle contacts vessel. Note the advancing introducer needle is not directly visualized.

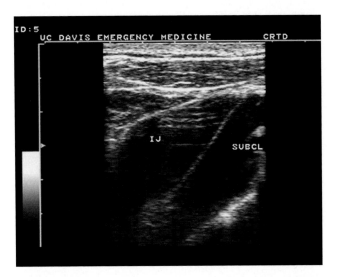

Figure 15–13. Transverse view of the "venous lake" created by the combined subclavian vein and internal jugular vein.

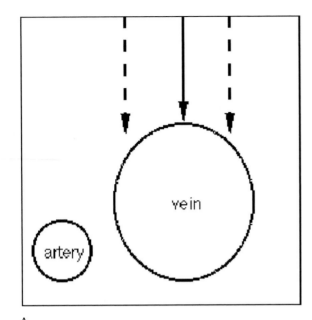

A

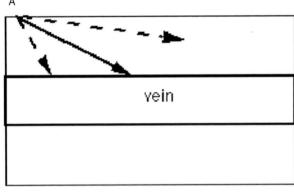

B

Figure 15–14. (A) Demonstrates the concept of lateral orientation seen with a transverse view of the vessel. (B) Demonstrates the concept of longitudinal orientation, which provides information regarding slope and depth of needle approach.

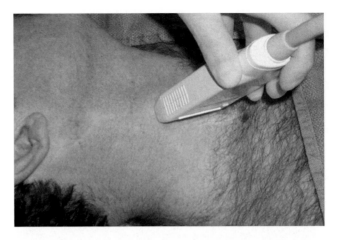

Figure 15–15. Probe placement to provide longitudinal orientation for internal jugular vein.

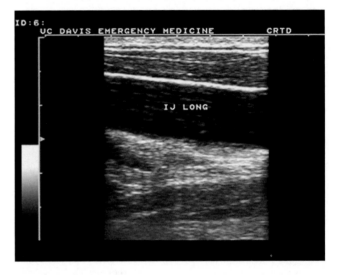

Figure 15–16. Sonographic image of internal jugular vein in long axis.

allows for real-time observation of the needle position and target vascular structures. However, it may require that a second individual be responsible for maintaining probe placement or sterility during the procedure. The logistical simplicity of the static technique may be advantageous in the case where the landmark-based anatomy is straightforward. Thus, the static technique allows a brief inspection and confirmation of the vessel location without having to rely on a second operator.

STERILE TECHNIQUE.
There are several different options for maintaining operative sterility. The optimal, though most expensive, option

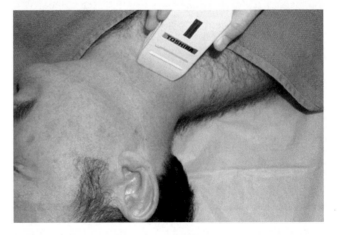

Figure 15–17. Transducer placement for initial vascular survey preceding "static" technique for venous cannulation.

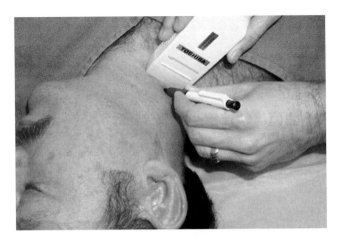

Figure 15–18. Skin marking for "static" technique of venous cannulation.

be taken to avoid compromising sterility by puncturing one of the "extra" fingers of the glove during the process of venipuncture. Sterile examination lubricant, readily available in the emergency department, is sufficient as a conductive medium between the sleeve and the skin.

▶ COMMON VARIANTS AND OTHER ABNORMALITIES

Variability of Normal Venous Anatomy

The large central venous structures of the body have fairly constant anatomy, whereas the peripheral veins are extremely variable in their position. It is helpful, however, to keep in mind the typical course of the veins and the important adjacent structures while using ultrasound to assist in vessel identification and cannulation.

Effect of Patient Positioning

The usual considerations apply for patient preparation for central or peripheral venous cannulation. The Trendelenburg position is useful to provide slight venous distention in the veins of the head and neck. Furthermore, the use

is to use prepackaged sterile probe sleeves that are manufactured solely for the purpose of handling the probe and transducer cord in a sterile fashion. A less expensive option is to use a large sterile glove; adequate amounts of conductive gel should be squeezed into the thumb of the glove (Figure 15–19). If using the glove option, care must

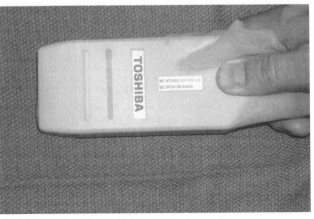

A

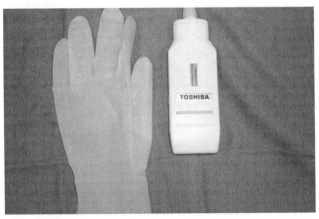

B

C

Figure 15–19. (A) Sterile glove used as a sterile cover for linear transducer. (B) Transducer with conductive gel placed into thumb of sterile glove. (C) Transducer covered and readied by holding extra glove fingers away from operating field.

of ultrasound may help to determine optimal patient position with respect to surrounding arterial anatomy. It is apparent in individual patients that rotation or abduction of a limb will significantly alter the relationship of the vein and artery with respect to the skin. It merits emphasizing that in certain individuals, leg position alone can cause the femoral artery to directly overlie the femoral vein. Hence, the use of a standard (non-ultrasound assisted) technique, given certain patient positioning, may result in arterial injury or failed venous cannulation (see Figure 15–3).

▶ PITFALLS

There are no absolute contraindications to the use of ultrasound for vascular access; however, there are a few common pitfalls.

1. *Failure to identify the needle in tissue.* When using ultrasound for dynamic venous access, it is important to accurately view the needle ring-down artifact or venous tenting to confirm position. Whether using the transverse or longitudinal approach, it is important to identify the needle with ultrasound visualization prior to advancing into deeper structures. This is important to ensure successful cannulation while minimizing complications. Transverse orientation allows for better lateral positioning of the needle. Longitudinal orientation provides better depth and needle-slope positioning.
2. *Failure to distinguish between vein and artery through compression testing or color-flow Doppler.* Since arterial pulsations at times may be subtle, veins and arteries may initially appear very similar (especially in the hypotensive patient). In the absence of color-flow Doppler capability, the vessel should be confirmed that it is a vein by using compression maneuvers. A vein will easily collapse with gentle external pressure.
3. *Locating the vessel with the static approach prior to the patient being in proper position.* The vessel should be located *after* the clinician has the patient properly positioned for the cannulation attempt. As emphasized earlier, many vessels will move slightly and change relationship depending on the patient's position.
4. *Failure to angle the transducer beam into the needle puncture area.* Since ultrasound provides a two-dimensional image, the beam should be angled toward the needle where it will enter the vessel. Occasionally, fanning the transducer beam may be required to identify the optimal location.

▶ CASE STUDIES

Case 1

Patient Presentation

A 50-year-old man who is morbidly obese presents complaining of chest pain. On examination, he is hypotensive and diaphoretic. A 12-lead ECG reveals him to be in complete heart block. Multiple attempts at peripheral access fail. The transcutaneous pacemaker is intermittently capturing but has little effect on the patient's hemodynamic status. There are no good external anatomic landmarks due to his adiposity.

Management Course

The patient's right internal jugular vein is easily visualized under ultrasound guidance using a 7.5 MHz linear transducer. A dynamic real-time ultrasound-guided cannulation of the right internal jugular vein is successful on the first attempt. An intravenous pacemaker wire is then successfully placed (also under ultrasound visualization). Upon improved ventricular capture, the patient's blood pressure normalizes.

Case 2

Patient Presentation

An 18-year-old woman, who is severely scarred and contractured from old burns to the neck, chest, arms, and legs, presents after ingesting a lethal quantity of a tricyclic antidepressant in a suicide attempt. On examination, the patient is hypotensive and lethargic. Numerous attempts at peripheral access have failed. There are no appreciable anatomic landmarks for central access due to her old scars.

Management Course

Although a femoral arterial pulsation was difficult to palpate for the landmark-based approach, the femoral vein was easily visualized under ultrasound guidance. An ultrasound-guided femoral vein catheter is inserted on the first attempt. The patient is then administered induction agents for orotracheal intubation and successfully resuscitated.

Case 3

Patient Presentation

A 40-year-old man with a long history of intravenous drug use presents for drainage of a deltoid abscess. It is determined that the abscess can be drained as an outpatient with the use of systemic sedation and analgesia. Numerous attempts at routine peripheral venous access have failed. The patient is refusing a central venous line.

Management Course

The patient has a large right basilic vein easily visualized with ultrasound. A 2-in. 18-gauge catheter is inserted without difficulty. The patient's abscess is successfully drained after receiving adequate intravenous sedation and analgesia.

Commentary

Anatomic landmarks in patients may be distorted, obscured, or non-existent. In the three cases, each patient presented with anatomic variations that made it difficult to obtain rapid peripheral venous access or landmark-based central venous access. Venous access was facilitated by the use of ultrasound in each case, thereby expediting patient resuscitation and care. Ultrasound use allowed the clinicians to obtain venous access on the first attempt and helped prevent complications associated with delays in obtaining venous access or multiple attempts to obtain central venous access.

REFERENCES

1. Denys BG, Uretsky BF. Anatomical variations of internal jugular vein location: impact on central venous access. Crit Care Med 1991;19:1516–1519.
2. Conz PA, Dissegna D, Rodighiero MP, La Greca G. Cannulation of the internal jugular vein: comparison of the classic Seldinger technique and an ultrasound guided method. J Nephrol 1997;10:311–313.
3. Lee W, Leduc L, Cotton DB. Ultrasonographic guidance for central venous access during pregnancy. Am J Obstet Gynecol 1989;161:1012–1013.
4. Trottier SJ, Veremakis C, O'Brien J, Auer AI. Femoral deep vein thrombosis associated with central venous catheterization: results from a prospective, randomized trial. Crit Care Med 1995;23:52–59.
5. Bagwell CE, Salzberg AM, Sonnino RE, Haynes JH. Potentially lethal complications of central venous catheter placement. J Pediatr Surg 2000;35:709–713.
6. Farrell J, Gellens M. Ultrasound-guided cannulation versus the landmark-guided technique for acute hemodialysis access. Nephrol Dial Transplant 1997;12:1234–1237.
7. Gallieni M, Cozzolino M. Uncomplicated central vein catheterization of high-risk patients with real time ultrasound guidance. Int J Artif Organs 1995;18:117–121.
8. Hudson PA, Rose JS. Real-time ultrasound guided internal jugular vein catheterization in the emergency department. Am J Emerg Med 1997;15:79–82.
9. Meredith JW, Young JS, O'Neil EA, et al. Femoral catheters and deep venous thrombosis: a prospective evaluation with venous duplex sonography. J Trauma 1993;35:187–190.
10. Vucevic M, Tehan B, Gamlin F, et al. The SMART needle. A new Doppler ultrasound-guided vascular access needle. Anaesthesia 1994;49:889–891.
11. Caridi JG, Hawkins IF, Wiechmann BN, et al. Sonographic guidance when using the right internal jugular vein for central vein access. AJR 1998;171:1259–1263.
12. Slama M, Novara A, Safavian A, et al. Improvement of internal jugular vein cannulation using an ultrasound-guided technique. Intensive Care Med 1997;23:916–919.
13. Teichgraber UK, Benter T, Gebel M, Manns MP. A sonographically guided technique for central venous access. AJR 1997;169:731–733.
14. Denys BG, Uretsky BF, Reddy PS. Ultrasound-assisted cannulation of the internal jugular vein. A prospective comparison to the external landmark-guided technique. Circulation 1993;87:1557–1562.
15. Hilty WM, Hudson PA, Levitt MA, Hall JB. Real-time ultrasound-guided femoral vein catheterization during cardiopulmonary resuscitation. Ann Emerg Med 1997;29:331–336.
16. Nee PA, Picton AJ, Ralston DR, Perks AG. Facilitation of peripheral intravenous access: an evaluation of two methods to augment venous filling. Ann Emerg Med 1994;24:944–946.
17. Parkinson R, Gandhi M, Harper J, Archibald C. Establishing an ultrasound guided peripherally inserted central catheter (PICC) insertion service. Clin Radiol 1998;53:33–36.
18. Keyes LE, Frazee BW, Snoey ER, et al. Ultrasound-guided brachial and basilic vein cannulation in emergency department patients with difficult intravenous access. Ann Emerg Med 1999;34:711–714.

CHAPTER 16
Soft Tissue Applications

Andreas Dewitz and Bradley W. Frazee

Beyond the well-known primary and secondary indications for emergency ultrasound lie a rich assortment of clinically useful soft tissue ultrasound applications. These offer the emergency care provider the ability to rapidly evaluate and better manage a wide array of common clinical problems. This chapter focuses on six areas where the use of these soft tissue techniques can be of considerable value in the care of the emergency or ambulatory care patient. These include: (1) evaluation of soft tissue infections, particularly for detection and accurate localization of subcutaneous or peritonsillar abscesses prior to drainage; (2) identification, localization, and removal of soft tissue foreign bodies; (3) evaluation and aspiration of fluid collections in the pleural and peritoneal cavities, as well as in the knee, ankle, and hip joints, for diagnostic and/or therapeutic purposes; (4) evaluation of suspected musculotendinous injuries; (5) assessment of bony cortices for rapid fracture diagnosis; and (6) evaluation of the eye for various ocular emergencies.

SOFT TISSUE INFECTIONS

▶ CLINICAL CONSIDERATIONS

Emergency and ambulatory care physicians are called upon to evaluate patients with soft tissue infections on a daily basis. These infections include cellulitis or subcutaneous abscess, peritonsillar abscess, and, on rare occasions, necrotizing fasciitis. The diagnosis of cellulitis is usually easily made by the physical examination alone when findings of erythema, warmth, and tenderness of the soft tissue are present. Similarly, determining that a soft tissue abscess exists is simple when focal erythema,

tenderness, and fluctuance are present. Where clinical findings can be misleading, however, are in the case of abscesses that are early, small, or deep, where previous incision and drainage have left residual scar tissue, or in patients presenting with obvious cellulitis, where the presence of a coexisting abscess may be overlooked. Because of ambiguous clinical findings in these situations, the clinician may be led away from performing an incision and drainage when pus is in fact present. Ultrasound has emerged as an extremely valuable diagnostic tool for the assessment of these soft tissue infections and is being used with increasing frequency in the emergency setting to assist with the diagnosis and localization of these occult abscesses.

▶ CLINICAL INDICATIONS

The clinical indications for the use of ultrasonography in the management of soft tissue infections include:

- Detection of an occult subcutaneous abscess when ambiguous clinical findings are present.
- Localization of an optimal site for incision and drainage (or aspiration) of an abscess, especially when there is scar tissue from prior surgical intervention.
- Detection of a peritonsillar abscess.

Detection of Occult Abscess

Ultrasound's ability to detect soft tissue abscesses and its utility in helping guide subsequent incision and drainage have been appreciated since the 1980s.[1-5] In reports focusing on injection drug users, particularly those with inflammatory lesions of the groin, ultrasonography has been shown to successfully differentiate not only between cellulitis and abscess, but also adenitis, septic thrombophlebitis, and pseudoaneurysm.[2,3] Ultrasound has additionally been found to be of value in the diagnosis and treatment of odontogenic facial abscesses.[6] One study of 56 emergency department patients with soft tissue infections sought to determine if ultrasound improved or changed patient management. Based on the history and physical examination alone, patients were stratified into one of three groups with regard to clinical pretest probability of having an abscess (low, indeterminate, or high probability). Among the 12 "low probability" cases, fluid was identified by ultrasound in seven and pus drained in six (50%). Among the 32 "indeterminate probability" cases, fluid was identified in 25 and pus drained in 23 (72%). Providers participating in the study believed that the use of ultrasound influenced their management in 66% of the "low probability" cases and 56% of the "indeterminate" cases. The investigators emphasized that pus was commonly identified when it was not clinically expected and, therefore, that the use of ultrasound in this setting often significantly altered patient management.[7]

Detection of a Peritonsillar Abscess

Ultrasonography is also of considerable value in the assessment and management of suspected peritonsillar abscess. A peritonsillar abscess is the most common deep infection of the face and neck.[8] The pathophysiologic process begins with tonsillitis, then progresses to peritonsillar cellulitis, and finally to peritonsillar abscess formation. Peritonsillar cellulitis is usually treated with antibiotics and analgesics alone; however, a peritonsillar abscess generally requires aspiration or incision and drainage for definitive therapy. Because physical examination findings are occasionally unreliable in differentiating between these two entities,[9] the traditional management approach has been to perform a diagnostic needle aspiration of the peritonsillar swelling to search for pus.[10] This procedure is not without risk because the abscess cavity is frequently located within a few mm of the carotid artery. Furthermore, blind needle aspiration has been reported to be falsely negative in as many as 10 to 12% of aspirations.[8] Computed tomography (CT) has been used as a gold standard diagnostic test for peritonsillar abscess, but it is expensive and often too time-consuming to obtain in the emergency setting. The use of intraoral sonography for the diagnosis of peritonsillar abscess was first described in 1993,[11] and the advantages of ultrasound for this indication have been recognized ever since. It is noninvasive, can be rapidly performed at the bedside, and, if a fluid collection is found, knowledge of its size and location can then be used to guide aspiration or incision and drainage. Subsequent studies of ultrasound for diagnosis of peritonsillar abscess in the

otolaryngology literature reported a sensitivity of 89 to 90% and a specificity of 83 to 100% compared to CT, magnetic resonance imaging (MRI), or surgical follow-up.[9,12] The use of intraoral sonography by emergency physicians for diagnosing peritonsillar abscess was reported to be well tolerated by patients.[13]

► ANATOMIC CONSIDERATIONS

A thorough understanding of the regional anatomy of the area being sonographically evaluated is essential for the clinician. Subcutaneous abscesses may be encountered anywhere and are commonly seen on the face, peritonsillar region, hand, antecubital fossa, neck, back, buttocks, and perianal region. They may be found in close proximity to veins, arteries, nerves, tendons, or muscles. An awareness of the anatomic proximity of these adjacent structures, familiarity with their normal sonographic appearance, and an understanding of the preferred location for lines of elective incision is mandatory.

The anatomy in the region of a peritonsillar abscess is complex. Structures that may be visualized by intraoral ultrasound include the palatine tonsil, the margin of the bony hard palate and styloid process of the temporal bone, the medial pterygoid muscle, various fascial planes, the internal jugular vein, and the internal carotid artery. In the sonographic evaluation of peritonsillar abscess, only the carotid artery need be identified in every case. It courses anterior to the jugular vein within the carotid sheath and is normally located posterolateral to the tonsil and within 5 to 25 mm of a peritonsillar abscess.[11]

► TECHNIQUE AND NORMAL ULTRASOUND FINDINGS

Sonographic evaluation of the skin and subcutaneous tissue for a suspected subcutaneous abscess should be performed with a 5.0 to 7.5 MHz linear array, annular array, or sector transducer. An acoustic standoff pad may improve image resolution if a lower frequency transducer is being used or if the abscess is very superficial. Electronic focusing should be adjusted to place the area of interest within the transducer's optimal focal zone. Normal subcutaneous tissue is composed primarily of subcutaneous fat, which is hypoechoic (Figure 16–1). Echogenic linear streaks representing strands of connective tissue may be seen within this hypoechoic fatty tissue. Adjacent arteries or veins may be noted as hypoechoic linear or circular structures, depending on the orientation of the transducer relative to the vessel; use of color flow may aid in their identification. Transducer pressure should be kept to a minimum to avoid collapse and subsequent non-visualization of superficial veins. The soft tissue area

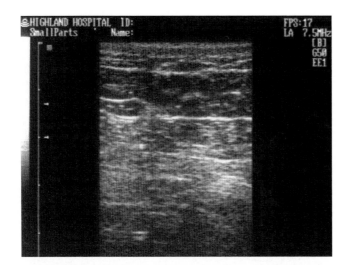

Figure 16–1. Normal subcutaneous tissue with well-visualized, brightly hyperechoic fascial planes. (7.5-MHz linear array probe.)

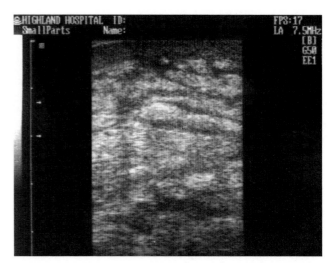

Figure 16–2. Cellulitis. Note the hypoechoic strands traversing the diffusely hyperechoic subcutaneous tissue in a reticular or cobblestone pattern. (7.5-MHz linear array probe.)

being evaluated should be systematically scanned in two perpendicular planes.

Sonographic evaluation of a suspected peritonsillar abscess can be undertaken with a 5.0 to 10.0 MHz curved array intracavitary probe or a dedicated flexible endoscopic transducer. Anesthesia does not appear to be necessary prior to intraoral examination of the peritonsillar region,[12,14] but preapplication of topical anesthetic spray is nonetheless recommended, particularly to reduce gagging. The examination is reportedly well tolerated, even in the setting of trismus.[13] A primary consideration in the ultrasound evaluation of a suspected peritonsillar abscess is the identification of the carotid artery and its relationship to the abscess cavity. The internal carotid artery is identified sonographically by its anechoic and tubular shape. Its location should become evident with systematic scanning of the peritonsillar region in both sagittal and transverse imaging planes. Unlike the internal jugular vein, which is also visualized in this region, the internal carotid artery is pulsatile and relatively noncompressible.

► COMMON AND EMERGENT ABNORMALITIES

Cellulitis

Cellulitis is a diffuse infection of the skin and subcutaneous tissue. The ultrasound findings considered typical of cellulitis likely arise from edema formation in the subcutaneous tissue and are nonspecific.[15] Best appreciated with a 7.5 MHz or higher frequency transducer, the findings can include: (1) diffusely swollen and hyperechoic skin, (2) diffusely increased echogenicity of the subcutaneous tissue, and (3) appearance of hypoechoic strands that randomly traverse the subcutaneous fat in a reticu-

lar or cobblestone pattern (Figure 16–2).[15–17] Comparison to the unaffected side may aid in the recognition of these subtle findings (Figures 16–3 and 16–4). Due to the nonspecific nature of these sonographic findings, their diagnostic utility is limited.

Subcutaneous Abscesses

Subcutaneous abscesses can have a variety of sonographic appearances.[3,15,17,18] Furthermore, they are often located within an area of induration or cellulitis that alters the

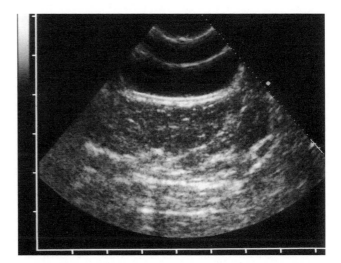

Figure 16–3. Normal soft tissue. Skin and fascial planes of the lateral chest wall appear brightly hyperechoic and the superficial subcutaneous tissue is hypoechoic. [5.0-MHz sector probe with acoustic standoff (note reverberation ring artifacts in the near field.)]

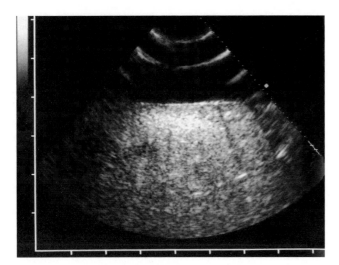

Figure 16–4. Cellulitis of the chest wall (same patient as Figure 16–3). Diffusely hyperechoic soft tissue without evidence of focal abscess collection.

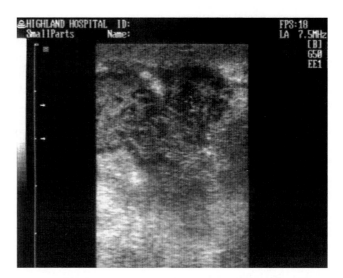

Figure 16–6. Soft tissue abscess with anechoic, hyperechoic, and isoechoic material within the abscess cavity. (7.5-MHz linear array probe.)

sonographic appearance of the surrounding subcutaneous tissue (Figure 16–5). The most common appearance of an abscess is that of a spherical- or elliptical-shaped mass, although it may be lobulated or appear to interdigitate between tissue planes. The mass is usually hypoechoic relative to the surrounding tissues, or entirely anechoic. It may be surrounded by a hyperechoic rim and often contains hyperechoic debris (Figure 16–6), septae, or gas within it (the latter causing a ring-down or reverberation artifact). Less commonly, abscesses are diffusely and homogenously hyperechoic, simulating a solid mass. Rarely, they may be isoechoic or only slightly hypoechoic when compared to surrounding tissue, such that a distinct mass

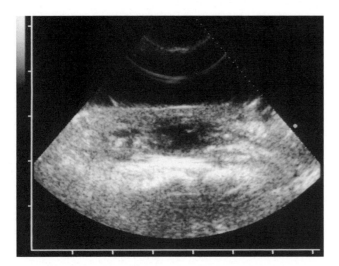

Figure 16–5. Dorsal foot cellulitis with a clinically unsuspected coexistent abscess confirmed by incision and drainage. Note the hypoechoic abscess cavity with posterior acoustic enhancement and hyperechoic surrounding tissues. (5.0-MHz sector probe with acoustic standoff.)

is difficult to appreciate sonographically. In the latter two cases, important clues pointing to the presence of a liquefied abscess are the sonographic finding of posterior acoustic enhancement (Figures 16–7 and 16–8) and the ability to induce motion of purulent material with palpation or with compression of the transducer.[17] If available, color-flow Doppler may show hyperemia adjacent to the abscess cavity and absence of flow within it.[15] If a hypoechoic fluid collection is seen adjacent to a long bone, then the diagnosis of osteomyelitis should be entertained (Figure 16–9).

Peritonsillar Abscess

Sonographically, a peritonsillar abscess most commonly appears as a hypoechoic or complex cystic mass, typical of most abscesses (Figure 16–10). In two studies that describe the spectrum of sonographic findings associated with peritonsillar abscesses, a less common homogenous and isoechoic form was encountered in 13 to 33% of cases.[13,14] Other characteristics that may be of use in identifying peritonsillar abscesses include posterior acoustic enhancement, which was found in all nine abscesses described in one report,[13] and medial and caudal displacement of the tonsil by the adjacent abscess.[14]

▶ COMMON VARIANTS AND SELECTED ABNORMALITIES

Necrotizing Fasciitis

Necrotizing fasciitis is a rare soft tissue infection defined by tissue necrosis (particularly involving fascia) and a fulminant course. While rapid recognition and treatment can favorably affect outcome,[19] making the diagnosis of necrotizing fasciitis on clinical grounds alone is often dif-

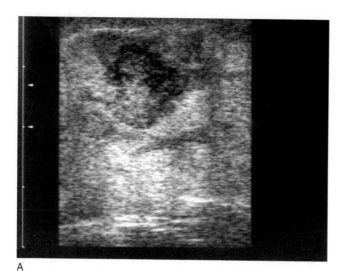

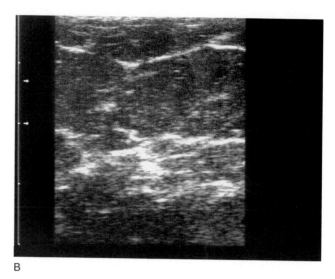

A

B

Figure 16–7. (A) Large thigh abscess in an injection drug user. Hypo- and hyperechoic material is noted in the abscess cavity. Posterior acoustic enhancement is also present. Surrounding soft tissue is diffusely hyperechoic with loss of the normal sonographically apparent tissue planes. (B) Normal subcutaneous tissue at an equivalent location in the contralateral thigh of the same patient is shown for comparison. (7.5-MHz linear array probe.)

ficult. The role of ultrasound as a diagnostic test for necrotizing fasciitis has never been studied systematically, and it should not be used to exclude the diagnosis. However, sonographic findings thought to be characteristic of the disease were described in a report of four cases in children. Invariably, the subcutaneous fascia, normally seen as a thin, brightly hyperechoic line, was greatly thickened and edematous-appearing, as was the overlying subcutaneous tissue. Discrete masses were seen in and around the fascial plane from which pus was aspirated in three of four cases.[20] In some cases, the presence of subcutaneous gas

(seen as areas of "dirty" acoustic shadowing and reverberation artifact) may be rapidly confirmed with bedside ultrasound.

▶ PITFALLS

For most patients, subcutaneous abscesses can be successfully aspirated or incised in the emergency or ambulatory care setting with either local anesthesia or conscious sedation (Figure 16–11). Some abscesses, however, by virtue of size, location (such as in the perineum or perianal area), or close proximity to vital adjacent anatomic structures, are best left to a surgical specialist to drain in the operating room, where adequate anesthesia and lighting are available.

FOREIGN BODY LOCALIZATION AND REMOVAL

▶ CLINICAL CONSIDERATIONS

Management of a wound with a known or suspected soft tissue foreign body can be challenging, especially when the foreign body is radiolucent. To further complicate matters, these wounds often occur in the hand or foot, where the likelihood for iatrogenic injuries from blind wound exploration and for subsequent infectious complications are high. Even with strong clinical index of suspicion, liberal use of radiography, and careful wound exploration, a soft tissue foreign body can easily be missed. The possible infectious and medicolegal consequences of this missed diagnosis can be disastrous for patient and provider alike. While metal and glass are

Figure 16–8. Soft tissue abscess with hypo and hyperechoic material within the abscess cavity and prominent posterior acoustic enhancement. Hyperechoic fascial planes are noted deep to the abscess. (7.5-MHz linear array probe.)

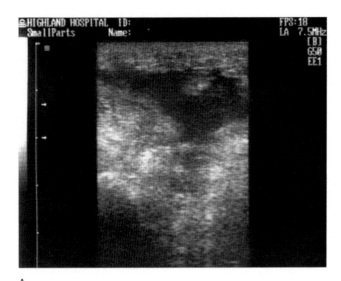

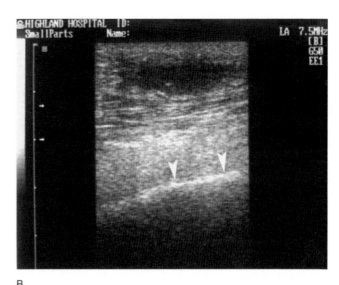

A   B

Figure 16–9. Transverse (A) and long axis (B) views of a thigh abscess. The abscess cavity is predominantly anechoic with some internal debris noted. The echogenic cortex of the femur (arrowheads) is noted in the far field. (7.5-MHz linear array probe.)

radiopaque and usually apparent on standard two-view radiographs of the injured area, other commonly encountered foreign bodies, such as wood or thorns, are nearly always radiolucent. Imaging studies, such as CT or MRI, may be useful in the assessment of such wounds but are expensive, time-consuming, and not always readily obtainable. Furthermore, the sensitivity of CT for the detection of a wooden foreign body is low, reported to range from 0 to 60%.[1]

Ultrasound imaging in this clinical setting offers several decided advantages. Foremost, its excellent sensitivity and specificity as a test for detecting wooden foreign bodies (nearly always missed with radiography) makes it

especially valuable in the assessment of a wound suspected of containing a fragment of wood. Sensitivities reported for this application range as high as 79 to 95%, with specificities as high as 86 to 97%.[1-3] With bedside ultrasound readily available in many emergency departments and a reported steep learning curve for this application, sonographic assessment of wounds suspected of harboring a wooden foreign body should become routine.

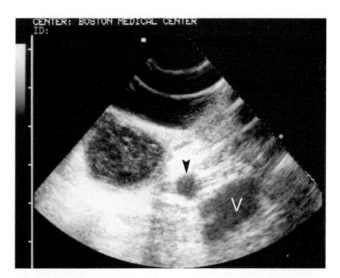

Figure 16–11. Large groin abscess with mixed internal echogenicity, an echogenic rind, as well as posterior acoustic enhancement. The location of the adjacent saphenous (arrowhead) and common femoral veins (V) are noted. Incision and drainage were greatly facilitated with the knowledge of the precise location of adjacent vascular structures. (5.0-MHz sector probe with acoustic standoff.)

Figure 16–10. Peritonsillar abscess. Note the echogenic rind and prominent posterior acoustic enhancement. (6.5-MHz endocavitary probe.)

Whether radiopaque or radiolucent, once a soft tissue foreign body has been identified, the next question to be addressed is how best to remove it. As most clinicians dealing with such cases may confirm, removal of a foreign body can turn into an enormous exercise in frustration. Here again, ultrasound imaging can be used for both a precise pre-operative three-dimensional localization of the foreign body and, if necessary, retrieval of the foreign body under direct sonographic guidance.

▶ CLINICAL INDICATIONS

The clinical indications for the use of ultrasound in the management of a soft tissue foreign body include the following:

- Detection of a radiolucent foreign body
- Localization of a radiolucent or radiopaque foreign body
- Foreign body removal

Detection and Localization of a Foreign Body

The literature on sonographic detection of soft tissue foreign bodies encompasses a range of specialties and methodologies.[1–15] The types of foreign bodies investigated range from isolated wood fragments to multiple materials, including metal, wood, plastic, gravel, sand, and thorns or cactus spines. Sonographers with widely varying degrees of skill performed the ultrasound examinations in these studies, including emergency physicians with no prior formal training, emergency medicine residents who had just completed a 16-h introductory training course in ultrasound, credentialed sonographers, and radiologists specially trained in musculoskeletal ultrasound. What emerges from this body of literature is the following.

1. *Success in detecting a soft tissue foreign body varied widely in the experimental literature, depending on the tissue model and foreign body type(s) employed.* Using a homogenous beef cube model, a 98% sensitivity and specificity for detecting a foreign body were reported in one study.[8] With a chicken thigh model (which more closely mimics the hand and where more confounding acoustic interfaces are present), the overall sensitivity for detecting a wooden foreign body was reported to be 79%.[2] In a study using a "freshly thawed" cadaver foot, an overall sensitivity and specificity of 90 and 97%, respectively, were reported for the detection of wooden foreign bodies.[5] In a study using a fresh frozen cadaver hand, 156 out of 166 foreign bodies were detected, with ultrasound resulting in a sensitivity and specificity of 94 and 99%, respectively.[14] In contradistinction to

the excellent results noted above, one investigation evaluating the use of ultrasound for the detection of various foreign bodies in chicken thighs reported an overall sensitivity and specificity of 43 and 70%, respectively. Sensitivity for detection of a 1-cm wooden foreign body was only 50% in this report. Review of the methods in this study revealed that all the chicken thighs were incised and systematically opened with a hemostat prior to foreign body placement.[12] Such tissue disruption, including introduction of air into the wound, probably far exceeds that found in most puncture wounds, and could have had an unpredictable effect on the results of subsequent imaging.

2. *Success in the detection of a foreign body depended upon the size of the foreign body imaged.* Foreign bodies such as small glass fragments and cactus thorns were difficult to detect and may have exceeded the limits of the ultrasound transducer's resolution. Comparison of test characteristics reported in various studies must be interpreted with an awareness of the size of the foreign body employed in that study model. In two experimental studies where wooden foreign bodies were included,[8,2] the wood fragments were all 1.5 cm long; another study[5] evaluated the use of ultrasound in the detection of 2.5 mm and 5.0 mm wooden foreign bodies. Sensitivities and specificities in this latter report varied as a function of foreign body size, with an 87% sensitivity and 97% specificity reported for the detection of the 2.5 mm wooden foreign bodies and a 93% sensitivity and 96% specificity reported for the detection of the 5.0 mm wooden foreign bodies.[5]

3. *Transducer type varied among studies.* Linear array transducers of 5.0, 7.5, 8.0, and 10.0 MHz were variously employed in these studies. Some researchers also advocated the use of sector transducers. The relative advantages and disadvantages of each transducer type are addressed below.

4. *The type of training and experience of sonographers varied considerably among studies.* Ultrasound imaging was performed variously by radiologists, sonographers, and emergency physicians. Only one study directly compared the ability of various types of sonographers to find foreign bodies by ultrasound.[2] The difference in test accuracy between a board-certified radiologist, whose practice was limited to ultrasonography, two sonographers, and three emergency medicine residents was not statistically significant in this study. Test accuracy for each group was reported as 83%, 85%, and 80%, respectively.

5. *In clinical studies, hand and foot injuries predominated.* For example, in one review of 50 patients

evaluated for a non-radiopaque foreign body, 45 of the 50 injuries were confined to the hand or foot.[3]

6. *In clinical studies, most foreign bodies were found to be superficial in location.* Of 10 wooden foreign bodies retrieved from foot wounds in one series, all were located 0.4 to 1.4 cm from the skin surface. In another clinical review, all of the 21 foreign bodies retrieved at surgery were noted to be less than 2 cm from the skin surface.[1,3]

▶ ANATOMIC CONSIDERATIONS

Patients evaluated for a suspected or known soft tissue foreign body will typically present with either a hand or a foot injury. A thorough familiarity with the anatomic complexity of these areas is essential for the clinician. Given the relatively shallow depth of the soft tissues in these anatomically intricate regions and the multiple acoustic interfaces present, clinicians should practice scanning on normal hands and feet to gain familiarity with the normal sonographic appearance of these commonly injured areas. The utility of examining the contralateral, uninjured extremity for comparison when a confusing sonographic finding is encountered cannot be overemphasized.

▶ TECHNIQUE AND NORMAL ULTRASOUND FINDINGS

Typically, a high-frequency linear array transducer, in the 7.5 to 10.0 MHz range, should be used when scanning for foreign bodies in superficial soft tissues. A 7.5 MHz annular array probe may function adequately in this capacity and has the advantage of a smaller skin contact footprint. A 5.0 MHz transducer may be useful when searching for a deeper foreign body. Higher frequency transducers, in the 10.0 to 13.0 MHz range, offer the ability to discern smaller foreign bodies (e.g., a 12.0 MHz transducer can reportedly detect a 1- to 2-mm foreign body), but transducers of this type are not commonly available in emergency departments. Although linear array transducers may be technically superior for image acquisition, the smaller skin contact footprint of a sector transducer should be advantageous in difficult-to-scan areas (such as the webspace between fingers) and when performing ultrasound-guided retrieval of a foreign body.[13] As a general rule, one should use the highest frequency transducer available since the foreign body will be more clearly delineated and more brightly echogenic. Most foreign bodies encountered should reside at relatively superficial tissue depths (less than 2 cm) where high frequency transducers excel at imaging.

Use of an acoustic standoff pad will usually be necessary in order to adequately image the superficial soft tissues. Standoff pads are acoustically sonolucent and serve to raise the transducer approximately 2 cm above the skin surface, thereby allowing the skin and superficial subcutaneous tissues to be moved well away from the transducers near field "dead zone." Although incorporation of standoff pads into the ultrasound examination requires some additional technical agility, this skill is rapidly acquired and the effort is amply rewarded with improved image quality in the near field. Use of inexpensive, commercially available acoustic gel pads developed just for this purpose is recommended. Small pieces (size based on the transducer's skin contact footprint) can be cut for single patient use and then be discarded. Other standoff pad options include the use of a gel-filled finger of a glove or a small (50 cc) intravenous fluid bag. These are generally more cumbersome to use, however, and image quality may suffer.

In the case of a small or inapparent puncture wound, ultrasound gel can be applied directly to the site of injury, followed by a piece of the gel pad, then additional gel, and finally, the transducer. The wound should be thoroughly irrigated after the ultrasound examination. In the case of a large open wound, sterile surgical gel can be applied onto the wound itself, and the transducer covered by a sterile sheath or glove.

As with all ultrasound imaging, appropriate adjustment of the ultrasound machine's depth and electronic focus settings should be made to position the soft tissue area being investigated within the transducer's optimal focal zone. For optimal image quality, the transducer should be held perpendicular to the skin surface and the area should be scanned systematically in two perpendicular planes. A foreign body will be most clearly visualized when the plane of the transducer beam is aligned parallel to the long axis of the foreign body. Rotating the transducer so the beam plane is increasingly oblique to the long axis of the foreign body diminishes the intensity of the echoes returning to the transducer. If available, color-flow Doppler may be used to establish if an adjacent echo-free structure is vascular in nature.

For ultrasound-guided retrieval of a foreign body, several techniques have been advocated. Most employ ultrasound-guided introduction of a sterile needle, which should be advanced to the foreign body. Needle position should be noted on the monitor from the reverberation artifact it produces. One report suggested guiding the needle tip directly to the foreign body and then incising down to the needle tip to retrieve the foreign body.[7] Another report compared three slightly different retrieval techniques using a pork model.[17] Once the foreign body was positioned on the monitor in its best long axis plane, under direct ultrasound guidance: (1) a needle was advanced to the foreign body until it just touched the foreign body, (2) a needle was passed just under the foreign body, or (3) two small-gauge needles were inserted directly under the foreign body at a 90° angle from one another. Retrieval of the foreign body required more than 10 min using methods #1 and #2 and further opening of the initial 1.5 cm wound was required in five of six cases. Using method #3 (where two needles were used to localize the foreign body), retrieval was accomplished in less than 4 min in six of six and no further widening of the initial 1.5 cm wound was required.

Yet another accepted retrieval technique relies on the use of a hemostat. The foreign body should be positioned on the monitor in its best long axis orientation. After injection of local anesthetic, the hemostat should then be advanced toward the foreign body under direct sonographic guidance, keeping the instrument within the plane of the transducer's beam. If the removal attempt fails, the transducer can be rotated 90° until the tip of the foreign body is seen in cross section. With the hemostat now held in a horizontal plane, the slightly opened jaws of the hemostat can then be guided toward the echogenic tip of the foreign body for retrieval. The opened jaws of the hemostat should be apparent on the monitor as two echogenic structures with posterior acoustic shadowing. The investigators stated that this procedure was most easily and quickly accomplished when both the sonography and hemostat removal of the foreign body were performed simultaneously by a single physician.[16]

Because of the numerous anatomic structures found in the hand and foot, where most foreign bodies will be encountered, a wide array of normal sonographic findings will be seen (Figure 16–12). The most anterior echogenic structure noted on the sonogram will be the skin surface. If a standoff pad is used, the skin surface will be seen immediately below the sonolucent region in the near field that corresponds to the acoustic standoff pad. Muscle

has a characteristic hypoechoic echotexture traversed by hyperechoic internal striations and brightly echogenic fascial planes. In long axis orientation, tendons appear as echogenic linear structures with a characteristic fibrillar echotexture. In short axis orientation, they have a characteristic ovoid to flat profile. When assessed dynamically, they can be seen gliding within a tendon sheath or in the subcutaneous tissue, thus establishing both the nature and function of the particular tendon being imaged. The bright echo representing the anterior cortex of underlying bone should be identified. Joint spaces can be readily identified by a V-shaped discontinuity in the bright cortical echo. Bony shadowing of the multiple carpal and metacarpal bones (or tarsal and metatarsal bones) and phalanges should not be confused with a foreign body. The course and proximity of adjacent vascular structures should be noted where relevant.

► COMMON AND EMERGENT ABNORMALITIES

Soft Tissue Foreign Bodies

The sonographic appearance of soft tissue foreign bodies is variable. All soft tissue foreign bodies will exhibit a hyperechoic acoustic profile and may additionally demonstrate acoustic shadowing, reverberation echoes, or comet-tail artifacts. Larger linear metallic foreign bodies (e.g., a needle or needle fragment) (Figures 16–13 and 16–14) usually produce a prominent reverberation artifact; whereas, a small rounded metallic foreign body (such as a small BB or metal fragment) (Figure 16–15) usually produces a comet-tail artifact. Glass fragments may exhibit a comet-tail artifact, but are more likely to cause a diffuse

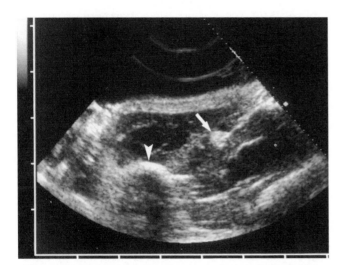

Figure 16–12. Normal hand, thenar eminence. Note the hypoechoic muscles of the thenar eminence, the brightly hyperechoic flexor pollicis longus tendon (arrow), and shadowing from the first metacarpal (arrowhead). (7.5-MHz sector probe with acoustic standoff pad.)

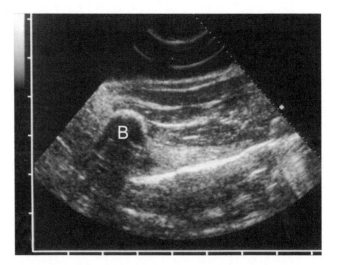

Figure 16–13. Normal chicken thigh. Similar to the hand in its acoustic profile; note the acoustic shadowing from the thighbone (B) and the brightly echogenic fascial plane in the far field. 5.0-MHz sector probe with acoustic standoff pad.

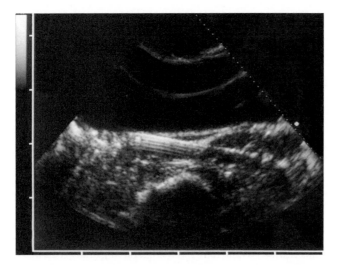

Figure 16–14. Metal sewing needle. Note the brightly echogenic reverberation artifact. Chicken thigh tissue model and a 7.5-MHz sector probe with an acoustic standoff pad.

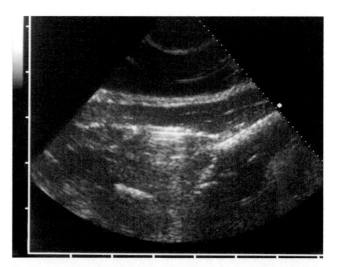

A

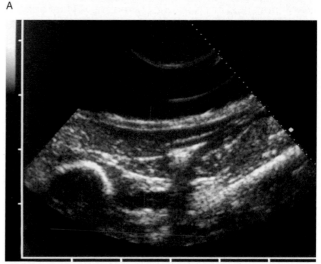

B

Figure 16–16. Glass shard. Reverberation artifact noted on long axis (A) and dirty shadowing on short axis. (B). Chicken thigh tissue model and a 7.5-MHz sector probe with an acoustic standoff pad.

scattering of the ultrasound beam (Figures 16–16). This is due to the irregular acoustic interfaces of the glass fragment and "dirty" shadowing caused by air that has entered the soft tissues along with the foreign body. A gravel fragment will typically demonstrate a bright echo return from its anterior surface and dense posterior acoustic shadowing, similar to a gallstone (Figure 16–17). Wood, thorns, and plastic typically exhibit a hyperechoic acoustic profile (Figure 16–18). With a wooden foreign body, a posterior acoustic shadow is frequently but not always observed. In one clinical review, nine of ten wooden foreign bodies removed from injured feet exhibited posterior acoustic shadowing; the one that did not was "very small." However, in another clinical series,

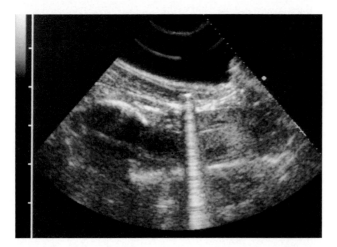

Figure 16–15. BB pellet. Typical comet tail reverberation artifact, this pattern is also seen with most bullets. Shadowing from thighbone on left of image. Chicken thigh tissue model and a-7.5 MHz sector probe with an acoustic standoff pad.

only 11 of 17 wooden foreign bodies retrieved surgically from hand or foot wounds exhibited acoustic shadowing on the preoperative sonogram.[3] Of additional note, the intensity of the hyperechoic acoustic profile of wooden foreign bodies does not appear to change with time and remains similar in acute, subacute, and chronic wounds.[1]

Except in the case of acute injuries, where inflammatory changes have not yet had time to occur, the clinician evaluating a wound with a foreign body will often encounter a hypoechoic halo surrounding the foreign body. The host response to the foreign body, whether it is edema, granulation tissue, or abscess formation, results in a hypoechoic region of varying size surrounding the hyperechoic foreign body. This hypoechoic halo can actually assist with the detection and localization of the foreign body (Figures 16–19). In a clinical review of wooden

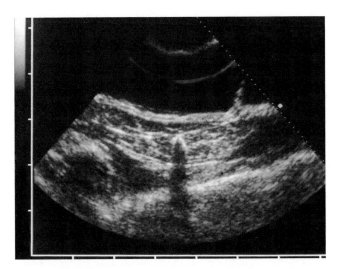

Figure 16–17. Gravel fragment with a brightly echogenic anterior surface and dense posterior acoustic shadowing similar to a gallstone. Shadowing from thighbone on left of image. Chicken thigh tissue model and a 7.5-MHz sector probe with an acoustic standoff pad.

foreign bodies removed from injured feet, seven of ten demonstrated an associated hypoechoic halo on the preoperative sonogram. As expected, two of the three without such a halo were acute injuries.[1]

▶ COMMON VARIANTS AND SELECTED ABNORMALITIES

A number of wound characteristics can complicate the sonographic evaluation of the injured area. Air introduced

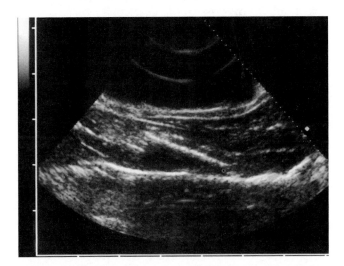

Figure 16–18. Wooden toothpick fragment in long axis with a brightly echogenic anterior surface and dense posterior acoustic shadowing. Chicken thigh tissue model and a 7.5-MHz sector probe with an acoustic standoff pad.

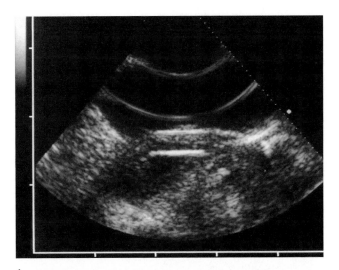

A

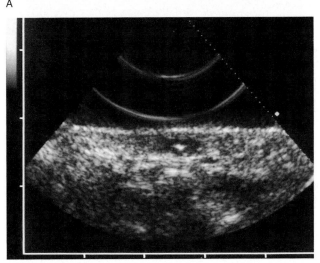

B

Figure 16–19. Clinical history: Patient with a wooden splinter lodged in the volar proximal phalangeal region for 2 weeks. Long (A) and short (B) axis views. Note the wooden splinter's hyperechoic acoustic profile and the surrounding hypoechoic halo, which aids in its localization. (7.5-MHz sector probe with acoustic standoff pad.)

into the wound by either the injury itself, prior wound irrigation, or wound exploration can create significant and misleading artifacts. Such sonographic artifacts may either completely obscure the foreign body or may be mistakenly interpreted as representing a foreign body when none is actually present. Small air pockets can sometimes be obliterated by slight compression with the transducer, dramatically improving image quality. Ultrasound examination of a large, open wound may be altogether impractical because of associated tissue distortion and the technical demands of trying to maintain sterile technique while simultaneously scanning and making adjustments on the ultrasound machine.

▶ PITFALLS

1. *Inadequate knowledge of the regional anatomy.* Lack of familiarity with the normal sonographic anatomy of the part of the body being imaged, particularly the hand or foot, can make accurate interpretation of the ultrasound image difficult. Normal bony shadows, brightly echogenic tissue interfaces and fascia, echogenic muscle striations, and shadowing from vascular calcifications can all lead to potential misinterpretation of the image obtained. Also, tissue interfaces in close proximity to one another may distort the image. Adjacent bone and its associated acoustic shadow may hide a foreign body, particularly smaller ones.

2. *Other pitfalls.* Small foreign bodies may also test the limits of the transducer's resolution. Sesamoid bones, whether typical or atypical in location, may be falsely interpreted as signifying the presence of a foreign body. Scar tissue from prior surgery in the area can also give rise to a hyperechoic signal that may be mistaken for a foreign body. Additionally, air, fresh hematoma, ossified cartilage, and keratin plugs may all give rise to hyperechoic acoustic images that may be falsely interpreted as representing a foreign body. Finally, certain anatomic areas such as the webspace between digits may be technically difficult or impossible to image if a transducer with a large skin contact footprint is used.

3. *Foreign body removal.* Once a soft tissue foreign body has been located, an important clinical decision must be made as to whether retrieval is appropriate or even technically feasible. Various factors to consider include the skill of the operator, the body part injured, the time available, and the size and type of foreign body involved. In the case of a deep wound, a poorly accessible foreign body or closely adjacent neurovascular structures, consultation or referral to an appropriate surgical specialist should be sought.

BODY FLUID LOCALIZATION AND ASPIRATION

The utility of ultrasound for identifying fluid collections has long been recognized; that, combined with its ease of use at the bedside makes it particularly well suited for guiding diagnostic or therapeutic aspiration. This section will focus on emergency ultrasound's use in assisting with three procedures commonly performed in the emergency setting: thoracentesis, paracentesis, and arthrocentesis.

▶ THORACENTESIS

▶ CLINICAL CONSIDERATIONS

Ultrasound allows for rapid identification and precise localization of pleural effusions, and has been shown to be an excellent diagnostic and procedural aid when thoracentesis is performed. While percussion, tactile fremitus, and landmark identification have their role, there is no question that ultrasound guidance permits a much safer performance of a procedure that is associated with a complication rate as high as 20 to 50%.[1] Additionally, ultrasound is much more sensitive than standard chest radiography for identifying small pleural fluid collections. It has been noted that even 300 to 400 mL collections may not be visible on a routine chest radiograph.[2] In clinical settings where prolonged delays in obtaining an inpatient bed are common, thoracentesis is frequently performed in the emergency department. With the widespread use of portable ultrasound units by specialists of all types, and given the significantly improved safety of performing thoracentesis under direct ultrasound guidance,[3] sonographic mapping of a pleural effusion prior to aspiration should become routine.

▶ CLINICAL INDICATIONS

Thoracentesis may be performed for diagnostic or therapeutic purposes. Aspiration of pleural fluid is usually undertaken to determine if a transudate or exudate is present, and, occasionally, to determine if the fluid collection is due to a hematoma or empyema. Analysis of the fluid obtained allows for further diagnostic differentiation as to its potential etiology. Thoracentesis may be performed therapeutically in patients with large pleural effusions to relieve dyspnea or mediastinal shift.

In a report on 85 patients with small pleural effusions (defined as obliterating less than one-half of the hemidiaphragm on an upright chest radiograph), chest sonography was demonstrated to be significantly superior to the decubitus chest radiograph for detecting pleural fluid and assisting in collection of an adequate fluid sample for analysis.[2] In another study of 52 patients undergoing thoracentesis of large free-flowing pleural effusions (defined as obliterating more than one half of the hemidiaphragm on an upright chest radiograph), the sonographically guided procedure was associated with significantly fewer complications. While the rate of pneumothoraces was 19% overall, none occurred in the sonographically guided group.[4] In another review of 26 patients who had undergone at least one prior failed attempt at blind thoracentesis, subsequent ultrasound-guided thoracentesis was successful in 88% of cases. The sonographers in this study began their examination at the site of the failed blind thoracentesis attempt and made the disturbing discovery that in 18 of 26 patients (69%) the initial thoracentesis attempt had been misdirected either below the hemidiaphragm or above the pleural effusion. In 15 cases (58%), the failed thoracentesis needle entry site was noted to be directly over the spleen, liver, or kidney; in three cases (11%), the needle had been directed above the site of the effusion.[5]

One study provided data supporting the use of ultrasound for thoracentesis in mechanically ventilated patients. In a series of 45 procedures in 40 mechanically ventilated patients, thoracentesis was safely and easily performed with a 97% success rate for obtaining more than 5 mL of fluid, usually in less than 10 sec. No pneumothorax or hemoptysis was observed. The researchers recommended that these guidelines be followed: the width of the fluid collection as measured by the interpleural distance (parietal to visceral) should be at least 15 mm and the fluid should be visible over at least three intercostal spaces. Of incidental note, pleural fluid was considered to be "absent" on the chest radiograph in 17 patients, in whom fluid was subsequently identified and obtained by ultrasound.[6]

▶ TECHNIQUE AND NORMAL ULTRASOUND FINDINGS

In a supine patient, pleural fluid is readily detected as an anechoic collection just above the brightly echogenic diaphragm (Figure 16–20). If thoracentesis is contemplated and the patient is able to cooperate, scanning of the posterior thorax should be performed immediately prior to the procedure with the patient sitting up to determine the extent and limits of the pleural fluid collection. In the mechanically ventilated patient, scanning takes place along the long axis of the accessible intercostal spaces with the patient in either a dorsal decubitus position (on their back,

face up) or in an oblique to complete lateral decubitus position (turned on their side, pleural fluid side up).[6]

Ideally, a 3.5 or 5.0 MHz transducer should be used. Once a pleural effusion has been detected, its location and size should be systematically mapped out to determine whether aspiration is feasible, and, if so, where the point of puncture should occur. In the sitting patient, the relevant hemithorax should be scanned from the anterior axillary line to the paravertebral region, and the superior and inferior extent of the fluid collection should be mapped out. Scanning should be performed over and parallel to the rib interspaces, requiring that the ultrasound beam be turned somewhat oblique to the transverse scan plane. The location of the diaphragm and underlying liver or spleen (Figure 16–21) should be clearly noted, as well as the changes in their position that occur with respiration. The optimum depth of needle insertion should be predetermined either by directly measuring the distance from skin to the center of the fluid collection or by estimation using the depth-scale markers located on the ultrasound screen. Use of M-mode imaging through several respiratory cycles can provide additional useful information on the variation in the depth of the fluid pocket as well as the variation in the proximity of adjacent structures. Lung tissue is frequently seen as an echogenic wedge-shaped structure undulating within the anechoic pleural fluid (Figure 16–22). In the left hemithorax, the heart is often seen beating in the far field of the fluid collection, usually in short axis orientation (Figure 16–23).

In the mechanically ventilated patient, a similar technique should be employed. While at the anticipated puncture site, the transducer should be angled slightly in all four directions, checking specifically for the absence of interposed lung, heart, liver, or spleen during the respiratory cycle (Figure 16–24). Again, the distance from skin to parietal pleura (Figure 16–25) as well as the depth

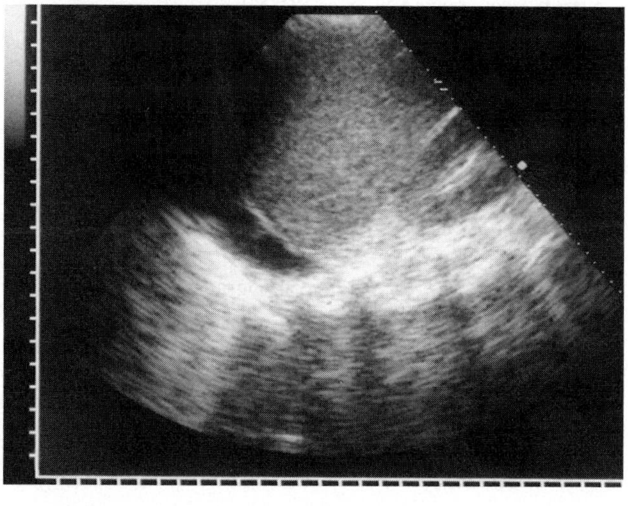

Figure 16–20. Small right pleural effusion seen in a supine patient. (All pleural fluid images taken with a 3.5-MHz sector probe.)

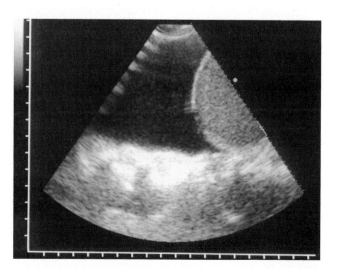

Figure 16–21. Large left pleural effusion with spleen and echogenic diaphragm.

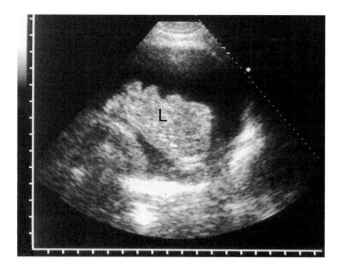

Figure 16–22. Echogenic atelectatic lung parenchyma (L) within a large right pleural effusion.

of the fluid collection itself should be noted and the needle length and puncture depth adjusted accordingly.[6]

Standard caveats for thoracentesis apply[7]: needle puncture should not be performed through a site of skin infection; needle insertion should occur above the rib margin and not below it to avoid the neurovascular bundle; and the needle should not penetrate too deeply into the chest cavity. A significant coagulopathy or thrombocytopenia should be corrected prior to thoracentesis. Standard landmark technique recommends that thoracentesis be attempted only between the mid-scapular line and posterior axillary line and never below the eighth intercostal space. However, real-time sonographic visualization of the fluid collection at the anticipated puncture site throughout the respiratory cycle will frequently permit aspiration outside these traditionally defined borders.

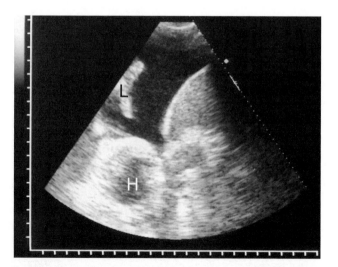

Figure 16–23. Large left pleural effusion imaged from the back with the heart seen in short axis (H) and echogenic lung noted at left of image (L).

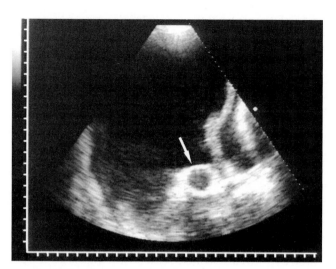

Figure 16–24. Large right pleural effusion imaged from the back with the vena cava noted in the far field (arrow).

▶ PITFALLS

Specific pitfalls of ultrasound-guided thoracentesis are: (1) failure to use it for all anticipated thoracentesis procedures, regardless of the size of the effusion, (2) failure to systematically map out the deepest portion of the fluid collection and an appropriate site for aspiration, and (3) not noting the changes in fluid depth or the changes in lung, diaphragm, or organ position with changes in the phase of respiration.

Complications of thoracentesis include: pneumothorax (one-third of which will reportedly require a thoracostomy tube), unilateral pulmonary edema with lung reexpansion (reportedly limited by removal of no more than 1000 to 1500 mL of pleural fluid at a given time), tran-

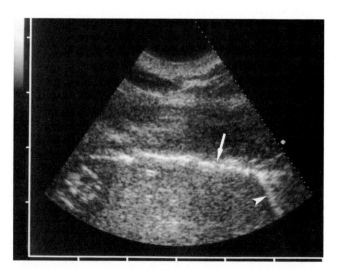

Figure 16–25. Brightly echogenic pleura (arrow) with gliding comet-tail artifacts (arrowhead) seen real-time. 7.5-MHz sector probe.

sient hypoxia from ventilation/perfusion mismatches, hemothorax, hemoperitoneum, infection, air embolus, and shearing of a catheter tip. A preceding sonographic evaluation of the thorax to determine the best location for safe aspiration and a thorough familiarity with the components and use of the thoracentesis kit can help avoid many of these complications.

▶ PARACENTESIS

Sonographic evaluation of the abdominal cavity for detection of hemoperitoneum is becoming routine in the trauma setting. Evaluation of the abdomen for localization of nontraumatic peritoneal fluid prior to paracentesis should become an extension of this technique.

▶ CLINICAL CONSIDERATIONS

The most common cause of ascites in the United States is alcoholic cirrhosis;[1] thus, the frequency with which paracentesis will be performed in a given emergency department or medical center will depend largely on the patient population being served. Presence of ascitic fluid should always be established before paracentesis is performed. Whereas the presence of ascitic fluid is obvious in some patients with advanced cirrhosis, establishing the presence and location of ascitic fluid by the history and physical examination alone may be difficult.[3] Moreover, the potential complications of the procedure itself—including abdominal wall hematoma, intraperitoneal hemorrhage, bowel perforation (particularly in the setting of unsuspected bowel obstruction), and peritonitis—all argue strongly against abdominal paracentesis being routinely performed in a blind fashion.

▶ CLINICAL INDICATIONS

Indications for performing abdominal paracentesis include: diagnostic evaluation of suspected new-onset ascites, evaluation of a patient with suspected spontaneous bacterial peritonitis, and as a therapeutic intervention in symptomatic patients with large volume ascites.[1,2]

Ultrasonography is considered a gold standard test for detecting ascites, reliably identifying as little as 100 mL of free fluid.[4] Many experts recommend ultrasound guidance whenever the physical examination is not definitive, such as in an obese patient or when multiple abdominal scars are present.[1,5,6] However, there are several compelling reasons to recommend routine bedside ultrasonography prior to every paracentesis that is performed in the emergency department. First and foremost, the presence of free-flowing ascites can be rapidly and definitively established and bowel obstruction, as the cause of a patient's abdominal distention, can be simultaneously excluded. Also, an accessible fluid pocket and a

safe puncture site for the planned paracentesis can be rapidly identified. In a study of 27 patients with more than 300 mL of documented ascites, ultrasound of the left lower quadrant—long considered a "standard" location for blind paracentesis—revealed that there was no fluid present at this location in 19 of the 27 patients (70%) and that there were air-filled loops of bowel between the fluid pocket and abdominal wall in three patients (11%).[7]

▶ TECHNIQUE AND NORMAL ULTRASOUND FINDINGS

The ultrasound examination for ascites should usually be performed with a 3.5 MHz transducer. The approach to the examination is somewhat dependent on the volume of ascites present. In patients with large volume ascites, where the goal of the ultrasound examination is simply to establish the presence of an accessible pocket of fluid, a single view at the expected site of paracentesis (usually in the infraumbilical midline or the left lower quadrant) may be all that is required. Optimally, paracentesis should be performed with the patient in the same position as when the ultrasound images were obtained. The location of the superior portion of the bladder should be noted, particularly when the planned site of paracentesis is inferior to the umbilicus in the midline (Figure 16–26).

To detect small collections of intraperitoneal fluid, the ultrasound examination should begin with the patient in a supine position. Based on a study of the use of ultrasound to detect intraperitoneal fluid in cadavers,[4] it appears that small fluid collections are normally first seen in Morison's pouch (Figure 16–27). Scanning the patient in the right lateral decubitus position or placing the patient in Trendelenburg can improve detection of small volumes of fluid.

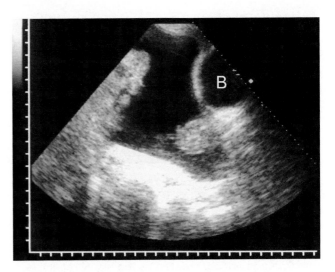

Figure 16–26. Ascites, midline infraumbilical view. Note the bladder (B) and bladder dome on the right side of the sonogram.

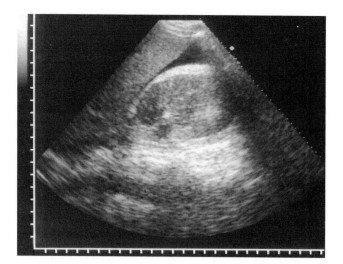

Figure 16–27. Ascites noted in the right upper quadrant in a supine patient. (3.5-MHz sector probe for all ascites images.)

Ascitic fluid usually appears anechoic on ultrasound (Figure 16–28). Echogenic fibrinous strands may also be noted within the fluid collection. Gain settings should be appropriately adjusted to make the fluid appear black. Loops of small bowel may be seen moving slowly within the ascitic fluid (Figure 16–29A and B). A mesenteric stalk attached to the loops of bowel may also be seen. The location of the bladder and its muscular dome should be routinely noted.

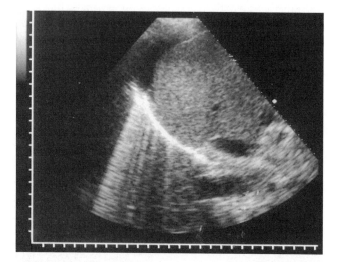

Figure 16–28. Large amount of ascites resulting in fluid above the liver in this right upper quadrant scan. Note and compare the location of this hypoechoic fluid collection with that of the right pleural effusion (see Figure 16–20). The region above the diaphragm exhibits an echotexture similar to liver because of the mirror image artifact created by the highly reflective and echogenic diaphragm. Prominent gliding comet-tail artifacts can also be seen arising from the pleura adjacent to the diaphragm.

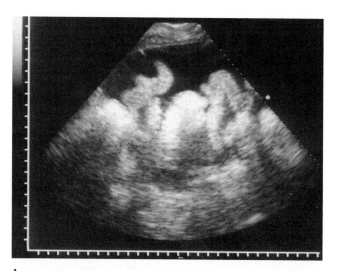

A

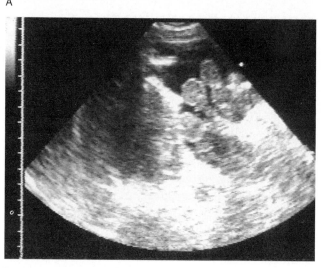

B

Figure 16–29. (A, B) Ascites with floating loops of small bowel.

▶ PITFALLS

Complications of paracentesis include abdominal wall hematoma, intraperitoneal hemorrhage, bladder and bowel perforation (particularly in the setting of unsuspected bowel obstruction), and peritonitis.

ARTHROCENTESIS

▶ CLINICAL CONSIDERATIONS

Emergency and acute care providers are regularly called upon to evaluate a patient with a painful or swollen joint where the ultimate diagnosis depends on obtaining joint fluid for analysis. Multiple processes may cause joint effusions. The most common processes are by crystal deposition or degenerative arthritis, but infection, trauma, and intraarticular fracture or hematoma, as well as a host of connective tissue disorders may also be responsible. Although typically performed for diagnostic purposes, arthrocentesis may be performed as a therapeutic intervention to relieve the pain associated with a tense joint effusion. Arthrocentesis also is used occasionally to clarify whether painful joint swelling is articular or periarticular in nature.[1] While arthrocentesis of most joints can be performed using standard landmark techniques alone, successful localization and aspiration of fluid in the hip and ankle, and occasionally even small effusions in the knee or elbow, can be challenging. In these circumstances, the ability of ultrasound to readily locate the joint space and the most accessible pocket of fluid can be extremely helpful.

▶ CLINICAL INDICATIONS

Ultrasound-guided arthrocentesis can be performed at the hip, ankle, knee, and various other joints.

Hip Joint

When physical examination findings suggest that an inflammatory process involving the hip joint might be present, ultrasound can be used to rapidly determine the presence or absence of an effusion. If an effusion is present, ultrasound can also be used to precisely guide the needle tip to the fluid collection for aspiration. In one review where ultrasound-guided hip aspirations were performed to exclude infection, joint fluid was readily aspirated in 10 of 13 patients in whom capsular distention was apparent on the sonogram.[2] The investigators noted that ultrasound-guided arthrocentesis also could be performed in patients with a total hip prosthesis. The use of ultrasound-guided arthrocentesis by an emergency physician was illustrated in a case report involving a patient with hip pain and a low-grade fever in whom the diagnosis of a septic hip was entertained.[3] After several failed attempts at blind aspiration by the consulting orthopedist, plans were made for hip arthrotomy and irrigation in the operating suite. However, joint fluid was obtained after bedside ultrasound examination was performed by the emergency physician to visualize the hip effusion and to guide the needle aspiration. Joint fluid analysis revealed calcium pyrophosphate crystals, consistent with pseudogout, which ultimately spared the patient an unnecessary operation.

Ankle Joint

While the use of landmark techniques is usually adequate to locate the ankle joint for arthrocentesis, precise localization of the joint line can at times be difficult. For most clinicians, the failure rate of ankle arthrocentesis is considerably higher than in the knee. The use of bedside ultrasound by emergency physicians has been reported in the work-up of a patient with ankle pain and a fever in whom arthrocentesis was necessary to exclude a septic ankle joint.[4] After multiple blind attempts to obtain synovial fluid were unsuccessful, ultrasound was used to precisely determine the location of the tibiotalar joint. The ankle joint was then successfully aspirated and the patient was ultimately diagnosed with acute gouty arthritis.

Knee Joint

Although aspiration of a knee effusion is usually accomplished with landmark techniques alone, successful aspiration can be elusive when the effusion is small or the synovium thickened by chronic inflammation. As the aspirating needle encounters the thickened synovium, the pressure required to penetrate it may collapse the underlying fluid collection resulting in a "dry tap." A similar phenomenon can occur with small joint effusions. In patients in whom standard landmark-guided knee aspiration is unsuccessful for whatever reason, a brief sonographic "mapping" of the effusion to find the area of maximum fluid depth (often at the suprapatellar bursa) will frequently result in a successful tap. In morbidly obese patients, ultrasound can be used to locate the joint space and assist in identifying an effusion that may be difficult to appreciate clinically. With the ready availability of bedside ultrasound in many emergency care settings and the brief time required for this examination (usually less than one min), an ultrasound-guided aspiration should be routinely considered after any failed attempt at blind knee arthrocentesis.

Other Joints

The ultrasound-guided technique should apply to a failed blind arthrocentesis of the elbow joint as well as to unsuccessful attempts to aspirate fluid from the olecranon, prepatellar or calcaneal bursae.

▶ TECHNIQUE AND NORMAL ULTRASOUND FINDINGS

Sonographic evaluation of the hip joint for an effusion has been successfully accomplished with a variety of transducers, ranging from 3.0, 5.0, and 10.0 MHz linear array transducers to a 3.0 MHz sector transducer. The best view for establishing the presence of a hip effusion is a ventral oblique view oriented parallel to the long axis of the femoral neck (Figure 16–30).

The transducer orientation marker should be aimed superomedially so that the distal femoral neck will be located on the right side of the image (this assumes that presets are set to abdominal or vascular imaging orientation). The brightly echogenic cortex of the femoral head and neck will usually be apparent 3 to 4 cm below the skin surface (Figure 16–31). The articular capsule of the hip

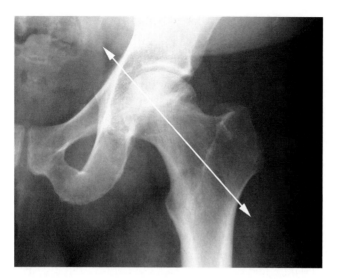

Figure 16–30. Hip X-ray demonstrating the axis for imaging the hip for an effusion. The transducer is placed parallel to the long axis of the femoral neck.

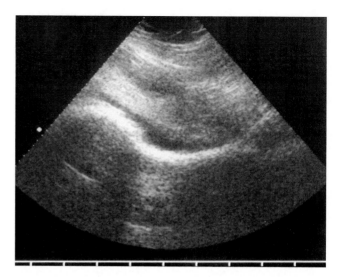

Figure 16–32. Opposite hip of Figure 16–31. Sonogram of a hip effusion. Hypoechoic fluid collection noted in the anterior synovial recess. (7.5 MHz sector probe.)

joint extends from the acetabular labrum to the base of the femoral neck. A hip effusion will appear as a convex anechoic stripe, adjacent to the anterior bony echo of the femoral neck in an area called the anterior synovial recess (Figure 16–32). This region can be found near field on the sonogram at the concave region of the femoral neck beginning just distal to the femoral head and tracking further distally to the lower femoral neck. The relationship of the joint space to the femoral artery and vein should be carefully noted and is best seen on a transverse view of the hip joint. Criteria for defining an effusion include: (1) a convex bulging joint capsule with a fluid stripe greater than 5 to 6 mm; or (2) when compared to the asymptomatic joint, a greater than 2 mm increase in

the distance from the cortical echo to the joint capsule.[2,5] Comparison to the contralateral hip can be very helpful and should be routinely performed.

Once a fluid collection is identified, needle aspiration of the effusion may be undertaken with ultrasound guidance. Aspiration can be performed with a lumbar puncture needle, either freehand or with a needle guide. The needle should be advanced within the long axis plane of the transducer's beam, where its characteristic reverberation artifact can be visualized and used to guide the needle into the sonolucent effusion.

When performing ankle arthrocentesis, bedside ultrasound can be extremely useful to precisely identify the space between the distal tibia and the talar dome, where the arthrocentesis needle should be directed (Figure 16–33). Sagittal scanning of the distal tibia should be performed with a 5.0 to 7.5 MHz linear or annular array transducer. With screen depth set at 3 to 4 cm, the brightly echogenic anterior cortex of the distal tibia will be seen. While still in a sagittal plane, the transducer should be moved distally to the approximate middle of the ankle joint. The bony echo of the distal tibia will be seen to curve slightly anteriorly, then dive posteriorly, revealing the narrow echo-free space that corresponds to the joint space. Just distal to this echo-free space, the bright ascending echo that represents the dome of the talus will be noted. A large ankle effusion will appear as a prominent sonolucency at the base of the V-shaped recess. It should be noted that fluid in the tibiotalar recess is common. It has also been noted that neither the amount nor the sonographic appearance will reliably identify which effusions are pathologic, however.[7] Therefore, although sonography can reliably identify the presence or absence of an ankle effusion, clinical judgment must guide the need for arthrocentesis of this joint.

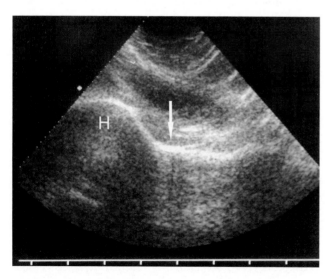

Figure 16–31. Sonogram of a normal hip, showing anterior recess (arrow) and head of the femur (H). (5.0-MHz sector probe.)

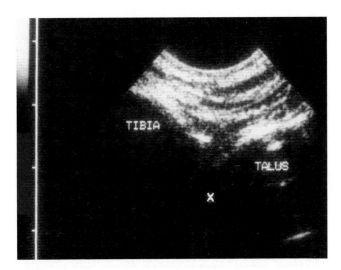

Figure 16–33. Ankle sonogram. X marks the location of the tibiotalar recess. (5.0-MHz sector probe.)

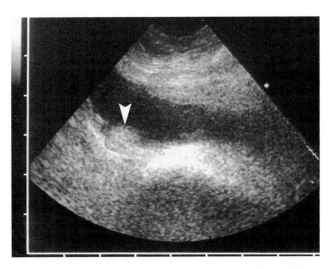

Figure 16–35. Sagittal view of a large suprapatellar effusion. (arrowhead) points to a synovial polyp. (5.0-MHz sector probe.)

With the transducer positioned so that the deepest portion of this V-shaped recess is located in the exact center of the sonogram, a mark is made on the skin adjacent to the center of the transducer. The acoustic shadow of a pen tip placed under the edge of the transducer can be used to precisely mark the location of this recess as well. The angle of the transducer relative to the skin surface, and the degree of ankle plantar flexion, should be noted. The aspiration can subsequently be performed freehand using this information to aim the needle in the appropriate direction.

Occasionally, as noted above, knee arthrocentesis using standard landmark techniques is unsuccessful due to a small effusion (Figure 16–34), synovial thickening, or patient obesity. In this setting, a rapid ultrasound evalua-

tion is recommended to establish if joint fluid is present and, if so, to identify a more appropriate site for aspiration (Figures 16–35 and 16–36). Fluid will usually best be found at the medial or lateral suprapatellar bursa. A 3.5 to 5.0 MHz transducer can be used. The knee is optimally scanned with the patient supine and the slightly flexed knee supported from behind with a sheet or towel for patient comfort. Scanning is most easily performed in a longitudinal plane just above the patella.

With small effusions, care should be taken to apply as little pressure to the transducer as possible to avoid causing collapse of the fluid collection. Additional sonographic findings commonly encountered in the knee

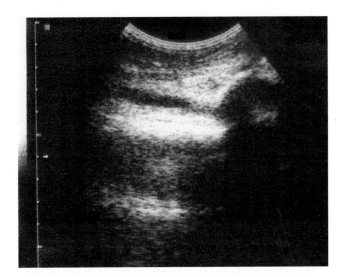

Figure 16–34. Sagittal view of a small suprapatellar effusion. Curved echo of patella noted at right and bright echo of femur below the anechoic effusion. (3.5-MHz linear array probe.)

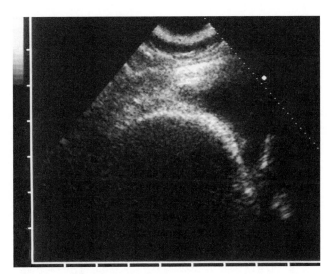

Figure 16–36. Transverse view of a suprapatellar effusion. Curvilinear echo and shadow from the femur noted in the far field. The effusion is above and slightly lateral to the femur in this view. (5.0 MHz sector probe.)

include: (1) thickened, hyperechoic synovium; (2) hemarthrosis, initially echo-free and indistinguishable from an effusion, but later acquiring a homogenous, mid-level echogenicity when coagulation has occurred; (3) lipohemarthrosis (Figure 16–37), similar to hemarthrosis but with the addition of a fat/blood level within the effusion, signifying the presence of an associated fracture, and finally; (4) freely mobile loose bodies that exhibit a hyperechoic acoustic profile with posterior acoustic shadowing. These are usually found in the suprapatellar pouch, and can be seen to move with either gentle palpation of the effusion or pressure on the transducer.[6] On a cautionary note, aspiration in the popliteal fossae should generally be avoided because popliteal (Baker's) cysts, popliteal artery aneurysms, and varicose veins can all appear as echo-free fluid collections.

Sonographic detection of a joint effusion in the elbow is usually easily accomplished. The elbow should be held in 90° of flexion if possible with the palm resting on the table or stretcher. Scanning is most easily performed along the posterior aspect of the distal humerus, just above the olecranon, with the transducer aligned parallel to the long axis of the humerus. An effusion will appear as an echo-free collection within the olecranon fossa just anterior to the bright echo from the distal humerus and trochlea (Figure 16–38). Aspiration is performed along the lateral aspect of the humerus in order to stay well away from the ulnar nerve.

Small bursal fluid collections in the olecranon, prepatellar and calcaneal bursae may be imaged if blind aspiration has failed or if the presence of bursal fluid is in question, as may occasionally occur with a prepatellar bursitis (Figure 16–39). Again, gentle transducer pressure

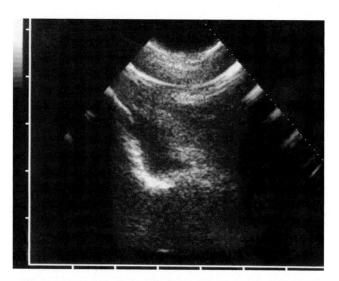

Figure 16–38. Elbow effusion. Posterior approach, demonstrating an echo free effusion in the olecranon fossa.

should be employed to avoid collapse of the underlying bursal sac.

MUSCULOSKELETAL APPLICATIONS

▶ CLINICAL INDICATIONS

Numerous musculoskeletal applications for diagnostic ultrasound have been described in the ultrasound literature. These include: (1) evaluation of suspected partial

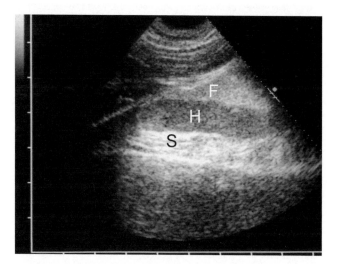

Figure 16–37. Lipohemarthrosis. Sagittal view of a large, several days old posttraumatic knee effusion with layering fat in near field (F), echogenic hematoma below (H), and thickened echogenic synovium (S) noted just above the femur. (5.0 MHz sector probe.)

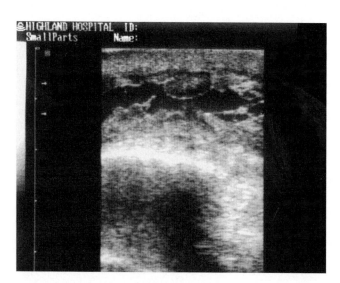

Figure 16–39. Prepatellar bursitis. Echo free fluid collection with fibrinous stranding noted just below the skin. Bright cortical echo from the patella is noted in mid-field. (7.5 MHz linear array probe.)

or complete tendon tears in the rotator cuff, triceps tendon, distal biceps tendon, Achilles tendon, quadriceps tendon, patellar tendon, and flexor tendons of the hand; (2) evaluation for tears of the rectus femoris or gastrocnemius muscles; (3) diagnosis of occult ganglion cysts in the wrist; (4) dynamic evaluation of flexor tendons of the hand to diagnose a disruption of an annular pulley ligament; and (5) assessment of the ulnar nerve in cubital tunnel syndrome. Some of these applications require expertise in ultrasound scanning beyond that of most sonographers or require specialized transducers that are not generally available in the emergency department. However, some of these musculoskeletal applications are potentially extremely useful in the emergency or ambulatory care setting and these are discussed as follows.

A number of clinical studies have investigated the use of ultrasound to image rotator cuff tears.[1-3] Using arthrography as a gold standard, one study of 100 patients, evaluated with ultrasound for suspected rotator cuff injury, reported 95% sensitivity and 100% specificity for identifying a complete rotator cuff tear.[1] However, the protocol in this study required that the joint be imaged in ten different planes. In another review of 81 patients with shoulder injuries, ultrasound was 67% sensitive for the diagnosis of rotator cuff tear.[2] A study of ultrasound to detect subscapularis tears reported a sensitivity of 86%.[3] In an attempt to explain the wide range of reported accuracy of ultrasound for diagnosing rotator cuff tears (60 to 95%), Fornage identified the following factors: the technical difficulty involved, the considerable experience required to perform the examination, the complex anatomy of the shoulder, and prominent beam propagation artifacts in the shoulder.[4] Because of these difficulties, only a few centers use ultrasound commonly to evaluate rotator cuff tears. MRI, with its excellent image quality and lack of operator dependence, has become the most commonly employed imaging technique for this injury. With recent improvements in ultrasound imaging technology, however, the use of ultrasonography in the evaluation of the rotator cuff will likely increase.

A careful clinical evaluation will usually reveal whether a tendon injury or disruption is likely. Complete disruptions of the rotator cuff, or the triceps, quadriceps, or Achilles tendons, are usually not difficult to detect on physical examination. Where ultrasonography can play a useful role is in the diagnosis of certain partial tendon ruptures that might otherwise be misdiagnosed on clinical examination alone. Ultrasound imaging of tendons and the dynamic assessment of their function in real time offers important additional diagnostic information that cannot be discerned by physical examination or plain radiography. Where this technique may be of particular value to the emergency care provider is with injuries of the patellar tendon, Achilles tendon, and flexor or extensor tendons of the hand.

Ultrasonography can also play a useful role in the evaluation of the athlete with chronic localized knee pain suggestive of partial rupture of the proximal patellar tendon ("jumper's knee"). In a review of 25 surgically proven cases of "jumper's knee," ultrasound correctly identified the lesion in all patients. The investigators advocated the use of ultrasound as "the method of choice for the evaluation of jumper's knee, as it is cheap, noninvasive, repeatable and accurate."[5] Sonography of the knee joint may also be useful for identification of an occult effusion, demonstration of synovial thickening, and assessment of popliteal masses. It is generally considered unsuitable for evaluation of meniscal or other ligamentous injuries; MRI has become the imaging technique of choice for these injuries.

As with the patellar tendon, the superficial location of the Achilles tendon makes it an excellent candidate for ultrasound evaluation. While a complete tear is usually reliably diagnosed clinically, a partial tear can present more of a diagnostic challenge; here, ultrasound may clarify the nature and extent of the injury.

The dynamic, real-time imaging of tendon movement can be valuable for assessing both tendon integrity and function. It may also be of use for establishing the precise location of a tendon prior to draining an adjacent abscess cavity or removing a foreign body.

► TECHNIQUE AND NORMAL ULTRASOUND FINDINGS

Most formal musculoskeletal ultrasound imaging should be performed with high-frequency linear array or small parts transducers in the 7.5 to 13.0 MHz range. Sector transducers are generally not recommended for this application because the diverging beam of sector transducers can create undesirable beam scattering artifacts that leave only a small central portion of the image unaffected.[4] This drawback can be somewhat compensated for by narrowing the sector angle and using a standoff pad. When imaging very superficial structures, such as the Achilles tendon, patellar tendon, or structures within the finger, use of an acoustic standoff pad is recommended. The patellar tendon should be scanned in longitudinal and transverse planes (Figure 16–40) with the knee held in 30° of flexion to avoid this "false hypoechogenicity" artifact. The contralateral knee should always be scanned for comparison.[5] For evaluation of the Achilles tendon, the patient should be scanned prone with the foot hanging over the edge of the examining table. Use of a standoff pad is recommended, and the foot should be plantar and dorsiflexed in order to observe tendon movement (Figure 16–41).

Skeletal muscle is readily identified by its characteristic hypoechoic echotexture with echogenic internal striations and brightly echogenic fascial planes (Figure 16–42). Fiber movement is visible with muscle contraction.

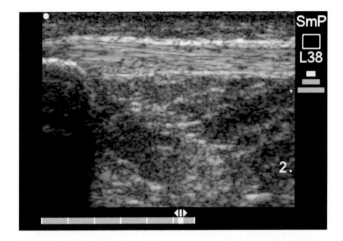

A

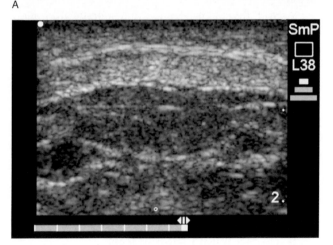

B

Figure 16–40. (A) Normal patellar tendon. Longitudinal view shows characteristic fibrillar structure. Inferior border of patella is on the left. Image obtained with 7.5 MHz linear array probe. (B) Patellar tendon. Transverse view through the mid-portion of the tendon. *(Courtesy of James Mateer, MD.)*

Tendons will appear as hyperechoic linear (in long axis) or ovoid (in short axis) structures with a fibrillar echotexture (Figure 16–43).

► COMMON AND EMERGENT ABNORMALITIES

Patellar Tendon Rupture

Partial rupture of the proximal patellar tendon is apparent sonographically as a characteristic cone-shaped hypoechoic lesion, exceeding 0.5 cm in length, located close to the origin of the patellar tendon (near the inferior border of the patella). This hypoechoic lesion represents both a focal discontinuity of the ligament at that area and an associated hematoma. An underlying tendonitis is often associated with this injury and is identified by thickening

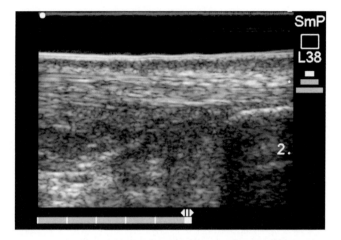

Figure 16–41. Normal Achilles tendon. Long-axis view with the calcaneal reflection and shadow on the right side of the image. Image obtained with a standoff and a 7.5 MHz linear array probe. *(Courtesy of James Mateer, MD.)*

of the tendon and overall hypoechogenicity in the area of inflammation. A complete tear will appear as a total disruption of the tendon.

Other Musculoskeletal Findings

With biceps femoris, rectus femoris, or gastrocnemius muscle tears, a "clapper in the bell sign" may be seen where the retracted, ruptured upper portion of the muscle (the clapper) is surrounded by a hypoechoic hematoma (the bell). Ganglion cysts reportedly represent 50 to 75% of all soft tissue masses of the hand; they commonly appear as a sonolucent cystic or ovoid structure adjacent to a tendon sheath or the wrist joint. Typically, an anechoic linear duct

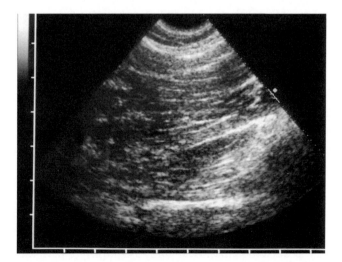

Figure 16–42. Normal hypoechoic thigh musculature with echogenic internal striations and fascial planes. The echogenic cortex of the femur in long axis is seen in the far field. (5.0 MHz sector probe.)

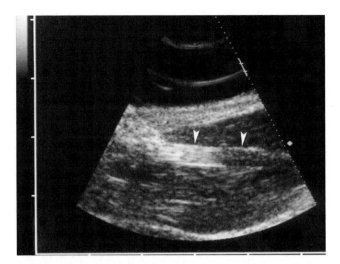

Figure 16–43. Long-axis view of the flexor pollicis longus tendon (arrowheads) demonstrating both the characteristic fibrillar echotexture of tendons and the false hypoechogenicity artifact that occurs with any obliquity of the tendon relative to the ultrasound beam. (7.5 MHz sector probe with acoustic standoff).

will be seen extending from the ganglion cyst to the tendon sheath or joint giving the structure a "tadpole" appearance.[7] Gouty tophi demonstrate posterior acoustic shadowing, much like gallstones. Inflamed bursae (see Figure 16–39) may be apparent as superficial hypoechoic fluid collections. Care should be taken to limit transducer pressure on the smaller bursae to avoid causing them to collapse and displace the fluid out of the field of view.

▶ PITFALLS

One potentially misleading artifact deserves particular mention. Fornage noted that the most significant artifact in tendon sonography is the false hypoechogenicity that results from the slightest obliquity of the ultrasound beam in relation to the tendon fibers (see Figure 16–43).[4] This optical characteristic is also referred to as anisotropy. Since areas of focal or complete tendon hypoechogenicity are sonographic clues to true tendon disruption, scanning must be performed with the transducer as parallel to the tendon being imaged as possible to avoid this significant pitfall.

EVALUATION OF BONY CORTICES AND FRACTURES

▶ CLINICAL INDICATIONS

The bright echo return from the anterior cortex of any bony structure imaged with ultrasound is usually readily identifiable. It is this bright cortical echo and the associated acoustic shadow behind it that helps identify the vertebral column in abdominal scanning, and the bony margins of the joint space in ultrasound-guided arthrocentesis. This section will focus on ultrasound applications for the evaluation of bony structures, particularly rib and sternal fractures.

In several clinical series, ultrasound has been shown to be considerably more sensitive at diagnosing rib fracture than standard chest radiography.[1-3] In one review of 50 patients with suspected rib fractures, only eight rib fractures were identified with standard chest radiographs, whereas 83 fractures were diagnosed with ultrasound. The majority of these fractures (89%) were located on the rib itself, with costochondral junction and costal cartilage fractures accounting for only 5 and 6% of the total, respectively.[1] In another series of 103 patients with suspected rib injury, rib fractures were diagnosed about twice as often with ultrasound when compared to standard chest radiography.[2] Also noted in this series was that ultrasound detected coexisting small pleural effusions that were not demonstrated on chest radiograph. The investigators stated that the ability to provide a definitive diagnosis of rib fracture and thus better estimate the duration of work disability, were important advantages that support the use of ultrasound in this setting. Of additional note in this review, no difference was found between ultrasound and radiography in the ability to diagnose a sternal fracture.

Although the sensitivity of chest radiography and ultrasound may be similar for establishing a diagnosis of a sternal fracture, the time required to reach this diagnosis can be considerably shortened using bedside ultrasound. In a study of 16 patients with radiologically documented sternal fractures, an examiner unfamiliar with the chest radiograph results was able to locate and diagnose the sternal fracture with bedside ultrasound in all 16 patients within one minute.[4]

Several additional novel applications involving ultrasound imaging of bony cortices have been proposed. In the initial assessment of the blunt trauma patient following the focused assessment with sonography for trauma (FAST) examination, a standard 3.5 MHz probe may be used for rapid evaluation of a suspected long bone fracture. Sometimes not clinically apparent during the secondary survey, a long bone fracture (such as the femur) may be rapidly diagnosed with ultrasound by sliding the transducer axially along the affected extremity. Such an extension of the FAST examination, requiring little additional time to perform, may yield timely and valuable diagnostic information.

Ultrasound has also been reported to be useful as a procedural aid when lumbar puncture must be performed in an obese patient with unidentifiable bony landmarks. Sonographic identification of the spinous processes is used to locate the midline. Ultrasound guidance can be of great clinical utility in this setting, permitting successful completion of a lumbar puncture that might otherwise require fluoroscopy to perform.

Additional bony diagnostic applications reported in the ultrasound literature include: intraoperative post-reduction confirmation of the position of zygomatic arch fracture fragments,[5] diagnosis of infant hip dislocation, diagnosis of infant posterior shoulder dislocation,[6] and diagnosis of posterior sternoclavicular dislocation.[7,8] With each of these techniques, the identification of the bright bony cortical echo on the sonogram establishes if the bony contour is normal or if the bone being imaged has a normal or abnormal relationship to adjacent structures. Some of these applications or permutations thereof (such as rapid bedside confirmation of a shoulder or jaw dislocation) may eventually play a role in the care of emergency or ambulatory patients. The use of sonography for pediatric forearm fracture reduction is discussed in Chapter 17.

▶ TECHNIQUE AND NORMAL ULTRASOUND FINDINGS

Transducers commonly used for evaluation of rib and costochondral cartilage fractures include 7.5, 9.0, and 12.0 MHz linear array transducers. Scanning should be performed parallel to the long axis of the rib at the area(s) of maximal tenderness. The superficial cortex of normal rib and costal cartilage should appear as a thin echogenic line on the sonogram (Figure 16–44).

The time-consuming nature of the examination (from 10 to 15 min/patient reported in one study) and the inability to visualize retroscapular and infraclavicular rib injuries are some of the disadvantages reported for this particular ultrasound application.[1] On the other hand, the potential utility of this rapid, bedside application for the work-up of the ambulatory patient with a suspected cough fracture or isolated rib injury is undeniable.

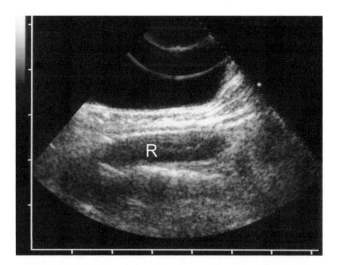

Figure 16–44. Long-axis view of a normal rib (R) with brightly echogenic rib cortex in near field, acoustic shadowing, followed by hyperechoic gliding pleura noted real-time just below the rib. (5.0 MHz sector probe with acoustic standoff.)

A 5.0 to 7.5 MHz linear array transducer is recommended for evaluation of a suspected sternal fracture. The sternum should be imaged in both long and short axis views, although the long axis view is reported to be the most fruitful (Figure 16–45). As with the evaluation for suspected rib fractures, scanning at the area of maximal tenderness can help to locate the fracture site quickly. An acoustic standoff pad may be used to bring the sternum into an optimal focal zone.

▶ COMMON AND EMERGENT ABNORMALITIES

Rib Fractures

Fractures of the rib or costochondral junction will be recognized either by a clear discontinuity of the anterior cortical echo of the rib(s), costochondral junction or costal

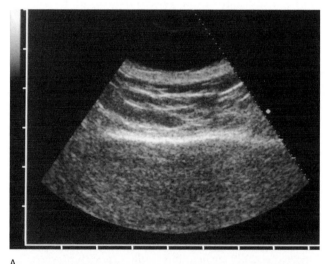

A

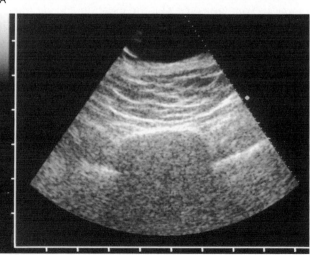

B

Figure 16–45. Normal sternum in long axis (A) at 7.5 MHz and short axis (B) at 5.0 MHz.

cartilage being scanned, or by real-time visualization of widening of the fracture line with local transducer pressure (Figure 16–46). In the latter case, a comet-tail artifact may be noted to emanate posteriorly from the mobile fracture site, a finding that has been termed the "lighthouse phenomenon."[2] An associated hypoechoic hematoma is commonly noted adjacent to the fracture site.

Sternum Fractures

Movement of the sternum fracture fragments with respiration may be observed, and a hypoechoic fracture hematoma may be noted adjacent to the bone.

▶ PITFALLS

1. *Identifying a pseudofracture.* A "pseudofracture" may be seen if the transducer is located partly over the rib and partly over an intercostal space (or over a portion of the scapula). Costal cartilage calcifications may also give rise to a "pseudofracture."
2. *Misidentifying pleura for a rib.* The brightly echogenic pleural surface (seen when scanning in an intercostal space) should not be mistaken for the cortex of the rib. Scanning the ribs in cross section first can help quickly clarify the location and depth of the anterior rib margin (with its associated posterior acoustic shadowing) relative to the deeper echo from the pleural surface (Figure 16–47). Careful observation during real-time scanning will also reveal the to-and-fro gliding movements of this brightly echogenic pleural margin (the "gliding sign"). Gliding comet-tail artifacts (arising from the visceral pleural surface

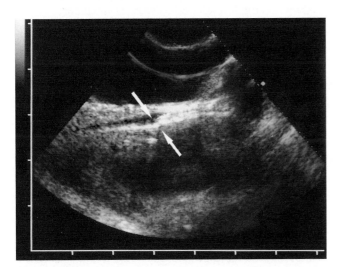

Figure 16–46. Long axis view of a rib fracture with a cortical step-off noted and a small adjacent hypoechoic fracture hematoma (arrows). (5.0 MHz sector probe with acoustic standoff.)

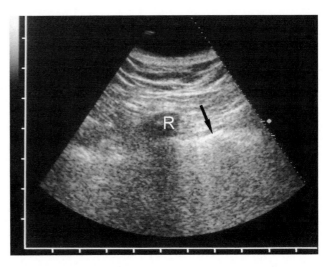

Figure 16–47. Transverse image of a normal rib (R) with posterior acoustic shadowing and hyperechoic pleura noted just below the rib (arrow). Gliding comet tail artifacts help distinguish this echo from the rib. (7.5 MHz sector probe.)

and the adjacent alveoli) are usually apparent at this interface and aid in its identification. Both these findings are reported to be absent if a pneumothorax is present.
3. *Sternum fracture pitfalls.* One pitfall is confusing the hypoechoic sternomanubrial junction with a fracture site on the long axis view. Another is mistaking the hypoechoic pectoralis muscles as a hematoma on the short axis view.[4]
4. *General pitfalls.* A potentially important pitfall of fracture sonography was illuminated in an experimental study examining the sonographic profile of fractured cadaver bones. It was observed that fractures and bony defects were not visualized when the transducer was oriented parallel to the fracture line or zone of bony impaction. For optimal imaging of a fracture and any associated bony displacement, therefore, the ultrasound transducer should be oriented axially along the bone and, ideally, perpendicular to the fracture line. Characteristically, an interruption of both the normal cortical echo reflection and its distal acoustic shadow will be visible, in addition to a dorsal band of comet-tail echoes at the fracture site (Figure 16–48).[9]

OCULAR APPLICATIONS

▶ CLINICAL INDICATIONS

In the setting of a busy emergency department, where the delays in obtaining a CT scan or ophthalmologic consultation may be significant, the ability to rapidly and

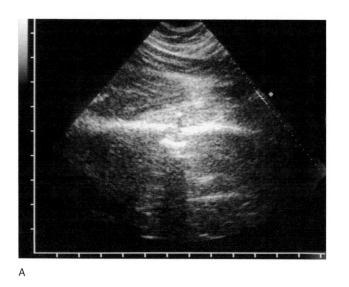

A

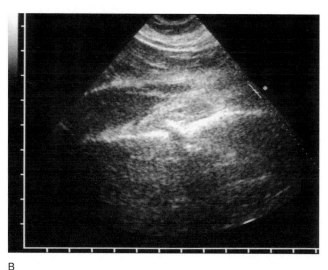

B

Figure 16–48. (A, B) Humerus fracture. The cortical defect and approximate axial location of the fracture is readily apparent on a rapid bedside-screening exam. (5.0 MHz sector probe.)

accurately evaluate an injured eye at the bedside is clearly appealing. Ultrasound evaluation of the globe can potentially expedite the diagnostic work-up of a patient with suspected traumatic globe perforation, retrobulbar hematoma, intraocular foreign body, or a posteriorly subluxed lens. Ocular ultrasound can also play an important diagnostic role when the light-conducting media of the eye are opaque due to hyphema, vitreous hemorrhage, or lens opacification where direct evaluation of the posterior segment of the eye may be impossible.[1] Finally, the diagnosis of a retinal detachment may also be facilitated with ocular ultrasound.

As many as 67% of patients with a periorbital fracture will have associated ocular trauma. Although rarely encountered, patients who develop a retrobulbar hematoma can tolerate only 90 to 120 min of ischemia prior to developing irreversible visual loss. Prompt diagnosis and immediate medical or surgical treatment (with mannitol, acetazolamide, corticosteroids, and timolol, or lateral canthotomy) is required.[2]

The use of ultrasound in the emergency department evaluation and management of two ocular emergencies, ruptured globe and vitreous hemorrhage, has been reported[3]. In both cases, the diagnosis was made rapidly at the bedside. The use of ultrasound for detecting a retrobulbar hematoma has been studied in a bovine model. A 10-mL mixture of blood/contrast material was injected into the retro-orbital space in 18 of 22 bovine orbits, with the other four serving as normal controls. Ultrasound performed by a blinded emergency physician was compared to CT as the gold standard. Ultrasound correctly identified 15 of the 18 positive studies as well as all four normal orbits. The investigators concluded that bedside ultrasound evaluation of the orbit might aid in making a rapid diagnosis of a retro-orbital hematoma.[4]

Ultrasound can also play a useful role in the detection of intraocular foreign bodies. Ultrasound biomicroscopy using ultra-high frequency transducers has been successfully used clinically for detection and localization of small anterior segment intraocular foreign bodies (average size, 516 μm).[5] In an experimental report investigating the use of ultrasound for the evaluation of intraocular foreign bodies, 117 foreign bodies of varying sizes and compositions (metal, wood, glass, plastic, and graphite) were inserted into fresh porcine eyes and subsequently evaluated with ultrasound. The overall intraocular foreign body detection rate was reported as 93%. Ultrasound was found to be a considerably more sensitive investigative tool than plain roentgenograms (the latter demonstrating only 40% sensitivity) for the imaging of intraocular foreign bodies, especially when the foreign bodies were nonmetallic.[6]

► TECHNIQUE AND NORMAL ULTRASOUND FINDINGS

Formal ocular sonography is usually performed with a dedicated high-frequency ocular transducer (usually 10.0 MHz) that has a small skin contact footprint. Ultrasound evaluation of the eye is also occasionally performed with specialized 50.0 MHz probes that permit imaging of the subsurface ocular structures in the anterior segment at the equivalent of low power microscopic resolution.[5] While probes of this type usually are not available in emergency departments, standard high-frequency (7.5 to 10.0 MHz) linear array transducers are generally adequate for emergency ocular imaging. The use of a non-dedicated scanner for ultrasound imaging of the eye has been investigated in a clinical series of 200 ocular examinations on 184 patients. Ocular imaging was performed with a 5.0 MHz probe through the closed lid with coupling gel placed on the eyelid. Of the 200 referrals, 172 were because of opaque media (110 with cataracts, 62 with vitreous hemorrhage). Abnormalities diagnosed included 70 retinal detachments, 38 vitreous hemorrhages, 14 ocular tumors, 9 foreign bodies, and 4 subluxed lenses. Overall sensitivity and specificity in the "detection and exclusion of intraocular disease" was reported as 92% and 99%, respectively.[1]

Standard water-soluble ultrasound transmission gel should be applied to the patient's closed eyelid and the globe should be scanned in both a sagittal and transverse plane. Pressure on the globe should obviously be avoided in the patient with a suspected globe perforation; fortunately, little to no pressure is required for adequate imaging, providing that a thick pool of transmission gel is utilized.

On the ocular sonogram, the normal eye appears as a circular hypoechoic structure with the lens sometimes visible anteriorly (Figure 16–49), the echo-free vitreous occupying the majority of the cystic structure, and the optic nerve visible posteriorly as a linear region of hypoechogenicity radiating away from the globe.

► COMMON AND EMERGENT ABNORMALITIES

Retrobulbar Hematoma

A retrobulbar hematoma may appear as a large hypoechoic region posterior to the globe and anterior to the bony orbit; the posterior aspect of the globe may also ex-

hibit some degree of distortion. A scleral fold signifies that the globe has been ruptured.

Intraocular Foreign Bodies

Intraocular foreign bodies will be apparent by their hyperechoic acoustic profile and either shadowing or reverberation artifacts seen in the usually echo-free vitreous.

Retinal Detachment

A retinal detachment will be apparent on the sonogram as a hyperechoic linear structure in the posterior to lateral globe; in large (complete) detachments, the retina will still remain attached to the ora serrata anteriorly and the optic disk posteriorly (Figure 16–50). High gain settings are recommended. Even with this technique, it is not always easy to differentiate between the image of a vitreous hemorrhage and that of a detached retina when using a non-dedicated scanner.[1]

► PITFALLS

Unique to ophthalmic ultrasound are exposure limit guidelines that are almost 50% below the maximum suggested for fetal imaging (50 mW/cm^2 vs. 94 mW/cm^2). Therefore, when performing emergency ultrasound of the eye, power settings should be kept low, no Doppler or color flow imaging should be employed, and lower frequency transducers (less than 5.0 MHz), with their corresponding higher power output, should not be used.

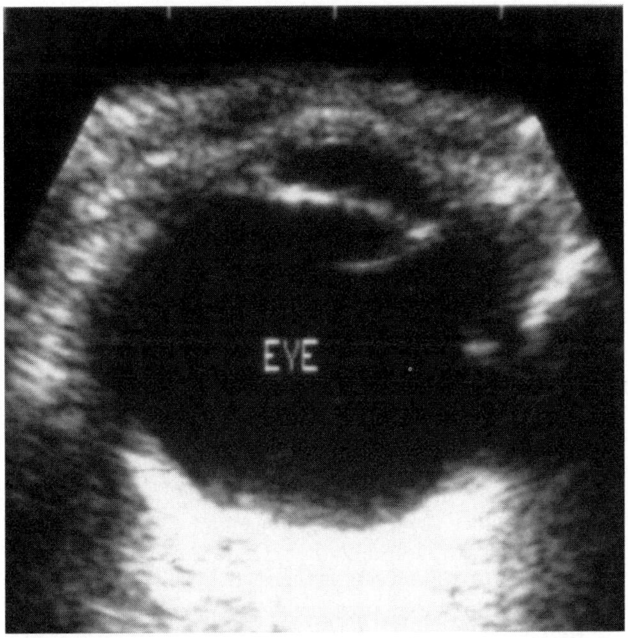

Figure 16–49. Normal eye (7.5 MHz sector probe with standoff). A portion of the posterior lens reflection is visible. *(Courtesy of James Mateer, MD.)*

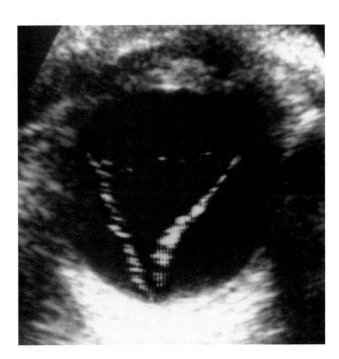

Figure 16–50. Ultrasound illustration of a complete retinal detachment. *(Courtesy of James Mateer, MD.)*

► CASE STUDIES

Case 1

Patient Presentation

A 68-year-old man presented to the emergency department at 9 p.m. with a 3-d history of worsening right lower extremity pain, redness, and swelling. He denied any fever, chills, chest pain, or dyspnea. Past medical history was significant for a "mild" hemorrhagic stroke that he suffered 1 month ago. He stated that since his stroke he had been mostly "a couch potato" except for attending physical therapy sessions 3 times per week.

On physical examination, his blood pressure was 175/90 mm Hg, heart rate 96 beats per min, respiratory rate 18 per min, and temperature 99.8°F. He was in no acute distress. His lungs were clear and his cardiovascular examination revealed regular rhythm and rate with no murmurs, gallops, or rubs. His left lower extremity was unremarkable. His right lower extremity revealed posterior edema, erythema, and tenderness to palpation.

Management Course

Based on the patient's history and physical examination, the emergency physician's differential diagnosis included deep venous thrombosis and cellulitis. The patient's pulse oximetry was 95% on room air. His white blood cell count was 11,000. Since the hospital's medical imaging department was unable to provide sonography services after 5 p.m. on weekdays, the emergency physician performed an ultrasound examination of the right lower extremity. The examination revealed diffusely increased echogenicity of the subcutaneous tissue and the appearance of hypoechoic strands that traversed the subcutaneous fat in a reticular pattern. These findings were consistent with a cellulitis. Also, there was no evidence of deep venous thrombosis on the ultrasound examination. Blood cultures were obtained, the patient was administered IV antibiotics, and admitted into the hospital.

Commentary

Case 1 was an example of how emergency ultrasound could assist with the expeditious and safe management and disposition of a patient in the emergency department. Based on this patient's recent history of a hemorrhagic stroke, the emergency physician obviously did not want to empirically administer heparin for a presumed deep venous thrombosis. The bedside ultrasound examination rapidly helped him make the correct diagnosis and initiate the proper therapy.

Case 2

Patient Presentation

A 43-year-old man presented to the emergency department with a 2-week history of progressively worsening abdominal pain, fullness, and distention. This was associated with low grade fever, rigor, hematemesis, and melena. The patient had a significant history of alcohol abuse but denied other medical problems.

On physical examination, his blood pressure was 102/54 mm Hg, heart rate 124 beats per min, respiratory rate 20 per min, and temperature 101°F. He was toxic in appearance. His sclerae were icteric. His chest examination was unremarkable except for tachycardia. Abdominal examination revealed a morbidly obese man with moderate diffuse tenderness throughout. He demonstrated some moderate guarding. His abdomen appeared distended but a fluid wave was difficult to appreciate. His rectal examination had guaiac-positive melena.

Management Course

The emergency physician initiated the standard work-up for an acute gastrointestinal (GI) bleed. The patient's hematocrit was 28 and his INR was 3.5. The emergency physician also was concerned that the patient might have spontaneous bacterial peritonitis. Her ultrasound examination revealed a profuse amount of free intraperitoneal fluid that she presumed to be ascites. After clearly identifying a large amount of fluid in the left lower quadrant of the abdomen, she expeditiously performed a paracentesis and aspirated 1 L of ascitic fluid on the first pass. Laboratory analysis of the ascitic fluid was consistent with spontaneous bacterial peritonitis and the patient was started on IV antibiotic therapy prior to admission into the hospital.

Commentary

Case 2 was an example of a patient with undiagnosed alcoholic liver disease and ascites presenting with a GI bleed, coagulopathy, and possible spontaneous bacterial peritonitis. This case demonstrated how the clinician's ultrasound examination was able to assist her with making the diagnosis of ascites in this clinical setting. It also assisted her with locating a safe site to perform the invasive procedure in a patient with obesity and a coagulopathy.

REFERENCES

Soft Tissue Infections

1. VanSonnenberg E, Wittich GR, Casola G, et al. Sonography of thigh abscess: detection, diagnosis and drainage. AJR 1987;149:769–772.
2. Yiengpruksawan A, Ganepola AP, Freeman HP, et al. Acute soft tissue infection in intravenous drug abusers: its differential diagnosis by ultrasonography. J Nat Med Assoc 1986;78:1193–1196.
3. Sandler MA, Alpern MB, Madrazo BL, et al. Inflammatory lesions of the groin: ultrasonic evaluation. Radiology 1984;151:747–750.
4. Yeh H, Rabinowitz JG. Ultrasonography of the extremities and pelvic girdle and correlation with computed tomography. Radiology 1982;143:519–525.

5. Gitschlag KF, Sandler MA, Madrazo BL, et al. Disease in the femoral triangle: sonographic appearance. AJR 1982; 39:515–519.

6. Peleg M, Heyman Z, Ardekian L, et al. The use of ultrasonography as a diagnostic tool for superficial fascial space infections. J Oral Maxillofacial Surg 1988;56:1129–1131.

7. Page-Wills C, Simon BC, Christ D, et al. Utility of ultrasound on emergency department management of suspected cutaneous abscess. Acad Emerg Med 2000;7:493.

8. Spires JR, Owens JJ, Woodsen GE, et al. Treatment of peritonsillar abscess: a prospective study of aspiration versus incision and drainage. Arch Otolar Head Neck Surg 1987;113:984–986.

9. Scott PMJ, Loftuss WK, Kew J, et al. Diagnosis of peritonsillar infections: a prospective study of ultrasound, computerized tomography and clinical diagnosis. J Laryng Otol 1999;113:229–232.

10. Manthey DE, Harrison BP. Otolaryngologic procedures. In: Roberts JR, Hedges JR, eds. Clinical procedures in emergency medicine, 3rd ed. Philadelphia: W.B. Saunders, 1998:1124.

11. Haegstrom A, Gustafsson O, Engquist S. Intraoral ultrasonography in the diagnosis of peritonsillar abscess. Otolaryngol Head Neck Surg 1993;108:243–247.

12. Strong EB, Woodward PJ, Johnson LP. Intraoral ultrasound evaluation of peritonsillar abscess. Laryngoscope 1995;105: 779–782.

13. O'Brien E. Intraoral sonography of peritonsillar abscesses: feasibility and sonographic appearance. Ann Emerg Med 1999;34:26.

14. Kew J, Loftus WK, Scott PMJ, et al. Peritonsillar abscess appearance on intra-oral ultrasonography. Clin Radiol 1998;53:143–146.

15. Bureau NJ, Chhem RK, Cardinal E. Musculoskeletal infections: ultrasound manifestations. Radiographics 1999;19: 1585–1592.

16. Craig JG. Infection: ultrasound-guided procedures. Radiol Clin North Am 1999;37:669–678.

17. Loyer EM, Dubrow RA, David CL, et al. Imaging of superficial soft-tissue infections: sonographic findings in cases of cellulitis and abscess. AJR 1996;166:149–152.

18. Loyer EM, Kaur H, David CL, et al. Importance of dynamic assessment of soft tissues in the sonographic diagnosis of echogenic superficial abscesses. J Ultrasound Med 1995;14:669–671.

19. Lille ST, Sato TT, Engrave LH, et al. Necrotizing soft tissue infections: obstacles in diagnosis. J Am Coll Surg 1996;182:7–11.

20. Chao H, Kong M, Lin T. Diagnosis of necrotizing fasciitis in children. J Ultrasound Med 1999;18:277–281.

Foreign Body Identification, Localization, and Removal

1. Rockett MS, Gentile SC, Gudas CJ, et al. The use of ultrasonography for the detection of retained wooden foreign bodies in the foot. J Foot Ankle Surg 1995;34: 478–484.

2. Orlinsky M, Knittel P, Feit T, et al. The comparative accuracy of radiolucent foreign body detection using ultrasonography. Am J Emerg Med 2000;18:401–403.

3. Gilbert FJ, Campbell RSD, Bayliss AP. The role of ultrasound in the detection of non-radiopaque foreign bodies. Clin Radiol 1990;41:109–112.

4. Fornage BD, Schernberg FL. Sonographic diagnosis of foreign bodies of the distal extremities. AJR 1986;147:567–569.

5. Jacobson JA, Powell A, Craig JG, et al. Wooden foreign bodies in soft tissue: detection at US. Radiology 1998; 201:45–48.

6. Crawford R, Matheson AB. Clinical value of ultrasonography in the detection and removal of radiolucent foreign bodies. Injury 1989;20:341–343.

7. Schlager D. The use of ultrasound in the emergency department. Emerg Med Clin North Am 1997;15:895–912.

8. Schlager D, Sanders AB, Wiggins D, et al. Ultrasound for the detection of foreign bodies. Ann Emerg Med 2000; 20:189–191.

9. Banerjee B, Das RK. Sonographic detection of foreign bodies of the extremities. Br J Radiol 1991;64:107–112.

10. Hill R, Conron R, Greissinger P, et al. Ultrasound for the detection of foreign bodies in human tissue. Ann Emerg Med 1997;29:353–356.

11. Ginsburg MJ, Ellis GL, Flom LL, et al. Detection of soft-tissue foreign bodies by plain radiography, xerography, computed tomography, and ultrasonography. Ann Emerg Med 1990;19:6:701–703.

12. Manthey D, Storrow AB, Milbourn JM, et al. Ultrasound versus radiography in the detection of soft-tissue foreign bodies. Ann Emerg Med 1996;28:7–9.

13. Turner J, Wilde CH, Hughes KC, et al. Ultrasound-guided retrieval of small foreign objects in subcutaneous tissue. Ann Emerg Med 1997;29:731–734.

14. Bray PW, Mahoney JL, Campbell JP, et al. Sensitivity and specificity of ultrasound in the diagnosis of foreign bodies in the hand. J Hand Surg 1995;20:661–666.

15. Bonatz E, Robbin ML, Weingold MA. Ultrasound for the diagnosis of retained splinters in the soft tissue of the hand. Am J Orthop 1998;27:445–459.

16. Shiels II WE, Babcock DS, Wilson JL, et al. Localization and guided removal of soft-tissue foreign bodies with sonography. AJR 1990;155:1277–1281.

17. Teisen HG, Torfing KF, Skjodt T. Sonographische Feinlokalisation von Fremdkörpern. Ultraschall 1988;9: 135–137.

Body Fluid Localization and Aspiration

Thoracentesis

1. Quershi N, Momin ZA, Brandstetter RD. Thoracentesis in clinical practice. Heart Lung 1994;23;376–383.

2. Kohan JM, Poe RH, Israel RH, et al. Value of chest ultrasonography versus decubitus roentgenography for thoracentesis. Am Rev Respir Dis 1986;133:1124–1136.

3. O'Moore PV, Mueller PR, Simeone JF, et al. Sonographic guidance in diagnostic and therapeutic interventions in the pleural space. AJR 1987;149:1–5.

4. Grogan DR, Irwin RS, Channick R, et al. Complications associated with thoracentesis. Arch Intern Med 1990;150:873–877.

5. Weingart JP, Guico RR, Nemcek AA, et al. Ultrasound findings following failed, clinically directed thoracenteses. J Clin Ultrasound 1994;22:419–426.

6. Lichtenstein D, Hulot JS, Rabiller A, et al. Feasibility and safety of ultrasound-aided thoracentesis in mechanically ventilated patients. Intensive Care Med 1999;25: 955–958.
7. Ross DS. Thoracentesis. In: Roberts JR, Hedges JR, eds. Clinical procedures in emergency medicine, 3rd ed. Philadelphia: W.B. Saunders, 1998:130–147.

Paracentesis

1. Runyan BA. Care of patients with ascites. N Engl J Med 1994;330: 337–342.
2. Sullivan MJ, Davis C. Outpatient treatment of ascites with large-volume paracentesis. Am J Emerg Med 1994;12:509–510.
3. Williams JW, Simel DL. Does this patient have ascites? How to divine fluid in the abdomen. JAMA 1992;267: 2645–2648.
4. Goldberg BB, Goodman GA, Clearfield HR. Evaluation of ascites by ultrasound. Radiology 1970;96:15–22.
5. Runyon BA. Paracentesis of ascitic fluid. A safe procedure. Arch Intern Med 1986;146:2259–2261.
6. Lipsky MS, Sternback MR. Evaluation and initial management of patients with ascites. Am Fam Phys 1996;54:1327–1333.
7. Bard C, Lafortune M, Breton G. Ascites: ultrasound guidance or blind paracentesis? Can Med Assoc J 1986;135: 209–210.

Arthrocentesis

1. Benjamin GC. Arthrocentesis. In: Roberts JR, Hedges JR, eds. Clinical procedures in emergency medicine, 3rd ed. Philadelphia: W.B. Saunders, 1998:919–932.
2. Mayekawa DS, Ralls PW, Kerr RM, et al. Sonographically guided arthrocentesis of the hip. J Ultrasound Med 1989;8:665–667.
3. Smith SW. Emergency physician-performed ultrasonography-guided hip arthrocentesis. Acad Emerg Med 1999;6:84–86.
4. Roy S, Dewitz A, Paul I. Ultrasound-assisted ankle arthrocentesis. Am J Emerg Med1999;17:300–301.
5. Harcke HT. Hip in infants and children. Clin Diagn Ultrasound 1995;30:179–199.
6. Tran TK, Vogel H. Der suprapatellare Raum des Kniegelenkes im Sonogram. Roentgen-Bl 1988;41:31–35.
7. Valley VT, Stahmer SA. Targeted musculoarticular sonography in the detection of joint effusions. Acad Emerg Med 2001;8:361–367.

Musculoskeletal Applications

1. Taboury J. Etude echographique des tendons des muscles rotateurs de l'epaule. Ann. Radiologie 1995;38:275–279.
2. Vick CW, Bell SA. Rotator cuff tears: diagnosis with sonography. AJR 1990;154:121–123.
3. Farin P, Jaroma H. Sonographic Detection of tears of the anterior portion of the rotator cuff (subscapularis tendon tears). J Ultrasound Med 1996;16:221–225.
4. Fornage BD. Musculoskeletal evaluation. In: Mittelstaedt CA, ed. General ultrasound. New York: Churchill Livingstone, 1992:157.

5. Kalebo, P, Sward, L. Karlsson J, et al. Ultrasonography in the detection of partial patellar ligament ruptures (jumper's knee). Skeletal Radiol 1991;20:285–289.
6. Hoglund M, Tordai P, Engkvist O. Ultrasonography for the diagnosis of soft tissue conditions in the hand. Scand J Plast Reconstr Hand Surg 1991;25:225–231.
7. Hashimoto BE, Kramer DJ, Wiitala L. Applications of musculoskeletal sonography. J Clin Ultrasound 1999;27:293–318.

Evaluation of Bony Cortices and Fractures

1. Griffith JF, Rainer TH, Ching ASC, et al. Sonography compared with radiography in revealing acute rib fracture. AJR 1999;173:1603–1609.
2. Bitschnau R, Gehmacher O, Kopf A, et al. Ultraschalldiagnostik von Rippen-und Sternumfrakturen. Ultraschall Med 1997;18:158–161.
3. Wischhofer E, Fenkl R, Blum R. Sonographischer Nachweis von Rippenfrakturen zur Sicherung der Frakturdiagnostik. Unfallchirurg 1995;98:296–300.
4. Fenkl R, Garrel T, Knaepler H. Notfalldiagnostik der Sternumfraktur mit Ultraschall. Unfallchirurg 1992;95:375–379.
5. Akizuki H, Yoshida H, Michi K. Ultrasonographic evaluation during reduction of zygomatic arch fractures. J Cranio-Maxillo-Facial Surg 1990;18:263–266.
6. Hunter JD, Franklin K, Hughes PM. The ultrasound diagnosis of posterior shoulder dislocation associated with Erb's palsy. Pediatr Radiol 1998;28:510–511.
7. Benson LS, Donaldson JS, Carrol NC. Use of ultrasound in management of posterior sternoclavicular dislocation. J Ultrasound Med 1991;10:115–118.
8. Pollock RC, Bankes MJK, Emery RJH. Diagnosis of retrosternal dislocation of the clavicle with ultrasound. Injury 1996;27:670–671.
9. Grechenig W, Clement HG, Fellinger M, Seggl W. Scope and limitations of ultrasonography in the documentation of fractures–an experimental study. Arch Orthop Trauma Surg 1998;117:368–371.

Ocular Applications

1. Fielding JA. Ultrasound imaging of the eye through the closed lid using a non-dedicated scanner. Clin Radiol 1987;38:131–135.
2. Rosdeutscher JD, Stadelmann WK. Diagnosis and treatment of retrobulbar hematoma resulting from blunt periorbital trauma. Ann Plastic Surg 1998;41:618–622.
3. Blaivas M. Bedside emergency department ultrasonography in the evaluation of ocular pathology. Acad Emerg Med 2000;7:947–950.
4. Estevez A, Deutch J, Sturmann K, et al. Ultrasonographic evaluation of retrobulbar hematoma in bovine orbits. Ann Emerg Med 2000;36:21.
5. Barash D, Goldenberg-Cohen, Tzadok D, et al. Ultrasound biomicroscopic detection of anterior ocular segment foreign body after trauma. Am J Opthalmol 1988;126:197–202.
6. Bryden, FM, Pyott AA, Bailey M, et al. Real time ultrasound assessment of intraocular foreign bodies. Eye 1990;4:727–731.

CHAPTER 17

Pediatric Applications

Daniel D. Price and Michael A. Peterson

Ultrasonography is an especially appealing imaging modality in children. Examinations can be performed at the bedside, at times with the child being held by a parent. The diagnostic test is noninvasive, involves no contrast or ionizing radiation, and is considered virtually risk free. Also, pediatric patients generally have less body fat and thinner abdominal walls, which enhances the ultrasound examination.

PEDIATRIC TRAUMA

Trauma remains the most common cause of morbidity and mortality in children. Traumatic injuries result in hospital admission for approximately 600,000 children each year.[1] In the pediatric age group, blunt trauma is more prevalent than penetrating injuries. Twenty to 30% of pediatric trauma cases involve the abdomen.[1] Timely, accurate, and cost-effective evaluation of children suffering from blunt abdominal trauma remains a challenge for trauma physicians.

The history and physical examination form the foundation of patient evaluation; however, they may be difficult or impossible to obtain in children who have altered mental status, central nervous system trauma, or distracting injuries. In one study of children with blunt abdominal trauma, an initial physical examination was considered reliable in only 41% of cases.[2] The physical examination has been reported to be misleading in up to 45% of injured children.[3-4] Although the physical examination is an important piece in the diagnostic puzzle, the clinician must resort to other modalities to adequately evaluate and treat the pediatric blunt abdominal trauma patient.

► CLINICAL CONSIDERATIONS

In the 1960s, diagnostic peritoneal lavage became a popular procedure for detecting blood or bowel contents in the peritoneal cavity. It can be performed at the bedside and is relatively rapid and safe, with a complication rate of approximately 1%.[5-7] Studies of diagnostic peritoneal lavage in children have demonstrated a high sensitivity in detecting injury (96%), but have noted the findings to be too nonspecific. Positive diagnostic peritoneal lavage studies do not provide information on which organ is injured or how severely, and have led to nontherapeutic laparotomy rates between 13 and 19%.[8-9] Since these studies were published, the trend toward nonoperative management of pediatric abdominal injuries has advanced significantly.[10-23] In the 1980s, the direction shifted away from the use of diagnostic peritoneal lavage and toward the use of abdominal computed tomography (CT).

CT is now the most commonly used modality in evaluating pediatric abdominal injuries.[24-33] The primary advantage of CT is that it identifies and characterizes most abdominal injuries and provides important information to guide the management of the patient. CT scanning is noninvasive and can evaluate intraperitoneal and retroperitoneal structures. The primary disadvantage of CT is that the test requires the transport of the patient to the medical imaging department; consequently, its use is inadvisable in the hemodynamically unstable patient.[34] Additionally, CT often requires sedation of pediatric patients. CT involves the administration of intravenous (IV) and oral contrast. This results in filling the stomach in a patient already at risk for vomiting, and possibly necessitates insertion of a nasogastric tube. CT scans also expose patients to significant doses of ionizing radiation. CT interpretation may be more difficult in children because they lack the adipose tissue that helps differentiate anatomic planes. Furthermore, CT can be an expensive screening tool.[35] These considerations have led some trauma surgeons to advocate for the use of ultrasound in evaluating pediatric blunt abdominal trauma patients.[36–37]

The focused assessment with sonography for trauma (FAST) examination is a noninvasive, diagnostic tool for detecting hemoperitoneum, hemopericardium, and hemothorax.[38] The examination can be performed at the bedside in 3 min or less[39–41] and is easily repeatable. Use of the FAST examination has been well established in adults (see Chapter 4). Although the examination is less sensitive than CT for identifying solid organ injuries, the immediate identification of free fluid provides a useful operative triage tool.[42–43]

Unlike adults, over one-third of pediatric solid organ injuries are not associated with free intraperitoneal fluid[47,49] and may not be identified by ultrasonography. When solid organ injuries are identified, they are more commonly managed nonoperatively. However, the diagnosis of solid organ injuries is important in determining the need for hospitalization, duration of bed rest, resumption of activity, and need for follow-up. Additionally, one study demonstrated that results of CT scanning led to changes in management in 44% of patients.[48]

The sensitivity of the FAST examination in detecting intraperitoneal fluid and solid organ injury is difficult to determine (Table 17–1). Studies supporting the use of ultrasound have demonstrated sensitivities ranging from 71 to 100%.[37,49–52,57,59,73–74] Some of these studies evaluated only for free fluid, and they often lacked a gold standard by which to compare ultrasound results. Other

studies have demonstrated sensitivities ranging from 31 to 65%,[2,53–56] but they often focused on detection of all injures and included injuries one would not expect to be detected by ultrasound, such as pneumoperitoneum.[53] When investigators focused on hypotensive patients, ultrasound was found to be very sensitive in identifying free intraperitoneal fluid.[53,57] Investigators in studies showing low sensitivity for detecting injury have also endorsed a potential role for ultrasound in hemodynamically unstable pediatric blunt trauma patients.[55]

► CLINICAL INDICATIONS

A limited bedside ultrasound examination is indicated in children with:

- Significant blunt abdominal or thoracic trauma
- Significant penetrating abdominal or thoracic trauma

An algorithm developed in Denver is useful for delineating an appropriate role for the FAST examination in the emergency evaluation of pediatric blunt trauma patients (Figure 17–1).[49] Viewing the FAST examination as a triage tool is the key to understanding the role of ultrasound in the evaluation of children. The FAST examination helps determine which patients should go directly to the operating suite, which are less likely to decompensate during CT scanning, and which stable patients can be observed without CT scanning. Since the FAST examination lacks sensitivity for identifying specific solid organ injuries, the FAST examination cannot replace CT scanning for stable patients with clinical findings suggestive of intraabdominal injury.

TABLE 17–1. STUDIES OF ULTRASOUND IN PEDIATRIC TRAUMA

Year	Lead Investigator	Patients	Sonographer	Sensitivity (%)
2001	Holmes	224	Rad tech	82
2000	Corbett	47	EM res/faculty	75
2000	Benya	51	Rad tech/faculty	59
2000	Coley	107	Rad faculty	55
1999	Mutabagani	46	Rad faculty	44
1999	Patel	94	Rad res	45
1998	Partrick	230	Surg/EM res	71
1998	Thourani	192	Surg res/faculty	80
1997	Richardson	26	Rad faculty	86
1997	Akgur	217	Rad res/faculty	100
1997	Krupnick	32	Rad tech	80
1996	Katz	121	Rad	91
1993	Luks	81	Rad res/faculty	89
1993	Akgur	109	Rad res	95
1987	Filiatrault	170	Rad	80

EM = emergency medicine, Rad = radiology, res = resident, surg = surgery, tech = technologist.

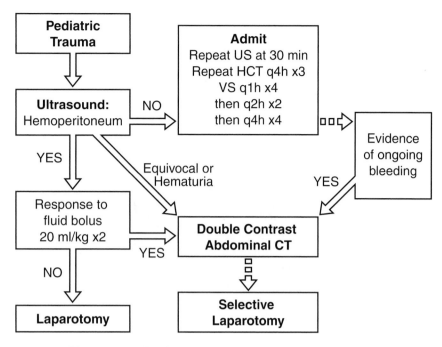

Figure 17–1. Pediatric trauma management algorithm.

The FAST examination should be performed in all patients with significant blunt abdominal trauma as part of the secondary survey. If free intraperitoneal fluid is identified, and the patient remains hypotensive after a 20-mL/kg bolus of crystalloid, the decision to perform exploratory laparotomy should be made. If the patient's vital signs respond to the fluid bolus, double contrast abdominal CT scanning can be performed and is used to guide selective laparotomy. Patients who are hemodynamically stable and have a negative FAST examination should undergo abdominal CT scanning if they demonstrate peritoneal signs, abdominal distention, seat belt abrasion, hematuria, or persistent tachycardia. Patients who have sustained a significant mechanism of trauma but who have normal vital signs, a normal abdominal examination, and a negative FAST examination should be admitted for observation. These patients should receive serial abdominal examinations and FAST examinations.

The FAST examination may also be applied in cases of penetrating trauma. In one study, six children who sustained penetrating trauma were evaluated with a FAST examination, and then followed by CT or laparotomy as part of a larger study.[59] Ultrasound identified one of two cases of intraperitoneal fluid and confirmed negative results in four cases. The missed injury involved a small hemoperitoneum noted on laparotomy in a 17-year-old gunshot wound victim who required a partial small bowel resection. Although virtually all patients who sustain a gunshot wound to the abdomen will be explored, blood in the abdomen, thorax, or around the heart may be detected by ultrasound and help guide the surgeon.

▶ ANATOMIC CONSIDERATIONS

The FAST examination was designed to assess the three primary dependent areas of the peritoneal cavity in the supine trauma patient: right upper quadrant, left upper quadrant, and pelvis. The location of the fluid depends primarily upon the source of the bleeding but may be affected by the position of the patient. Some investigators refer to seven dependent spaces in the abdomen.[60] For the purpose of understanding the anatomy as it relates to the FAST examination, the abdomen should be thought of being divided into quadrants by the mesentery of the transverse colon horizontally and by the spine vertically (Figure 17–2).

In the right upper quadrant, Morison's pouch is the potential space between the liver and the right kidney and represents the most dependent supramesocolic area. Blood from a liver laceration will accumulate in this area; blood from a splenic injury may also spill over the lumbar spine into Morison's pouch. Blood from an inframesocolic injury can spread over the sacral promontory into Morison's pouch as well via the right paracolic gutter. Since most major blunt abdominal injuries involve the liver and spleen, the right upper quadrant view of Morison's pouch is regarded as the most important of the four views in the FAST examination.[60] Alone, it has been found to be 51 to 82% sensitive in detecting free fluid.[61–63]

Blood from a splenic injury will accumulate first in the subphrenic space. It may then spread to the potential space between the spleen and kidney (splenorenal recess), which is analogous to Morison's pouch. Blood from this

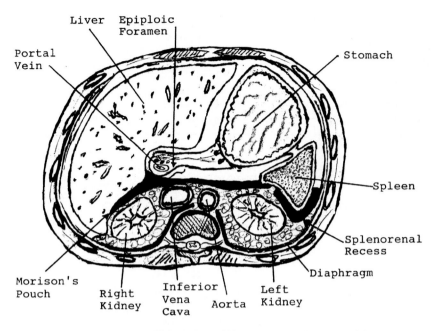

Figure 17–2. Transverse illustration of the upper abdomen, which demonstrates the dependent compartments where free intraperitoneal fluid may collect. *(Courtesy of Mark E. Hoffmann, MD.)*

area can flow into Morison's pouch, and it will preferentially reach the pelvis by spilling down the right paracolic gutter because the left upper quadrant is separated from the left paracolic gutter by the phrenicocolic ligament.[64]

Blood from inframesocolic injuries will accumulate first in the rectovesicular pouch in boys and the retrouterine pouch of Douglas in girls. These areas are the most dependent portions of the peritoneal cavity.[64] One study found an isolated pelvic view to be 68% sensitive in detecting free intraperitoneal fluid.[61]

▶ TECHNIQUE AND NORMAL ULTRASOUND FINDINGS

The classic FAST examination consists of right and left upper quadrant, suprapubic, and subxiphoid views (Figure 17–3). Time permitting, views of the hemidiaphragms and caudal thorax can be examined for blood. A 3.5 MHz transducer can be used in both children and adults. Some researchers recommend using a 5.0 MHz (or even 7.5 MHz) transducer for finer resolution.[37,55] Because children tend to have less body fat and a thinner abdominal wall, the focus may be appropriate for a 5.0 MHz transducer, which will provide a higher quality image. The FAST examination should be performed with the patient supine, which is how the patient is transported on a long backboard after blunt trauma. By convention, the index marker on the transducer should be directed cephalad or to the patient's right. The transducer may be moved up or down one or more rib spaces to optimize the view. Though not imperative, a partially darkened room will aid the sonologist's ability to discern subtler findings.

Hemoperitoneum results from splenic or hepatic injuries 74% of the time in pediatric blunt trauma.[65] The right upper quadrant view can be performed first in pediatric blunt trauma patients because it will be the most sensitive in detecting free fluid. With the index marker cephalad, the transducer should be placed in a coronal

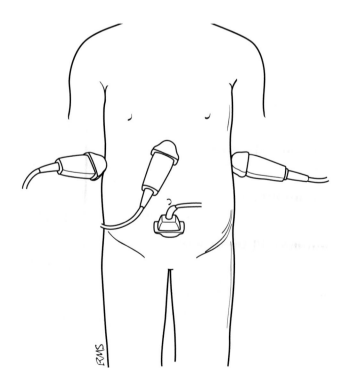

Figure 17–3. FAST exam transducer placement.

plane in the mid to anterior axillary line at the tenth inter-costal space or below (see Figure 17–3). The kidney lies retroperitoneal, so the transducer should be directed dorsally to maximize the view of the liver to right kidney interface (Figure 17–4). The transducer can be rotated 45° counterclockwise to fit between the ribs and mini-mize shadowing. Sliding the transducer cephalad should bring the lower thorax into view where blood may ap-pear on the monitor as a dark area cephalad to the bright, hyperechoic hemidiaphragm.

The left upper quadrant view is generally more diffi-cult to obtain. The goal is to examine the potential space between the spleen and the diaphragm and the spleno-renal recess where blood may accumulate (Figure 17–5). With the index marker cephalad, the transducer should be placed in the posterior axillary line in the coronal plane at the ninth intercostal space or below (see Figure 17–3). The transducer may be rotated 45° clockwise to minimize rib shadows. The diaphragm and lower thorax can be in-spected for intrathoracic blood, as described previously.

The solid organs, liver, spleen, and kidneys, should be quickly examined by rotating the transducer in a fan-ning motion to image through the entire organ. Although the goal of the FAST examination is to detect free in-traperitoneal fluid, evidence of organ injury is helpful when identified.

An attempt should be made to obtain the suprapubic view prior to insertion of a Foley catheter. Urine in the bladder provides an important acoustic window through which to view the pelvic anatomy more accurately. The transducer should be placed just superior to the symph-ysis pubis and in the midline sagittal plane with the index marker cephalad, or in the transverse plane with the index marker to the patient's right (see Figure 17–3). Urine ap-pears dark and is well circumscribed by the bladder wall (Figure 17–6). The uterus in girls and prostate in boys can be seen dorsal to the bladder. The transition in tissue den-

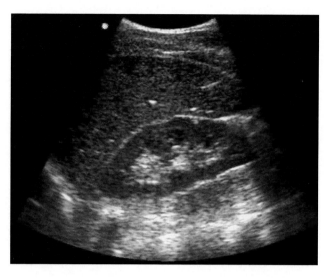

Figure 17–5. Ultrasound: normal LUQ view.

sities between urine in the bladder and the surrounding soft tissue can produce bright echoes, so reducing the far gain will enhance subtle soft tissue details and help avoid missing free fluid in this area.

The subxiphoid view of the heart completes the clas-sic four-view FAST examination. Some sonologists rec-ommend obtaining this view first. It certainly should be the initial view obtained in penetrating trauma patients in whom cardiac tamponade is suspected. The transducer should be placed in the coronal plane adjacent and de-pressed below the xiphoid process with the index marker to the patient's right. It should be directed toward the left shoulder with as flat an angle as possible (relative to the abdominal skin) using the liver as an acoustic window. This provides a four-chamber view of the heart surrounded by a hyperechoic pericardium (Figure 17–7). Pericardial fluid will appear as a dark stripe between the bright peri-cardium and the contracting, gray myocardium.

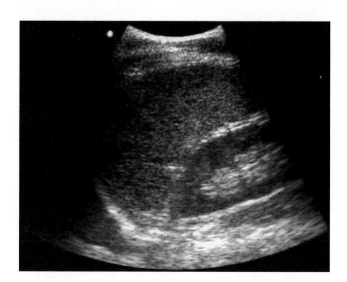

Figure 17–4. Ultrasound: normal RUQ view.

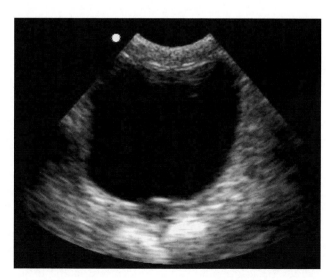

Figure 17–6. Ultrasound: normal suprapubic view.

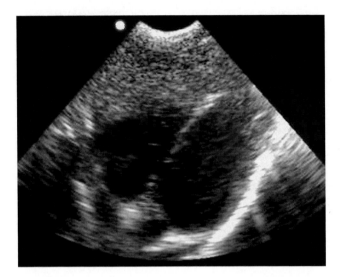

Figure 17–7. Ultrasound: normal subxiphoid view. The right ventricle is closest to the probe and left ventricle is below with a bright posterior pericardial reflection. Only a portion of the posterior atria on are seen in this example.

Some sonologists' include views of the left and right paracolic gutters in their FAST examinations. These views can be obtained by placing the transducer, with index marker pointing cephalad, in the coronal plane below the 11th rib in the mid to posterior axillary line. Transverse views can also be obtained.

The amount of fluid that can be reliably detected in children has not been studied. In adults, 400 mL is a fair estimate.[66-67] One study suggests that placing the patient in Trendelenburg or decubitus positions allows sonographers to detect intraperitoneal fluid with only two-thirds of the amount of fluid required in the supine position.[68] The reverse Trendelenburg position may help with identification of pleural or pelvic free fluid.

▶ COMMON AND EMERGENT ABNORMALITIES

Hemoperitoneum

An anechoic stripe of blood separates the liver from the right kidney in Morison's pouch (Figure 17–8). This may extend to separate the liver from the overlying abdominal wall if large amounts of blood are present (Figure 17–9). Similarly, an anechoic stripe of blood may separate the spleen from the left kidney; however, blood more often accumulates between the spleen and diaphragm. Blood in the pelvic region may be seen floating above and outlining the loops of bowel (Figure 17–10) or it may assume a dependent position in the pelvis. On paracolic gutter views, free fluid appears as an anechoic pocket of fluid below the lower pole of the kidney and lateral to the psoas muscle. Also, free fluid in the pararenal retroperi-

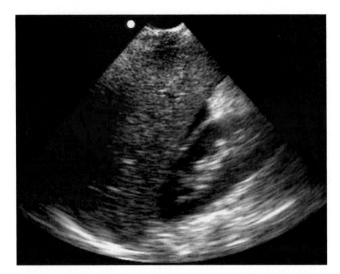

Figure 17–8. Ultrasound: RUQ hemoperitoneum. A thin echolucent stripe of fluid is seen in Morison's pouch.

toneum can be identified as an echolucent stripe between the psoas muscle and medial renal border in this view.

Hemopericardium

Unclotted blood in the pericardial space will appear as an anechoic stripe lying between the two brightly, echogenic layers of the pericardium (Figure 17–11). Clotted blood is more complex and gray, but can generally be distinguished from the contracting myocardium and the thin, white layers of the pericardium.

Hemothorax

Blood in the chest appears as an anechoic area cephalad to the bright echogenic hemidiaphragm (Figure 17–12).

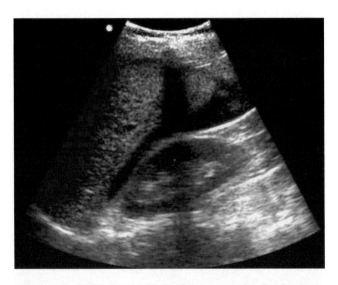

Figure 17–9. Ultrasound: RUQ hemoperitoneum. A large fluid collection is noted that extends inferior to the liver edge. A rib shadow is projecting down the center of the image.

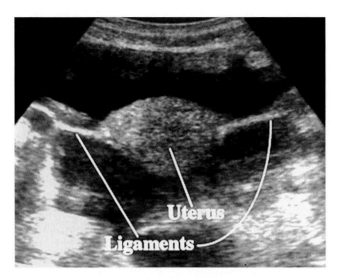

Figure 17–10. Ultrasound: suprapubic transverse view reveals hemoperitoneum. The broad ligaments are usually not seen unless outlined with fluid.

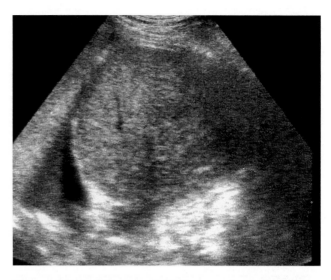

Figure 17–12. Ultrasound: RUQ view. A small pleural fluid collection is noted superior to the diaphragm. Lung artifact is present on the left side of the image.

► COMMON VARIANTS AND SELECTED ABNORMALITIES

Certain aspects of normal anatomy can be easily mistaken for positive findings. In the upper quadrant views, dark rib shadows must not be interpreted as anechoic blood. Since all fluid appears black (anechoic) on ultrasound, bile in the gallbladder and blood in the inferior vena cava can be erroneously interpreted as intraperitoneal free fluid. In each of the abdominal views, and especially in the suprapubic view, fluid-filled loops of bowel can be mistaken for free intraperitoneal fluid.[56] If viewed carefully, peristaltic movements often help to identify the bowel. Perinephric adipose tissue may be

hypoechoic relative to surrounding structures and can be mistaken for free fluid or clotted blood. Comparison with the area around the other kidney may help distinguish this; also, perinephric fat does not move with respirations and is more homogenous than clotted blood.

A subcapsular hematoma may be visible between the bright reflection of the splenic capsule and the homogenous parenchyma, which may be disrupted by injury. Blood is often clotted, appearing more echogenic, but may be distinguished from the splenic parenchyma (Figure 17–13). Intraparenchymal blood is often isoechoic with the splenic parenchyma on initial evaluation (Figure 17–14).[69] Over time, a hematoma will become primarily hypoechoic.

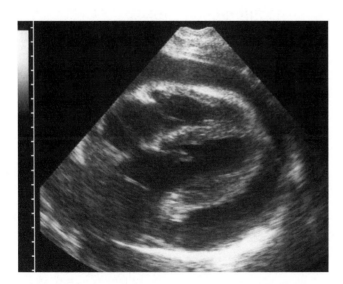

Figure 17–11. Ultrasound: subxiphoid view demonstrates a large fluid collection within the pericardium. *(Courtesy of James Mateer, MD.)*

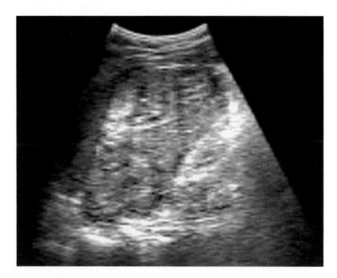

Figure 17–13. Ultrasound: LUQ subcapsular hematoma. A wide hyperechoic hematoma is located along the lateral border of the spleen (area closest to the probe).

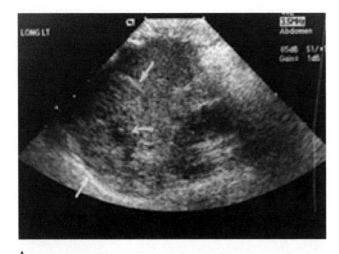

A

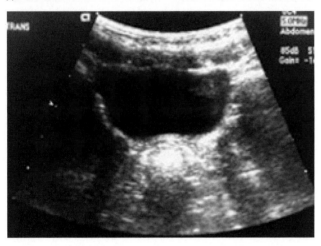

B

Figure 17–14. Splenic laceration associated with intraparenchymal hematoma. (A) Longitudinal view through the spleen demonstrates a linear hypoechoic region (curved arrow), representing a splenic laceration associated with an adjacent area of parenchymal heterogeneity (straight arrows) representing an intraparenchymal hematoma. (B) Transverse view through the pelvis in the same child demonstrates absence of associated peritoneal fluid. There were no fluid pockets noted anywhere in the abdomen or pelvis.

▶ PITFALLS

1. *Contraindications.* The only absolute contraindication to performing the FAST examination is when immediate surgical management is clearly indicated. Findings, such as subcutaneous emphysema, gas-filled bowel, or morbid obesity, may render the examination indeterminate.

2. *Over-reliance on the FAST examination.* The FAST examination is one data point in clinical decision making. The initial FAST examination

(and often repeat examinations) may not detect intraperitoneal bleeding or significant injury. CT is generally needed to characterize abdominal injuries, since most of them will be managed non-operatively in children. The algorithm (see Figure 17–1) provides a guideline for the appropriate utilization of trauma ultrasound in the pediatric population.

3. *Limitations.* Air and adipose tissue reflect sound waves and make the ultrasound image more difficult to interpret. Ascites is rarely a problem in children, and free fluid identified in the chest or abdomen in an injured child should be regarded as blood until proven otherwise. Ultrasound has not been found to be as accurate as CT for identifying solid organ injuries or hollow viscus injuries.[36,70] When the FAST examination is used solely to evaluate for intraperitoneal fluid, it suffers from limitations similar to diagnostic peritoneal lavage and has been regarded simply as a noninvasive diagnostic peritoneal lavage.[71]

4. *Technical difficulties with the FAST examination.* The view of Morison's pouch is generally the easiest for sonographers to locate and interpret. In children, however, this view is often more caudad than compared to an adult. For the left upper quadrant view, sonologists often fail to place the transducer far enough posteriorly (dorsally). The splenorenal recess is also more cephalad than the Morison's pouch view. Missed subcapsular hematomas and blood between the spleen and diaphragm are often the causes of false negatives scans. It is recommended that at least 50% of the left hemidiaphragm be visualized to avoid missing blood in this area. The suprapubic view may yield the most errors.[56,59,72] A bladder containing little urine provides no acoustic window. Sterile normal saline in quantities appropriate for the patient's age can be introduced into the bladder through the Foley catheter, if necessary. Finally, it can also be difficult to adequately visualize the heart in the subxiphoid view, especially when the child is obese or their abdomen is tender. Flattening the angle of the probe and having the patient breathe deeply can bring the heart into view. If adequate visualization is still not possible, parasternal long or short axis views of the heart are recommended (see Chapter 5).

▶ CASE STUDIES

Case 1

Patient Presentation

A 2-year-old boy was unbelted in a child seat when his car was struck on the side, throwing him against the driver's seat. He lost consciousness briefly and had a Glasgow Coma Scale (GCS) score of 12 on arrival to the emergency department. His initial blood pressure was 90/60 mm Hg, with a heart rate of 140 beats per min, respiratory rate of 20 per min, and an oxygen saturation of 94% on room air.

On physical examination, the patient's skin was red as he cried for his mother. He opened his eyes and localized to painful stimuli. Pupils were equal and reactive, and an abrasion was noted on his forehead. His neck, lung, and heart examinations were normal except for tachycardia. His abdomen was firm as he cried, and it was difficult to discern tenderness because of his agitation.

Management Course

A 20-mL/kg bolus of normal saline was administered for his tachycardia, and CT scans of his head and abdomen were ordered. However, his GCS score dropped to 7, and his next systolic blood pressure read 70 mm Hg. He underwent rapid sequence intubation, and the FAST examination revealed free intraperitoneal fluid in the left upper quadrant with suspected disruption of the splenic parenchyma. After the FAST examination, he was taken directly to the operating room where a portion of his lacerated spleen was removed and a 1-cm tear in the small bowel was repaired. His hospital course was uncomplicated and he recovered completely.

Commentary

Case 1 demonstrated the difficulty in adequately examining young children during the initial trauma resuscitation. The abdominal examination was unreliable in the face of a severe injury. His acute decline in mental status was due to hypovolemia, not a head injury. His postoperative head CT scan was normal. This patient was unstable and could not be transported to the medical imaging department for abdominal CT scanning. Bedside emergency ultrasound rapidly revealed the cause of his hypotension and directed his care toward appropriate surgical intervention.

Case 2

Patient Presentation

A 7-year-old girl riding her bicycle was hit by a car traveling 20 miles per hour. She was thrown 25 ft and cracked her helmet but did not lose consciousness. She was alert and complained of abdominal pain.

On arrival in the emergency department, her blood pressure was 100/60 mm Hg, heart rate 105 beats per min, respiratory rate 16 per min, and oxygen saturation 98% on room air. Her head, neck, and chest examinations were normal. Her abdomen was soft with mild, diffuse tenderness, but no peritoneal signs. The left side of her body exhibited superficial abrasions.

Management Course

Cervical spine, chest, and pelvis radiographs were normal. The FAST examination detected no intraperitoneal fluid. An abdominal CT scan was ordered because of the patient's pain, tenderness, and abrasions. The nurse noted gross hematuria on placing a Foley catheter. The patient vomited after drinking the oral contrast, and her abdominal pain and tenderness worsened. A repeat FAST examination revealed no intraperitoneal fluid. CT confirmed the absence of hemoperitoneum but identified a perinephric hematoma. Intravenous pyelography (IVP) further identified the renal pedicle injury, which was surgically repaired.

Commentary

One of the limitations of the FAST examination is that it often misses renal and retroperitoneal injuries. The patient's abdominal pain, tenderness, and the abrasion guided the physician toward ordering the CT scan. The hematuria would also have led to further study with CT and IVP. Ultrasound represents one piece in the clinical puzzle. The emergency physician understood the limitations of the FAST examination, did not rely on it solely, and moved forward with further studies based on the patient's signs and symptoms.

Case 3

Patient Presentation

An 8-year-old boy showed a classmate his father's handgun stored in the nightstand drawer. The gun discharged, and his classmate was shot in the abdomen. The patient's systolic blood pressure was 80 mm Hg in the ambulance and he complained of abdominal pain. He received a bolus of normal saline en route, and on arrival to the emergency department his systolic blood pressure was 90 mm Hg, heart rate was 120 beats per min, respiratory rate was 22 per min, and oxygen saturation 96% on room air. The patient was agitated, but his lung sounds were clear and equal. His heart was tachycardic with a regular, distinct S_1 and S_2. An entrance wound was noted in his epigastrium and this area was tender. The rest of his examination was normal.

Management Course

During the secondary survey, while the operating room was preparing for an exploratory laparotomy, a FAST examination quickly identified hemopericardium but no free intraperitoneal fluid. Shortly thereafter, the patient lost pulses and consciousness. A thoracotomy was performed in the emergency department while the patient was intubated. The pericardium was incised and the tamponade relieved. Closure of a large hole in the right atrium was quickly attempted with pledgeted, horizontal mattress sutures. The patient was rushed to the operating room, but died during surgery.

Commentary

Although the bullet entered the abdomen, it traveled cephalad, penetrating the diaphragm and injuring the heart. The FAST examination identified the true cause of the patient's cardiac arrest, which was pericardial tampo-nade, and directed the trauma team away from its focus on the abdomen as the source of possible exsanguinating injury.

APPENDICITIS

Acute appendicitis is the most common indication for emergency surgery in children, representing approximately 80% of emergent cases. The diagnosis is made in 60,000 to 80,000 children each year in the United States.[78,79] Appendicitis is thought to result from luminal obstruction by hard concretions, fecal impaction, or appendiceal calculi. The lumen becomes distended, leading to ischemia and bacterial infection. Left untreated, this leads to necrosis, perforation, and abscess formation in 36 to 48 h.[80]

Delays in diagnosis have been associated with higher rates of perforation and an increase in the rate of overall morbidity from 6 to 36%.[81] Studies of preschool-aged children report a perforation rate of 30 to 60% at laparotomy.[82,83] If the diagnosis is delayed, the perforation rate is greater than 65%, and mortality increases.[84] The long-term sequelae are not well characterized, but a history of ruptured appendix has been shown to convey a three- to fivefold increased risk of infertility.[85] Failure to diagnose appendicitis is one of the most frequently successful malpractice claims against emergency physicians.[86] Timely diagnosis is the only proven means of decreasing morbidity and mortality.[87] In the pediatric patient, the diagnosis is often elusive for even the most astute clinician.

▶ CLINICAL CONSIDERATIONS

The classic presentation of appendicitis includes right lower quadrant abdominal pain associated with peritoneal signs, fever, vomiting, and anorexia. Together, these signs and symptoms have been found to be highly sensitive for appendicitis.[88] Younger children are often unable to adequately express themselves, and the physical examination may be nondiagnostic. Although frequently requested, the white blood cell (WBC) count[89] and plain abdominal radiograph[90,91] are neither sensitive nor specific for appendicitis. In light of the risks of misdiagnosis and subsequent perforation, pediatric surgeons have been quick to proceed to operation. Negative laparotomy rates as high as 20% have been reported, and rates of 10 to 15% widely accepted.[92–94] Negative laparotomies come at significant costs, both financially and in terms of morbidity. Morbidity includes adhesions, hospitalization, and time away from school. Children with equivocal findings represent 25 to 30% of all cases of acute appendicitis.[95–96] This diagnostic challenge forces clinicians to rely on ancillary studies in equivocal cases.

Multiple ancillary studies have been used to help diagnose acute appendicitis, but each have their limitations. Barium enema has been used in the past, but is limited in an unprepared bowel. Barium enema's limitations include nonvisualization of the appendix, patient discomfort, time consumption, and radiation exposure. The barium enema is neither sensitive nor specific, except for the occasional appendicolith.[91] Leukocyte scintigraphy is also time consuming and difficult to perform.[97] Recently, the advent of laparoscopy has made minimally invasive surgery another tool for both the diagnosis and treatment of appendicitis in children.[98,99] However, laparoscopy requires general anesthesia and is an invasive study. Currently, ultrasound and CT are most commonly used to help diagnose appendicitis in patients with equivocal presentation.

Deutsch and Leopold reported the first demonstration of an inflamed appendix by ultrasound in 1981.[100] Development of the graded compression examination by Puylaert in 1986 established a technique and criteria for the diagnosis of appendicitis.[93] Ultrasound has several advantages, including lower cost, widespread availability, and no patient exposure to ionizing radiation. Ultrasound is noninvasive and there is no need for sedation or contrast material.

Studies of ultrasound use in children for detecting appendicitis have sensitivities ranging from 44 to 90% and specificities from 88 to 100% (Table 17–2).[93,101–110] The wide range in sensitivity likely reflects the operator-dependent nature of ultrasound, particularly for this examination. The right lower quadrant examination for signs of appendicitis is one of the more technically difficult examinations for emergency ultrasonography. It may be difficult for a physician or part-time sonographer to gain the skills and experience necessary to reliably locate the appendix and recognize findings consistent with appendicitis.[111] To date, no studies have evaluated the accuracy of right lower quadrant ultrasound examinations in the hands of emergency physicians or surgeons, although Hahn and associates used "specially trained pediatricians" and achieved 90% sensitivity.[105] Clinicians who are trained in right lower quadrant ultrasound examinations should not allow findings of a normal appendix, or inability to identify the appendix, to influence their clinical decision making.

Studies of the use of helical CT for the diagnosis of appendicitis in children have produced sensitivities of 84 to 97% and specificities of 89 to 98%.[101–102,104,112] Although these ranges of sensitivity and specificity overlap with those of ultrasonography, the reliability of sonography is less consistent. When CT and ultrasonography are compared directly, CT has been superior in each study.[96,101,102,104] Sivit and associates found that in 20 out of 84 (24%) patients who had discordant CT and ultrasound readings, the CT diagnosis was correct 85% of the time.[104] When radiologists were asked to rate their confidence in reading ultrasound and CT images evaluating

TABLE 17–2. STUDIES OF ULTRASOUND IN PEDIATRIC APPENDICITIS

Year	Investigator	Patients	Ultrasound Sensitivity (%)	Ultrasound Specificity (%)	CT Sensitivity (%)	CT Specificity (%)
2000	Karakas	360	74	94	84	99
2000	Sivit	386	78	93	95	93
2000	Horton	106	76	90	97	100
1999	Garcia Pena	139	44	93	97	94
1999	Rice	103	87	88		
1999	Lessin	99	88	96		
1998	Roosevelt	231	88	95		
1998	Hahn	3859	90	97		
1994	Zaki	56	67			
1993	Crady	98	85	94		
1991	Siegel	178	82			
1988	Jeffrey	245	90	96		
1986	Puylaert	60	89	100		

for appendicitis in children, sonography was interpreted with very low, low, or medium confidence in 59 of 139 (42.4%) patients. This is in comparison to 9 of 108 (8.3%) patients with CT.[113] In comparing ultrasound to CT for the diagnosis of appendicitis, Horton and co-workers asserted that a key to managing patients is the negative predictive value of each study. This was 56% for an ultrasound examination compared to 92% for CT scan.[96] Patients with negative CT scans were sent home from the emergency department, whereas those with negative ultrasound examinations required further testing and observation.

▶ CLINICAL INDICATIONS

An ultrasound examination is indicated when a clinician suspects a child might have appendicitis, the physical examination is equivocal, and the patient is not sent directly to the operating room. Signs and symptoms typically last less than 48 h and may include:

1. Abdominal pain—especially pain that migrates from the periumbilical area to the right lower quadrant with accompanying peritoneal signs
2. Fever
3. Vomiting
4. Anorexia

Garcia Pena and associates described a protocol for managing children with suspected appendicitis.[114] In their study, this protocol led to a beneficial change in management (i.e., a child with appendicitis who would have been discharged from the hospital or admitted for inpatient observation but was instead taken directly to the operating room) in 86 out of 139 (62%) of their patients with equivocal clinical presentations. Roughly one-third of patients who clinically appeared to have appendicitis were taken

directly to the operating room for appendectomy. Another one-third of patients for whom appendicitis was doubtful were discharged if no other diagnosis was identified other than nonspecific abdominal pain. The remaining one-third, who had equivocal clinical presentations, underwent graded compression ultrasonography. When findings consistent with appendicitis were identified, patients were taken to the operating room. If the ultrasound results were negative or equivocal, context-limited CT with rectal contrast was performed. Patients with positive findings on CT underwent appendectomy, and patients with normal findings were discharged from the emergency department. This resulted in a cost savings of $565 per patient.

▶ ANATOMIC CONSIDERATIONS

The vermiform (*Latin* worm-shaped) appendix is a hollow lymphoid organ whose function is not well understood. The blind-ended appendix typically arises from the cecum, 1- to 2-cm distal to the ileum in the right lower quadrant (Figure 17–15). It is rarely congenitally absent.[115] Clinically, maximum pain from an inflamed appendix may localize to McBurney's point, which is the midpoint of an imaginary line between the umbilicus and the anterior-superior iliac crest. This should not be used as a rigid anatomic landmark because the appendix and the umbilicus are too variable in position. The appendix lies anterior to the psoas muscle.[115] A 1933 study reported a classic pelvic orientation of the appendix in only 31% of 10,000 autopsies.[116] The appendix was retrocecal in 65% of cases; in this position, the ultrasound view is frequently obscured by overlying bowel gas.

The appendix averages 6 to 9 cm in length, but it can be twice as long. The normal diameter is less than 6 mm.[80] The appendiceal wall is composed of the serosa, muscularis, submucosa, and mucosa. These layers are typical of

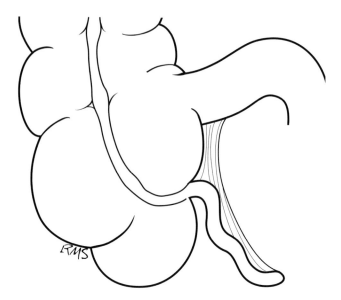

Figure 17–15. Normal appendix.

the intestinal wall, except that, in the appendix, the submucosa is heavily infiltrated with lymphoid tissue. The appendix is partially covered by a peritoneal fold known as the mesoappendix, which contains the appendicular artery, a branch of the ileocolic artery. The fold is often short, so the appendix may be folded or kinked.[115]

► TECHNIQUE AND NORMAL ULTRASOUND FINDINGS

A 5.0 MHz or 7.5 MHz linear array transducer should be used, depending on the child's body habitus and need for penetration. The index marker should point cephalad or to the patient's right by convention. The graded compression technique is now the standard technique for the evaluation of appendicitis. It improves the quality of the examination and minimizes patient discomfort.[93]

With the patient supine, the transducer should be placed at the lateral edge of the right lower quadrant in a sagittal plane. It should be moved gently toward the midline to find the area of maximum tenderness. Gradual, gentle compression should be applied in the area of maximum tenderness, slowly advancing during expiration. Graded compression helps displace gas out of the cecum and ascending colon and moves the transducer closer to the appendix. Adequate compression has been achieved when the iliac vessels and psoas muscle are visualized, as the appendix will always be anterior to those structures.[80] Once the appendix is identified, the diameter should be measured in both transverse and longitudinal planes with electronic calipers.[105] A normal appendix will collapse with compression and should be observed for peristaltic activity.

► COMMON AND EMERGENT ABNORMALITIES

Appendicitis is diagnosed when the following findings are present.

- *Target shape:* Inflammation gives the appendix a classic targetoid or "bull's eye" appearance when viewed transversely (Figure 17–16). This results from anechoic fluid in the lumen, surrounded by an echogenic ring of mucosa and submucosa, and an outer ring of hypoechoic muscularis externa.[97]
- *Diameter larger than 6 mm:* The diameter will be greater than 6 mm (see Figure 17–16) due to inflammation.
- *Noncompressible:* Inflammation and appendicoliths impede change in the shape of the appendix during graded compression.
- *No peristaltic activity:* The inflamed appendix is no longer able to contract sequentially.

► COMMON VARIANTS AND SELECTED ABNORMALITIES

The most important variant is that a normal appendix is rarely seen on ultrasound examination, which would render that study indeterminate. In his original work, Puylaert never identified a normal appendix.[93] One study reported that only 2% of normal appendices were seen

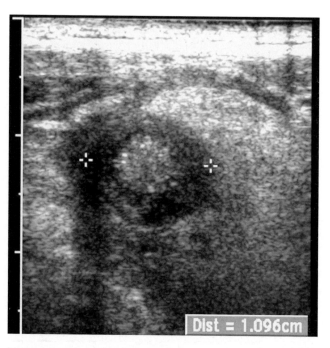

Figure 17–16. Ultrasound RLQ: short axis view shows appendicitis with targetoid appearance. *(Courtesy of Phillip J. Silberberg, MD, Oregon Health and Science University.)*

on ultrasound.[101] Hahn and colleagues were able to identify a normal appendix in 36/54 (67%) of healthy controls; however, 98% (49/50) of histologically proven cases of appendicitis were not visualized on ultrasound. Consequently, they cautioned against concluding that a nonvisualized appendix is not inflamed.[105]

An appendicolith, when seen, helps make the diagnosis of appendicitis (Figure 17–17). An appendicolith resembles gallstones. They are dense, brightly echogenic, and produce acoustic shadowing.

The appendix loses its targetoid appearance when it perforates and is more difficult to identify. It may be surrounded by anechoic fluid or a developing abscess. A pericecal abscess usually demonstrates anechoic fluid with bright, hyperechoic debris (Figure 17–18). The appearance often varies, and the abscess may be loculated and more complex.

► PITFALLS

1. *Contraindications.* Children with a high clinical suspicion for appendicitis should be evaluated immediately by a pediatric surgeon in anticipation of expeditious appendectomy. They should not incur a delay in the emergency department or elsewhere for any unnecessary tests.
2. *Over-reliance.* As discussed, an ultrasound examination for this diagnosis has a limited sensitivity. A positive examination is an indication for

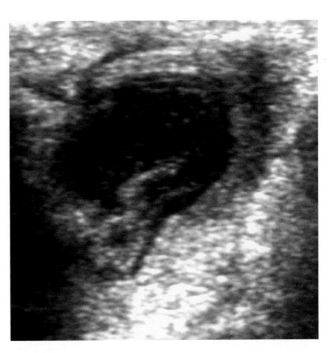

Figure 17–18. Ultrasound RLQ: pericecal abscess. *(Courtesy of Paul A. Nancarrow, MD, Children's Hospital, Oakland, CA.)*

operative management. A negative examination is not adequate to rule out appendicitis and further evaluation with CT should be obtained.
3. *Perforation.* Sonography has a much lower sensitivity for recognizing appendicitis once perforation has occurred.[117–119] Peritonitis associated with perforation may inhibit adequate compression, and necrosis of the appendix may render it difficult to visualize.[119]
4. *Technical difficulties.* Air and adipose tissue reflect sound waves and make the ultrasound image difficult or impossible to distinguish. In an obese child, a 5.0 MHz transducer should be used to improve tissue penetration. An ultrasound study may be complicated by an overlying gas-filled cecum and ascending colon or a location that is difficult to visualize, such as the retrocecum. While Sivit asserts that if the psoas muscle is visualized on graded compression, even a retrocecal appendix should be seen,[80] this has not been conclusively demonstrated.

► CASE STUDIES

Case 1

Patient Presentation

An 18-month-old boy was brought into the emergency department by his mother complaining of four episodes of

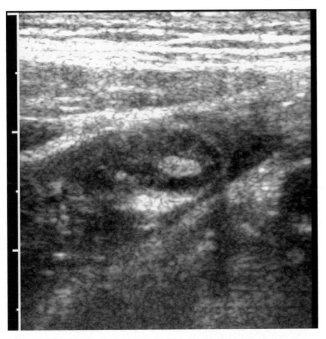

Figure 17–17. Ultrasound RLQ: An appendicolith is visible within the appendix (middle of the image). *(Courtesy of Phillip J. Silberberg, MD, Oregon Health and Science University.)*

emesis and increased irritability since lunch. She stated he did not eat dinner, and she was concerned he may have a fever. In triage, his blood pressure was 87/50 mm Hg, heart rate 130 beats per min, respiratory rate 24 per min, oxygen saturation 97% on room air, and temperature 38.5°C. His mucous membranes were mildly dry, and his heart and lungs sounds were normal. His abdomen was firm while crying.

Management Course

The child was administered a 20 mL/kg bolus of normal saline. A complete blood count (CBC) and basic metabolic panel were sent to the lab. The patient was re-examined after IV hydration and, without crying, exhibited guarding on abdominal examination. The pediatric surgeon was called in from home. While she drove in, the emergency physician performed a graded compression ultrasound examination of the right lower quadrant. The emergency physician identified a classic targetoid appendix that measured 8 mm in diameter. The appendix was noncompressible, though the patient was not able to cooperate optimally with the examination. She relayed these results to the pediatric surgeon on arrival, and the patient was taken to the operating room where an inflamed appendix was resected.

Commentary

In Case 1, there was ample clinical evidence of appendicitis, and the patient could have been taken directly to the operating room. In this case, it was reasonable to perform an ultrasound examination while waiting for the pediatric surgeon. This did not delay definitive care. The positive results may have helped reassure the pediatric surgeon of the diagnosis. Graded compression can be difficult in children, especially younger children who understand only the pain.

Case 2

Patient Presentation

An 8-year-old girl was brought to the emergency department by her father with a "tummy ache" after eating dinner. She had not been febrile or nauseated. Her last bowel movement occurred in the morning and was normal. Her blood pressure was 95/55 mm Hg, heart rate 100 beats per min, respiratory rate 22 per min, oxygen saturation 98% on room air, and temperature 38°C. She did not appear ill. Her mucous membranes were moist, and her heart and lung examinations were normal. Her abdomen was soft but diffusely tender to palpation. No peritoneal signs were appreciated.

Management Course

The emergency physician sent blood to the laboratory for CBC, metabolic panel, liver function tests, and lipase. Urine was dip negative for infection or blood, but was sent for urinalysis and culture. The emergency physician performed a bedside ultrasound examination but was unable to confidently identify the appendix. Still concerned with the patient's abdominal pain, he administered broad-spectrum antibiotics and ordered an abdominal CT with oral, IV, and rectal contrast. The CT showed possible stranding in the periappendiceal fat. The child was thin, and the radiologist recommended clinical correlation. The pediatric surgeon decided to admit the patient for observation. Her pain worsened overnight, and she was taken to the operating room where a focally inflamed appendix was resected.

Commentary

In Case 2, the emergency physician recognized the limits of the ultrasound examination in detecting appendicitis and his limited experience in using this imaging modality. Because of his concern and these limitations, it was important that he followed up with a more definitive test. A formal ultrasound evaluation of the right lower quadrant could have been ordered, but CT is arguably a better study because it is more sensitive and specific. In this case, the CT showed possible signs of early inflammation but was not conclusive. The emergency physician ordered triple contrast for the CT, which is standard in many institutions. However, research by Garcia Pena suggests that rectal contrast alone is sufficient to produce a highly sensitive study. It is faster and exposes the patient to less contrast material and ionizing radiation.[101]

PYLORIC STENOSIS

Idiopathic hypertrophic pyloric stenosis (IHPS) is an infrequent but serious problem encountered in any emergency department or pediatric clinic. Although there is usually no doubt about the need to hospitalize infants with symptoms suggestive of IHPS regardless of the cause, the need to diagnose this entity rapidly stems from the desire to involve surgical consultants as early as possible in the course of the disease. A reduction in the severity of complications associated with IHPS has been documented in recent years, which is presumably due to earlier intervention.

▶ CLINICAL CONSIDERATIONS

Most experts agree that the diagnosis of IHPS can be made on clinical grounds alone by palpation of the classic olive-shaped mass in the right upper quadrant in combination with the typical history of vomiting in the appropriate age group.[120–122] The positive predictive value of this combination of findings is nearly 100%. Though the number of patients presenting with these classic findings has declined somewhat over the last few decades, possibly due to patients presenting earlier in the course of the disease, it is still estimated that from 70 to 90% of cases meet the criteria for clinical diagnosis,[122] and these patients could be referred directly for surgery without any imaging studies. Despite these recommendations, the majority of patients with suspected IHPS receive some type of imaging study prior to surgery.

The choice of imaging for IHPS is generally between an upper gastrointestinal (GI) series and ultrasound. Neither study seems to be clearly superior from a sensitivity or specificity standpoint. Sensitivities for ultrasound range from 85 to 100%[120,123] and for upper GI series range from 90 to 100%. One approach is to start with an ultrasound examination followed by an upper GI series if the ultrasound examination is nondiagnostic or the patient's signs and symptoms persist despite a negative initial study. Sensitivity with this approach is 100%. Another approach is to perform an ultrasound examination, and repeat the diagnostic test later if the initial study is nondiagnostic or symptoms persist. This approach has a sensitivity of 97%.[124]

The pros and cons of an upper GI series and ultrasound examination should be considered when deciding which imaging study to request for evaluation of the infant with projectile emesis. An upper GI series does involve administration of contrast and exposure to small amounts of radiation,[122] which can be avoided with ultrasound examination. An upper GI series is a safe procedure and, despite concerns over potential complications, such complications were found to be nonexistent in one large study involving 666 patients.[120] One advantage of an upper GI series is that it more frequently defines other etiologies of vomiting when IHPS is not the cause, the most common being gastroesophageal reflux. In one study, when upper GI series was the initial imaging study, only 6% of patients needed a second study (ultrasound) as part of their evaluation, as opposed to 17% when sonography was the first imaging study.[120] Despite the apparent advantage of using an upper GI series as the initial diagnostic study, ultrasound predominates as the study of choice for suspected IHPS.[121,125,126]

Ultrasound is a rapid and non-invasive means of assessing for a hypertrophic pyloric segment using measurements of the pyloric width and length. Unlike an upper GI series, which only implies a hypertrophied muscle by visualization of a thinned channel of barium through the pylorus, the ultrasound examination actually views the hypertrophied muscle itself. Infants are good candidates for ultrasound imaging because of their small size and limited body fat, which allows for the use of a higher frequency transducer and, thus, produces higher resolution examinations. The examination is well tolerated by the ill infant and can be done at the bedside with the parent holding the infant, if necessary. No sedation is usually required.

▶ CLINICAL INDICATIONS

The ultrasound examination for IHPS should be performed in any patient, aged 10 d to 20 weeks, who presents with persistent painless, nonbilious vomiting and who may or may not have a palpable olive-sized mass in the right upper quadrant or peristaltic stomach waves.

IHPS is the pathologic hypertrophy of the muscle of the pylorus that occurs for unknown reasons. It is not a congenital disease.[121] The hypertrophied muscle obstructs outflow from the stomach, leading to persistent vomiting, classically projectile in nature. The disease occurs in 1:200 to 300 births,[120,122,125] with the typical age range of presentation between 4 and 6 weeks. IHPS has been reported as early as 10 d and as late as 20 weeks of age. The mean age of presentation is around 5 weeks, with males affected 3 to 6 times more than females. Of infants presenting with symptoms suggesting IHPS, about one-third will be found to have the disease.[120,122] Anywhere from 50 to 90% of patients with IHPS will have the classic olive-sized right upper quadrant mass,[121,122,124] which is pathognomonic for the disease in the correct clinical setting. In some patients, no mass can be felt, possibly due to a stomach distended with air or tense abdominal wall musculature due to crying. When the diagnosis is not clear clinically, imaging should be employed.

Treatment consists of a pylorotomy, in which a segment of the hypertrophied muscle is removed. This treatment is curative and long-term sequelae are rare.[121] Atropine has been successfully used in Japan to reverse pyloric stenosis non-operatively, but this treatment has not been widely used in the United States.[128]

▶ ANATOMIC CONSIDERATIONS

The pylorus is contiguous with the stomach and usually lies just to the right of the midline and just caudal to the gallbladder (Figure 17–19). The stomach lies just to the left of the pylorus. Due to the inability of the stomach to pass fluid through the pylorus, the stomach may be distended with fluid making its identification even easier. The hypertrophic pylorus itself is usually a linear structure lying along a line passing roughly from the right shoulder to the left hip (Figure 17–20).

▶ TECHNIQUE AND NORMAL ULTRASOUND FINDINGS

The ultrasound examination for IHPS consists of identifying the hypertrophied pyloric wall muscle and measuring the muscle wall thickness (MWT). The examination should be performed with a 5.0 to 7.5 MHz linear or sector probe from an anterior approach on the supine patient. A warmed standoff pad (a latex glove with water or

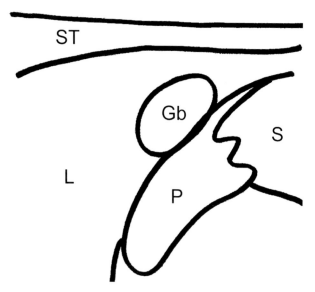

Figure 17–19. Oblique cross section as depicted in Figure 17–20: location of pylorus in abdomen. Gb = gallbladder; L = liver; P = pylorus; S = stomach; ST = soft tissue.

intravenous fluid bag will work) may be used if necessary to place the area of interest in the focal zone of the transducer. The pylorus is a cylindrical structure with an echogenic center surrounded by a sonolucent wall and is found between the gastric antrum and the duodenal bulb. The stomach is often filled with fluid from the obstruction, which facilitates its localization. If not, it may be filled orally with up to 100 mL of clear fluid. Only the hypoechoic muscle layer should be measured, not the mucosa, and measurements should be taken only on a perpendicular cross-section of the pylorus, or in the midline on a longitudinal section. The pylorus should be observed for

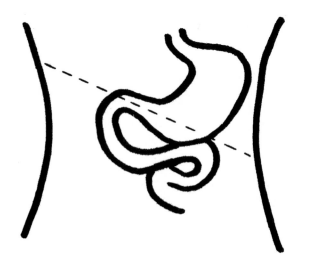

Figure 17–20. Orientation line for pylorus. The plane for imaging the pylorus along its length (dotted line) is intermediate between the transverse and sagittal planes.

at least 5 min to ensure that the MWT does not change. A changing MWT indicates pylorospasm and not IHPS.

► COMMON AND EMERGENT ABNORMALITIES

A MWT greater than 3 mm that does not vary with time is considered diagnostic for IHPS (Figure 17–21). Although several more complicated measurements that take into account patient weight, pyloric length, or pyloric volume have been used to diagnose IHPS, the fact remains that the pyloric muscle width remains the most widely accepted diagnostic standard and has a very high accuracy rate.[126,129]

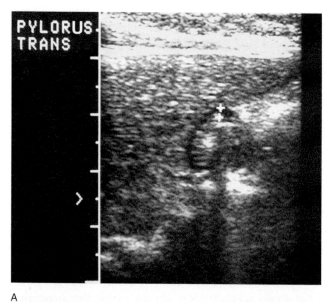

A

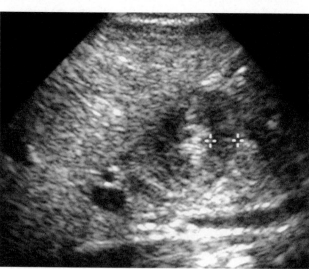

B

Figure 17–21. Ultrasound: normal pylorus in cross section (A). The MWT was measured as 1.5 mm. Transverse view of pylorus in IHPS (B). The MWT was measured at 4.7 mm.

In addition, a functional assessment may support or refute the diagnosis of IHPS. In IHPS, no gastric contents should be seen transiting to the duodenum during the ultrasound examination. Strong gastric peristaltic contractions may also be observed. The "antral nipple sign" has also been described with IHPS. The nipple-shaped mass found protruding into the gastric antrum is formed by thickened gastric mucosa adjacent to the pylorus (Figure 17–22).

► COMMON VARIANTS AND SELECTED ABNORMALITIES

When performing the IHPS ultrasound examination, it is essential to recognize common normal variants that may mimic positive findings. The most important normal variant to exclude is pylorospasm. The MWT in pylorospasm may exceed 3 mm initially, but if observed over time, the MWT will vary, often dropping below 3 mm. Pylorospasm resolves without any surgical intervention.[130] Fluid in the colon or small bowel may appear to represent the stomach, leading to the presumption that a portion of the bowel is the pylorus. A normal pylorus viewed tangentially instead of in true cross-section may give falsely elevated muscle thickness measurements simulating IHPS.

If the cause of vomiting in the infant is not IHPS, clues to an alternate diagnosis may be seen. In malrotation with midgut volvulus, obstruction occurs past the pylorus, so that a fluid-filled dilated proximal duodenum is present.[121] Other rare causes of vomiting, such as duodenal duplication[120] or duodenal stenosis, may be visualized as well. When the examination is negative for IHPS, the most likely alternate diagnosis is gastroesophageal reflux disease.

► PITFALLS

1. *Measurement error.* The difference between normal and abnormal may be 1 mm in size or less, so accurate measurement is key. In one study, seven of eight false negative examinations were due to inaccurate measurements from poor technique.[124] Only the hypoechoic muscle layer should be measured, not the mucosa. Measurements should be taken only on a perpendicular cross-section of the pylorus, or in the midline on a longitudinal section (Figure 17–23). A tangential cut on cross-section will exaggerate the muscle thickness, as will a longitudinal view taken off the midline.
2. *Bilious vomiting.* Bilious vomiting suggests obstruction more distally than the pylorus, and malrotation with midgut volvulus should be considered in such cases. An upper GI series, and not ultrasound, would be the study of choice.
3. *Pylorospasm.* A thickened MWT should be observed for over 5 to 10 min to ensure that it does not vary.

► CASE STUDIES

Case 1

Patient Presentation

A one-month-old male infant was brought to the emergency department by his mother after the infant vomited everything he had eaten four times over the last 12 h, and had been crying more than usual. The mother reported

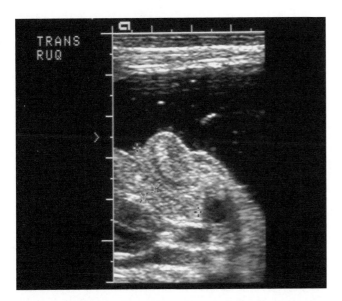

Figure 17–22. Ultrasound: antral nipple sign. The nipple-shaped mass protruding into the fluid-filled gastric antrum, is formed by thickened gastric mucosa adjacent to the pylorus.

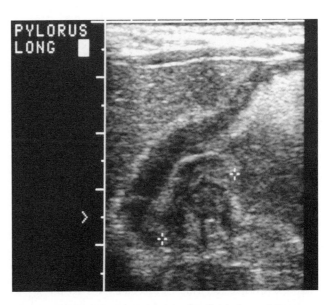

Figure 17–23. Ultrasound: longitudinal view of the pylorus in IHPS. Measurement cursors are locating the overall width of the pylorus (not MWT).

the child had otherwise acted normally, had an unremarkable birth history, and was on no medications. She had been bottle feeding the infant milk-based formula.

On physical examination, vital signs were normal for his age although the infant did appear mildly dehydrated. He was alert and active. His head, neck, pulmonary, and cardiovascular examinations were unremarkable. The abdomen was soft, slightly distended and tympanitic, nontender, and had good bowel sounds. No right upper quadrant mass was palpated.

Management Course

An intravenous line was established and 10 mL/kg of crystalloid was infused. A CBC and an electrolyte panel were sent, and an ultrasound examination was performed to evaluate the patient for IHPS. A 3.5-mm pyloric MWT was detected. The pylorus was observed for 5 min and did not demonstrate any passage of gastric contents or change in MWT. The diagnosis of IHPS was confirmed and the patient was admitted to the hospital for intravenous hydration and surgical consultation for pylorotomy.

Commentary

The ultrasound examination was necessary only because the classic right upper quadrant mass was lacking on physical examination. Had this mass been present it would have been reasonable to proceed directly to surgical consultation.

Case 2

Patient Presentation

A 20-day-old female infant presented to the emergency department with 2 d of profuse vomiting, described as projectile. The grandmother (the patient's caretaker) reported that the infant had been well prior to the start of the vomiting and other than being a 36-week premature infant the birth history was unremarkable. The infant fed on breast milk from a bottle since her mother worked full time.

On physical examination, the child's vital signs included a blood pressure of 75/50 mm Hg, heart rate 160 beats per min, respiratory rate 36 per min, and temperature 37°C rectally. The infant was alert and active though appearing mildly dehydrated. Her head, neck, and pulmonary examinations were unremarkable. Cardiovascular examination showed capillary refill time of 3 sec but was otherwise normal. Abdominal examination was normal and no mass could be palpated.

Management Course

An intravenous line was established and 20 mL/kg of crystalloid was administered. An ultrasound examination of the abdomen for IHPS was performed by the medical imaging department and was negative. Serum chemistries

and CBC were unremarkable as was the urinalysis. After fluid hydration, the patient vomited a challenge of oral electrolyte solution and was admitted to the hospital for continued hydration and observation.

The patient was observed for 6 h and, when the vomiting persisted, the patient's primary physician ordered a repeat ultrasound examination. The repeat ultrasound examination was positive for IHPS and surgical consultation was then obtained for pylorotomy.

Commentary

Case 2 was an example of the imperfect negative predictive value of a single ultrasound examination. Repeat imaging was indicated with either an ultrasound or upper GI series if symptoms consistent with IHPS did not resolve over time. Most infants with a significant history of vomiting and dehydration deserve a period of observation in the hospital regardless of the cause.

INTUSSUSCEPTION

Intussusception is a rare but serious diagnosis in children. Delays in diagnosis can lead to increasing bowel wall edema, ischemia, possible bowel perforation, and may make the need for surgical intervention more likely. Prior to this century, intussusception was usually a fatal disorder, but with current diagnostic and treatment tools, mortality has been reduced to less than 1%. If diagnosed early, intussusception can be easily treated through radiographic reduction.

▶ CLINICAL CONSIDERATIONS

The imaging modalities commonly used in the evaluation of intussusception include plain abdominal radiographs, contrast enemas, and ultrasound. Plain films are appropriate in clinical situations suggestive of obstruction or perforation, and may demonstrate some abnormality consistent with intussusception in 45 to 73% of cases, including a "target" or "crescent" lucency soft tissue mass, lack of cecal gas, or small bowel obstructive pattern.[131–133] Plain radiographs are nonspecific and further imaging studies are needed when intussusception is suspected. Plain films are helpful if free air is detected since liquid contrast studies are contraindicated when perforation occurs, and surgical exploration is necessary.

The gold standard for the diagnosis of intussusception has been the barium or air-contrast enema. Not only is this procedure diagnostic for the condition but it can be curative as well. Despite being mildly invasive, the procedure is relatively safe. Radiation exposure is quite low, on the order of 4 to 7 rads. Although perforation of the bowel can occur, unless the bowel is completely obstructed or the patient is unstable, the risk of perforation is less than 1%.[134] Currently, the use of air enemas seems to be favored over barium or other liquid enemas. Air enemas are less messy and require less radiation.[135] Although they have a slightly higher perforation rate than barium enemas (1.4% versus 0.2%),[131] this may be countered by the fact that perforation associated with air enemas are smaller, and leakage of air into the peritoneal space causes fewer problems than barium leakage. The disadvantages of contrast enemas are their invasive nature, radiation exposure, and the requirement to move patients to the medical imaging suite. The major advantage to contrast enemas is that should intussusception be diagnosed, it can usually be reduced during the same procedure. The procedure of reducing the intussusception involves infusing fluid or air rectally under fluoroscopic guidance, and pushing the telescoped segment out of the bowel into which it is invaginated.

Ultrasound has recently gained favor over contrast enemas as the initial diagnostic study for suspected intussusception. It has the distinct advantage of being entirely noninvasive, requiring no radiation exposure, and can be performed at the bedside if needed. The sensitivity of an ultrasound examination for intussusception ranges from 98 to 100%.[121,131,132,134,136] In addition, an ultrasound examination can locate the pathologic lead points responsible for the intussusception; contrast enemas cannot. Ultrasound can also assess blood flow to the involved segment, though the clinical utility of this information has not yet been determined. The major disadvantage of an ultrasound examination is that if intussusception is diagnosed, then the patient still requires a contrast enema for reduction. There are reports of ultrasound-guided reduction, but this technique is not generally used in the United States.

There exists some controversy as to whether an ultrasound examination or contrast enema study should be done as the initial imaging choice. In one study, 20% of patients with suspected intussusception did not have the disease.[132] If an ultrasound examination is employed as the initial imaging modality, 20% of these patients will have been spared the radiation and invasiveness of a contrast enema. On the other hand, the 80% of patients diagnosed with intussusception would be subjected to both an ultrasound examination and a contrast enema study.

► CLINICAL INDICATIONS

An ultrasound examination is indicated in any patient suspected of intussusception. These patients usually present with severe, intermittent abdominal pain, possibly associated with vomiting, a right upper quadrant mass, or guaiac-positive stool.

Intussusception occurs when one piece of bowel invaginates and telescopes into a more distal segment, causing intermittent pain whenever the bowel peristalses on

itself. Ages at the time of presentation typically range from 6 weeks to 1 year, but intussusception has been reported up to age 7 years.[136] The incidence peaks at 10 to 14 months,[135] with 65% of patients under 1 year of age.[125] Intussusception in children is usually idiopathic, occurring without a definable pathologic lead point. Patients present with a history of severe, intermittent abdominal pain. In the younger age group, a depressed level of alertness may be present. Up to 20% of younger children may present with vomiting as the only symptom. Although up to 75% of patients have some blood in the stool,[135] the classic triad of intermittent abdominal pain, vomiting, and "currant jelly" stools occurs in less than 20% of cases.[132,134] Half of these patients have a palpable abdominal mass,[132] usually in the right upper quadrant. Ninety-four percent of all pediatric patients with intermittent abdominal pain suspicious for intussusception that had a right upper quadrant mass on physical examination proved to have intussusception.[134] Most cases of intussusception involve invagination of the terminal ileum into the cecum, though some involve ileum into ileum. When a lead point is present, it is most commonly a Meckel's diverticulum or lymphoma.[132]

► ANATOMIC CONSIDERATIONS

Most cases of pediatric intussusception involve the terminal ileum invaginating into the cecum. The cecum is located in the right lower quadrant and is the gas-filled structure sandwiched between the anterior abdominal musculature and the large posterior psoas muscle. Continued pulling of the terminal ileum into the cecum pulls the cecum up into the right upper quadrant, giving rise to the classically described mass.

► TECHNIQUE AND NORMAL ULTRASOUND FINDINGS

The highest frequency ultrasound probe, preferably linear, that still has the depth of penetration to focus on the area of interest should be used. In older children, this may be as low as 3.5 MHz; in smaller children, up to a 7.5 MHz probe may be used. The child should be examined supine. As with all children, a warmed conducting gel should be applied. If an abdominal mass can be palpated, this should be imaged in multiple planes. If no mass is palpated, then the path of the colon should be followed from the cecum and terminal ileum to as far distally as possible. On an ultrasound examination, normal bowel appears as a hypoechoic ring (bowel wall) around a hyperechoic center (bowel contents often have small gas bubbles causing a bright reflection and shadowing). Normal bowel should show peristalsis if observed for a short period of time. Imaging of the bowel may be more difficult in patients who have copious bowel gas due to bowel obstruction.

▶ COMMON AND EMERGENT ABNORMALITIES

When imaged along its longitudinal plane, the segment of intussuscepted bowel may appear to have multiple thick hypoechoic layers that are distinctly different from normal proximal and distal bowel, or may have the general appearance of a kidney ("pseudokidney sign") (Figure 17–24). Another well-described finding is of a sonodense center (bowel contents) surrounded by a sonolucent ring (bowel wall), which is known as the "target sign." This is seen on transverse cuts of the bowel (Figure 17–25). Thickened bowel from a variety of causes, including inflammatory bowel disease, may give a similar appearance; however, if the bowel wall shows multiple echolucent layers, then intussusception must be suspected.

▶ COMMON VARIANTS AND SELECTED ABNORMALITIES

In up to 20% of cases of suspected intussusception, another diagnosis is made. In a quarter of these cases, the ultrasound examination will find alternate abnormalities,[134] including nonspecific bowel wall thickening (Crohn's, Henoch-Schönlein purpura, or enterocolitis), dilated loops of bowel filled with fluid, free intraabdominal fluid, enlarged mesenteric lymph nodes, ovarian cysts, or volvulus.[125,134,136] Free fluid does not necessarily imply perforation as long as no debris is seen in the free fluid.[125]

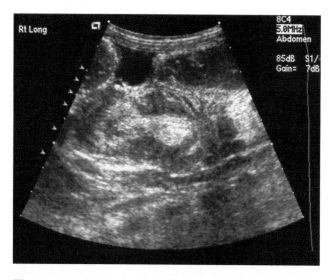

Figure 17–24. Longitudinal image of intussusception (arrows) demonstrating the "pseudokidney sign". Hypodense areas of intussusception are edematous bowel wall. Hyperechoic central area is caused by bowel contents (and possibly intussuscepted mesenteric fat).

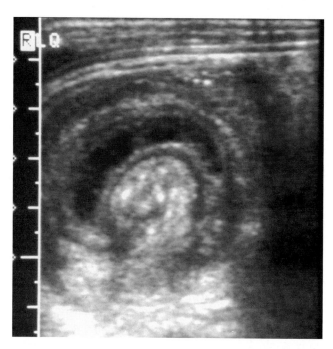

Figure 17–25. A transverse scan through ascending colon demonstrates the "donut" appearance of intussusception. The outer ring (arrows) is the intussuscipiens, while the central echoes are the intussusceptum. *(Reproduced from Cohen HJ, Sivit CJ: Fetal and pediatric ultrasound. New York: McGraw-Hill, 2001;287.)*

In 10 to 20% of intussusception cases, a lead point exists and may be seen on an ultrasound examination. Meckel's diverticula, duplication cysts, polyps, or lymphoma may serve as lead points.[121] An ultrasound examination may pick up other masses, such as a polycystic kidney, IHPS, and Wilms' tumor, or identify complications such as pneumoperitoneum.

▶ PITFALLS

False positive ultrasound examinations are usually due to sonologist inexperience. In one study, the most common imitator of intussusception was fecal matter in the colon.[136] Other reported false positive findings include hematoma of the bowel wall associated with Henoch-Schönlein purpura and nonspecific bowel wall edema or inflammation (such as with inflammatory bowel disease).

▶ CASE STUDIES

Case 1

Patient Presentation

A 2-year-old boy was brought to the emergency department by his parents after a 2-h history of severe intermittent abdominal pain during which the patient squats to partially relieve the pain. The parents reported that the episodes lasted for 10 min and then subsided. He had vomited four times. He was otherwise healthy.

On physical examination, his vital signs were normal. He was alert and appeared in no distress. His head, neck, pulmonary, and cardiovascular examinations were unremarkable. The abdominal examination was soft and without tenderness, but with a palpable right upper quadrant mass. Rectal examination was guaiac negative. Just after the examination, the patient exhibited another episode of severe distress secondary to abdominal pain that lasted 5 min and then resolved.

Management Course

A complete blood count, chemistry panel, and urinalysis were ordered and an intravenous line was established. The patient was administered a 10 mL/kg bolus of normal saline. An ultrasound examination demonstrated the mass to have the typical multilayered hypodense rings consistent with intussusception (see Figure 17–25). A subsequent fluoroscopic hydrostatic reduction was successful. The patient was admitted to the hospital overnight for observation.

Commentary

Case 1 was an example of a patient presenting to the emergency department with a history suggestive of intussusception and an abdominal mass on physical examination. The differential diagnosis of abdominal pain with an abdominal mass in children is lengthy and includes various tumors, adrenal pathology, pancreatitis, enteric duplication, various cysts, pyloric stenosis, polycystic kidneys, and hydronephrosis. Ultrasound is helpful in differentiating these general categories in a rapid and noninvasive manner.

PROCEDURAL USES

URINE COLLECTION

Clinical Indications

Both urethral catheterization and suprapubic aspiration for collection of urine can be considered in situations where sterile urine collection for urinalysis and culture is paramount to patient evaluation. Both techniques have been shown to be safe and accurate, and both may be performed rapidly.[137] Without the use of ultrasound to assist with the procedure, suprapubic aspiration has a reported success rate of approximately 50%[138–140]; whereas blind urethral catheterization has a success rate of near 100%.[137] Most providers prefer urethral catheterization because not only is it somewhat less invasive, especially for female infants, but the procedure can be performed by nursing personnel. Complications of urethral catheterization are rare and consist primarily of microhematuria, which usually resolves spontaneously, and introduction of infection into the bladder. An ultrasound examination can be used to as-

sist with the collection of urine by urethral catheterization by viewing the bladder just prior to the procedure to ensure that an adequate volume of urine exists in the bladder. An empty bladder is the most common reason for failure to collect urine by catheterization. Because of the high-success rate of blind urethral catheterization, bladder volume assessment by an ultrasound examination prior to this procedure is generally unnecessary except in cases where there is a high suspicion of an empty bladder (such as evidence of recent voiding or significant dehydration).

In certain instances, however, urethral catheterization may be contraindicated (urethral pathology) or unsuccessful (unable to locate meatus or pass catheter). Ultrasound-assisted or guided suprapubic aspiration of urine may be the procedure of choice in such cases. Use of an ultrasound examination to assist or guide suprapubic aspiration can increase the procedure success rate from 50 to 70 to 90%.[137–139,141] Ultrasound-assisted means that ultrasound is used primarily to determine if sufficient urine exists in the bladder to perform a successful suprapubic aspiration, and secondarily to confirm the best location to insert the needle; ultrasound is not used during the actual procedure. An ultrasound examination can also be used to guide the procedure by continuous visualization of the needle during the placement. Complication rates with either procedure are very low. The most common complication in suprapubic aspiration is microhematuria, which occurs in up to 4% of cases and clears spontaneously within 24 h.[140] Bowel perforation during suprapubic aspiration is rare, and these tend to resolve without further sequelae. There appears to be no significant advantage of an ultrasound-guided over an ultrasound-assisted suprapubic aspiration as far as success rates are concerned.[139]

Anatomic Considerations

The bladder is located in the midline of the lower abdomen, and is mostly hidden behind the symphysis pubis when empty, though it grows spherically and becomes exposed above the symphysis when filled with urine. Notably, in younger infants, the bladder enlarges more posteriorly as it fills (as opposed to cephalad), which may account for some of the low success rates in blind suprapubic aspiration. The bladder is anterior to the peritoneal space and, when full or partially full, is the first abdominal structure encountered when passing from anterior to posterior at a level just above the symphysis. This relationship makes it possible to insert a needle into the bladder from the anterior abdomen without placing any of the other abdominal organs at risk for inadvertent puncture.

Technique and Normal Ultrasound Findings

Bladder Volume Assessment

This technique takes very little training and can be learned in less than 10 min.[138] The bladder is imaged using a 5.0

Figure 17–26. Probe position for bladder imaging in the infant.

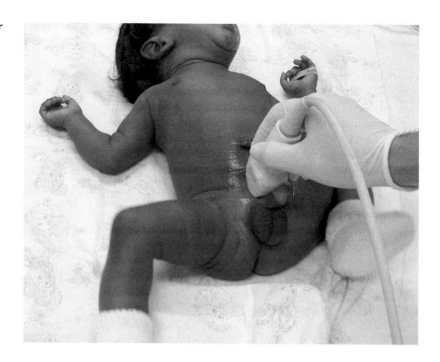

to 7.5 MHz sector probe (a standoff pad may be used if necessary) in a sagittal orientation in the midline of the lower abdomen The probe should be placed just above the symphysis pubis (Figure 17–26). The probe is correctly placed if by moving the probe farther toward the patient's feet, the symphysis begins to shadow most of the screen. The bladder can be identified as a triangular-shaped (if mostly empty) or more spherically shaped (if mostly full) midline cystic structure (Figure 17–27). The amount of urine in the bladder can be qualitatively estimated as "none" (bladder cannot be seen), "small amount" (less than 2 cm diameter), or "more than a small amount" (greater than 2 cm diameter). Bladders measuring less than 2 cm diameter generally contain less than 5 mL of urine and have a lower suprapubic aspiration success rate.[138] If urine volume is insufficient, at least 30 min should elapse before attempting to rescan the bladder. The bladder should also be scanned in the transverse plane to confirm midline position. If there is sufficient urine volume, then suprapubic aspiration may be attempted.

A urethral catheterization will be successful as long as the bladder is not empty, but may not return a sufficient amount of urine if the bladder volume is "small."

Suprapubic Aspiration

Equipment

- Povidone-iodine solution
- 22- or 23-gauge needle, 1 in. length
- 3 to 10 mL syringe

Procedure

Once it has been determined that the bladder has sufficient volume, the suprapubic area should be swabbed with an iodine-based solution. Under sterile conditions,

the needle should be inserted into the abdomen perpendicularly to the skin, one fingerbreadth above the symphysis pubis (Figure 17–28). While the needle is slowly advanced, constant negative pressure should be maintained on the syringe. If no urine is aspirated, then the needle should continue to be slowly advanced all the way to the hub. If unsuccessful, then the needle should be backed out until the tip is just under the skin and redirected 30° more caudad, again with negative pressure maintained as the needle is inserted slowly to the hub. If unsuccessful again, another attempt should be made with

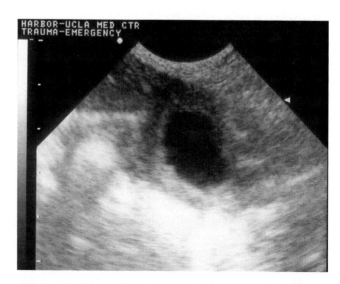

Figure 17–27. Sagittal midline image of the bladder in an infant. Note that the bladder is about 1 cm in diameter (compare to centimeter scale to left of image), probably holding less than 1 cc of urine. SPA in this situation is less likely to be successful.

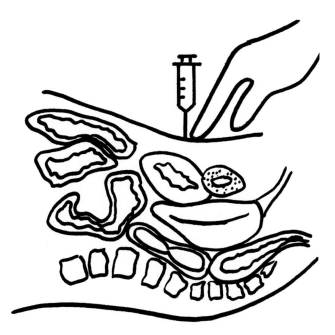

Figure 17–28. For suprapubic aspiration the needle is initially directed perpendicularly to the skin one finger-breadth above the symphysis pubis.

30° of cephalad angulation. If no urine is returned after this third attempt, the patient should receive further hydration and the procedure should be performed under ultrasound guidance.

Pitfalls

1. *Complications.* Although a procedure with a very low complication rate, suprapubic aspiration does present the potential for serious misadventure if careful attention is not paid to the insertion site and direction of needle advancement.
2. *Other fluid.* Although unlikely, it is possible that another fluid-filled structure may be misidentified as the bladder. Fluid collections that are off the midline or more posterior in the abdomen should be regarded with suspicion. Free intraabdominal fluid collections tend to have acute angles with "sharp edges" created by the fluid tracking around organs, as opposed to the more rounded edges of fluid inside a walled structure such as the bladder. Bowel will show intermittent peristalsis if observed for a short time, and usually will display a more heterogeneous content, often with gas bubbles.

FOREARM FRACTURE REDUCTION

Clinical Indications

Pediatric forearm fractures are a common problem encountered in the emergency or acute care setting. Closed reduction of forearm fractures in children can be a te-

dious process, requiring multiple trips to the medical imaging suite to assess the adequacy of the reduction by plain radiographs. More recently, orthopedists have begun using bedside fluoroscopy to obtain immediate feedback on the adequacy of each reduction attempt. Because of the relative infrequency with which non-orthopedic physicians would use such equipment, combined with the expense and the regulation associated with any radiation-producing device, emergency and acute care physicians rarely have access to bedside fluoroscopy. For physicians performing pediatric forearm reductions in a setting where ultrasound use has already been established for other indications, ultrasound represents an attractive alternative for assessment of fracture reduction.[142]

Anatomic Considerations

Although the interior structures of bones cannot be imaged with an ultrasound examination, the exterior surface can be. The bones of the forearm are very superficial structures, which can be seen easily through the soft tissues. The surface contours of both the ulna and radius are directly beneath the skin and are easy to follow. Using an ultrasound examination to visualize forearm fracture reduction is based on demonstrating vertical displacement and angulation of one surface of the bone relative to another. The degree of displacement and angulation can be visualized and measured as well.

Technique and Normal Ultrasound Findings

Equipment

- 5.0 to 7.5 MHz linear array transducer
- Standoff pad (preferable)

Procedure

Patients should receive conscious sedation in the usual manner. After reduction of the fracture, the ultrasound probe should be placed directly over the site of the fracture with the plane of the beam along the long axis of the bone and the indicator on the probe oriented toward the proximal extremity. This places the distal segment on the right of the monitor screen as the examiner would view it. A standoff pad may be used to place the area of interest in the middle of the focal zone. Displacement and angulation between the proximal and distal segments can easily be seen, and can be measured if desired (Figure 17–29). If the reduction is inadequate, the ultrasound gel should be removed and the reduction modified. This process should be repeated until an adequate reduction is achieved.

Pitfalls

1. *Probe curvature.* If a curved transducer is used, it may be difficult to create a full screen image due

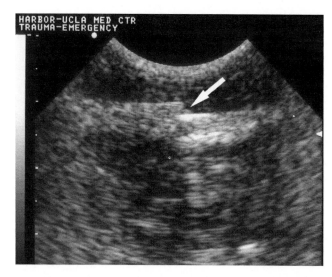

Figure 17–29. Fractured proximal ulna. Longitudinal view of the surface of the ulna. There is an obvious step-off at the fracture site (arrow). The displacement at the fracture was only 2 mm but was clearly visible on ultrasound.

to lack of contact at the curved edges of the probe. In addition, the bone may appear to "curve" on the screen even though it is straight, which may interfere with correction of bony angulation. This should not distort the interpretation or measurement of any fracture displacement.

2. *Orientation.* The probe should be oriented correctly so that on further reduction, the distal fragment is moved in the appropriate direction.

▶ ACKNOWLEDGMENT

The authors would like to express their appreciation to Ellen Benya, MD, of the Department of Radiology, Children's Memorial Hospital in Chicago, Illinois, for her review of the content of this chapter.

REFERENCES

1. Division of Injury Control, Center for Environmental Health and Injury Control. Childhood injuries in the United States. Am J Dis Child 1990;144:627–646.
2. Patel JC, Tepas JJ. The efficacy of focused abdominal sonography for trauma (FAST) as a screening tool in the assessment of injured children. J Pediatr Surg 1999;34:44–47.
3. Jaffee D, Wesson D. Emergency management of blunt trauma in children. N Engl J Med 1991;324:1477–1482.
4. Rodriquez A, Dupriest RW, Shatney CH. Recognition of intra-abdominal injury in blunt trauma victims: a prospective study comparing physical examination with peritoneal lavage. Am Surg 1982;48:456–459.
5. Davis JW, Hoyt DB, Mackersie RC, et al. Complications in evaluating abdominal trauma: diagnostic peritoneal lavage versus computerized axial tomography. J Trauma 1990;30:1506–1509.
6. Fischer RP, Beverlin BL, Engrav LH, et al. Diagnostic peritoneal lavage: fourteen years and 2,586 patients later. Am J Surg 1978;136:701–704.
7. Soderstrom CA, DuPriest RW, Cowley RA. Pitfalls of peritoneal lavage in blunt abdominal trauma. Surg Gynecol Obstet 1980;151:513–518.
8. Rothenberg S, Moore EE, Marx JA, et al. Selective management of blunt abdominal trauma in children: the triage role of peritoneal lavage. J Trauma 1987;27:1101–1106.
9. DuPriest RW, Rodriguez A, Shatney CH. Peritoneal lavage in children and adolescents with blunt abdominal trauma. Am Surg 1982;48:460–462.
10. Trunkey DD, Federle MP. Computerized tomography in perspective. J Trauma 1986;26:660.
11. Oldham KT, Guice KS, Ryckman F, et al. Blunt liver injury in childhood: evolution of therapy and current perspective. Surgery 1986;100:545–549.
12. Wisner DH, Blaisdell FW. When to save the ruptured spleen. Surgery 1992;111:121–122.
13. Taylor GA, Guion CJ, Potter BM, et al. CT of blunt abdominal trauma in children. AJR 1989;153:555.
14. Knudson MM. Definitive care phase: pediatric trauma. In: Greenfield LJ, Mulholland M, Oldham KT, et al, eds. Surgery: scientific principles and practice, 2nd ed. Philadelphia: JB Lippincott, 1997:377–386.
15. Karp MP, Cooney DR, Pros GA, et al. The nonoperative management of pediatric hepatic trauma. J Pediatr Surg 1983;18:512–518.
16. Kohn JS, Clark DE, Isler RJ, et al. Is computer tomographic grading of splenic injury useful in the nonsurgical management of blunt trauma? J Trauma 1994;36:385–389.
17. Brick SH, Taylor GA, Potter BM, et al. Hepatic and splenic injury in children: role of the CT in the decision for laparotomy. Radiology 1987;165:643–646.
18. Bensard DD, Beaver BL, Besner GE, et al. Small bowel injury in children after blunt abdominal trauma: is diagnostic delay important? J Trauma 1996;41:476–483.
19. Haller JA, Papa P, Drugas G, et al. Nonoperative management of solid organ injuries in children: is it safe? Ann Surg 1994;219:625–631.
20. Le-Neel JC, Guiberteau B, Khosrovani C, et al. Traumatic hemoperitoneum of splenopancreatic origin. Appropos of 155 cases. Can a non-surgical treatment be proposed? Chirurgie 1991;117:437–444.
21. Rossi D, de Ville de Goyet J, Clement de Clety S, et al. Management of intra-abdominal organ injury following blunt abdominal trauma in children. Intensive Care Med 1993;19:415–419.
22. Giacomantonio M, Filler RM, Rich RH. Blunt hepatic trauma in children: experience with operative and non-operative management. J Pediatr Surg 1984;19:519–522.
23. Luna GK, Dellinger EP. Nonoperative observation therapy for splenic injuries: a safe therapeutic option? Am J Surg 1987;153:462.
24. Taylor GA, Kaufman RA. Commentary: emergency department sonography in the initial evaluation of blunt

abdominal injury in children. Pediatr Radiol 1993; 23:161–164.

25. Taylor GA, Fallat ME, Potter BM, et al. The role of computed tomography in blunt abdominal trauma in children. J Trauma 1988;38:1660–1664.

26. Meyer DM, Thal ER, Coln D, et al. Computed tomography in the evaluation of children with blunt abdominal trauma. Ann Surg 1993;217:272–276.

27. Turrock RR, Sprigg A, Lloyd DA. Computed tomography in the management of blunt abdominal trauma in children. Br J Surg 1993;80:982–984.

28. Feliciano DV. Diagnostic modalities in abdominal trauma. Surg Clin North Am 1991;71:241.

29. Goldstein AS, Sclafani SJ, Kupferstein NH, et al. The diagnostic superiority of computerized tomography. J Trauma 1985;25:938.

30. Mohamed G, Reyes HM, Fantus R, et al. Computed tomography in the assessment of pediatric abdominal trauma. Arch Surg 1986;121:703–707.

31. Richardson MC, Hollman AS, Davis CF. Comparison of computed tomography and ultrasonographic imaging in the assessment of blunt abdominal trauma in children. Br J Surg 1997;84:1144–1146.

32. Sivit CJ, Kaufman RA: Commentary. Sonography in the evaluation of children following blunt abdominal trauma: is it to be or not to be? Pediatr Radiol 1995;25:326–328.

33. Stylianos S. The role of sonography in the initial evaluation of children after blunt abdominal trauma. Pediatr Radiol 1993;23:164.

34. Davis JW, Hoyt DB, Mackersie RC, et al. Complications in evaluating abdominal trauma: diagnostic peritoneal lavage versus computerized axial tomography. J Trauma 1990;30:1506–1509.

35. Taylor GA, Eichelberger MR. Abdominal CT in children with neurologic impairment following blunt trauma. Ann Surg 1989;210:229–233.

36. Agkur FM, Tanyel FC, Akhan O, et al. The place of ultrasonographic examination in the initial evaluation of children sustaining blunt abdominal trauma. J Pediatr Surg 1993;28:78–81.

37. Akgur FM, Aktug T, Olguner M, et al. Prospective study investigating routine usage ultrasonography as the initial diagnostic modality for the evaluation of children sustaining blunt abdominal trauma. J Trauma 1997;42:626–628.

38. Bioeffects and safety of diagnostic ultrasound. Baltimore, MD: American Institute of Ultrasound in Medicine, 1993.

39. Boulanger B, McLellan B, Brenneman F, et al. Emergent abdominal sonography as a screening test in a new diagnostic algorithm for blunt trauma. J Trauma 1996; 40:867–874.

40. Rozycki GS, Ochsner MG, Jaffin JH, et al. Prospective evaluation of surgeons' use of ultrasound in the evaluation of trauma patients. J Trauma 1993;24:516–526.

41. Price DD, Wilson SR, Murphy TG. Trauma ultrasound feasibility during helicopter transport. Air Med J 2000; 19:144–146.

42. Tso P, Rodriquez A, Cooper C, et al. Sonography in blunt abdominal trauma: a preliminary progress report. J Trauma 1992;33:39–42.

43. Liu M, Lee C, P'eng F. Prospective comparison of diagnostic peritoneal lavage, computed tomography scanning and ultrasonography for the diagnosis of blunt abdominal trauma. J Trauma 1993;35:267–270.

44. Hoffman R, Nerlich M, Muggia-Sullam M, et al. Blunt abdominal trauma in cases of multiple trauma evaluated by ultrasonography: a prospective analysis of 291 patients. J Trauma 1992;32:452–458.

45. Goletti O, Ghiselli G, Lippolis PV. The role of ultrasonography in blunt abdominal trauma: results in 250 consecutive cases. J Trauma 1994;36:178–181.

46. Gruessner R, Mentges B, Duber C, et al. Sonography versus peritoneal lavage in blunt abdominal trauma. J Trauma 1989;29:242–244.

47. Taylor GA, Sivit CJ. Posttraumatic peritoneal fluid: is it a reliable indicator of intraabdominal injury in children? J Pediatr Surg 1995;30:1644–1648.

48. Neish AS, Taylor GA, Lund DP, et al. Effect of CT information on the diagnosis and management of acute abdominal injury in children. Radiology 1998;206:327–331.

49. Partrick DA, Bensard DD, Moore EE, et al. Ultrasound is an effective triage tool to evaluate blunt abdominal trauma in the pediatric population. J Trauma 1998;45:57–63.

50. Akgur FM, Aktug T, Kovanlikaya A, et al. Initial evaluation of children sustaining blunt abdominal trauma: ultrasonography vs. diagnostic peritoneal lavage. Eur J Pediatr Surg 1993;3:278–280.

51. Katz S, Lazar L, Rathaus V, et al. Can ultrasonography replace computed tomography in the initial assessment of children with blunt abdominal trauma? J Pediatr Surg 1996;31:649–651.

52. Luks FI, Lemire A, Dickens St.–VII, et al. Blunt abdominal trauma in children: the practical value of ultrasonography. J Trauma 1993;34:607–311.

53. Mutabagani BD, Coley N, Zumberge N, et al. Preliminary experience with focused abdominal sonography for trauma in children: is it useful? J Pediatr Surg 1999;34:48–54.

54. Benya EC, Lim-Dunham JE, Landrum O, Statter M. Abdominal sonography in examination of children with blunt abdominal trauma. AJR 2000;174:1613–1616.

55. Krupnick AS, Teitelbaum DH, Geiger JD, et al. Use of abdominal ultrasonography to assess pediatric splenic trauma potential pitfalls in the diagnosis. Ann Surg 1997;225:408–414.

56. Coley BD, Mutabagani KH, Martin LC, et al. Focused abdominal sonography for trauma (FAST) in children with blunt trauma. J Trauma 2000;48:902–906.

57. Holmes JF, Brant WE, Bond WF, et al. Emergency department ultrasound in the evaluation of hypotensive and normotensive children with blunt abdominal trauma. J Pediatr Surg 2001;36:968–973.

58. Sizer JS, Wayne ER, Fedrick PL. Delayed rupture of the spleen: review of the literature and report of 6 cases. Arch Surg 1966;92:362–366.

59. Corbett SW, Andrews HG, Baker EM, et al. ED evaluation of the pediatric trauma patient by ultrasonography. Am J Emerg Med 2000;18:244–249.

60. Hilty W, Snoey ER. Trauma ultrasonography. In: Simon BC, Snoey ER, eds. Ultrasound in emergency and ambulatory medicine, 1st ed. St. Louis: Mosby, 1997:151–189.

61. Ma OJ, Kefer MP, Mateer JR, et al. Evaluation of hemoperitoneum using a single- vs multiple-view ultrasonographic examination. Acad Emerg Med 1995;2:581–586.

62. Jehle D, Guarino J, Karamanoukian H. Emergency department ultrasound in the evaluation of blunt abdominal trauma. Am J Emerg Med 1993;11:342–346.

63. Hilty W, Wolfe R, Moore E, et al. Sensitivity and specificity of ultrasound in the detection of intraperitoneal fluid (abstract). Ann Emerg Med 1993;22:921.

64. Meyers MA. The spread and localization of acute intraperitoneal effusion. Radiology 1970;94:547–554.

65. Taylor GA, Sivit CJ. CT imaging of abdominal trauma in children. Semin Pediatr Surg 1992;1:253–259.

66. Branney S, Wolfe R, Moore E, et al. Quantitative sensitivity of ultrasound in detecting free intraperitoneal fluid. J Trauma 1995;39:375–380.

67. Frezza E, Solis R, Silich R, et al. Competency-based instruction to improve the surgical resident technique and accuracy of the trauma ultrasound. Am Surg 1999;65:884–888.

68. Adams B, Sukumvanich P, Seibel R, et al. Ultrasound for the detection of intraperitoneal fluid: the role of Trendelenburg positioning. Am J Emerg Med 1999;17:117–120.

69. Lupien C, Sauerbrei EE. Healing in the traumatized spleen: sonographic investigation. Radiology 1984;151:181–185.

70. Filiatrault D, Longpre D, Patriquin H, et al. Investigation of childhood blunt abdominal trauma: a practical approach using ultrasound as the initial diagnostic modality. Pediatr Radiol 1987;17:373–379.

71. Givre S, Kessler S. The evaluation of blunt abdominal trauma: the evolving role of ultrasound. Mt Sinai J Med 1997;64:311–315.

72. Ingemen JE, Plewa MC, Okasinski RE, et al. Emergency physicians use of ultrasonography in blunt abdominal trauma. Acad Emerg Med 1996;3:931–937.

73. Thourani VH, Pettitt BJ, Schmidt JA, et al. Validation of surgeon-performed emergency abdominal ultrasonography in pediatric trauma patients. J Pediatr Surg 1998;33:322–328.

74. Richardson MC, Hollman AS, Davis CF. Comparison of computed tomography and ultrasonographic imaging in the assessment of blunt abdominal trauma in children. Br J Surg 1997;84:1144–1146.

75. Hoelzer, DJ, Brian MB, Balasara VJ, et al. Selection and nonoperative management of pediatric blunt trauma patients: the role of quantitative crystalloid resuscitation and abdominal ultrasonography. J Trauma 1986;26:57–62.

76. Ochsner MG, Knudson MM, Pachter HL, et al. Significance of minimal or no intraperitoneal fluid visible on CT scan associated with blunt liver and splenic injuries: a multicenter analysis. J Trauma 2000;49:505–510.

77. Shanmuganathan K, Mirvis SE, Sherbourne CD, et al. Hemoperitoneum as the sole indicator of abdominal visceral injuries: a potential limitation of screening abdominal ultrasound for trauma. Radiology 1999;212:423–430.

78. Lund DP, Folkman J. Appendicitis. In: Walker WA, Durie PR, Hamilton JR, et al., eds. Pediatric gastrointestinal disease: pathophysiology, diagnosis and management, 2nd ed. St Louis: Mosby, 1996:907–915.

79. Lund DP, Murphy EU. Management of perforated appendicitis in children. J Pediatr Surg 1994;29:1130–1134.

80. Sivit CJ. Acute appendicitis. In: Cohen HL, Sivit CJ, eds. Fetal and pediatric ultrasound: a casebook approach, 1st ed. New York: McGraw-Hill, 2001:444–449.

81. Savrin RA, Clatworthy HW. Appendiceal rupture: a continuing diagnostic problem. Pediatrics 1979;63:37–43.

82. Graham JM, Pokorny WJ, Harberg FJ. Acute appendicitis in preschool age children. Am J Surg 1980;139:247.

83. Jess P, Bjerregaard B, Bryntz S, et al. Acute appendicitis: prospective trial concerning diagnostic accuracy and complications. Am J Surg 1981;141:232.

84. Hartman GE. Acute appendicitis. In: Behrman RE, Kliegman RM, Alvin AM, eds. Nelson textbook of pediatrics, 16th ed. Philadelphia: WB Saunders, 1996;1109–1111.

85. Meuller BA, Daling JR, Moore DE, et al. Appendectomy and the risk of tubal infertility. N Engl J Med 1986;315:1506–1508.

86. Trautlein JJ, Lambert RL, Miller J. Malpractice in an emergency department: review of 200 cases. Ann Emerg Med 1984;13:709–711.

87. Ravitch MM. Review article appendicitis. Pediatrics 1982;70:414–419.

88. Reynolds SL, Jaffe DM. Diagnosing abdominal pain in a pediatric emergency department. Pediatr Emerg Care 1992;8:126–128.

89. Bolton JP, Craven ER, Croft RJ, et al. Assessment of the value of the white blood count in the management of suspected acute appendicitis. Br J Surg 1975;62:906–908.

90. Fee HJ Jr, Jones PC, Kadell B, et al. Radiologic diagnosis of appendicitis. Arch Surg 1977;112:742–744.

91. Lewis FR, Holcroft JW, Boe J, et al. Appendicitis: a critical review of diagnosis and treatment in 1000 cases. Arch Surg 1975;110:677–684.

92. White JJ, Santillana M, Haller JA. Intensive in hospital observation: a safe way to decrease unnecessary appendectomy. Am Surg 1975;41:793–798.

93. Puylaert JB. Acute appendicitis: ultrasound evaluation using graded compression. Radiology 1986;158:335–360.

94. Bell MJ, Bower RJ, Ternberg JL. Appendectomy in childhood. Analysis of 105 negative explorations. Am J Surg 1982;144:335–337.

95. Rothrock SG, Skeoch G, Rush JJ, et al. Clinical features of misdiagnosed appendicitis in children. Ann Emerg Med 1991;20:68–73.

96. Horton MD, Counter SF, Florence MG, et al. A prospective trial of computed tomography and ultrasonography for diagnosing appendicitis in the atypical patient. Am J Surg 2000;179:379–381.

97. Abu-Yousef JB, Rutgers PH, Lalisang RI, et al. High-resolution in the diagnosis of acute appendicitis. Am J Radiol 1987;149:53–58.

98. Blewett CJ, Krummel TM. Perforated appendicitis: past and future controversies. Semin Pediatr Surg 1995;4:234–238.

99. Lobe TE. Acute abdomen: the role of laparoscopy. Semin Pediatr Surg 1997;33:681–687.

100. Deutsch AA, Leopold GR. Ultrasonic demonstration of the inflamed appendix: case report. Radiology 1981;140:163–164.

101. Garcia Pena BM, Mandl KD, Draus SJ, et al. Ultrasonography and limited computed tomography in the diagnosis and management of appendicitis in children. JAMA 1999;282:1041–1046.

102. Karakas SP, Guelfguat M, Leonidas JC, et al. Acute appendicitis in children: comparison of clinical diagnosis

with ultrasound and CT imaging. Pediatr Radiol 2000; 30:94–98.

103. Roosevelt GE, Reynolds SL. Does the use of ultrasonography improve the outcome of children with appendicitis? Acad Emerg Med 1998;5:1071–1075.

104. Sivit CJ, Applegate KE, Stallion A, et al. Imaging evaluation of suspected appendicitis in a pediatric population: effectiveness of sonography versus CT. AJR 2000; 175:977–980.

105. Hahn HB, Hoepner FU, von Kalle T, et al. Sonography of acute appendicitis in children: 7 years experience. Pediatr Radiol 1998;28:147–151.

106. Crady SK, Jones JS, Wyn T, et al. Clinical validity of ultrasound in children with suspected appendicitis. Ann Emerg Med 1993;22:1125–1129.

107. Siegel MJ, Carel C, Surratt S. Ultrasonography of acute abdominal pain in children. JAMA 1991;266:1987–1989.

108. Rice HE, Arbesman M, Martin DJ, et al. Does early ultrasonography affect management of pediatric appendicitis? A prospective analysis. J Pediatr Surg 1999;34: 754–759.

109. Lessin MS, Chan M, Catallozzi M, et al. Selective use of ultrasonography for acute appendicitis in children. Am J Surg 1999;177:193–196.

110. Zaki AM, MacMahon RA, Gray AR. Acute appendicitis in children: when does ultrasound help? Aust NZ J Surg 1994;64:695–698.

111. Promes SB. Miscellaneous applications. In: Simon BC, Snoey ER, eds. Ultrasound in emergency and ambulatory medicine. St. Louis: Mosby, 1997:151–189.

112. Sivit CJ, Dudgeon DL Applegate KE, et al. Evaluation of suspected appendicitis in children and young adults: helical CT. Radiology 2000;216:430–433.

113. Pena BM, Taylor GA. Radiologists' confidence in interpretation of sonography and CT in suspected pediatric appendicitis. AJR 2000;175:71–74.

114. Garcia Pena BM, Taylor GA, Fishman SJ, et al. Costs and effectiveness of ultrasonography and limited computed tomography for diagnosing appendicitis in children. Pediatrics 2000;106:672–676.

115. O'Rahilly R, Muller F. Anatomy: a regional study of human structure, 5th ed. Philadelphia: WB Saunders, 1986:401.

116. Wakely CPG. The position of the vermiform appendix as ascertained by an analysis of 10,000 cases. J Anat 1933;67:277.

117. Puylaert JB, Rutgers PH, Lalisang RI, et al. A prospective study of ultrasonography in the diagnosis of appendicitis. N Engl J Med 1987;317:666–669.

118. EM, Cronan JJ. Compression ultrasonography as an aid in the differential diagnosis of appendicitis. Surg Gynecol Obstet 1989;169:290–298.

119. Borushok KF, Jeffrey RB, Laing FC, et al. Sonographic diagnosis of perforation in patients with acute appendicitis. Am J Radiol 1990;154:275–278.

120. Hulka F, Campbell JR, Harrison MW, et al. Cost–effectiveness in diagnosing infantile hypertrophic pyloric stenosis. J Pediatr Surg 1997;32:1604–1608.

121. Morrison SC. Controversies in abdominal imaging. Pediatr Clin North Am 1997;44:555–574.

122. Olson AD, Hernandez R, Hirschl RB. The role of ultrasonography in the diagnosis of pyloric stenosis: a decision analysis. J Pediatr Surg 1998;33:676–681.

123. Leonidas JC. The role of ultrasonography in the diagnosis of pyloric stenosis: a decision analysis. J Pediatr Surg 1999;34:1583–1584.

124. Godbole P, Sprigg A, Dickson JA, et al. Ultrasound compared with clinical examination in infantile hypertrophic pyloric stenosis. Arch Dis Child 1996;75:335–337.

125. Mendelson KL. Emergency abdominal ultrasound in children: current concepts. Med Health R I 1999;82:198–201.

126. Rohrschneider WK, Mittnacht H, Darge K, et al. Pyloric muscle in asymptomatic infants: sonographic evaluation and discrimination from idiopathic hypertrophic pyloric stenosis. Pediatr Radiol 1998;28:429–434.

127. Heller RM, Hernanz-Schulman M. Applications of new imaging modalities to the evaluation of common pediatric conditions. J Pediatr 1999;135:632–639.

128. Nagita A, et al. Management and ultrasonographic appearance of infantile hypertrophic pyloric stenosis with intravenous atropine sulfate. J Ped Gastroent Nutr 1996;23:172.

129. Lowe LH, Banks WJ, Shyr Y. Pyloric ratio: efficacy in the diagnosis of hypertrophic pyloric stenosis. J Ultrasound Med 1999;18:773–777.

130. Cohen HL, Zinn HL, Haller JO, et al. Ultrasonography of pylorospasm: findings may simulate hypertrophic pyloric stenosis. J Ultrasound Med 1998;17:705–711.

131. Littlewood Teele R, Vogel SA. Intussusception: the pediatric radiologist's perspective. Pediatr Surg Int 1998;14:158–162.

132. Shanbhogue RL, Hussain SM, Meradji M, et al. Ultrasonography is accurate enough for the diagnosis of intussusception. J Pediatr Surg 1994;29:324–327.

133. Stanley A, Logan H, Bate TW, et al. Ultrasound in the diagnosis and exclusion of intussusception. Ir Med J 1997;90:64–65.

134. Harrington L, Connolly B, Hu X, et al. Ultrasonographic and clinical predictors of intussusception. J Pediatr 1998;132:836–839.

135. Brown L, Gerardi MJ. Acute abdominal pain in children: "Classic" presentations vs. reality. Emerg Med Pract 2000;2:12.

136. Verschelden P, Filiatrault D, Garel L, et al. Intussusception in children: reliability of ultrasound in diagnosis: a prospective study. Radiology 1992;184:741–744.

137. Pollack CV Jr, Pollack ES, Andrew ME. Suprapubic bladder aspiration versus urethral catheterization in ill infants: success, efficiency and complication rates. Ann Emerg Med 1994;23:225–230.

138. Gochman RF, Karasic RB, Heller MB. Use of portable ultrasound to assist urine collection by suprapubic aspiration. Ann Emerg Med 1991;20:631–635.

139. Kiernan SC, Pinckert TL, Keszler M. Ultrasound guidance of suprapubic bladder aspiration in neonates. J Pediatr 1993;123:789–791.

140. Ozkan B, Kaya O, Akdag R, et al. Suprapubic bladder aspiration with or without ultrasound guidance. Clin Pediatr 2000;39:625–626.

141. Ramage IJ, Chapman JP, Hollman AS, et al. Accuracy of clean-catch urine collection in infancy. J Pediatr 1999;135:765–767.

142. Durston W, Swartzentruber R. Ultrasound guided reduction of pediatric forearm fractures in the ED. Am J Emerg Med 2000;18:72–77.

INDEX

Note: Page numbers followed by f and t indicate figures and tables, respectively.